T0183689

Emergency Neurology

Karen L. Roos

Editor

Emergency Neurology

Second Edition

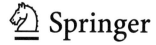 Springer

Editor
Karen L. Roos
The John and Nancy Nelson Professor of Neurology
Indiana University School of Medicine
Indianapolis, IN
USA

ISBN 978-3-030-75780-9   ISBN 978-3-030-75778-6   (eBook)
https://doi.org/10.1007/978-3-030-75778-6

This Springer imprint is published by the registered company Springer Nature Switzerland AG
The registered company address is: Gewerbestrasse 11, 6330 Cham, Switzerland

This book is dedicated to Daphne, Ari and Molly with love.

Preface

The evaluation and management of neurological emergencies are shared by neurologists, emergency medicine physicians, internists, hospitalists, neurosurgeons, family practitioners, and advanced practice providers. The way we care for these patients is defined by the scholarly work of those who are the experts. Their work guides us in the care of our patients.

When Springer asked me to edit a second edition of *Emergency Neurology*, I asked the authors of the first edition if they would be willing to write for a second edition. I was overwhelmed by the generosity and the kindness of the authors and their willingness to write for the second edition. There are also a few new authors who have joined this distinguished group.

Although this book is intended for neurologists, emergency medicine physicians, internists, family practitioners, and hospitalists, it is so much more than an ordinary textbook. It is a collection of the scholarly work of those who have spent their careers doing the work they love, advancing knowledge for the care of patients in their area of expertise. They are Living Legends. This book is also a reunion of friends. What has made my career so meaningful to me is my colleagues whose work I greatly admire and whose friendship I dearly cherish.

Indianapolis, IN, USA   Karen L. Roos

Contents

Contributors

Clotilde Balucani, MD, PhD Division of Neurocritical Care, The Johns Hopkins School of Medicine, Baltimore, MD, USA

J. D. Bartleson Jr., MD Department of Neurology, Mayo Clinic, Rochester, MN, USA

Valérie Biousse, MD Neuro-Ophthalmology Unit, Emory University School of Medicine, Atlanta, GA, USA

Cynthia Bodkin, MD Indiana University School of Medicine, Indiana University Health, Indianapolis, IN, USA

Rachel Calix, MD Department of Neurology, New York University Langone Medical Center, New York, NY, USA

Mark D. Carlson, MD, MA Case Western Reserve University, Department of Medicine, Case Western Reserve University School of Medicine, Cleveland, OH, USA

David Dornbos III, MD Department of Neurosurgery, Semmes-Murphey Clinic and University of Tennessee Health and Science Center, Memphis, TN, USA

Lucas Elijovich, MD Department of Neurology and Neurosurgery, Semmes-Murphey Clinic, University of Tennessee Health Sciences Center, Memphis, TN, USA

Amjad Elmashala, MD The University of Iowa Carver College of Medicine, Iowa City, IA, USA

Luca Farrugia, MD Department of Neurology, Division of Epilepsy, Mayo Clinic, Phoenix, AZ, USA

Jane H. Lock, FRANZCO Neuro-Ophthalmology Unit, Emory University School of Medicine, Atlanta, GA, USA

Department of Ophthalmology, Royal Perth Hospital, Perth, WA, Australia

Department of Ophthalmology, Sir Charles Gairdner Hospital, Nedlands, WA, Australia

Romergyko Geocadin, MD Division of Neurocritical Care, The Johns Hopkins School of Medicine, Baltimore, MD, USA

Christopher L. Groth, MD Neurology Department, Roy J. and Lucille A. Carver College of Medicine, University of Iowa, Iowa City, IA, USA

Kendrick Johnson, MD Department of Neurosurgery, Semmes-Murphey Clinic and University of Tennessee Health and Science Center, Memphis, TN, USA

Kevin A. Kerber, MD Department of Neurology, University of Michigan Health System, Ann Arbor, MI, USA

Cédric Lamirel, MD Service d'ophtalmologie, Fondation Ophtalmologique Adolphe Rothschild, Paris, France

Steven L. Lewis, MD Division of Neurology, Lehigh Valley Health Network, Allentown, PA, USA

Greta B. Liebo, MD Department of Radiology, Mayo Clinic, Rochester, MN, USA

Chris Marcellino, MD Department of Neurologic Surgery, Mayo Clinic, Rochester, MN, USA

Department of Neurology, Mayo Clinic, Rochester, MN, USA

Rohan Mathur, MD, MPA Division of Neurocritical Care, The Johns Hopkins School of Medicine, Baltimore, MD, USA

Tim Maus, MD Department of Radiology, Mayo Clinic, Rochester, MN, USA

Nancy J. Newman, MD Neuro-Ophthalmology Unit, Emory University School of Medicine, Atlanta, GA, USA

Pratik V. Patel, MD Department of Anesthesiology and Pain Medicine, Harborview Medical Center, University of Washington School of Medicine, Seattle, WA, USA

Alejandro A. Rabinstein, MD Department of Neurology, Mayo Clinic, Rochester, MN, USA

Carrie E. Robertson, MD Department of Neurology, Mayo Clinic College of Medicine and Science, Rochester, MN, USA

Robert L. Rodnitzky, MD Neurology Department, Roy J. and Lucille A. Carver College of Medicine, University of Iowa, Iowa City, IA, USA

Karen L. Roos, MD The John and Nancy Nelson Professor of Neurology, Indiana University School of Medicine, Indianapolis, IN, USA

Christian Rosenow, MD Department of Neurology, Division of Epilepsy, Mayo Clinic, Phoenix, AZ, USA

Janet C. Rucker, MD Departments of Neurology and Ophthalmology, New York University Langone Medical Center, New York, NY, USA

Kelsey Satkowiak, MD Department of Neurology, Division of Neuromuscular Medicine, Virginia Commonwealth University, Richmond, VA, USA

Richard V. Scheer, MD Indiana University School of Medicine, Indianapolis, IN, USA

William F. Schmalstieg, MD Department of Neurology, University of Minnesota, Minneapolis, MN, USA

Jennifer Siriwardane, MD Department of Neurology, Indiana University School of Medicine, Indianapolis, IN, USA

Joseph I. Sirven, MD Department of Neurology, Division of Epilepsy, Mayo Clinic, Jacksonville, FL, USA

A. Gordon Smith, MD, FAAN, FANA Department of Neurology, Division of Neuromuscular Medicine, Virginia Commonwealth University, Richmond, VA, USA

Jerry W. Swanson, MD Department of Neurology, Mayo Clinic College of Medicine and Science, Rochester, MN, USA

Laura M. Tormoehlen, MD Neurology and Emergency Medicine, Indiana University School of Medicine, Indianapolis, IN, USA

Brian G. Weinshenker, MD, FRCP(C) Department of Neurology, Mayo Clinic, Rochester, MN, USA

Mark A. Whealy, MD Department of Neurology, Mayo Clinic College of Medicine and Science, Rochester, MN, USA

Headache in the Emergency Department

Mark A. Whealy, Carrie E. Robertson, and Jerry W. Swanson

Introduction

Headache is an extremely common malady that causes numerous sufferers to present to the emergency department for relief and diagnosis. While some headaches are symptomatic of a serious underlying disorder, fortunately, most are of benign origin. Headaches can be classified within two major categories as outlined by the International Headache Society Headache Classification of Headache Disorders (ICHD 3) [1]: (1) primary headache disorders and (2) secondary headache disorders. Primary headache disorders include such diagnoses as migraine, cluster headache, and tension-type headache. These are thought to represent an abnormal activation of the intrinsic pain system that may include both central and/or peripheral mechanisms. The predisposition to such disorders depends on both genetic and environmental factors.

A primary headache is diagnosed based on the patient's history and the absence of an identifiable underlying etiology. Imaging and laboratory investigations are most often used to help exclude secondary causes for headache. There is an extensive and varied list of possible sources of secondary headache, which include intracranial neoplasms, infections, hemorrhage, physiologic abnormalities such as hypothyroidism, toxic exposure such as carbon monoxide poisoning, and many others.

This chapter will address the differential diagnosis of headache disorders likely to be seen in the emergency department as well as various diagnostic approaches utilized in the evaluation of secondary causes of headache. It will also outline several treatments for primary headache disorders. Therapeutic options for many secondary headache disorders are covered in other chapters of this book and are beyond the scope of this chapter. For an exhaustive list of all headache disorders and their diagnoses, the reader should see the ICHD-3 [1] classification.

Epidemiology

The symptom of headache is a frequent reason for visits to the emergency department (ED). In the National Hospital Ambulatory Medical Care Survey in 2017, headache was the seventh most common reason that patients sought care in an emergency department. It was the third most common reason among adult (age 15 or older) women. Overall, headache accounted for over 3.5 million emergency department visits which represented 2.5% of a total of over 138 million visits [2].

M. A. Whealy (✉) · C. E. Robertson · J. W. Swanson
Department of Neurology, Mayo Clinic College of Medicine and Science, Rochester, MN, USA
e-mail: whealy.mark@mayo.edu;
robertson.carrie@mayo.edu; swanson.jerry@mayo.edu

K. L. Roos (ed.), *Emergency Neurology*, https://doi.org/10.1007/978-3-030-75778-6_1

In the largest study of its kind, Goldstein and colleagues evaluated a representative sample of all of the adult ED visits for headache between 1992 and 2001 and found that approximately two-thirds of the visits were for a primary headache disorder [3]. Of those that presented with a secondary headache disorder, the vast majority were benign. In fact, only 2% of visits were found to be due to a serious pathologic etiology [3]. Previous studies also found that the majority of patients presenting to the emergency department with headache had primary headaches, with rates of secondary causes as low as 4% [3]. Certain clinical characteristics such as sudden onset, older age, and marked severity increase the probability of finding an underlying cause [3, 4].

Pathophysiology

A detailed discussion of the pathophysiology of all primary headache disorders is beyond the scope of this chapter; nevertheless, a brief overview of the pathophysiology of migraine is appropriate. Migraine headache likely is a result of alterations in central pain nociception regulation with consequential activation of meningeal and blood vessel nociceptors. Headache and its related neurovascular changes occur as a result of activation of the trigeminal system. Reflex links to the cranial parasympathetics comprise the trigeminoautonomic reflex. Activation leads to vasoactive intestinal polypeptide release and vasodilation [5].

Substance P, calcitonin gene-related peptide (CGRP), and neurokinin A are contained in trigeminal sensory neurons [6]. Excitation leads to release of substance P and CGRP from sensory C-fiber terminals [7], which contribute to neurogenic inflammation [8]. These substances interplay with blood vessels, causing dilation, plasma protein extravasation, and platelet activation [9]. Neurogenic inflammation is thought to sensitize nerve fibers (peripheral sensitization) resulting in responses to formerly innocuous stimuli, like blood vessel pulsations [10], leading to, in part,

the pain of migraine [11]. Central sensitization can also take place. After meningeal receptors are activated, neuronal activation takes place in the trigeminal nucleus caudalis [12] and in the dorsal horn in the upper cervical spinal cord [13, 14]. Positron emission tomography has demonstrated brainstem activation during migraine headache in areas approximating nociceptive pathways as well as in systems that modulate pain [15].

Clinical Features

Primary headaches are defined by their onset, duration, and associated features such as nausea/ vomiting, visual aura, conjunctival tearing, rhinorrhea, etc. These discriminating features are broken down in detail under the differential diagnosis section. Some secondary headaches have classic presentations as well. The following is a list of clinical features on the history and exam that may be seen with particular headache etiologies.

History of Trauma

A history of trauma increases the chance of intracranial hemorrhage (subarachnoid, subdural, epidural, intraparenchymal) and may also precede a carotid or vertebral dissection. Cerebral venous thromboses are another uncommon but serious complication of closed head injury [16]. Trauma to the dural sleeve could result in a cerebrospinal fluid (CSF) leak causing a low-pressure headache. Trauma resulting in fractures to the skull base or cervical vertebra can contribute to severe posterior head and neck pain. Minor head injuries can trigger a migraine in patients with a migraine history. Headaches following closed head injury may mimic migraine or tension headaches and may have associated symptoms such as cervical pain, dizziness, cognitive impairment, and psychologic/somatic complaints such as irritability, anxiety, depression, fatigue, and sleep disturbance [17].

Fever or Known Infection

The presence of an infection elsewhere in the body should raise suspicion that the infection could have spread to the central nervous system. Patients should be assessed for the presence of neck stiffness/meningismus (resistance to passive movement of the neck), fever, or altered level of consciousness. Recent medications for headache should be noted, as nonsteroidal anti-inflammatory drugs and acetaminophen may mask fever. Fever may also occur in the setting of vasculitis, malignancy, thrombosis, and subarachnoid hemorrhage. In subarachnoid hemorrhage, however, the fever tends to be delayed and is therefore less likely to be present on assessment in the ED.

Immunocompromised (HIV or Immunosuppression)

Patients with compromised immune defenses are at increased risk for CNS infections, including meningitis, encephalitis, or abscess. In addition, patients with AIDS are at increased risk of opportunistic CNS neoplasms, such as lymphoma. Certain immunosuppressants, such as cyclosporine, tacrolimus, and gemcitabine, are associated with an increased risk of posterior-reversible leukocncephalopathy. Other immunosuppressive agents, such as liposomal cytarabine, IVIG, intrathecal methotrexate, and azathioprine, can present with headache in the context of aseptic meningitis.

Concurrent Headache in Close Friends, Family, or Coworkers

If people with whom the patient has had contact have also developed new headaches, this should raise suspicion for an infectious or toxic exposure. Infectious meningitis may present with isolated headache or may have associated neck stiffness, meningismus, photophobia, nausea/vomiting, fever, or rash. If the symptomatic group of people have been in an enclosed environment (especially in winter), consider carbon monoxide poisoning. Carbon monoxide poisoning may have associated confusion, nausea/vomiting, chest pain, weakness, or dizziness. Tachypnea and tachycardia are the most frequent physical findings [18]. At carboxyhemoglobin levels greater than 31%, a cherry pink coloring of skin is almost always seen [19]. However, a patient presenting mainly with headache would be expected to have milder levels and would only rarely present with this classic skin color [20].

History of Cancer

A history of malignancy should raise concern for metastases to brain parenchyma or meninges. The most common malignancies to metastasize to the brain are lung (36–46%), breast (15–25%), and skin (melanoma) (5–20%). Almost any systemic tumor can metastasize to the brain, however, including kidney, colon, testes, and ovaries [21]. Headache in the setting of metastases may be nonspecific but may be associated with nausea/vomiting, focal neurologic deficits, or seizures. The headache may be described as getting progressively worse in frequency or intensity and may worsen in the supine position, with straining, or with cough. A malignancy-associated hypercoagulable state puts the patient at an increased risk of cerebral infarction and cerebral venous thrombosis (CVT). Headache may also occur as a side effect of chemotherapy (such as fluorouracil, procarbazine, or temozolomide). Associated anemia, hypercalcemia, or dehydration may also precipitate headaches.

Pregnancy

Primary headaches, such as tension-type headaches and migraine, often improve or remain unchanged during pregnancy [22–24]. Therefore, if a pregnant patient presents to the emergency department with her first-ever headache or a change in her headaches, the physician should be aggressive in the search for secondary causes.

For pregnant women after 20 weeks gestation, it is necessary to exclude preeclampsia/eclampsia. The presentation may be similar to migraine and may even be accompanied by a visual aura. Associated altered mental status and seizures are concerning for eclampsia. Cerebral venous thrombosis and reversible cerebral vasoconstriction may both occur during pregnancy and in the first few weeks after delivery [25]. Both carotid and vertebral dissections have been reported during pregnancy and following prolonged delivery [26–29]. Furthermore, the risk for ischemic stroke, intracerebral hemorrhage, and subarachnoid hemorrhage appears to be the greatest during the two days prior to, and one day following, delivery. This risk remains somewhat elevated for 6 weeks postpartum [30, 31]. Stimulation of the pituitary gland during pregnancy can increase the risk of pituitary apoplexy, and this should be considered if the patient presents with a new severe headache with visual changes. If the patient is presenting in the post-partum period with an orthostatic headache, a post-dural puncture headache should be considered.

Visual Loss

There is a large differential for headaches presenting with associated visual loss. Bilateral visual loss may occur in the setting of papilledema with increased intracranial pressure from a mass or cerebral venous thrombosis. A pituitary mass can compress the optic chiasm and cause varying degrees of bilateral visual loss, especially in peripheral vision. Posterior reversible leukoencephalopathy syndrome (PRES) may present with both headache and bilateral visual loss, possibly associated with hypertension, and sometimes seizures. An ischemic stroke or mass in one hemisphere may present with headache and associated visual loss in one visual field (homonymous hemianopsia).

Monocular visual loss (amaurosis) with headache in a patient over age 50 is immediately concerning for giant cell arteritis. Associated features may include temple tenderness, reduced temporal artery pulse, jaw claudication, increased erythrocyte sedimentation rate, fever, weight loss, or shoulder and hip girdle aching and stiffness (polymyalgia rheumatica). Idiopathic intracranial hypertension is often accompanied by transient visual obscurations which are episodes of visual loss lasting seconds; these are often monocular. Acute angle-closure glaucoma can present with rapidly progressive visual loss and associated eye pain or headache.

Headache Induced by Valsalva Maneuver

Exertion, cough, strain (Valsalva), bending over, or lifting heavy objects, all tend to increase intracranial pressure. If a headache is precipitated by these maneuvers, consider structural processes affecting the posterior fossa, such as a Chiari malformation [32]. Patients with increased intracranial pressure may also have papilledema, nausea/vomiting, and worsening of their headache in a supine position. Disorders associated with intracranial hypertension such as CNS infection, masses, and hematomas may also worsen with these maneuvers. Cerebral venous thrombosis can be associated with increased intracranial pressure due to venous hypertension. Idiopathic intracranial hypertension (pseudotumor cerebri) may present similarly, although this is a diagnosis of exclusion. Although they are associated with low rather than high intracranial pressure, spontaneous cerebrospinal fluid leaks may present with Valsalva induced headaches as well. It is important to note that there are benign headaches, such as cough headache, that may be triggered by cough or strain. Furthermore, migraineurs most often describe their headaches as worsening (but not generally triggered) with activity in general, frequently including Valsalva maneuvers.

Pupillary Abnormalities

Patients presenting with a headache in the ED should routinely be examined for a Horner's syndrome (small pupil that does not dilate well in the dark with associated mild eyelid ptosis). Although a Horner's syndrome may occur in primary headaches such as trigeminal autonomic cephalalgias (TACs) and rarely migraine headaches, the presence of a Horner's syndrome should alert the clinician to the possibility of a carotid or vertebral dissection. A lung/neck malignancy can also cause a Horner's syndrome and could be associated with headache in the setting of brain metastases. A larger pupil that reacts sluggishly to light may be seen with acute-angle glaucoma or a lesion along the pupillary pathway (including optic neuropathy, cranial nerve III palsy, or a brainstem lesion). Anisocoria can also occur as part of a typical migraine.

Red Flags

A helpful mnemonic to remember the clinical "red flags" during evaluation of headache is [33] SNNOOP10, which stands for:

- Systemic symptoms including fever
  → Think infectious, inflammatory, or neoplastic etiologies
- Neoplasm in history
  →Think brain metastasis
- Neurologic deficit or dysfunction (including decreased consciousness)
  →Think of structural intracranial disorders
- Onset of headache is sudden or abrupt
  →Think subarachnoid hemorrhage, reversible cerebral vasoconstriction syndrome, or other vascular/structural disorders
- Older age (after 50 years)
  → Think giant cell arteritis, other vascular or non-vascular intracranial disorder
- Pattern change or recent onset of headache
  → Think neoplasms, vascular, or nonvascular intracranial disorders
- Positional headache
  →Think intracranial hypotension due to CSF leak
- Precipitated by sneezing, coughing, or exercise
  →Think posterior fossa malformations, including Chiari malformation, cervical or cranial vascular disorders, intracranial

hypertension, non-vascular intracranial structural disorders, or CSF leak
- Papilledema
  →Think neoplasms and other nonvascular intracranial disorder or intracranial hypertension
- Progressive headache and atypical presentations
  →Think neoplasms, vascular, or nonvascular intracranial disorders
- Pregnancy or puerperium
  →Think post-dural puncture headache; hypertension-related disorders (e.g., pre-eclampsia); cerebral sinus thrombosis; pituitary apoplexy (if abrupt); reversible cerebral vasoconstriction syndrome; stroke; hypothyroidism; anemia; diabetes
- Painful eye with autonomic features
  →Think pathology in posterior fossa, pituitary region, or cavernous sinus; Tolosa-Hunt syndrome; ophthalmic causes
- Posttraumatic onset of headache
  → Think subdural hematoma, subarachnoid hemorrhage, epidural hematoma, or acute and chronic posttraumatic headache
- Pathology of the immune system such as HIV
  →Think opportunistic infections
- Painkiller overuse or new drug at onset of headache
  →Think medication overuse headache; drug induced headache

When any of these are present, further labs, imaging, and/or spinal fluid analysis should be considered to investigate for a secondary cause of headache.

Approach to Diagnosis

The clinical history is the most valuable tool the clinician has to efficiently and accurately diagnose and treat a patient suffering from headache in the emergency department. The suddenness of onset and whether the patient has had similar headaches in the past can help guide differential diagnoses and management. A severe and unexpected headache that reaches peak intensity within seconds, often referred to as a "thunder-clap headache," should be considered a neuro-logic emergency and requires a systematic work-up (Fig. 1.1). It is tempting to assume that patients with a chronic history of headaches are presenting to the emergency department for treatment only. However, if the headache has changed dramatically in pattern, a more thorough diagnostic evaluation should be performed. Answers to the following questions should be sought:

- Previous headache history/pattern? How does this headache compare with previous experiences?

- Onset and progression of this headache?
- Location and quality of pain?
- Radiation?
- Severity?
- Duration?
- Any fluctuation in intensity? If so, what makes it better or worse? Specifically, is the severity affected by certain positions, times of day, cough, Valsalva, or sleep?
- Any associated symptoms such as:
  - Nausea/vomiting
  - Photophobia/phonophobia
  - Visual changes (blurring, diplopia, flashing/colorful lights)

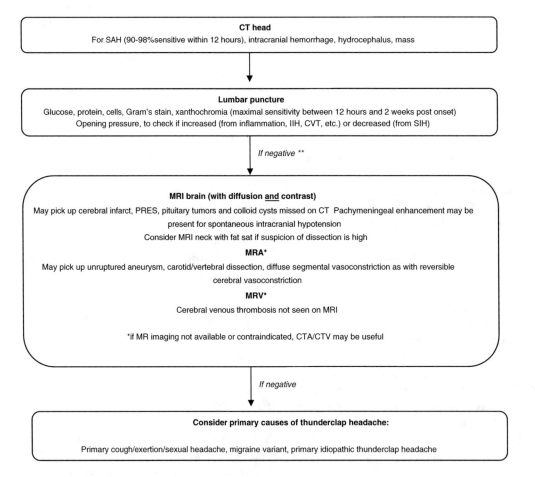

CT head
For SAH (90-98%sensitive within 12 hours), intracranial hemorrhage, hydrocephalus, mass

Lumbar puncture
Glucose, protein, cells, Gram's stain, xanthochromia (maximal sensitivity between 12 hours and 2 weeks post onset)
Opening pressure, to check if increased (from inflammation, IIH, CVT, etc.) or decreased (from SIH)

If negative **

MRI brain (with diffusion <u>and</u> contrast)
May pick up cerebral infarct, PRES, pituitary tumors and colloid cysts missed on CT Pachymeningeal enhancement may be present for spontaneous intracranial hypotension
Consider MRI neck with fat sat if suspicion of dissection is high

MRA*
May pick up unruptured aneurysm, carotid/vertebral dissection, diffuse segmental vasoconstriction as with reversible cerebral vasoconstriction

MRV*
Cerebral venous thrombosis not seen on MRI

*if MR imaging not available or contraindicated, CTA/CTV may be useful

If negative

Consider primary causes of thunderclap headache:

Primary cough/exertion/sexual headache, migraine variant, primary idiopathic thunderclap headache

**If headache has resolved, consider observation. If headache
persists or if suspicion for secondary headache is high, can proceed
with further work up

Fig. 1.1 Proposed work-up for sudden-onset headache

- Whooshing/roaring tinnitus
- Weakness, numbness, or difficulty walking
- Autonomic features (tearing, conjunctival injection, rhinorrhea, flushing/sweating)
- Seizures
- Current pregnancy, infection/fever, immuno-compromised state?
- Current medications (anticoagulants, nitrates) and any recent medication changes?
- Past medical history of recent trauma, cancer, previous blood clots/miscarriages, or polycystic kidney or connective tissue disease (last two may increase chance of aneurysm and therefore subarachnoid hemorrhage)?
- Family history of migraines, clots, bleeding?
- Any family members, friends, or coworkers also suffering from new headache?

A general examination with special attention to vital signs is necessary, followed by a careful examination for any focal neurologic findings. This should include:

- Detailed eye exam (for papilledema, pupillary abnormalities, and visual field abnormalities)
- Auscultation for carotid, temple, or orbital bruits
- Palpation of bilateral temple regions to assess for prominent superficial temporal arteries with reduced pulsation
- Identification of any reported areas that increase or cause pain such as the "trigger zones" in trigeminal neuralgia
- Examination of cranial nerves, strength, and sensation, with special attention to symmetry
- Deep tendon reflexes and plantar reflexes (Babinski sign)
- Unless impossible, the gait should be observed for subtle ataxia/weakness. This may also help elicit positional changes in headache severity

Labs and Imaging

Given the wide variability of secondary headache presentations, it is often difficult to identify which patients require more evaluation than a history and physical examination. As mentioned previously, if there are any associated red flags such as immunocompromised state, older age, or a change in the pattern of headache, further work-up should be considered. A sudden onset, extremely severe, "worst headache of my life" presentation should be treated as a medical emergency and be evaluated in a systematic fashion for subarachnoid hemorrhage or alternative etiologies (see Fig. 1.1).

Serologic Testing

Initial blood tests for headache might include a CBC to look for leukocytosis or glucose/electrolytes to look for metabolic derangements and any evidence of dehydration (especially if vomiting). Sedimentation rate should be considered in any patient older than age 50 with a new type of headache, to screen for giant-cell (temporal) arteritis. Coagulation factors (PT and PTT) should be considered if there is concern for hemorrhage, such as with a thunderclap presentation or if the patient is on anticoagulants. If the headache has associated altered mentation, consider liver function tests and a drug/toxicology screen. If carbon monoxide poisoning is suspected, testing for carboxyhemoglobin may also be useful.

ECG

Although rare, cardiac ischemia may present with isolated headache and is referred to as "cardiac cephalalgia." If a patient has cardiac risk factors, associated shortness of breath, or a new headache that is precipitated by exertion, consider an ECG and/or stress test to look for ischemia [34].

Computed Tomography of the Head

Computed tomography (CT) is the most widely available brain imaging technique in the emergency department and in most cases is adequate to rule out mass effect (from a tumor, abscess, stroke, or other lesion) and acute blood (sub-arachnoid, epidural, subdural, or intraparenchymal). It is important, however, to understand that CT has its limitations. CT of the head will miss subtle, early, or small infarcts and may also miss small subarachnoid and subdural hemorrhages. With a well-read head CT, the sensitivity for sub-arachnoid hemorrhage in the first 12 h is around 90–98% [35–37]. CT becomes less sensitive with increasing time from the onset of headache, with a sensitivity of about 58% at 5 days and about 50% at 1 week [35]. Sensitivity for any type of hemorrhage is reduced if the hematocrit is less than 30% [38]. Lesions and mass effect in the posterior fossa can also be difficult to visualize, especially with a poor-quality CT, given the artifact from surrounding bone structures.

A CT head is normally performed without contrast in the emergency room. However, it may be reasonable to add contrast if there is suspicion for CVT or metastases.

Lumbar Puncture

When infection is suspected, it is necessary to analyze spinal fluid for inflammatory cells, protein and glucose concentrations, Gram's stain, and culture. Ideally the patient should have this procedure in the lateral decubitus position, and opening pressure should be measured. Normal opening pressure is about 5–22 cm H_2O (up to 25 in obese adults). Care must be taken to relax the patient with legs extended when measuring the opening pressure, to avoid a spurious elevation of the measurement.

The opening pressure may be elevated with many pathologic processes, including infection or inflammation of the meninges. It may also be elevated with mass effect, increased venous pressure (such as from CVT), idiopathic intracranial hypertension, or metabolic disorders causing cerebral edema (anoxia, hypertensive encephalopathy, hepatic encephalopathy). If there is a concern for a mass lesion, a head CT should be performed prior to lumbar puncture. If a mass lesion is present, the lumbar puncture should be deferred due to the risk of herniation. It may be

reasonable to skip the head CT if the following are not present: age greater than 50, immuno-compromised state, previous brain injury (stroke, infection, mass), seizures, altered mentation, or focal neurologic findings [39].

If subarachnoid hemorrhage is a consideration and the head CT is negative for blood, a lumbar puncture is required to look for xanthochromia, a yellowish appearance to the CSF. In subarach-noid hemorrhage, xanthochromia is caused by blood breakdown products, such as oxyhemoglobin and bilirubin. Xanthochromia may also be positive if the CSF protein concentration is more than 150 mg/dL, if there are more than 400 red blood cells (RBCs), or with hyperbilirubinemia. Xanthochromia may be undetectable if tested too early (less than 12 h after a hemorrhage) or too late (longer than 2 weeks) [38]. If available, spec-trophotometry is significantly more sensitive than visual inspection for xanthochromia [40, 41], though specificity seems to be lower [42].

In the event of a "traumatic spinal tap," RBCs may be elevated in the CSF. To try and differenti-ate whether the RBCs are from the lumbar punc-ture or an acute hemorrhage, it is reasonable to compare the number of RBCs in the first tube to the last tube of CSF. Usually, if the red blood cells are from the procedure, the blood will become progressively dilute, and there will be fewer RBCs in the last tube drawn. Keep in mind, however, that if the number of RBCs in the last tube is not zero, it does not necessarily rule out subarachnoid hemorrhage [38].

MRI

MRI is not frequently available in the emergency department for evaluation of headache. Furthermore, there are limited instances where an MRI would be necessary in an emergent situation. One of the cases where a clinician might consider MRI is in a patient with persistent thunderclap headache with a negative head CT and lumbar puncture. If there are no other historical clues to diagnosis, an MRI provides the best visualization of the posterior fossa and may demonstrate cere-bral infarcts or posterior leukoencephalopathy

(PRES) missed on CT. It may also show changes on fat saturation images of a carotid or vertebral artery dissection. Pituitary tumors and colloid cysts that were not evident on CT may also be more conspicuous on MRI. Subdural fluid collections and pachymeningeal enhancement may be noted in spontaneous cerebrospinal fluid leaks from an incidental tear in the dura. If an MRI is to be performed in a patient with normal kidney function, it should be with diffusion and contrast imaging to increase sensitivity. If the patient has reduced kidney function, especially in the setting of hemodialysis or prior renal transplant, the benefits of using contrast (gadolinium) should be weighed against the risk of causing the rare, but sometimes fatal, condition of nephrogenic systemic fibrosis (NSF).

Vascular Imaging

If there is suspicion for dissection, the patient should be evaluated with carotid ultrasound, MRA, or CTA (of both the head and neck). If the emergency department is equipped to perform an MRI, MRI with fat saturation sequences may also identify the mural hematoma. An MRA or CTA will help delineate the extent of a dissection. MRA may also help identify unruptured aneurysms or diffuse vasoconstriction. If the patient has a contraindication to MR imaging, such as a pacemaker, then a CTA would be preferred. An MRV or CTV may be helpful in identifying cerebral venous thromboses that were not identified on CT or MRI.

Differential Diagnosis

Primary Headaches

As previously described, the majority of patients presenting to the emergency department with headache have a primary headache [3]. Thus, clinicians must have a basic understanding of the various types of primary headaches, their presentations, and their management. The following list is not comprehensive, but covers some of the more common primary headaches. Also listed are some rare, but uniquely presenting headaches that may mimic more serious conditions.

Migraine

According to the diagnostic criteria of the International Headache Society (ICHD-3), a diagnosis of migraine without aura requires at least five attacks lasting 4–72 h with nausea with or without vomiting or both photophobia and phonophobia. At least two of the following must also be present: unilateral location, pulsating quality, moderate to severe pain intensity, or worsening of pain with physical activity (or causing avoidance of physical activity). Migraine with aura is similar but is associated with focal neurologic symptoms that typically last for 5–60 min. Aura (when present) typically precedes the headache but may occur during the headache as well. Visual auras are most common and tend to occur unilaterally (hemianopia) with a combination of scotomas (blurred or graying visual areas) and positive phenomenon such as sparkling/flashing lights or colors. Sensory auras also tend to be a combination of negative features (numbness) and positive features (tingling) and may occur in a cheiro-oral (hand and face) distribution [43]. These tend to slowly march over 5–30 min. Unilateral weakness may accompany hemiplegic migraines, while brainstem symptoms, such as dysarthria, vertigo, and diplopia (with or without visual field defect) may be seen in migraine with brainstem aura. A reduced level of consciousness or transient loss of consciousness may also accompany migraine with brainstem aura.

In the emergency department, neurologic deficits should not be assumed to be related to migraine headache unless the patient has a clear history of the same symptoms with their typical migraine aura. Often the difficulty with migraineurs in the emergency department is not that of diagnosis but of treatment. This is especially true in patients with status migrainosus, a debilitating attack of an otherwise typical migraine that lasts longer than 72 h. See the treatment section for recommendations on managing migraine in the emergency department.

Tension-Type Headache

A tension-type headache is typically described as a bilateral, non-throbbing pressure or tightness that is mild to moderate in intensity and does not worsen with physical activity. It may last minutes to days and can have associated muscle spasm, especially in the cervical region. There may be photophobia or phonophobia, but usually no nausea or associated aura. Because of the lower intensity, this type of headache is unlikely to be the presenting complaint in the emergency department setting.

Cluster Headache and Other Trigeminal Autonomic Cephalalgias

The TACs are a group of headaches associated with autonomic symptoms, including conjunctival injection, tearing, nasal congestion, rhinorrhea, sweating, ptosis, eyelid edema, and miosis. They are divided into subcategories according to their duration.

Cluster Headache
- Patients with cluster headache present with severe attacks of unilateral pain in the orbital, supraorbital, or temporal areas, with typical autonomic features ipsilateral to the pain. Cluster headaches usually build in intensity, lasting 15 min to 3 h, and may recur up to eight times a day. During an attack, the pain is extremely severe and the patient may seem restless, and may pace back and forth, not wanting to lie down. These may occur at similar times of day and may recur for weeks or months (clusters), separated by remission periods. Cluster headaches are three times more prevalent in men and may be inherited in about 5% of cases [1].

Paroxysmal Hemicrania
- Episodic paroxysmal hemicrania is similar to cluster headache in that the patient has periods of repeated attacks separated by periods of remission. The attacks tend to be of shorter duration than cluster, lasting 2–30 min, and are described as severe unilateral orbital, supraorbital, or temporal pain accompanied by the autonomic symptoms described earlier. These typically occur more than five times a day from 7 days to 1 year, with pain-free periods of 1 month or longer [1]. In some patients, the attacks may be precipitated mechanically by bending or neck movement. If a patient has attacks for more than 1 year without remission, the headaches are referred to as chronic paroxysmal hemicrania [1]. By definition, attacks are prevented completely by therapeutic doses of indomethacin.

Short-Lasting Unilateral Neuralgiform Headache Attacks with Conjunctival Injection and Tearing/Cranial Autonomic Features (SUNCT/SUNA)
- Similar to the other TACs, SUNCT/SUNA headaches are described as unilateral stabbing or pulsating pain in the orbital, supraorbital, or temporal region associated with ipsilateral autonomic symptoms. As evidenced by their names, these headaches are the shortest in the group. They may last 1 sec to 10 min and occur 3–200 times per day [1]. Similar to trigeminal neuralgia, these paroxysmal pains may be triggered by chewing, smiling, light touch, or a cool breeze.

Hemicrania Continua
- Hemicrania continua is a persistent headache involving one side of the head, often fluctuating in intensity. This type of headache can be diagnostically challenging as patients may present with both migrainous and cluster headache characteristics. By definition, this type of headache is present continuously for

over three months and is associated with restlessness/agitation or worsening with routine physical activity and/or at least one autonomic symptom ipsilateral to the headache, such as ipsilateral lacrimation, eyelid edema or ptosis, conjunctival injection, nasal congestion, and/or rhinorrhea [1]. Also by definition, this headache responds absolutely to therapeutic doses of indomethacin. Because side-locked headaches are concerning for an underlying structural abnormality, neuroimaging with MRI is recommended for evaluation of these patients.

Benign Cough Headache

Benign cough headache is usually bilateral, is short lasting (1 sec to 30 min), and only occurs in association with coughing or straining. It occurs more often in men over the age of 40 [1]. Symptomatic cough headache may be caused by Arnold Chiari malformation (Fig. 1.2), posterior fossa mass lesions, cerebral aneurysms, spinal spontaneous cerebrospinal fluid leak, or other carotid/vertebral disease [1].

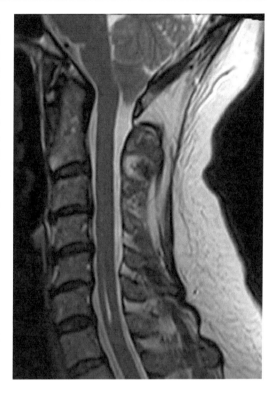

Fig. 1.2 Chiari I malformation. Sagittal unenhanced T2-weighted MRI demonstrates descent of the cerebellar tonsils >5 mm below the foramen magnum with an associated syrinx at C6. Note that without gadolinium and clinical screening, a patient with low CSF pressure from a CSF leak may be misdiagnosed as having a Chiari 1 malformation

Benign Sexual or Orgasmic Headache

Two types of headache may occur with sexual activity. One is a dull aching pain in the head and neck (similar to tension headache) that intensifies with increasing sexual excitement. The other is an explosive (or thunderclap) type of headache that occurs with orgasm. With an orgasmic headache, it is important to rule out subarachnoid hemorrhage, reversible cerebral vasoconstriction syndrome, and other sources of thunderclap headache [1].

Primary (Benign) Exertional Headache

It is not uncommon for headaches, especially migraine, to worsen with exertion. However, a throbbing headache lasting 5 min to 48 h, brought on by and occurring only with exertion, may represent benign exertional headache [1]. In the emergency department, such a patient should also be evaluated for exertional cardiac ischemia, as headache may sometimes be the only presenting symptom [34].

Secondary Headaches

While primary headaches present more often, the goal in the emergency department is not necessarily to diagnose which primary headache is present, but rather to rule out sources for secondary headache. Among the secondary headaches, the most concerning are those that present with an explosive, debilitating, or "thunderclap" presentation. When a patient presents in this way, the first goal is to rule out a subarachnoid hemorrhage. There are many other headaches in which the patient may describe "the worst headache of their life" with acute onset. These are outlined in Table 1.1. More detailed descriptions of some of these are included in the text below.

Subarachnoid Hemorrhage

While the classic thunderclap headache should not be missed, some patients with subarachnoid hemorrhage present with more subtle symptoms (Fig. 1.3). Any headache that is unusual for the patient, especially if there is associated neck pain or stiffness, should raise the possibility of a subarachnoid hemorrhage. Evaluation should include a head CT followed by a lumbar puncture if negative (see Section "Approach to Diagnosis").

Other Intracranial Hemorrhage

Hemorrhage into brain parenchyma may present similarly to a subarachnoid hemorrhage. If the blood tracks into the CSF, it may cause meningeal irritation and neck stiffness. Focal neurologic symptoms, including seizures and altered mentation, may be present depending on the size and location of the hematoma. Epidural and subdural hematomas may present with headache, often following trauma. A careful history must be taken as the associated trauma may be remote with subdural hematomas. Be concerned about hemorrhage in a patient on anticoagulation therapy with a new-onset headache, especially if they are older.

Cerebral Venous Thrombosis

Presentation depends on the size and location of the thrombosis (Fig. 1.4). The most frequent symptom is headache, which may be subacute over days or a more sudden "thunderclap" presentation. A large cerebral venous thrombosis may cause increased intracranial pressure, leading to blurred vision, nausea/vomiting, positional headache, pulsatile tinnitus, and occasionally cranial nerve VI palsy. This can progress into subacute mental status changes and coma. A small cortical venous thrombosis may present with focal neurologic findings or seizures [45]. Risk factors for CVT are similar to risk factors for other venous thrombosis and include infection, malignancy, oral contraceptives, pregnancy/postpartum, and history of a hypercoagulable state.

On a head CT with contrast, the classic appearance of a CVT is the "empty delta sign," which is the empty-appearing triangle created when the confluens sinuum fails to fill with contrast. This sign is present 25–30% of the time, but more often the CT shows nonspecific focal or generalized edema, gyral enhancement, or enhancement of the falx/tentorium [45]. Diagnosis relies on imaging of the cerebral venous system, with either an MRV or CTV (if MR imaging is contraindicated or difficult to obtain). Anticoagulation appears to be safe in these cases, and may even improve outcome. Even with anticoagulation, the mortality is around 5–10% [46].

Meningitis

The presence of fever, neck stiffness, meningismus, or altered mentation associated with headache is concerning for inflammation of the meninges, or meningitis. Unfortunately, the presentation may be subtle. In one study of bacterial meningitis, only 44% of patients presented with the classic triad of fever, neck stiffness, and change in mental status. However, 95% had at least two of the following four signs and symptoms: headache, fever, neck stiffness, and an altered level of consciousness [47].

Table 1.1   Differential for thunderclap headache

Diagnosis	What to look for	Testing
Subarachnoid hemorrhage	Sudden onset May have decreased consciousness, possible neck stiffness	CT without contrast. If no acute blood, check CSF for xanthochromia
Intracranial hemorrhage	Focal neurologic signs, altered mentation, possible seizures	CT without contrast
Cerebral venous sinus thrombosis	Headache may be postural (worse supine) and may worsen with Valsalva. May have whooshing tinnitus. Check for papilledema	MRV preferred. CT *with contrast* may reveal Delta sign. CSF may be normal or have increased pressure or elevated protein concentration
Cervicocephalic arterial dissection (carotid or vertebral)	May have associated neck pain Check for presence of Horner's sign and other neurologic deficits	MRI and MRA of head and neck. Can start with carotid ultrasound or get CTA if MRI not available
Pituitary apoplexy	Often have nausea May have change in consciousness, visual loss, or double vision May present with pituitary insufficiency	Start with CT if acute to look for blood. However, MRI may be required
Acute hypertensive crisis	Presence of hypertension, usually more than 180/110	Need to rule out other causes of headache with high BP ECG Consider CT head for blood, stroke, or PRES MRI is more sensitive for PRES
Spontaneous cerebrospinal fluid leak	Postural headache, better supine, worse upright	MRI to look for pachymeningeal enhancement and low-lying cerebellar tonsils Can check LP for opening pressure
Reversible cerebral vasoconstriction syndrome (RCVS)	May present with recurrent thunderclap headache or post-partum May have photophobia, nausea	Cerebral angiogram is gold standard; can check MRA or CTA
Ischemic stroke	New neurologic deficits, especially in a vascular distribution	MRI with diffusion-weighted imaging; if large or subacute/chronic, may show on CT
Third ventricular colloid cyst	Headache often positional, can be followed by syncope or even death if hydrocephalus is severe	CT often sufficient, but MRI may be required
Acute expansion of mass in posterior fossa	May have reduced consciousness, cerebellar signs, or asymmetric pupils if associated with herniation	CT head should show mass effect
Intracranial infection (e.g., bacterial meningitis)	Fever, chills, meningismus, leukocytosis	CSF studies; MRI may show meningeal enhancement
Primary sexual or exertional headache	Sudden onset before, during, or right after orgasm or peak of exertion. Look for previous episodes	Diagnosis of exclusion (especially if this is the first occurrence); specifically need to rule out aneurysm with SAH and RCVS
Primary cough headache	Sudden onset with cough or strain, lasting minutes (1 s to 30 min)	Diagnosis of exclusion
Glaucoma	Slowly responsive dilated pupil, with ipsilateral pain	Ophthalmology consult
Primary thunderclap headache	Maximum intensity in <1 min. Lasts 1 h to 10 days	Diagnosis of exclusion

Modified list from Schwedt et al. [44]

In the emergency department, it is necessary to first rule out infectious etiologies of meningitis, including bacteria, viruses, fungi, and mycobacteria. This should be done with a blood culture and spinal fluid analysis (with or without preceding CT, see Section "Lumbar Puncture"). Meningitis may be due to noninfectious etiologies as well and present with headache, with or

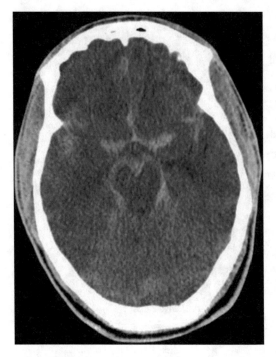

Fig. 1.3 Acute subarachnoid hemorrhage. Axial, unenhanced head CT demonstrates acute, high-attenuation subarachnoid blood products surrounding the brainstem, and filling the suprasellar cistern, sylvian fissures, and interhemispheric fissure

without fever. Etiologies for noninfectious meningitis include leptomeningeal metastases, systemic autoimmune diseases, or medications (NSAIDs, IVIG, intrathecal chemotherapy).

Cervicocephalic Dissection

Carotid and vertebral dissections are often associated with head or neck pain. In one study, 8% of 245 patients with cervical dissections presented with head and/or neck pain as their only symptom [48]. In all but one of these cases, the pain was different from their previous headaches. While it is difficult to recommend extensive testing for dissection in every new-onset headache, this should at least be on the differential. Investigations for dissection should be considered in an otherwise unexplained acute or thunderclap headache or with a new progressive headache (especially if side-locked) associated with neck pain, a Horner's syndrome, cranial nerve palsies, monocular vision loss (amaurosis fugax), or other focal neurologic signs. A history of preceding trauma to the neck, even minor trauma such as chiropractic neck manipulation or

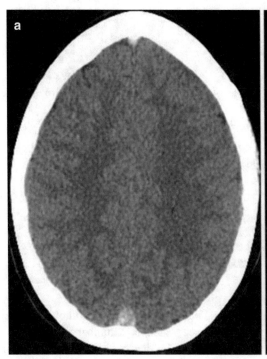

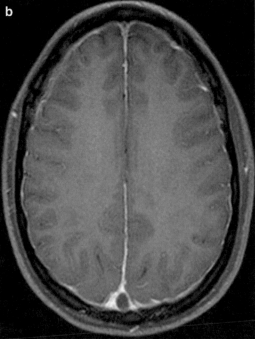

Fig. 1.4 Superior sagittal sinus thrombosis. Axial, unenhanced head CT (**a**) demonstrates high-attenuation material consistent with thrombus within posterior aspect of the superior sagittal sinus. T1-weighted, gadolinium-enhanced MRI (**b**) demonstrates a filling defect ("empty delta sign") within the superior sagittal sinus due to thrombus

whiplash from a roller coaster ride, increases the suspicion for dissection.

Ischemic Stroke

Headache is not uncommon in the setting of ischemic stroke, especially with large strokes. If a patient has a history of migraine headaches, the ischemic stroke may trigger one of their typical headaches. This can make diagnosis quite challenging as migraineurs can have neurologic symptoms as part of a migraine aura (see Section "Migraine"). If a migraine patient is presenting in the emergency department with a typical migraine, but has a new or changed neurologic aura, consider the possibility of ischemia or other focal neurologic injury.

Reversible Cerebral Vasoconstriction Syndrome

Reversible cerebral vasoconstriction syndrome (RCVS) is characterized by a sudden severe thunderclap headache associated with vascular narrowing in the vessels of the circle of Willis and its branches. Patients may present with recurrent thunderclap headaches, sometimes triggered by orgasm, exertion, or emotion [1]. The term represents a group of disorders including Call-Fleming syndrome, benign angiopathy of the CNS, postpartum angiopathy, drug-induced vasospasm, migrainous vasospasm, and migrainous angiitis [25, 49]. Headaches tend to last minutes to hours and may recur over a few days to weeks. Because of the vasoconstriction, most patients also have focal neurologic deficits, and one-third of patients have seizures. CSF is normal or near normal (protein <80 mg/dL, WBC < 10 cells mm^3) [25], and there may be a slight elevation of ESR [49]. The gold standard for diagnosis is conventional angiography which shows multifocal segmental vasoconstriction, reversible within 12 weeks after onset. MRA or CTA is the recommended first-line imaging procedure, however. MRI and CT may be normal, may show features similar to posterior reversible encephalopathy syndrome (PRES), or may show evidence of intracranial hemorrhage, especially cortical subarachnoid hemorrhage. Patients typically do well even without treatment, although cerebral infarction may occur [50]. There are some case reports suggesting possible benefit with calcium channel blockers such as nimodipine, but there has not been a well-designed trial to explore this further [49].

Headache Related to Spontaneous Spinal Cerebrospinal Fluid Leak

Spontaneous spinal cerebrospinal fluid leaks generally present as an orthostatic headache that is worse in the upright position and better while recumbent (Fig. 1.5). These headaches are often throbbing (not always) and either bilateral or holocephalic. These may occur as thunderclap headaches and occasionally present only with exertion or with valsalva. There may be a variety of associated symptoms, many of which are also orthostatic in nature. These include dizziness, hearing changes with a sense that sounds are muffled (from stretching of cranial nerve VIII or changes in perilymphatic pressure), visual blurring, reduced consciousness (from compression of the diencephalon), and ataxia or other gait disorders (from compression on the posterior fossa and spinal cord) [51].

The depletion of CSF may be from hypovolemia, overshunting of CSF, or a CSF leak. A history of recent lumbar puncture, epidural, spinal surgery, or motor vehicle accident suggests a persistent traumatic CSF leak. Spontaneous spinal cerebrospinal fluid leaks may occur through weak meningeal diverticula or weak dura and may be associated with connective tissue disorders [51]. A head CT is usually unremarkable, although subdural fluid collections are sometimes appreciated. On MRI, typical findings include pachymeningeal enhancement, descent of the cerebellar tonsils (resembling Chiari I malformation), engorgement of the pituitary, crowding of the posterior fossa, decreased ventricle size, and subdural fluid collections (typically bilateral). Lumbar puncture is not necessary for diagnosis, but when it is performed, the opening pressure may be normal to low and CSF protein

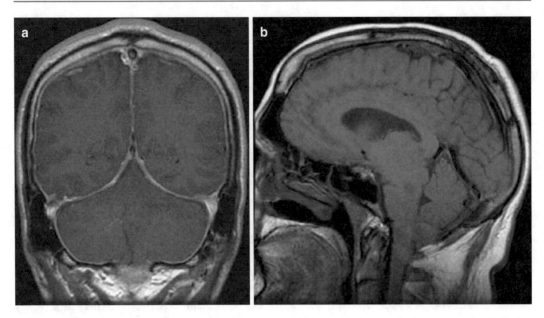

Fig. 1.5 Spontaneous cerebrospinal fluid leak. Coronal T1-weighted, gadolinium-enhanced MRI (**a**) demonstrates prominent pachymeningeal enhancement. Sagittal T1-weighted, unenhanced MRI (**b**) shows descent of the cerebellar tonsils through the foramen magnum with flattening of the pons against the clivus consistent with "brain sag"

concentration may be normal to high. Pleocytosis (WBC in the 10–50 cells/mm^3 range, rarely up to 220 cells/mm^3) may also occur [52, 53]. Most of these are self-limited and respond well to bed rest, caffeine, and increased fluid intake. However, a persistent headache may require an epidural blood patch by anesthesiology. Severe or persistent cases may need to be further evaluated with CT myelography to identify the leak for possible surgical repair.

Hypertensive Crisis and PRES

In a study of 50 patients presenting with hypertensive urgency (blood pressure greater than 180/110), the two most common presenting complaints were headache (42%) and dizziness (30%) [54] (Fig. 1.6). With hypertensive crisis, there is also evidence of end-organ damage such as stroke, hypertensive encephalopathy, or acute pulmonary edema. A patient presenting with headache and marked elevation of blood pressure presents a diagnostic dilemma. Severe hypertension may be a source for headache, but

severe headache pain may also result in secondary elevation of blood pressure. Furthermore, a patient may have an underlying process, such as a hemorrhagic or ischemic stroke, that is associated with both. The possibility of ischemic stroke is particularly worrisome because lowering blood pressure could potentially exacerbate cerebral ischemia. Before attempting to lower blood pressure, a careful neurologic examination should be performed to look for signs of ischemic stroke.

Posterior reversible leukoencephalopathy, also termed posterior reversible encephalopathy syndrome (PRES), is a syndrome involving vasogenic edema preferentially affecting the white matter of the posterior brain, including the occipital lobes and cerebellum. Symptoms may include headache, nausea/vomiting, seizures, altered mentation, and sometimes other focal neurologic signs, such as bilateral visual loss [55]. The name is somewhat misleading because PRES does not necessarily have to be posterior, reversible, or limited to white matter.

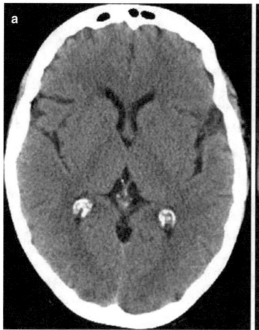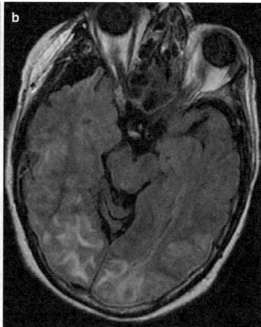

Fig. 1.6 Posterior reversible leukoencephalopathy syndrome (PRES). Axial unenhanced CT (**a**) shows subtle loss of differentiation between *gray and white matter* within the occipital lobes. Axial FLAIR MRI (**b**) demonstrates abnormal T2 signal in the posterior white matter

PRES may occur with hypertensive encephalopathy, as well as preeclampsia/eclampsia, and some immunosuppressive agents such as cyclosporine, tacrolimus, and IVIG. When diagnosing PRES, MRI is more sensitive than CT and demonstrates an increased T2 signal abnormality. Posterior reversible leukoencephalopathy may sometimes be noted as hypodense regions on a head CT.

Pituitary Apoplexy

Pituitary apoplexy occurs when a pituitary tumor (typically a benign adenoma) spontaneously hemorrhages or when it outgrows its blood supply (causing pituitary infarct) (Fig. 1.7). Patients may present with a sudden-onset severe headache, mimicking subarachnoid hemorrhage. They may have associated nausea, visual loss, or double vision. On occasion, they may present with a change in consciousness or adrenal failure. A head CT may show changes consistent with acute hemorrhage, but may miss subtle hemorrhage or infarct. If pituitary apoplexy is suspected and the CT is negative, consider MRI [56].

In addition to neurosurgery (for possible urgent trans-sphenoidal resection), an endocrinologist is often involved acutely and in recovery to help manage high dose corticosteroids and other hormonal replacements [57].

Idiopathic Intracranial Hypertension

The typical patient is an obese female presenting with headache that is daily, severe, and throbbing, lasts hours, and may wake the patient from sleep. Patients may have associated nausea/vomiting, transient visual obscurations or loss of vision (from papilledema), sparks/flashes in their vision, or horizontal diplopia. They may have associated tinnitus that is synchronized with their pulse [58]. Careful funduscopic examination should show evidence of papilledema or other changes consistent with

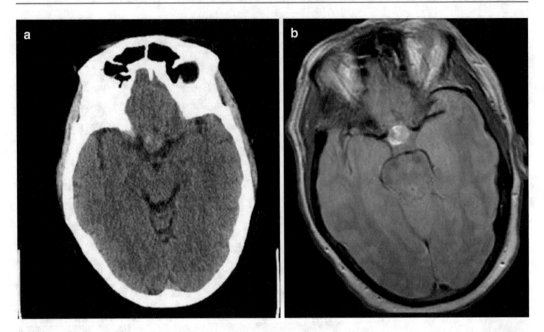

Fig. 1.7 Pituitary apoplexy. Unenhanced CT (**a**) and MRI (**b**) demonstrate acute hemorrhage into a pituitary adenoma

increased intracranial pressure [59]. Most work-up for idiopathic intracranial hypertension is performed as an outpatient. However, if the patient presents to the emergency department for evaluation, a head CT would need to be performed to exclude a mass lesion. A lumbar puncture should show normal composition and an elevated CSF pressure (>20 cm H_2O in the non-obese, >25 cm H_2O in the obese). As this is a diagnosis of exclusion, at some point the patient should have further testing such as an MRI and MRV to exclude sources for venous hypertension (from a dural venous thrombosis, AVM, or AV fistula) [60, 61]. In one study, 9.4% of 106 patients with presumed idiopathic intracranial hypertension had a CVT [62].

Management generally begins with treatment of obesity and discontinuing any medications associated with intracranial hypertension, such as nitrofurantoin, retinoic acid, excessive vitamin A, anabolic steroids, tetracycline, etc. [58]. Medical therapy with acetazolamide or furosemide may be attempted. If the patient fails therapy or has progressive visual loss, a surgical procedure such

as optic nerve sheath fenestration or shunting may be required [60, 61].

Headache Attributed to Traumatic Injury to the Head (Post Traumatic Headache)

Post traumatic headaches may mimic migraine or tension headaches. Furthermore, trauma may trigger a typical migraine in a migraineur. Sometimes post traumatic headaches are part of a syndrome of symptoms including cervical pain, dizziness, cognitive impairment, and psychologic/somatic complaints such as irritability, anxiety, depression, fatigue, or sleep disturbance [17]. Imaging performed on a patient with a headache following trauma is primarily done to rule out traumatic lesions such as intracranial hematomas. While subtle MRI changes may be seen later, there are no specific imaging findings to help diagnose a post traumatic headache [63]. As mentioned previously, dissection, cerebral venous thromboses, and CSF leaks with resulting intracranial hypotension should be considered in the differential for a headache following closed head injury and trauma.

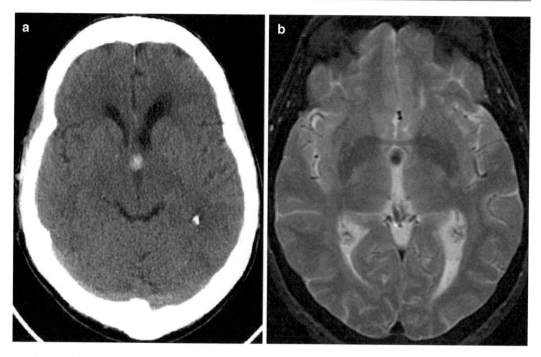

Fig. 1.8 Colloid cyst. Unenhanced CT (**a**) shows a hyperdense lesion anterior to the third ventricle that is seen as a low-signal lesion on T2-weighted MRI (**b**)

Third Ventricular Colloid Cyst

Colloid cysts are benign congenital cysts that arise in the anterior third ventricle (Fig. 1.8). They are usually asymptomatic and found incidentally on imaging in adulthood. However, if the cyst obstructs the foramen of Monro, it can disrupt CSF flow and lead to hydrocephalus. If both foramen of Monro are obstructed, this may lead to syncope, coma, or death. Occasionally, the tumor will act as a ball valve and only intermittently obstruct CSF flow. When this happens, the patient may complain of a severe positional headache, relieved in recumbency, sometimes associated with nausea and vomiting [64, 65].

Trigeminal Neuralgia

Classic trigeminal neuralgia presents as paroxysmal attacks of intense, sharp, and stabbing pain along one or more divisions of the trigeminal nerve. These attacks last from less than 1 second to 2 min and are often precipitated by stimulating certain "trigger zones." Chewing, talking, brushing teeth, cold air, or the slightest touch may trigger the paroxysmal pain [1]. Trigeminal neuralgia is most commonly due to compression of the trigeminal nerve by a blood vessel near its origin where it exits the brainstem. A demyelinating lesion or infarct at this so-called dorsal root entry zone may also cause trigeminal neuralgia and should be suspected in younger patients presenting with these symptoms. Much less commonly trigeminal neuralgia is due to compression by a mass lesion such as a meningioma or schwannoma or is idiopathic. Imaging is frequently performed to rule out a secondary etiology, but usually in an outpatient, rather than emergent, setting.

Glaucoma

Acute angle glaucoma may present with headache and associated eye discomfort, and there are also reports of subacute angle-closure glaucoma presenting with headache as the main presenting complaint [66]. If not identified and managed properly, either of these can result in permanent vision loss in the affected eye. Acute angle-closure glaucoma is an uncommon adverse effect of topiramate which is a common migraine preventative agent. Be concerned about glaucoma if the patient's headache pain came on suddenly when exposed to the dark. When going from light to dark, the sudden dilation of the pupil may block the outflow channels in the anterior chamber, leading to sudden increased intraocular pressure. The patient may complain of sudden severe unilateral headache and eye discomfort, associated with blurred vision in the affected eye and "halos" around lights. The affected eye is often red with a mid-dilated, sluggishly reactive pupil (may be irregularly shaped) and a hazy cornea [67]. Nausea and vomiting may be present. This is best evaluated by an emergent ophthalmology consult.

General Approach to the Management of Primary Headache in the Emergency Department

Once secondary headache disorders are excluded, the primary goal of the treating physician is to provide relief of headache pain and the accompanying symptoms such as nausea and vomiting. The majority of patients who present to the ED with headache will be diagnosed with a severe and/or prolonged migraine attack. Occasionally, patients with other diagnoses such as tension-type or cluster headache will present to the emergency department. Often the individual will have utilized her/his usual headache remedies without success. If the attack has lasted hours or longer and has been accompanied by poor oral intake of fluids with or without vomiting, the patient will likely be fluid depleted. If the patient is dehydrated, intravenous fluids need to be administered along with pharmacologic agents that treat the pain and other manifestations that accompany the pain. Often patients are quite distressed and anxious due to the duration and/or severity of the attack. The following general principles should be utilized:

- Place the patient in a darkened, quiet room.
- Provide reassurance.
- Provide IV rehydration.
- Treat nausea and vomiting quickly.
- Implement treatment with non-oral medication as soon as possible.
- Do not restrict antiemetics in patients with nausea, as many of the agents in this class are dopaminergic antagonists which have an anti-migraine action in addition to their antiemetic effect.
- Avoid drug-dependency-producing agents when possible (avoid butalbital and limit opioids, or at least use opioids with care).
- Rather than minimal dosing, use medication doses that are likely to be most effective.
- Use "migraine-specific" therapy when possible.
- Educate the patient regarding their condition.
- The patient should be counseled to make arrangements for follow-up as an outpatient for consideration of approaches that will optimally manage headaches.

Protocols for Acute Treatment of Migraine in the Emergency Department

There are several protocols employing a variety of agents that can be utilized for management of primary headache disorders in the emergency department. Again, most patients will be presenting with migraine and most of the protocols have been developed specifically for this disorder. Several of these have been shown to be effective in small prospective, controlled trials. To address the severe headaches that lead patients to seek care in the emergency department, many of these protocols focus on parenteral agents. Obviously, the treating care provider may elect to use an oral agent for management that can be self-administered by the patient.

The medications fall into relatively few categories of agents: (1) migraine-specific drugs (dihydroergotamine and sumatriptan); (2) dopamine (D_2)-blocking agents, such as neuroleptic drugs and metoclopramide; (3) other non-dependency-producing medications; and (4) opioid drugs.

It is important to note that drugs from different classes are often used together. This is done to maximize efficacy, to treat symptoms other than pain (e.g., nausea and vomiting), and, in some cases, to reduce the likelihood of side effects of another agent. For example, D_2 antagonists are always administered with intravenous dihydroer-gotamine to minimize its side effects of nausea and vomiting.

Evidence-based guidelines for the use of parenteral treatments in the treatment of migraine in the emergency department have been created by the American Headache Society and the Canadian Headache Society (Table 1.2). Note there are several differences in the recommendations, but many of the first-line treatment recommendations are similar.

Table 1.2 Summary of evidence based guidelines on parenteral treatment used in the treatment of migraine in the emergency department

Medication	American Headache Society Recommendations 2016	Canadian Headache Society Recommendations 2015
Sumatriptan SC	++	++
Ergotamine SC		+
Dihydroergotamine IM, SC, IV		+ (IM, SC)
Prochlorperazine IV	++	++
Metoclopramide IV	++	++
Chlorpromazine IV	+	+
Droperidol IM	+	Avoid
Haloperidol IV	+	Avoid
Trimethobenzamide SC,IV		Avoid (IV)
Lysine acetylsalicylic acid IV		++
Ketorolac IM, IV	+	++
Acetylsalicylic acid IV	+	
Dexketoprofen IV	+	
Diclofenac IM	+	Avoid
Lysine clonixinate IV		Avoid
Dexamethasone IV[a]	Avoid	Avoid
Acetaminophen IV	+	Avoid
Meperidine IM		+
Tramadol IM		Avoid
Hydromorphone IV	Avoid	
Morphine IV	Avoid	Avoid
Lidocaine IN, IV	Avoid (IV)	+ (IN); Avoid (IV)
Dipyrone IV[b]	+	
Valproic acid/sodium Valproate IV	+	Avoid
Magnesium sulfate IV		Avoid
Propofol IV		Avoid
Diphenhydramine IV	Avoid	
Octreotide IV, SC	Avoid (IV, SC)	Avoid (IV)
Gainsetron IV		Avoid

++ strong recommendation, + weak recommendation, *IM* intramuscular, *IN* intranasal, *IV* intravenous, *SC* subcutaneous [68, 69]

[a]Note these recommendations are for treatment of migraine; while dexamethasone has good evidence for preventing recurrence, there is no high quality evidence for treatment of migraine

[b]Banned in US and most of Europe due to possibility of agranulocytosis

Migraine-Specific Agents

Sumatriptan (5HT 1B/D/F Receptor Agonist)

Sumatriptan, 4 or 6 mg injected subcutaneously, has been shown to be both efficacious for treatment of acute migraine headache and for associated symptoms [70]. The dose can be repeated after an hour. Response rate at 1 h after a single dose of 6 mg is 70% [71]. Side effects include chest tightness, tingling, flushing, dizziness, and limb heaviness. Sumatriptan is the triptan of choice in the emergency department because it is the only triptan available in a subcutaneous formulation, which provides a rapid serum concentration and bypasses nausea, vomiting, and gastroparesis. Sumatriptan and eletriptan are at this time the only triptans to be considered "compatible" with breastfeeding by the American Academy of Pediatrics.

Contraindications for sumatriptan include:

- Pregnancy (relative contraindication)
- History or suspicion of ischemic heart disease
- History of coronary artery disease or Prinzmetal's angina
- Severe peripheral vascular disease
- Use of an ergot alkaloid (i.e., DHE, ergotamine) or other 5HT 1 agonist (i.e., another triptan) within 24 h
- Uncontrolled hypertension
- Previous adverse reaction
- Basilar or hemiplegic migraine
- Ischemic cerebrovascular disease

Dihydroergotamine

Dihydroergotamine mesylate (DHE) is an effective parenteral treatment for migraine attacks. The beneficial effects of DHE were initially attributed to vasoconstriction, but other mechanisms involving neurogenic inflammation and activity within central serotonergic systems provide a better explanation [72, 73]. It is important to note that headache resolution after treatment with IV DHE and metoclopramide has been reported in patients suffering headaches secondary to viral or carcinomatous meningitis; thus, response does not imply the diagnosis of a primary headache such as migraine or cluster headache [74]. Common side effects of DHE are nausea, vomiting, diarrhea, abdominal cramps, and leg pain.

DHE may be administered subcutaneously, intramuscularly, or intravenously. The intravenous route is the most rapidly effective. Unfortunately, the side effects of nausea and vomiting seem to be more prominent with intravenous administration.

The usual dose when administered subcutaneously or intramuscularly is 1.0 mg [75, 76]. In order to help prevent nausea, give an antiemetic such as 10 mg IV metoclopramide or 10 mg IV prochlorperazine approximately 10 minutes before giving DHE intravenously. The side effects and the utility of these D_2 blocking agents are outlined elsewhere in this chapter. DHE, 0.5 mg, is then slowly administered over a few minutes [77–79]. An additional 0.5 mg dose may be administered a few minutes later if no significant nausea or chest pain has developed. A 1.0 mg dose via subcutaneous, intramuscular, or intravenous routes may be repeated after one hour. In the case of status migrainosus or truly intractable migraine, the patient may require hospital admission and could be treated with repetitive or continuous DHE, using published protocols such as those of Raskin or Ford [80–82]. For instance, if the patient tolerates the medicine, IV DHE could be given as 0.5, 0.75, or 1.0 mg every 8 hours for 2–5 days along with an antiemetic such as metoclopramide 10 mg IV every 8 hours. Please see Fig. 1.9 for an example protocol. If extrapyramidal symptoms such as dystonia, akathisia, or oculogyric crisis develop from the metoclopramide, these could be addressed using parenteral benztropine mesylate or diphenhydramine. Alternatively, parenteral benztropine mesylate or diphenhydramine could be given as a pretreatment with each dose of DHE/metoclopramide to prevent these extrapyramidal side effects.

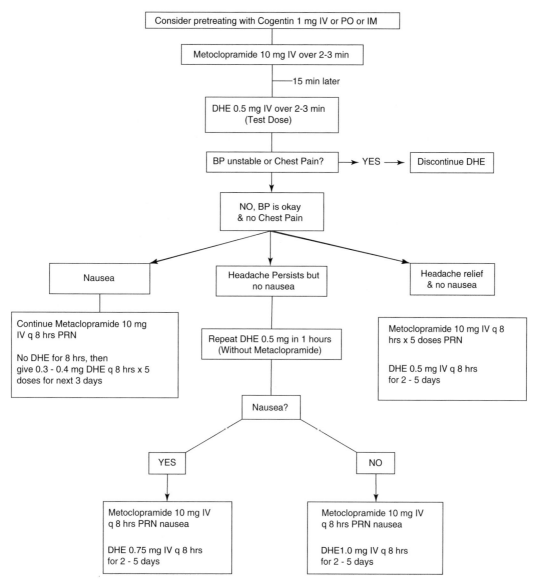

Fig. 1.9 Repetitive (every 8 hours) intravenous (IV) dihydroergotamine mesylate (DHE)–Raskin protocol. PO Orally, IM intramuscular, BP blood pressure, PRN as needed, q every. (Republished with permission of Thieme Medical Publishers, Inc. [TMP], from Management of Migraine Headache in the Emergency Department, Carrie E Robertson, Seminars in Neurology, 2010-03-29. Permission conveyed through Copyright Clearance Center, Inc. Adapted from *Raskin;* presented at: Headaches in the ED; AAN Annual Meeting; May 4, 2007; Boston, MA)

Contradictions for DHE include:

- Uncontrolled hypertension
- Ischemic heart disease
- Vasospastic angina
- Severe peripheral vascular disease
- MAO inhibitors within the last 2 weeks
- Prior use of a triptan within the last 24 h
- Significant hepatic disease
- Pregnancy
- Hemiplegic or basilar artery-type migraine

Antidopaminergic Agents

Antidopaminergic agents have well-recognized antiemetic and sedative effects which prove useful in the treatment of acute headache. In addition, there is significant clinical and experimental data suggesting that there is relative hyperactivity of dopaminergic neurotransmission in at least some migraineurs. These agents may have a specific antimigraine effect via blockade of D_2 dopamine receptors [83].

Common acute side effects of these agents include akathisia, acute dystonia, dizziness, and somnolence. Prolonged exposure (which is not an issue in the emergency department setting) may result in drug-induced tardive dystonia, parkinsonism, and tardive dyskinesia. The dizziness may be due to hypotension; therefore, carefully monitoring of vital signs, including a standing blood pressure prior to discharge, should be routine after administration of these agents.

The acute extrapyramidal side effects can be ameliorated by diphenhydramine, 25 mg, (intravenously or intramuscularly) or benztropine, 1 mg (intravenously or intramuscularly).

Rare but potentially fatal complications of these drugs include prolonged QT syndrome and *torsades de pointes*. Some individuals have an underlying genetic predisposition to the disorder, but it can also be acquired secondary to pharmacologic agents. For a list of agents which may produce a prolonged QT interval, see the online resource at Arizona Center for Education and Research on Therapeutics [84]. If a patient is taking one of these agents, treatment with a D_2 agent should be used with care. Prior to the parenteral administration of any of these agents, it is suggested that an ECG be obtained and the QT interval be carefully measured. If there is evidence of a prolonged QT interval, these agents should not be used.

Controlled trials show that a number of these drugs are effective in the acute management of migraine headache.

Prochlorperazine

Prochlorperazine has been shown to be an effective agent to relieve pain that can be used in repeated intravenous doses in a hospital or emergency department setting [85, 86]. Prochlorperazine, 10 mg per cc, can be diluted with 4 cc of normal saline to the concentration of 2 mg per cc. This is injected at a rate of 1 mg/min until the headache is relieved, or a maximum of 10 mg is administered [85–88]. Most often, a dose of 10 mg of intravenous prochlorperazine is injected over 2–5 min, and this is repeated every 20 min, up to a maximum dose of 30 mg. Prochlorperazine, administered as a 25-mg rectal suppository, is also effective for acute migraine therapy [89]. Its onset of action, however, is substantially slower than when administered intravenously.

Chlorpromazine

A number of studies demonstrate that chlorpromazine is an effective parenteral, acute treatment for migraine attacks. Prior to intravenous administration of this agent, the patient is often pretreated with 500 ml of normal saline to reduce the hypotensive side effect; more fluid may be appropriate if the patient has been vomiting or is dehydrated.

One of the most effective and easiest to use protocols is 12.5-mg chlorpromazine IV, which is repeated at 20-min intervals to a maximum of 37.5 mg [90]. Another protocol consists of chlorpromazine 0.1 mg/kg IV, which is repeated every 15 min as needed, up to a total of three doses [91]. Alternatively, chlorpromazine, 25 mg per cc, is diluted with 4 cc of normal saline to a concentration of 5 mg per cc. To reduce the risk of hypotension, chlorpromazine can be administered at a rate of 5 mg (1 cc) every 5 min until the headache is relieved, or the entire 25 mg is administered. An additional 10 mg (for a total of 35 mg) may be given in some cases. Chlorpromazine, 1 mg/kg intramuscularly, is also an effective headache treatment, but its action is slower in onset and the efficacy is less than by intravenous administration [92, 93]. Bigal et al. performed a double-blind randomized controlled study of 128 tension-type headache sufferers who either received placebo or 0.1 mg/kg of chlorpromazine IV as a one-time dose [94]. At 60 min, effects were statistically different from placebo for pain, nausea, photophobia, phonophobia, and need for rescue medication. Side effects included drowsiness and postural hypotension.

Haloperidol

In a small open study, haloperidol, 5 mg IV over a few minutes, resulted in headache relief [95]. Another randomized, controlled trial found that 5 mg of haloperidol in 500 cc of normal saline as a 20–30-min one-time infusion resulted in 16/20 (80%) of patients enjoying a marked relief from pain (a drop of greater than three on the visual analog pain scale) versus 15% in the placebo group measured between 1 and 3 h after infusion [96]. Side effects included 53% motor agitation (akathisia) and 53% sedation. Three of 20 patients treated with haloperidol returned to the emergency department with recurrent headache within 2–3 days. Haloperidol seems to cause less sedation and less hypotension than prochlorperazine or chlorpromazine. A more recent randomized, controlled trial comparing 5 mg IV haloperidol to 10 mg IV metoclopramide showed similar pain reduction at 80 minutes after receiving the medication [97]. However, those receiving haloperidol less frequently needed rescue treatment (3% vs 24%) as compared to those who received metoclopramide. The treatments were equally safe, but there was significantly more restlessness with haloperidol (43% vs 10%).

There is disagreement between the CHS and the AHS guidelines on whether haloperidol should be offered for treatment of migraine in the emergency department. This is possibly due to the fact that the most recent study comparing haloperidol and metoclopramide was not available when the Canadian guidelines were formulated. The CHS guidelines give a strong recommendation to avoid haloperidol based on the high likelihood of side effects of motor agitation and akathisia. The AHS guidelines report that haloperidol may be offered [68, 69].

Droperidol

Droperidol can be administered as 2.5 mg intravenously over 1 min and may be repeated every 30 min, up to a total of 7.5 mg [98]. Droperidol can also be effective when administered via the intramuscular route in doses ranging from 2.75 to 8.25 mg [99]. Though randomized controlled studies have demonstrated an effect equal to prochlorperazine, there is now a black-box warning for droperidol because it may provoke QT interval prolongation, *torsades de pointes*, or cardiac arrest. ECG monitoring should occur before, during, and for up to 2–4 h after administration, especially for those with congestive heart failure, bradycardia, cardiac hypertrophy, hypokalemia, and hypomagnesemia, or those patients using diuretics or other drugs known to cause QT interval prolongation [100]. As already noted, QT prolongation is a risk of all drugs in this class.

Metoclopramide

Metoclopramide, while not a neuroleptic agent, does have D_2 dopamine receptor-blocking properties [83]. It can be administered in a dose of 10 mg intravenously over a few minutes [101, 102]. Metoclopramide is generally less effective than the above neuroleptic agents, but efficacy can be substantially enhanced when used in combination with other antimigraine agents [103]. There have been eight randomized controlled trials of intravenous metoclopramide showing its efficacy [97, 104–110].

Sodium Valproate

Several preliminary or open-label studies found intravenous sodium valproate to be an effective, well-tolerated therapeutic agent for migraine in the emergency setting [111, 112]. Sodium valproate, 300–500 mg diluted in 100 cc of normal saline, is infused at a rate of 20 mg/min. Intravenous valproate has several advantages, including lack of cardiovascular side effects (no telemetry required), no interaction with triptans or ergot alkaloids, lack of sedation, and absence of dependence or habituation. Trials have used various dosing regimens. The half-life is 9–16 h, bioavailability is approximately 100%, and therapeutic blood levels are reached almost immediately [113].

There have been five randomized controlled trials of intravenous sodium valproate using different doses. The highest quality study was a randomized, controlled study comparing intravenous valproate (1000 mg) with metoclopramide (10 mg) and with ketorolac (30 mg). This study found that valproate was inferior to metoclopramide and to ketorolac with regard to pain reduction on a visual analog scale (2.8 vs 4.7 vs 3.9), need for rescue treatment (69% vs 22% vs 52%), and sustained headache freedom (4% vs 11% vs 16%) [109].

Another randomized, controlled study comparing intravenous valproate (500 mg) with IV prochlorperazine (10 mg) over 2 min found that prochlorperazine was statistically and clinically superior to IV valproate in reducing pain and nausea in migraine patients [114].

Sodium valproate (800 mg IV) was compared with lysine acetylsalicylic acid (1000 mg IV) in another randomized controlled study. Rates of pain relief at 1 hour and 24 hour sustained pain freedom were no different between groups [115]. In another randomized controlled trial, patients were given either sodium valproate 900 mg IV or dexamethasone 16 mg IV. There was no difference in reduction of the pain score between groups [116]. A similar randomized controlled trial of 400 mg IV sodium valproate compared to 16 mg IV dexamethasone also showed no difference between groups in pain reduction based on the visual analog scale, although sodium valproate appeared to perform better than dexamethasone [117].

It should be avoided in patients with hepatic disease. It is contraindicated in pregnancy; thus, women of childbearing age should have a negative pregnancy test before administration. Controlled trials need to be performed to confirm the efficacy of this agent.

Magnesium Sulfate

The evidence for magnesium sulfate's efficacy is far from overwhelming. One study concluded that 1 g of magnesium sulfate, given intrave-nously, resolved or improved acute migraine headaches (as well as cluster headaches) [118]. Improvement was more likely if basal serum ionized magnesium levels were low (less than 0.70 mmol/L). These results have not been confirmed in a placebo-controlled study. In this trial, magnesium sulfate had no significant side effects except mild flushing.

A study of 113 migraineurs compared 10-mg intravenous metoclopramide versus 2-g intravenous magnesium sulfate versus placebo. The study measured pain reduction at 30 min and found no difference compared to placebo for either magnesium or metoclopramide [105]. Another study found magnesium to be moderately helpful, but not as effective as prochlorperazine [86]. Yet another study showed that magnesium sulfate (1 g IV) was no better than placebo in pain relief when all patients with migraine were analyzed. However, in migraine with aura, there was significant improvement of pain and of all associated symptoms compared with controls with a therapeutic gain of nearly 37% at 1 h [119]. A recent systematic review of 7 randomized controlled trials in migraine ($n = 6$) and benign non-traumatic headache ($n = 1$) could not come to any firm conclusions on the efficacy of IV magnesium sulfate. Existing evidence shows potential benefits for the following endpoints: pain control beyond one hour, aura duration, and need for rescue analgesia [120].

Nonsteroidal Analgesics

Analgesics are widely used for acute treatment of headache. Ketorolac, a nonsteroidal anti-inflammatory drug which is available for injection, can be useful for treatment of some migraine attacks. The medication is given in a 30–60-mg IM injection [80, 121]. Intravenous ketorolac (0.4 mg/kg) can terminate both headache- and migraine-associated allodynia in up to 68% of patients within 1 h of treatment, even in those patients who have failed to respond to sumatriptan [105]. Ketorolac at a dose of 30-mg IV was beneficial but not as effective in reducing pain as

10-mg IV prochlorperazine [122]. Most patients should also be treated with an antiemetic. Drowsiness, dyspepsia, and nausea are potential side effects. Acute renal failure and gastrointestinal hemorrhage have been precipitated rarely by this agent.

In a small study comparing ketorolac 60-mg IM versus IV DHE/metoclopramide in various doses, only six of nine patients had moderate relief with ketorolac versus eight of nine who were given DHE/metoclopramide [80].

In a randomized controlled trial, ketorolac was shown to be superior to sodium valproate, and there was no difference when compared to metoclopramide [109].

The AHS provides a weak recommendation for the following parenteral NSAIDs: acetylsalicylic acid, ketorolac, dexketoprofen, and diclofenac []. The CHS provides a weak recommendation for lysine acetylsalicylic acid and ketorolac and provides weak recommendations against the use of lysine clonixinate and diclofenac [68].

Corticosteroids

Corticosteroids are typically given in combination with other antimigraine agents to enhance efficacy. Dexamethasone can be given IV or IM. Doses as high as 10–20-mg IV given over 10 min, followed by 4-mg IV every 6 h as needed, are very effective [123–125]. Alternatively, a one-time IM injection of 8 mg can also be employed [126].

A meta-analysis of studies that evaluated the efficacy of dexamethasone in addition to other therapy for acute migraine was performed. The analysis included studies that used randomized, double-blind, placebo-controlled methodology and that were performed in the emergency department. A pooled analysis of seven trials involving 742 patients suggested a modest but significant benefit when dexamethasone was added to standard antimigraine therapy. The analysis showed the addition of dexamethasone reduced the rate of patients with moderate or severe headache on 24- to 72-h follow-up evaluation (RR of 0.87,

95% CI of 0.80–0.95; absolute risk reduction of 9.7%). The treatment of 1000 patients with acute migraine headache using dexamethasone in addition to standard antimigraine therapy would be expected to prevent 97 patients from experiencing the outcome of moderate or severe headache at 24–72 h after emergency department evaluation [127].

Opioids

Despite multiple effective regimens of nonopioid medications, opioids continue to be commonly used for acute management of headache in the emergency department. In a nationwide survey of 811,419 adult migraine sufferers who visited an emergency department, 51% were treated with opioids and an alarming 77% of these had not received any nonopioid medications as a first-line attempt [128]. In a Canadian survey of 500 emergency department visits for headache, 59.6% of patients received narcotics as first-line treatment [129]. Opioids are not "migraine specific" and are generally not as effective as other agents. Further, in the setting of frequent emergency department or outpatient visits, their use raises concern about rebound and tolerance. Nevertheless, there are some patients for whom an opioid is the most effective and best-tolerated agent for acute, severe headaches, and opioids continue to play a role as rescue agents. Meperidine is the most commonly utilized agent in this setting. It may be administered intravenously or intramuscularly, most commonly in a dose of 75–150 mg. It should be accompanied by promethazine, 25–50 mg, or hydroxyzine, 25–100 mg, intramuscularly to treat nausea and vomiting; these also provide sedative and anxiolytic effects [130].

Because clinical trials assessing efficacy and side effects of meperidine performed to date have been small and have not arrived at consistent conclusions, Friedman et al. performed a systematic review and meta-analysis to determine the relative efficacy and adverse effect profile of opioids compared with nonopioid active comparators for the treatment of acute migraine [131]. Four trials (involving 254 patients) compared meperidine to dihydroergotamine, four trials (involving 248 patients) compared meperidine to an antiemetic, and three trials (involving 123 patients) compared meperidine to ketorolac. Meperidine was less effective than dihydroergotamine at providing headache relief (OR of 0.30; 95% confidence interval [CI] 0.09–0.97) and trended toward less efficacy than the antiemetics (OR of 0.46; 95% CI 0.19–1.11); however, the efficacy of meperidine was similar to that of ketorolac (OR of 1.75; 95% CI 0.84–3.61). Compared to dihydroergotamine, meperidine caused more sedation (OR of 3.52; 95% CI 0.87–14.19) and dizziness (OR of 8.67; 95% CI 2.66–28.23). Compared to the antiemetics, meperidine caused less akathisia (OR of 0.10; 95% CI 0.02–0.57). Meperidine and ketorolac use resulted in similar rates of gastrointestinal adverse effects (OR of 1.27; 95% CI 0.31–5.15) and sedation (OR of 1.70; 95% CI 0.23–12.72). The authors appropriately conclude that emergency department physicians should consider alternate parenteral treatments for migraine headaches.

Indeed, meperidine is losing favor among pain specialists for use as an analgesic, and many authorities argue that other opioids should be used for acute pain. This is due to meperidine's poor efficacy, toxicity, and multiple drug interactions [132]. The argument can be made that if a parenteral opioid is needed, then an opioid other than meperidine should be selected and administered in an equipotent dose [133].

Greater Occipital Nerve Blocks

Greater occipital nerve blocks with bupivacaine are a potentially attractive alternative to other IV treatments given their relative safety. Treatment of migraine in the emergency department with greater occipital nerve blocks has been studied in two small randomized clinical trials. One compared greater occipital nerve blocks vs sham intradermal bupivacaine injection, while the other compared greater occipital nerve blocks with bupivacaine vs saline injection vs IV dexketoprofen + metoclopramide [134, 135]. Both of these studies showed positive results, but given the small sample size, further study is needed prior to regular use of greater occipital nerve blocks for migraine in the emergency department.

Cluster Headache Treatment

Therapeutic options for cluster headache vary in some respects from other primary headache disorders and are therefore considered separately. Effective treatments include:

Oxygen

A range of 8–12 L/min of 100% oxygen through a closed face mask can resolve most cluster headache attacks if the sufferer can begin therapy at the onset of the attack. Sometimes, a flow rate of 15 L/min is effective when lower flow rates are not. Oxygen's effectiveness in cluster headache has been proven in a double-blind controlled trial [136].

Sumatriptan

In one study, 96% of cluster headache sufferers achieved pain relief in 15 min with 6-mg SC sumatriptan [137]. The maximal recommended dose per 24 h is 12 mg. Now that it comes in a 4-mg subcutaneous dosage, a cluster patient may use up to three doses a day. Some may break open the subcutaneous device and dole out only small quantities in order to make their medicine last longer and treat more attacks.

Dihydroergotamine

One milligram IV dihydroergotamine preceded by 10-mg metoclopramide can rapidly resolve cluster headache attacks in less than 15 min [138]. Subcutaneous or IM injections of 1 mg DHE up to 2–3 times a day can be used outside of the office or emergency department, but onset of relief is slower. Intranasal DHE is difficult to use and too slow to relieve individual attacks, but it may lessen attack severity.

Corticosteroids

Corticosteroids can provide a temporary reprieve lasting days to weeks in many patients with cluster headache. Corticosteroids have been used to treat cluster headache for over 50 years, and they have been shown to be more effective than placebo [139]. In a large, retrospective series, Kudrow found that 60 mg a day produced a complete remission in up to 77% of patients [140].

In one open-label study, 13 cluster headache patients used 30 mg/kg of IV methylprednisolone as a 3-h infusion in saline on the eighth day of the cluster period [141]. Only 3 of 13 patients had a complete remission of headache, and the mean interval until the next attack was 2–7 days indicating no advantage over prednisone.

In another study using IV methylprednisolone, 250-mg boluses over three consecutive days, followed by 90 mg per day of oral prednisone tapered off over 4 weeks, lowered attack frequency substantially for several weeks [142].

Greater Occipital Nerve Blocks

Ipsilateral greater occipital nerve blocks with corticosteroid have been shown to be superior to placebo in two randomized controlled trials for the treatment of cluster headache [143, 144]. These are helpful in the transitional treatment of cluster headache to obtain remission, while appropriate maintenance prophylaxis (i.e., verapamil) is initiated. The first study compared a combination of lidocaine and betamethasone

($n = 13$) with lidocaine and saline ($n = 10$). Eleven (85%) patients in the treatment group were headache free at one week with 8 remaining headache free at 4 weeks compared to none in the placebo group [143]. In the more recent study, subjects with cluster headache were randomized to receive either cortivazol ($n = 21$) or saline injections in the ipsilateral suboccipital region on 3 consecutive occasions (48–72 hours apart). The primary endpoint was reduction in frequency of attacks to 2 or fewer in the 72 hour period 2 to 4 days after the third suboccipital injection. Twenty of 21 subjects receiving cortivazol and 12 of 22 controls met the primary endpoint which was a significant difference. Mean number of attacks days 1 through 15 was also significantly lower in the cortivazol group, but 30 day remission and 30 day outcome of 2 or fewer cluster attacks was no different [144].

Special Circumstance: Treatment of Headache in the Pregnant Patient

As mentioned in the earlier headache history section, when evaluating a pregnant patient with new or worsening headaches in the emergency room, secondary causes must be ruled out first, including: preeclampsia/eclampsia, central venous thrombosis, reversible cerebral vasoconstriction syndrome, stroke, and pituitary apoplexy. Migraine headaches often improve during pregnancy, especially in the second and third trimesters. However, some pregnant migraineurs do notice worsening of their migraines.

Because home treatment options are somewhat limited, the pregnant migraine sufferer may be forced to come to the emergency department for management. There is general agreement that Tylenol, possibly combined with caffeine, is a good first-line choice for the acute migraine attack [23, 24, 145, 146], as both are felt to be generally safe during pregnancy. The drawback to Tylenol is that it is a short-acting analgesic and, if taken too frequently, could contribute to a potential rebound, or analgesic overuse, headache. Furthermore, by the time the patient arrives to the emergency department, there is a strong possibility that she has already tried this.

As mentioned early in the section on headache management, the initial approach should include conservative measures, such as making sure the patient is well hydrated. Ibuprofen and naproxen are generally considered safe during the second trimester, but should be avoided during the third trimester as they may cause premature closure of the ductus arteriosus [24, 147]. Some studies have shown a small risk of increased spontaneous abortion and congenital malformations when these NSAIDs are taken in the first trimester, so one might also be cautious early in pregnancy [148].

For nausea, metoclopramide has been used during all stages of pregnancy with no evidence of embryo, fetal, or newborn harm and is considered FDA class B (no evidence of risk in humans, but no controlled studies) [148]. Other antiemetics, such as prochlorperazine, remain class C due to limited information and therefore should be reserved for when the benefits are thought to outweigh the potential risks [147, 148].

Cranial nerve blocks, including blocks of the greater occipital, lesser occipital, and supraorbital nerves as well as blocks of the sphenopalatine ganglion (using lidocaine only), may be helpful in providing temporary headache relief during pregnancy.

As mentioned previously, narcotic medications should be avoided if at all possible, given the association with drug dependency and rebound headache. With prolonged use in pregnancy, especially in the third trimester, there is a risk of neonatal addiction and respiratory distress. Of the opiate medications, codeine has been associated with more reports of cleft lip/palate, cardiac, and respiratory defects and should therefore probably be avoided, especially during the first trimester [149]. Morphine, oxycodone, and meperidine are probably not teratogenic, but the data is somewhat limited [148]. Given the limited options during pregnancy, these may be considered for very short-term use, during status migrainosus, if necessary.

Sumatriptan was embryo lethal in rabbits when given in large doses intravenously and produced some vascular and skeletal anomalies when given in large doses orally [148]. The data in human fetuses is less clear. In the sumatriptan pregnancy registry, sumatriptan use has been associated with an increased risk of preterm delivery and low birth weight [150]. There have also been a small number of recorded birth defects, with any trimester exposure proportion of 4.4% (95% CI 2.8–6.8%) as compared to the prevalence of birth defects in migraineurs, which has been estimated at 3.4% [148]. In other retrospective and observational cohort studies, the risk has been even less [148]. Ultimately, there is not enough data on sumatriptan use in human fetuses to detect minor anomalies. Furthermore, some of the existing studies lack the long-term follow-up needed to detect late adverse effects. As there is insufficient data to rule out risk to the fetus, all triptans including sumatriptan remain FDA pregnancy class C.

Corticosteroids have been shown to increase major malformations when used in the first trimester. Therefore for the first trimester, they are FDA class D [148], showing positive risk to humans. One of these risks appears to be a small risk of orofacial defects [148]. For the second and third trimester of pregnancy, animal studies show clear risk to the fetus, but the human studies are less clear. Because of the limited information, they are considered FDA class C during the second and third trimesters. Of the corticosteroids, oral prednisone seems to have less risk than prednisolone [148] and has been advocated by some as an option for the short-term management of status migrainosus [23, 147].

Magnesium is no longer considered safe due to potential effects on bone development [151] US Food and Drug Administration (FDA): Drug Safety Communications: FDA recommends against prolonged use of magnesium sulfate to stop pre-term labor due to bone changes in exposed babies. U.S. Food and Drug Administration (FDA). Silver Spring, MD. 2013 https://www.fda.gov/media/85971/download; Accessed November 14, 2019]

Ergotamine/DHE should be avoided during pregnancy (FDA class X) as there have been idiosyncratic responses to treatment that have been associated with fetal toxicity and teratogenicity, possibly due to the disruption of maternal-fetal vascular supply [148]. Valproic acid (FDA class D, human data suggests risk) is also a known teratogen and should be avoided during pregnancy [148].

Summary of pregnancy list in the acute setting [24, 147, 148]:

- *Probably safe in the acute setting (FDA class B):* Tylenol, caffeine, NSAIDs during the second trimester, metoclopramide, morphine, oxycodone, and meperidine
- *Use if the benefit outweighs the risk (FDA class C):* NSAIDs during first trimester, triptans, prochlorperazine, oral prednisone, and codeine
- *Probably avoid (FDA class C but shows risk during first and third trimesters):* Aspirin
- *Avoid (FDA class D or X):* NSAIDs or aspirin during third trimester, sodium valproate, magnesium, and ergotamine/DHE

Because of the difficulty in management, the pregnant patient should receive counseling on how to minimize the frequency of future headaches. This would include avoidance of headache triggers and maintaining regular meals and sleep patterns. Physical therapy, exercise, relaxation, and biofeedback are nonmedication options to try. Thermal biofeedback, in particular, has been associated with headache reduction during pregnancy [147].

References

1. Headache classification committee of the international headache society (IHS) the international classification of headache disorders, 3rd edition. Cephalalgia. 2018;38:1–211.
2. Rui P, Kang K. National Hospital Ambulatory Medical Care Survey: 2017 Emergency Department summary tables. National Center for Health Statistics. Available from: https://www.cdc.gov/nchs/data/nhamcs/web_tables/2017_ed_web_tables-508.pdf. Accessed 17 Feb 2020.
3. Goldstein JN, Camargo CA Jr, Pelletier AJ, Edlow JA. Headache in United States emergency departments: demographics, work-up and frequency of pathological diagnoses. Cephalalgia. 2006;26(6):684–90.
4. Landtblom AM, Fridriksson S, Boivie J, Hillman J, Johansson G, Johansson I. Sudden onset headache: a prospective study of features, incidence and causes. Cephalalgia. 2002;22(5):354–60.
5. Pietrobon D, Striessnig J. Neurobiology of migraine. Nat Rev Neurosci. 2003;4(5):386–98.
6. Uddman R, Edvinsson L, Ekman R, Kingman T, McCulloch J. Innervation of the feline cerebral vasculature by nerve fibers containing calcitonin gene-related peptide: trigeminal origin and co-existence with substance P. Neurosci Lett. 1985;62(1):131–6.
7. Buzzi MG, Carter WB, Shimizu T. Heath 3 H. Moskowitz MA. Dihydroergotamine and sumatriptan attenuate levels of CGRP in plasma in rat superior sagittal sinus during electrical stimulation of the trigeminal ganglion. Neuropharmacology. 1991;30(11):1193–200.
8. Markowitz S, Saito K, Moskowitz MA. Neurogenically mediated plasma extravasation in dura mater: effect of ergot alkaloids. A possible mechanism of action in vascular headache. Cephalalgia. 1988;8(2):83–91.
9. Dimitriadou V, Buzzi MG, Theoharides TC, Moskowitz MA. Ultrastructural evidence for neurogenically mediated changes in blood vessels of the rat dura mater and tongue following antidromic trigeminal stimulation. Neuroscience. 1992;48(1):187–203.
10. Strassman AM, Raymond SA, Burstein R. Sensitization of meningeal sensory neurons on the origin of headaches. Nature. 1996;384(6609):560–4.
11. Moskowitz MA, Cutrer FM. SUMATRIPTAN: a receptor-targeted treatment for migraine. Annu Rev Med. 1993;44:145–54.
12. Nozaki K, Boccalini P, Moskowitz MA. Expression of c-fos-like immunoreactivity in brainstem after meningeal irritation by blood in the subarachnoid space. Neuroscience. 1992;49(3):669–80.
13. Kaube H, Keay KA, Hoskin KL, Bandler R, Goadsby PJ. Expression of c-Fos-like immunoreactivity in the caudal medulla and upper cervical spinal cord following stimulation of the superior sagittal sinus in the cat. Brain Res. 1993;629(1):95–102.
14. Goadsby PJ, Hoskin KL. The distribution of trigeminovascular afferents in the nonhuman primate brain Macaca nemestrina: a c-fos immunocytochemical study. J Anat. 1997;190(Pt 3):367–75.
15. Weiller C, May A, Limmroth V, et al. Brain stem activation in spontaneous human migraine attacks. Nat Med. 1995;1(7):658–60.
16. Matsushige T, Nakaoka M, Kiya K, Takeda T, Kurisu K. Cerebral sinovenous thrombosis after closed head injury. J Trauma. 2009;66(6):1599–604.
17. Lane JC, Arciniegas DB. Post-traumatic headache. Curr Treat Options Neurol. 2002;4(1):89–104.
18. Keles A, Demircan A, Kurtoglu G. Carbon monoxide poisoning: how many patients do we miss? Eur J Emerg Med. 2008;15(3):154–7.

19. Risser D, Bonsch A, Schneider B. Should coroners be able to recognize unintentional carbon monoxide-related deaths immediately at the death scene? J Forensic Sci. 1995;40(4):596–8.

20. Ernst A, Zibrak JD. Carbon monoxide poisoning. N Engl J Med. 1998;339(22):1603–8.

21. Soffietti R, Ruda R, Mutani R. Management of brain metastases. J Neurol. 2002;249(10):1357–69.

22. Melhado EM, Maciel JA Jr, Guerreiro CA. Headache during gestation: evaluation of 1101 women. Can J Neurol Sci. 2007;34(2):187–92.

23. Loder E. Migraine in pregnancy. Semin Neurol. 2007;27(5):425–33.

24. Menon R, Bushnell CD. Headache and pregnancy. Neurologist. 2008;14(2):108–19.

25. Calabrese LH, Dodick DW, Schwedt TJ, Singhal AB. Narrative review: reversible cerebral vasoconstriction syndromes. Ann Intern Med. 2007;146(1):34–44.

26. Gdynia HJ, Huber R. Bilateral internal carotid artery dissections related to pregnancy and childbirth. Eur J Med Res. 2008;13(5):229–30.

27. Oehler J, Lichy C, Gandjour J, Fiebach J, Grau AJ. Dissection of four cerebral arteries after protracted birth. Nervenarzt. 2003;74(4):366–9.

28. Tuluc M, Brown D, Goldman B. Lethal vertebral artery dissection in pregnancy: a case report and review of the literature. Arch Pathol Lab Med. 2006;130(4):533–5.

29. Wiebers DO, Mokri B. Internal carotid artery dissection after childbirth. Stroke. 1985;16(6):956–9.

30. Helms AK, Kittner SJ. Pregnancy and stroke. CNS Spectr. 2005;10(7):580–7.

31. Kittner SJ, Stern BJ, Feeser BR, et al. Pregnancy and the risk of stroke. N Engl J Med. 1996;335(11):768–74.

32. Corbett JJ, Brazis PW. The eye and headache. In: Silberstein SD, Lipton RB, Dodick DW, editors. Wolff's headache. 8th ed. Oxford: Oxford University Press; 2008. p. 571–94.

33. Do TP, Remmers A, Schytz HW, et al. Red and orange flags for secondary headaches in clinical practice: SNNOOP10 list. Neurology. 2019;92(3):134–44.

34. Wei JH, Wang HF. Cardiac cephalalgia: case reports and review. Cephalalgia. 2008;28(8):892–6.

35. Latchaw RE, Silva P, Falcone SF. The role of CT following aneurysmal rupture. Neuroimaging Clin N Am. 1997;7(4):693–708.

36. Perry JJ, Spacek A, Forbes M, et al. Is the combination of negative computed tomography result and negative lumbar puncture result sufficient to rule out subarachnoid hemorrhage? Ann Emerg Med. 2008;51(6):707–13.

37. Byyny RL, Mower WR, Shum N, Gabayan GZ, Fang S, Baraff LJ. Sensitivity of noncontrast cranial computed tomography for the emergency department diagnosis of subarachnoid hemorrhage. Ann Emerg Med. 2008;51(6):697–703.

38. Edlow JA. Diagnosis of subarachnoid hemorrhage. Neurocrit Care. 2005;2(2):99–109.

39. Hasbun R, Abrahams J, Jekel J, Quagliarello VJ. Computed tomography of the head before lumbar puncture in adults with suspected meningitis. N Engl J Med. 2001;345(24):1727–33.

40. Sidman R, Spitalnic S, Demelis M, Durfey N, Jay G. Xanthrochromia? By what method? A comparison of visual and spectrophotometric xanthrochromia. Ann Emerg Med. 2005;46(1):51–5.

41. Arora S, Swadron SP, Dissanayake V. Evaluating the sensitivity of visual xanthochromia in patients with subarachnoid hemorrhage. J Emerg Med. 2008;39:13.

42. Perry JJ, Sivilotti ML, Stiell IG, et al. Should spectrophotometry be used to identify xanthochromia in the cerebrospinal fluid of alert patients suspected of having subarachnoid hemorrhage? Stroke. 2006;37(10):2467–72.

43. Lipton RB, Scher AI, Silberstein SD, Bigal ME. Migraine diagnosis and comorbidity. In: Silberstein SD, Lipton RB, Dodick DW, editors. Wolff's headache. 8th ed. Oxford: Oxford University Press; 2008. p. 153–75.

44. Schwedt TJ, Matharu MS, Dodick DW. Thunderclap headache. Lancet Neurol. 2006;5(7):621–31.

45. Masuhr F, Mehraein S, Einhaupl K. Cerebral venous and sinus thrombosis. J Neurol. 2004;251(1):11–23.

46. de Bruijn SF, Stam J. Randomized, placebo-controlled trial of anticoagulant treatment with low-molecular-weight heparin for cerebral sinus thrombosis. Stroke. 1999;30(3):484–8.

47. van de Beek D, de Gans J, Spanjaard L, Weisfelt M, Reitsma JB, Vermeulen M. Clinical features and prognostic factors in adults with bacterial meningitis. N Engl J Med. 2004;351(18):1849–59.

48. Arnold M, Cumurciuc R, Stapf C, Favrole P, Berthet K, Bousser MG. Pain as the only symptom of cervical artery dissection. J Neurol Neurosurg Psychiatry. 2006;77(9):1021–4.

49. Gerretsen P, Kern RZ. Reversible cerebral vasoconstriction syndrome: a thunderclap headache-associated condition. Curr Neurol Neurosci Rep. 2009;9(2):108–14.

50. Ducros A, Bousser MG. Reversible cerebral vasoconstriction syndrome. Pract Neurol. 2009;9(5):256–67.

51. Mokri B, Schievink WI. Headache associated with abnormalities in intracranial structure or function: low-cerebrospinal fluid pressure headache. In: Silberstein SD, Lipton RB, Dodick DW, editors. Wolff's headache. 8th ed. Oxford: Oxford University Press; 2008. p. 513–31.

52. Mokri B, Piepgras DG, Miller GM. Syndrome of orthostatic headaches and diffuse pachymeningeal gadolinium enhancement. Mayo Clin Proc. 1997;72(5):400–13.

53. Mokri B. Spontaneous low cerebrospinal pressure/volume headaches. Curr Neurol Neurosci Rep. 2004;4(2):117–24.

54. Bender SR, Fong MW, Heitz S, Bisognano JD. Characteristics and management of patients presenting to the emergency department with hyper-

tensive urgency. J Clin Hypertens (Greenwich). 2006;8(1):12–8.

55. Matharu MS, Schwedt TJ, Dodick DW. Thunderclap headache: an approach to a neurologic emergency. Curr Neurol Neurosci Rep. 2007;7(2):101–9.

56. Sibal L, Ball SG, Connolly V, et al. Pituitary apoplexy: a review of clinical presentation, management and outcome in 45 cases. Pituitary. 2004;7(3):157–63.

57. Randeva HS, Schoebel J, Byrne J, Esiri M, Adams CB, Wass JA. Classical pituitary apoplexy: clinical features, management and outcome. Clin Endocrinol. 1999;51(2):181–8.

58. Wall M. Idiopathic intracranial hypertension (pseudotumor cerebri). Insight. 2008;33(2):18–25. quiz 26–17

59. Sengupta S, Eckstein C, Collins T. The Dilemma of diagnosing idiopathic intracranial hypertension without papilledema in patients with chronic migraine. JAMA Neurol. 2019;76(9):1001–2.

60. Brazis PW. Clinical review: the surgical treatment of idiopathic pseudotumour cerebri (idiopathic intracranial hypertension). Cephalalgia. 2008;28(12):1361–73.

61. Atkinson JL. Commentary on clinical review: the surgical treatment of idiopathic pseudotumour cerebri, by Paul Brazis. Cephalalgia. 2008;28(12):1374–6.

62. Lin A, Foroozan R, Danesh-Meyer HV, De Salvo G, Savino PJ, Sergott RC. Occurrence of cerebral venous sinus thrombosis in patients with presumed idiopathic intracranial hypertension. Ophthalmology. 2006;113(12):2281–4.

63. Solomon S. Post-traumatic headache: commentary: an overview. Headache. 2009;49(7):1112–5.

64. Humphries RL, Stone CK, Bowers RC. Colloid cyst: a case report and literature review of a rare but deadly condition. J Emerg Med. 2008;40:e5.

65. Spears RC. Colloid cyst headache. Curr Pain Headache Rep. 2004;8(4):297–300.

66. Nesher R, Epstein E, Stern Y, Assia E, Nesher G. Headaches as the main presenting symptom of subacute angle closure glaucoma. Headache. 2005;45(2):172–6.

67. Dennis WR, Dennis AM. Eye emergencies. In: Stone CK, Humphries RL, editors. Current emergency diagnosis & treatment. 5th ed. New York: McGraw-Hill; 2004. p. 599–625.

68. Orr SL, Aube M, Becker WJ, et al. Canadian headache society systematic review and recommendations on the treatment of migraine pain in emergency settings. Cephalalgia. 2015;35(3):271–84.

69. Orr SL, Friedman BW, Christie S, et al. Management of adults with acute migraine in the emergency department: the american headache society evidence assessment of parenteral pharmacotherapies. Headache. 2016;56(6):911–40.

70. Treatment of migraine attacks with sumatriptan. The subcutaneous Sumatriptan international study group. N Engl J Med. 1991;325(5):316–21.

71. IMITREX(R) injection, sumatriptan succinate injection. Research Triangle Park: GlaxoSmithKline; 2008.

72. Buzzi MG, Moskowitz MA. Evidence for 5-HT1B/1D receptors mediating the antimigraine effect of sumatriptan and dihydroergotamine. Cephalalgia. 1991;11(4):165–8.

73. Tfelt-Hansen P. Ergotamine, dihydroergotamine: current uses and problems. Curr Med Res Opin. 2001;17(Suppl 1):s30–4.

74. Gross DW, Donat JR, Boyle CA. Dihydroergotamine and metoclopramide in the treatment of organic headache. Headache. 1995;35(10):637–8.

75. Winner P, Ricalde O, Le Force B, Saper J, Margul B. A double-blind study of subcutaneous dihydroergotamine vs subcutaneous sumatriptan in the treatment of acute migraine. Arch Neurol. 1996;53(2):180–4.

76. Weisz MA, el-Raheb M, Blumenthal HJ. Home administration of intramuscular DHE for the treatment of acute migraine headache. Headache. 1994;34(6):371–3.

77. Callaham M, Raskin N. A controlled study of dihydroergotamine in the treatment of acute migraine headache. Headache. 1986;26(4):168–71.

78. Klapper JA, Stanton J. Current emergency treatment of severe migraine headaches. Headache. 1993;33(10):560–2.

79. Klapper JA, Stanton JS. Ketorolac versus DHE and metoclopramide in the treatment of migraine headaches. Headache. 1991;31(8):523–4.

80. Raskin NH. Treatment of status migrainosus: the American experience. Headache. 1990;30(Suppl 2):550–3.

81. Ford RG, Ford KT. Continuous intravenous dihydroergotamine in the treatment of intractable headache. Headache. 1997;37(3):129–36.

82. Robertson CE, Black DF, Swanson JW. Management of migraine headache in the emergency department. Semin Neurol. 2010;30(2):201–11.

83. Peroutka SJ. Dopamine and migraine. Neurology. 1997;49(3):650–6.

84. QT Drug Lists by Risk Groups. http://www.azcert.org/medical-pros/drug-lists/drug-lists.cfm. Accessed 22 Aug 2009.

85. Lu SR, Fuh JL, Juang KD, Wang SJ. Repetitive intravenous prochlorperazine treatment of patients with refractory chronic daily headache. Headache. 2000;40(9):724–9.

86. Ginder S, Oatman B, Pollack M. A prospective study of i.v. magnesium and i.v. prochlorperazine in the treatment of headaches. J Emerg Med. 2000;18(3):311–5.

87. Coppola M, Yealy DM, Leibold RA. Randomized, placebo-controlled evaluation of prochlorperazine versus metoclopramide for emergency department treatment of migraine headache. Ann Emerg Med. 1995;26(5):541–6.

88. Jones J, Sklar D, Dougherty J, White W. Randomized double-blind trial of intravenous prochlorperazine

for the treatment of acute headache. J Am Med Assoc. 1989;261(8):1174–6.

89. Jones EB, Gonzalez ER, Boggs JG, Grillo JA, Elswick RK Jr. Safety and efficacy of rectal prochlorperazine for the treatment of migraine in the emergency department. Ann Emerg Med. 1994;24(2):237–41.

90. Bell R, Montoya D, Shuaib A, Lee MA. A comparative trial of three agents in the treatment of acute migraine headache. Ann Emerg Med. 1990;19(10):1079–82.

91. Lane PL, McLellan BA, Baggoley CJ. Comparative efficacy of chlorpromazine and meperidine with dimenhydrinate in migraine headache. Ann Emerg Med. 1989;18(4):360–5.

92. Iserson KV. Parenteral chlorpromazine treatment of migraine. Ann Emerg Med. 1983;12(12):756–8.

93. McEwen JI, O'Connor HM, Dinsdale HB. Treatment of migraine with intramuscular chlorpromazine. Ann Emerg Med. 1987;16(7):758–63.

94. Bigal ME, Bordini CA, Speciali JG. Intravenous chlorpromazine in the acute treatment of episodic tension-type headache: a randomized, placebo controlled, double-blind study. Arq Neuropsiquiatr. 2002;60(3-A):537–41.

95. Fisher H. A new approach to emergency department therapy of migraine headache with intravenous haloperidol: a case series. J Emerg Med. 1995;13(1):119–22.

96. Honkaniemi J, Liimatainen S, Rainesalo S, Sulavuori S. Haloperidol in the acute treatment of migraine: a randomized, double-blind, placebo-controlled study. Headache. 2006;46(5):781–7.

97. Gaffigan ME, Bruner DI, Wason C, Pritchard A, Frumkin K. A randomized controlled trial of intravenous haloperidol vs. intravenous metoclopramide for acute migraine therapy in the emergency department. J Emerg Med. 2015;49(3):326–34.

98. Wang SJ, Silberstein SD, Young WB. Droperidol treatment of status migrainosus and refractory migraine. Headache. 1997;37(6):377–82.

99. Silberstein SD, Young WB, Mendizabal JE, Rothrock JF, Alam AS. Acute migraine treatment with droperidol: a randomized, double-blind, placebo-controlled trial. Neurology. 2003;60(2):315–21.

100. Weaver CS, Jones JB, Chisholm CD, et al. Droperidol vs prochlorperazine for the treatment of acute headache. J Emerg Med. 2004;26(2):145–50.

101. Tek DS, McClellan DS, Olshaker JS, Allen CL, Arthur DC. A prospective, double-blind study of metoclopramide hydrochloride for the control of migraine in the emergency department. Ann Emerg Med. 1990;19(10):1083–7.

102. Ellis GL, Delaney J, DeHart DA, Owens A. The efficacy of metoclopramide in the treatment of migraine headache. Ann Emerg Med. 1993;22(2):191–5.

103. Colman I, Brown MD, Innes GD, Grafstein E, Roberts TE, Rowe BH. Parenteral metoclopramide for acute migraine: meta-analysis of randomised controlled trials. BMJ. 2004;329(7479):1369–73.

104. Cameron JD, Lane PL, Speechley M. Intravenous chlorpromazine vs intravenous metoclopramide in acute migraine headache. Acad Emerg Med. 1995;2(7):597–602.

105. Cete Y, Dora B, Ertan C, Ozdemir C, Oktay C. A randomized prospective placebo-controlled study of intravenous magnesium sulphate vs. metoclopramide in the management of acute migraine attacks in the emergency department. Cephalalgia. 2005;25(3):199–204.

106. Friedman BW, Corbo J, Lipton RB, et al. A trial of metoclopramide vs sumatriptan for the emergency department treatment of migraines. Neurology. 2005;64(3):463–8.

107. Friedman BW, Esses D, Solorzano C, et al. A randomized controlled trial of prochlorperazine versus metoclopramide for treatment of acute migraine. Ann Emerg Med. 2008;52(4):399–406.

108. Talabi S, Masoumi B, Azizkhani R, Esmailian M. Metoclopramide versus sumatriptan for treatment of migraine headache: a randomized clinical trial. J Res Med Sci. 2013;18(8):695–8.

109. Friedman BW, Garber L, Yoon A, et al. Randomized trial of IV valproate vs metoclopramide vs ketorolac for acute migraine. Neurology. 2014;82(11):976–83.

110. Shahrami A, Assarzadegan F, Hatamabadi HR, Asgarzadeh M, Sarehbandi B, Asgarzadeh S. Comparison of therapeutic effects of magnesium sulfate vs. dexamethasone/metoclopramide on alleviating acute migraine headache. J Emerg Med. 2015;48(1):69–76.

111. Edwards KR, Norton J, Behnke M. Comparison of intravenous valproate versus intramuscular dihydroergotamine and metoclopramide for acute treatment of migraine headache. Headache. 2001;41(10):976–80.

112. Mathew NT, Kailasam J, Meadors L, Chernyschev O, Gentry P. Intravenous valproate sodium (depacon) aborts migraine rapidly: a preliminary report. Headache. 2000;40(9):720–3.

113. Norton J. Use of intravenous valproate sodium in status migraine. Headache. 2000;40(9):755–7.

114. Tanen DA, Miller S, French T, Riffenburgh RH. Intravenous sodium valproate versus prochlorperazine for the emergency department treatment of acute migraine headaches: a prospective, randomized, double-blind trial. Ann Emerg Med. 2003;41(6):847–53.

115. Leniger T, Pageler L, Stude P, Diener HC, Limmroth V. Comparison of intravenous valproate with intravenous lysine-acetylsalicylic acid in acute migraine attacks. Headache. 2005;45(1):42–6.

116. Foroughipour M, Ghandehari K, Khazaei M, Ahmadi F, Shariatinezhad K, Ghandehari K. Randomized clinical trial of intravenous valproate (orifil) and dexamethasone in patients with migraine disorder. Iran J Med Sci. 2013;38(2 Suppl):150–5.

117. Mazaheri S, Poorolajal J, Hosseinzadeh A, Fazlian MM. Effect of intravenous sodium valproate vs dexamethasone on acute migraine headache: a

double blind randomized clinical trial. PLoS One. 2015;10(3):e0120229.

118. Mauskop A, Altura BT, Cracco RQ, Altura BM. Intravenous magnesium sulfate rapidly alleviates headaches of various types. Headache. 1996;36(3):154–60.

119. Bigal ME, Bordini CA, Tepper SJ, Speciali JG. Intravenous magnesium sulphate in the acute treatment of migraine without aura and migraine with aura. A randomized, double-blind, placebo-controlled study. Cephalalgia. 2002;22(5):345–53.

120. Miller ACK, Pfeffer B, Lawson MR, Sewell KA, King AR, Zehtabchi S. Intravenous magnesium sulfate to treat acute headaches in the emergency department: a systematic review. Headache. 2019;59(10):1674–86.

121. Jakubowski M, Levy D, Goor-Aryeh I, Collins B, Bajwa Z, Burstein R. Terminating migraine with allodynia and ongoing central sensitization using parenteral administration of COX1/COX2 inhibitors. Headache. 2005;45(7):850–61.

122. Seim MB, March JA, Dunn KA. Intravenous ketorolac vs intravenous prochlorperazine for the treatment of migraine headaches. Acad Emerg Med. 1998;5(6):573–6.

123. Saadah HA. Abortive migraine therapy in the office with dexamethasone and prochlorperazine. Headache. 1994;34(6):366–70.

124. Rapoport AM, Silberstein SD. Emergency treatment of headache. Neurology. 1992;42(3 Suppl 2):43–4.

125. Silberstein SD. Evaluation and emergency treatment of headache. Headache. 1992;32(8):396–407.

126. Gallagher RM. Emergency treatment of intractable migraine. Headache. 1986;26(2):74–5.

127. Singh A, Alter HJ, Zaia B. Does the addition of dexamethasone to standard therapy for acute migraine headache decrease the incidence of recurrent headache for patients treated in the emergency department? A meta-analysis and systematic review of the literature. Acad Emerg Med. 2008;15(12):1223–33.

128. Vinson DR. Treatment patterns of isolated benign headache in US emergency departments. Ann Emerg Med. 2002;39(3):215–22.

129. Colman I, Rothney A, Wright SC, Zilkalns B, Rowe BH. Use of narcotic analgesics in the emergency department treatment of migraine headache. Neurology. 2004;62(10):1695–700.

130. Duarte C, Dunaway F, Turner L, Aldag J, Frederick R. Ketorolac versus meperidine and hydroxyzine in the treatment of acute migraine headache: a randomized, prospective, double-blind trial. Ann Emerg Med. 1992;21(9):1116–21.

131. Friedman BW, Kapoor A, Friedman MS, Hochberg ML, Rowe BH. The relative efficacy of meperidine for the treatment of acute migraine: a meta-analysis of randomized controlled trials. Ann Emerg Med. 2008;52(6):705–13.

132. Latta KS, Ginsberg B, Barkin RL. Meperidine: a critical review. Am J Ther. 2002;9(1):53–68.

133. Ashburn MA, Ready LB. Postoperative pain. In: Loeser JD, Butler SH, Chapman CR, Turk DC, editors. Bonica's management of pain. 3rd ed. Philadelphia: Lipincott Williams & Wilkins; 2001.

134. Friedman BW, Mohamed S, Robbins MS, et al. A randomized, sham-controlled trial of bilateral greater occipital nerve blocks with bupivacaine for acute migraine patients refractory to standard emergency department treatment with metoclopramide. Headache. 2018;58(9):1427–34.

135. Korucu O, Dagar S, Corbacioglu SK, Emektar E, Cevik Y. The effectiveness of greater occipital nerve blockade in treating acute migraine-related headaches in emergency departments. Acta Neurol Scand. 2018;138(3):212–8.

136. Fogan L. Treatment of cluster headache. A double-blind comparison of oxygen v air inhalation. Arch Neurol. 1985;42(4):362–3.

137. Treatment of acute cluster headache with sumatriptan. The Sumatriptan cluster headache study group. N Engl J Med. 1991;325(5):322–6.

138. Mathew NT. Cluster headache. Neurology. 1992;42(3 Suppl 2):22–31.

139. Jammes JL. The treatment of cluster headaches with prednisone. Dis Nerv Syst. 1975;36(7):375–6.

140. Kudrow L. Cluster headache. Mechanisms and management. Oxford: Oxford University Press; 1980.

141. Antonaci F, Costa A, Candeloro E, Sjaastad O, Nappi G. Single high-dose steroid treatment in episodic cluster headache. Cephalalgia. 2005;25(4):290–5.

142. Mir P, Alberca R, Navarro A, et al. Prophylactic treatment of episodic cluster headache with intravenous bolus of methylprednisolone. Neurol Sci. 2003;24(5):318–21.

143. Ambrosini A, Vandenheede M, Rossi P, et al. Suboccipital injection with a mixture of rapid- and long-acting steroids in cluster headache: a double-blind placebo-controlled study. Pain. 2005;118(1–2):92–6.

144. Leroux E, Valade D, Taifas I, et al. Suboccipital steroid injections for transitional treatment of patients with more than two cluster headache attacks per day: a randomised, double-blind, placebo-controlled trial. Lancet Neurol. 2011;10(10):891–7.

145. Goadsby PJ, Goldberg J, Silberstein SD. Migraine in pregnancy. BMJ. 2008;336(7659):1502–4.

146. Fox AW, Diamond ML, Spierings EL. Migraine during pregnancy: options for therapy. CNS Drugs. 2005;19(6):465–81.

147. Marcus DA. Managing headache during pregnancy and lactation. Expert Rev Neurother. 2008;8(3):385–95.

148. Briggs GG, Freeman RK, Yaffe SJ. Drugs in pregnancy and lactation. 8th ed. Philadelphia: Lippincott Williams & Wilkins; 2008.

149. Silberstein SD. Headaches and women: treatment of the pregnant and lactating migraineur. Headache. 1993;33(10):533–40.

150. Olesen C, Steffensen FH, Sorensen HT, Nielsen GL, Olsen J. Pregnancy outcome following prescription for sumatriptan. Headache. 2000;40(1):20–4.

151. U.S. Food and Drug Administration (FDA): Drug Safety Communications: FDA recommends against prolonged use of magnesium sulfate to stop preterm labor due to bone changes in exposed babies. U.S. Food and Drug Administration (FDA). Silver Spring, MD. 2013 https://www.fda.gov/media/85971/download; Accessed 14 Nov 2019.

Low Back Pain Emergencies

2

Chris Marcellino, Alejandro A. Rabinstein,
Greta B. Liebo, Timothy P. Maus, and J. D. Bartleson Jr.

Introduction

Low back pain is defined as pain located between the lower rib cage and the gluteal folds, often extending or radiating into the buttock, hip, thigh, and/or lower leg [1]. Acute low back pain usually lasts less than 3 months, and 90% of cases are resolved within 6 weeks. It is one of the most common medical problems in the adult population with an estimated 1-month prevalence of 23% [2, 3]. Low back pain is the second leading reason for visiting a primary care physician in the USA [3] and the second most common reason for recurrent utilization of emergency department services [4]. It is estimated that up to 90% of adults will experience low back pain at some time in their lives [5], and low back pain is the most

C. Marcellino (✉)
Department of Neurologic Surgery, Mayo Clinic, Rochester, MN, USA

Department of Neurology, Mayo Clinic, Rochester, MN, USA
e-mail: marcellino.christopher@mayo.edu

A. A. Rabinstein · J. D. Bartleson Jr.
Department of Neurology, Mayo Clinic, Rochester, MN, USA
e-mail: rabinstein.alejandro@mayo.edu; bartleson.john@mayo.edu

G. B. Liebo · T. P. Maus
Department of Radiology, Mayo Clinic, Rochester, MN, USA
e-mail: liebo.greta@mayo.edu; maus.timothy@mayo.edu

common cause of back and spine disability among young and middle-aged people [6].

Low back pain represents a substantial socio-economic challenge. The estimated annual US cost in 2011 for treatment and lost wages due to low back pain is $300 billion USD, after adjusting for inflation [7, 8]. About two-thirds of the total costs of low back pain are indirect, including the resources expended to address disability associated with the condition (e.g., lost wages, reduced productivity, compensation payments, and additional caregiving expenses). About 5% of Americans miss at least 1 day of work per year due to low back pain [8, 9].

In a randomly selected group of 2809 adults obtained from a cross-sectional telephone survey of North Carolina households, 26% reported impairing chronic low back pain [10]. Eighty-four percent of those with chronic back pain had at least one visit to a health-care provider in the previous year, almost half of whom saw an orthopedic or neurologic surgeon. Those who sought care had low back pain for a mean of 9.8 years and had a mean age of 53 years, and 62% were women [10]. Forty-six percent of the patients with chronic low back pain had plain radiographs in the preceding year, and 36% underwent a computed tomography (CT) scan or magnetic resonance imaging (MRI), half of whom had a second advanced imaging study within the year of reporting [10].

Although most low back disorders do not present as emergencies, recognition of those that do is critical to good outcomes. This chapter will focus on the evaluation and treatment of low back pain emergencies. The critical elements from the medical history and physical and neurological examinations will be identified for determining the etiology and directing appropriate use of ancillary studies, such as plain X-rays, CT, MRI, and medical and surgical consultations. Treatment for the serious causes of low back pain will be addressed.

Epidemiology

The interpretation of epidemiologic studies of low back pain can be confusing, mostly due to the use of different definitions for back pain, disparities in the ages of the populations studied, and physical and socioeconomic factors which could contribute to the development of back pain or influence symptoms [2].

The incidence of low back pain varies between studies [11, 12]. In a population-based, prospective cohort study of 308 patients free of low back pain for 6 months, Cassidy et al. reported a cumulative incidence of low back pain in 18.7% in the subsequent year [11]. Most of the cases were mild, and no differences were found between genders or across age groups, although other systematic reviews have suggested a slightly higher prevalence (23%) and the highest prevalence in females aged 40–69 years [3].

How often do patients present with a more serious pathology underlying their acute back pain? Winters et al. estimated that 5–10% of patients have underlying life-threatening problems, such as vascular catastrophes, malignancy, spinal cord compressive syndromes, and infectious diseases [13]. Deyo et al. estimated that in primary care, about 4% of patients with back pain will have compression fractures, 3% have spondylolisthesis (which can be and is often an incidental finding), 0.7% have spinal malignant neoplasms, 0.3% have ankylosing spondylitis, and 0.01% have spinal infection [14]. In contrast to these estimates, Henschke et al. reported the prevalence of serious spinal pathology in 1172 consecutive patients receiving primary care for acute low back pain from primary care clinics in

Sydney, Australia [15]. There were only 11 cases (0.9%) of serious pathology, 8 of whom had fractures. The likelihood of finding serious underlying pathology in the patient with acute low back pain will depend upon where they are seen (the likelihood of serious disease is higher in the emergency department compared to the outpatient clinic) and their presentation, including the presence of red flag symptoms.

Clinical Features and Evaluation

The evaluation and diagnosis of back pain is a challenge. Although most cases are presumed to be of musculoskeletal origin and benign, as noted, back pain can be caused by serious life-threatening conditions [16]. Approximately 85% of patients with isolated back pain cannot be given a precise pathoanatomical diagnosis [17].

The patient's history and findings from the physical and neurological examinations can be very helpful in determining the cause of a patient's back pain. Because an exact diagnosis is not possible in many patients, Deyo recommends answering these three questions: (1) Is a systemic disease causing the pain? (2) Is there social or psychological distress that may amplify or prolong the pain? (3) Is there neurological compromise that may require surgical evaluation [17]? Careful history taking and physical and neurological examinations are needed to answer these questions and determine the cause of an individual patient's low back pain. The role of the physician in the initial evaluation is to identify key elements or red flags that can indicate the possibility of significant spinal and nonspinal pathology. The presence of these indicators will help guide further diagnostic workup, and their absence can rule out the need for additional tests during the first 4 weeks of symptoms, since spontaneous recovery is expected within 1 month in 90% of patients lacking red flags [18].

Clinical practice guidelines from the US Agency for Healthcare Research and Quality (at http://www.ahrq.gov) and the Institute for Clinical Systems Improvement (at http://www.icsi.org) have determined a list of red flags that should be sought in patients with low back pain

Table 2.1 Red flags for potentially serious underlying cause of low back pain

Red flag item	Description	Rationale
Trauma	History of major trauma (e.g., motor vehicle accident, fall from height) or minor trauma in the setting of possible osteoporosis	Possible fracture, especially in an older or osteoporotic patient
Age	More than 50 years or less than 20 years	Increased risk of tumor, abdominal aortic aneurysm, fracture, infection
History of cancer	Past or present history of any type of cancer	History of cancer increases risk of back pain caused by metastatic tumors arising from the lung, breast, kidney, prostate, others
Fever, chills, night sweats	Oral temperature ≥37.8 °C (100 °F), chills, sweats, temperature changes at night	Constitutional symptoms increase risk of infection or cancer
Weight loss	Unexplained weight loss >4.5 kg (10 lbs) in 3 months, not directly related to a change in activity or diet	May indicate cancer or infection
Recent infection	Recent bacterial infection such as a urinary tract infection	Increases risk of infection
Immunosuppression	Immunosuppression for any reason (e.g., transplant, steroid use, IV drug abuse, HIV)	Increases risk of infection
Recumbency or night pain	Pain that is worsened by recumbency or awakens the patient from sleep, unrelated to movement or positioning	Increases risk of cancer, infection, or an abdominal aortic aneurysm
Saddle numbness	Reduced sensation in the second–fifth sacral dermatomes (perianal region)	May indicate cauda equina syndrome
Bladder or bowel dysfunction	Urinary retention, increased frequency of urination, incontinence of urine or stool, dysuria, hematuria	May indicate cauda equina syndrome or infection
Lower extremity neurological deficit	Progressive or severe neurological deficit in one or especially both lower extremities, weak anal sphincter	May indicate severe nerve root injury or cauda equina syndrome

(Table 2.1). The red flags raise a suspicion of serious underlying spinal conditions such as fracture, tumor, infection, or severe neurological deficits including the cauda equina syndrome. It is recommended that clinicians evaluating patients with acute or worsening low back pain routinely inquire about these red flags.

History

Similar to the evaluation of patients with chest and abdominal pain, a systematic approach should be used to identify low back pain red flags. With regard to the elements in the history, Winters et al. suggested using the mnemonic OLDCAAR (*O*nset, *L*ocation, *D*uration, *C*ontext, *A*ssociated symptoms, *A*ggravating factors, and *R*elieving factors) [13]. Onset includes how quickly the pain began, its course,

and the age at onset. Location of the pain includes what level of the spine and if there is any radiation of pain to the lower chest, abdomen, or extremities that might suggest a visceral origin or nerve root impingement. Pain in the distribution of the sciatic nerve (buttock, posterior thigh, posterior calf, and foot) is very suggestive of lumbosacral nerve root compression and has a sensitivity of 0.95 and a specificity of 0.88 that the patient harbors a herniated lumbar disc or another cause of nerve root impingement [14]. Deyo et al. estimate that the likelihood of a lumbar disc prolapse with a surgical indication in a patient without sciatica is only 1 in 1000 [14]. Duration of pain for more than 4–6 weeks is worrisome unless the pain is chronic. The context in which the pain begins is important. Trauma, a recent history of infection or intervention, and a history of cancer suggest fracture, spinal infection, and spinal metastasis, respectively. Current immunosuppression is associated with infection and tumors. Important associated symptoms include fever, chills, weight loss, and neurological symptoms. Significant aggravating factors which suggest nerve root compression include provocation or aggravation of pain by recumbency and positive cough, sneeze, and strain effect especially on radicular pain. Relieving factors include improvement with sitting or bending forward at the waist, which suggests spinal stenosis, and the assumption of certain postures such as a list or reluctance to bear weight on an extremity that may suggest neural compression but also may be related to musculoskeletal disease. In addition, the patient's past medical history may yield helpful clues, such as risk factors for aortic dissection or abdominal aortic aneurysm (AAA), previous immunosuppression, previous cancer, and diabetes. Psychosocial history can be valuable as in the cases of intravenous (IV) drug use, cigarette smoking, stress, and a history of other pains in the past.

Physical Examination

The physical examination of patients with acute low back pain should be guided by the history of present illness and the past medical history. The physical examination should include vital signs assessment [13], general observation of the patient, a regional back exam, and a thorough neurological screening [14, 18]. Findings suggestive of nonspinal pathology may warrant a careful evaluation of related organ systems (e.g., genitourinary) as many medical and surgical conditions can present with acute back pain.

General Observation

The general appearance of the patient may indicate the presence of serious disease [19]. Are they pale, cachectic, or jaundiced? Do they prefer to stand or lay down? In patients with back pain that does not change with movement, who cannot lie still, or appear to be in excruciating pain, the possibility of a ruptured AAA or renal colic should

be strongly considered [13]. Are there scars or needle marks that suggest IV drug use and possible vertebral column infection?

Fever in a patient with acute low back pain has been considered as an indicator of infection [19, 20]. However, its sensitivity varies considerably from 27% for tuberculous osteomyelitis [21] to 83% for spinal epidural abscess (SEA) [22]. It is crucial to note that the absence of fever does not rule out an infectious etiology of back pain [13]. Blood pressure measurement is also important. Hypotension in the patient with acute back or abdominal pain should alert the physician to the possibility of a ruptured AAA.

Regional Back Examination

Physical examination of the back should start with a careful inspection of the skin. Localized erythema (epidural abscess, inflammatory disease), hairy patches (spina bifida occulta, meningocele), and birthmarks and café-au-lait spots (neurofibromatosis) should be documented. The presence of bruises on the posterior torso, especially in the older patient, should alert the physician to physical elder abuse [23].

Observe the patient's posture while seated, standing, and walking. Patients with active radiculopathy may prefer to keep their weight on the unaffected limb; they may also flex the hip and knee and plantar flex the ankle of the affected limb to reduce tension on an impinged nerve root [24]. Palpate the back, paraspinal muscles, and the spine for bony abnormalities, shift of midline structures, muscle spasm, and tenderness. Vertebral tenderness with fist percussion has traditionally been associated with spinal infection, but is nonspecific and can be seen with other causes of low back pain including musculoskeletal etiologies [18].

Lumbosacral spine range of motion should be tested by assessing flexion, extension, lateral bending to both sides, and rotation of the spine to both sides while the pelvis remains stationary. Pain with forward flexion is associated with disc disorders, whereas pain with extension is associated with spinal stenosis [25]. Rigidity of the entire spine is observed in ankylosing spondylitis. While any limitation in range of motion should alert the physician to possible underlying spine pathology [26], given the marked variability between patients with and without symptoms, reduced spinal range of motion is of limited diagnostic value [18]. Possible causes of spinal rigidity include ankylosing spondylitis, infection, severe spondylosis, disc herniation with muscle spasm, and musculoskeletal injury.

Screening Tests for Lumbar Radiculopathy

Straight Leg Raising (Lasègue) Test

Straight leg raising or the Lasègue sign is commonly used in a patient with low back pain to confirm radiculopathy, usually affecting the L5 and/or S1 nerve roots, as they are involved in about 95% of lumbar disc herniations [14, 27]. The maneuver pulls on the sciatic nerve which in turn stretches the nerve roots which comprise the sciatic nerve (L4, L5, S1–3) [28]. Pain is provoked by compression of the nerve root against a structural abnormality, such as a herniated disc which restricts nerve root movement [28, 29]. In a systematic review, Devillé et al. reported a pooled sensitivity for the straight leg raising test of 0.91 but with a pooled specificity of 0.26 for surgically documented lumbar disc herniation [30].

In the Lasègue test, the patient lies supine and the examiner places one hand above the knee of the limb being examined. The examiner places his or her other hand under the patient's heel and gradually raises the patient's extended leg, flexing the thigh at the hip (Fig. 2.1). The test is considered positive if pain (sharp or burning) is elicited along the course of the sciatic nerve in the ipsilateral buttock, posterior thigh, posterior calf, or foot with elevations of 70° or less. It is important to note that provocation of low back pain alone does not indicate a positive straight leg raising test. A positive crossed straight leg raising sign in which pain in the affected lower limb is provoked by raising the contralateral lower extremity is thought to be highly suggestive of nerve root impingement by a herniated or extruded lumbar disc. Devillé et al. found a sen-

sitivity of 0.29 and a specificity of 0.88 for the crossed straight leg raising test [30]. Straight leg raising tests are also positive in patients with meningeal irritation (e.g., infection, malignant infiltration) in whom the finding is typically bilateral.

Kernig Sign

The Kernig sign is a variation of the straight leg raising test. While the patient lies supine the thigh is flexed at the hip to 90° with the knee in flexion. The examiner then extends the leg at the level of the knee. The test is considered positive if sciatica is elicited and the patient resists full extension of the knee.

Finally, while performing the Lasègue or Kernig test, dorsiflexing the foot or even the great toe increases the stretching of the tibial and sciatic nerves and can aggravate the pain in the patient with nerve root impingement (see Fig. 2.1). This maneuver is termed Spurling sign [31].

Seated Straight Leg Raising

The seated straight leg raising test is performed by extending the patient's knee while they are seated and assessing for the provocation of symptoms. It has the advantages of reducing the patient's discomfort by not performing straight leg raising with the patient in a supine position and also expediting the physical examination [32].

Several variants of the seated straight leg raising test have been developed. One is to ask the patient, while seated, to extend one knee then the other, or to ask them to perform heel to shin testing. This maneuver mimics the same position of the spine as 90° of straight leg raising when supine, but the degree of stretching of the sciatic nerve is less. It has been suggested that a positive straight leg raising test while seated is equivalent to a supine straight leg raising test that is positive at 65° of elevation [24].

Another variation is the slump test [33], a series of maneuvers designed to increase tension

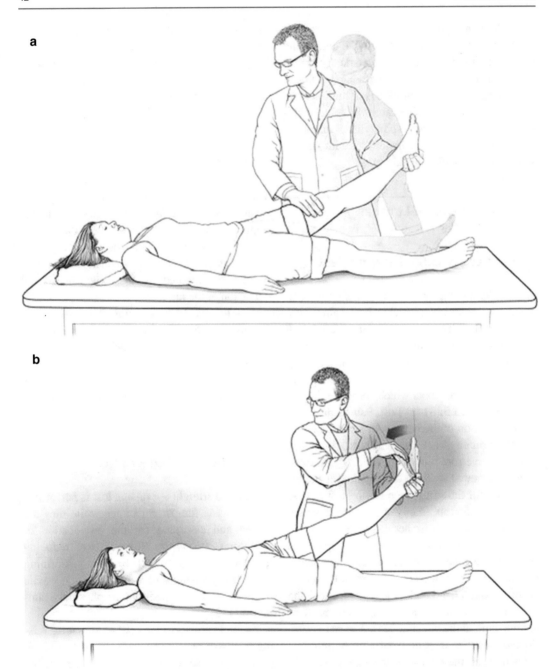

Fig. 2.1 The Lasègue test. The Lasègue sign is tested by passively flexing the hip with the knee extended (**a**). Provocation of ipsilateral radicular lower limb pain is highly suggestive of nerve root impingement. Dorsiflexing the patient's foot while performing a straight leg raising test (**b**) will increase tension on the sciatic nerve and the nerve roots which form the sciatic nerve. Exacerbation of the patient's radicular pain with this maneuver increases the likelihood of lumbosacral nerve root compression. This maneuver is termed Spurling sign. (From Bartleson and Deen [24], Chap. 4, pages 67 and 68. Reproduced with permission of Cambridge University Press. © Mayo Foundation for Medical Education and Research 2009)

on the lumbosacral nerve roots. Patients start in a seated position with their back straight, and they are encouraged to slump, relaxing and flexing the thoracic and lumbar spine, while looking straight ahead. The patient is then asked to flex their neck. The examiner can press on the back of their head to increase neck flexion. The patient is instructed to extend one knee (thus performing a seated straight leg raising maneuver) and then dorsiflex the foot on the same side. The maneuvers are repeated with the other lower extremity. With each movement, the patient is asked to report what they feel. Provocation of radicular lower limb pain suggests irritation of the sciatic nerve or one of the nerve roots that comprise the sciatic nerve. Subsequent extension of the neck into a neutral position should reduce tension on the lumbosacral nerve roots and lessen the patient's pain and enable them to extend the knee farther. In a prospective case-control study of 75 patients with low back pain who had undergone MRI for suspected lumbar disc herniation, sensitivity of the slump test was higher (84% versus 52%) than the traditional straight leg raising, but the specificity was slightly lower (83% versus 89%) [34].

Reverse Straight Leg Raising Test

The reverse straight leg raising test is performed with the patient in a prone position. One knee at a time is passively flexed as far as possible trying to touch the patient's heel to their buttock. If pain is elicited in the ipsilateral limb, typically in the anterior thigh, it suggests impingement of the L2, L3, or L4 nerve roots which contribute to the femoral nerve and are stretched by this maneuver. Additional extension of the hip after the knee is flexed may increase the sensitivity of this test.

Patrick or FABER Test

The Patrick or FABER (Flexion, ABduction, and External Rotation) test is used to evaluate for sacroiliac and hip joint pathology. It is performed while the patient is in a supine position. The heel or lateral ankle of the affected lower extremity is placed on top of the contralateral knee and the medial knee on the side of pain is pushed downward causing synchronized flexion, abduction, and external rotation of the ipsilateral hip. If pain is elicited in the groin (typically with slow downward pressure on the knee), this indicates possible hip joint disease. Pain in the sacroiliac area (usually with quick downward pressure on the knee) suggests sacroiliac joint pathology.

Neurological Examination

A careful neurological examination is paramount in patients with low back pain. The evaluation should search for evidence of spinal cord compression, nerve root impingement including the cauda equina syndrome, and peripheral nerve dysfunction. The examination should include (1) assessment of motor function, specifically lower limb strength and coordination; (2) reflexes including deep tendon reflexes, the Babinski sign, and the anal reflex; (3) sensation (pain and temperature, touch, vibration, and joint position sense); (4) gait; and (5) rectal tone and strength [13].

All of the lumbosacral spinal nerve roots should be assessed [19]. The signs and symptoms associated with specific lumbosacral nerve root injury are listed in Table 2.2.

Motor Function

Individual muscles can be assessed by testing their strength and tone and gauging their bulk. The L2–L4 nerve roots provide the motor innervation responsible for leg (knee) extension and thigh (hip) flexion and can be tested by having the patient arise from a seated position without the use of their upper limbs or ascend a step. The L5 root is largely responsible for ankle and toe dorsiflexion and foot eversion and inversion and can be tested by heel walk. The S1 nerve root innervates the muscles responsible for foot and toe plantar flexion (in conjunction with the S2 nerve root) and contributes to foot inversion (with the L5 root) and can be tested by toe walking and

Table 2.2 Symptoms and signs associated with lumbosacral radiculopathy

Root	Typical pain distribution	Dermatomal sensory distribution	Weakness	Affected reflex
L1	Inguinal region	Inguinal region	None	Cremasteric
L2	Inguinal region and anterior thigh	Proximal anterior and medial thigh	Hip flexion Hip adduction Some knee extension	Cremasteric Thigh adductor
L3	Anterior thigh and knee	Anterior and medial thigh	Knee extension Hip flexion Hip adduction	Knee Thigh adductor
L4	Anterior thigh, anteromedial leg	Anterior knee and medial leg	Knee extension Hip flexion Hip adduction	Knee
L5	Posterolateral thigh Lateral leg Medial foot	Anterolateral leg, top of foot, great toe	Foot dorsiflexion, inversion and eversion Knee flexion Hip abduction Toe extension and flexion	Possibly internal hamstring
S1	Posterior thigh and leg, heel, and lateral foot	Posterolateral leg, lateral foot, heel	Foot plantar flexion Toe flexion Knee flexion Hip extension	Ankle Possibly external hamstring
S2	Buttock	Posterior leg and thigh, buttock	Possibly foot plantar flexion Possibly hip extension	Anal reflex Possibly ankle

From Bartleson and Deen [24], Chap. 4, page 65. Copyright 2009 and reprinted with permission of the Mayo Foundation for Medical Education and Research

performing toe lifts while standing on one leg. The intrinsic foot musculature, the bladder, and the external anal sphincter are supplied by the S2–S4 nerve roots.

Reflexes

The knee reflex is supplied by the L2–L4 nerve roots. The ankle reflex is supplied chiefly by the S1 nerve root with some contribution from S2. The internal and external hamstring reflexes are supplied by the L4, L5, S1, and S2 nerve roots. The internal hamstring reflex is said to be supplied more by the L5 nerve root and the external hamstring more by the S1 nerve root, but asymmetries in the hamstring reflexes are hard to judge and correlation with a specific nerve root injury is unreliable. The plantar surface of the foot is innervated by L5, S1, and S2; plantar stimulation should provoke plantar flexion of the toes. Plantar stimulation resulting in extensor response with fanning of the toes is known as the Babinski sign. The Chaddock sign is present when there is extensor response to stimulation of the lateral

aspect of the foot. Babinski and Chaddock signs indicate upper motor neuron (corticospinal tract) damage typically above the L1 vertebral level (in most adults the spinal cord ends at the level of the L1 vertebral body). The cremasteric reflex is innervated by L1 and L2, and the superficial anal or anal wink reflex (contraction of the external sphincter in response to pricking or stroking the perianal skin) is supplied by S2–S4.

Sensation

Sensation is evaluated using light touch, pin prick, change in joint position, and vibration. Hot and cold stimuli can be used as substitutes for pin prick. The L1 nerve root supplies superficial sensation to the inguinal area. The L2 and L3 nerve roots provide sensation to the anterior and medial thigh. The L4 nerve root is responsible for sensation over the anterior knee and medial surface of the leg and foot (but not the first dorsal webspace). The L5 nerve root delivers sensation from the dorsal aspect of the foot, including the first dorsal webspace. The S1 dermatome covers the posterior and lateral aspect of the foot and leg. The S2–S4 nerve roots supply sensation to the posterior leg, posterior thigh, buttock, and peri-anal area.

Gait

Observation of casual gait can reveal significant abnormalities. Trendelenburg sign, due to hip abductor weakness (chiefly the gluteus medius muscle), is observed when the patient stands or walks on one leg and the pelvis on the opposite, non-weight-bearing side drops. The gluteus medius muscle receives innervation chiefly from the L5 and S1 nerve roots. Difficulty with heel walking suggests L5 distribution weakness or peroneal neu-ropathy or, if bilateral, a peripheral neuropathy. Difficulty with toe walking suggests S1 radiculop-athy. Bilateral difficulty with toe walking more than heel walking suggests bilateral S1 radiculopa-thies rather than peripheral neuropathy [35].

Rectal Exam

Rectal examination in the patient with low back pain is performed to assess rectal tone, anal sphincter strength, and sensation and can facili-tate testing the superficial anal reflex. It should be performed in patients with significant low back or lower limb pain, neurological complaints or deficits, and sphincter complaints and in associa-tion with any red flags [19]. Poor or absent rectal tone in the presence of saddle sensory loss strongly indicates neurological disease such as compression of the cauda equina or lower spinal cord (conus medullaris).

Diagnosis

The physician evaluating a patient with acute low back pain should consider two questions when ordering a diagnostic test. Can a diagnosis be established? And how will the information obtained influence management?

The American College of Radiology practice guidelines (as well as the American College of Physicians guidelines) state that imaging the acute low back pain patient is not indicated except in patients with red flags suggestive of cauda equina syndrome, malignancy, fracture, or infection [36, 37]. Red flags include recent sig-nificant trauma, minor trauma in a patient age >50, weight loss, fever, immunosuppression, his-tory of neoplasm, steroid use or osteoporosis, age >70, known IV drug abuse, or a progressive neu-rological deficit with intractable symptoms [38, 39]. However, the accuracy of each red flag inde-pendently is limited [40, 41]. In a consecutive group of 1172 patients receiving primary care for acute back pain, over 80% of patients with acute low back pain had at least one red flag symptom despite less than 1% having a serious disorder [15]. As such, patients without neurologic com-promise and only minor risk factors for cancer, inflammatory back disease, vertebral compres-sion fracture, or symptomatic spinal stenosis should only be considered for imaging after a trial of conservative therapy [37].

One reason to limit unnecessary imaging in patients with uncomplicated acute low back pain is because findings on plain radiographs and advanced imaging (CT or MR imaging) correlate poorly with symptoms [42–44]. In a large meta-analysis, the prevalence of asymptomatic degen-erative disc changes rose from 37% in 20-year-old patients to 96% in 80-year-old patients [45]. Authors concluded that the imaging features found in degenerative spines were likely part of the normal aging process and not associated with pain. Another recent meta-analysis of random-ized controlled clinical trials compared immedi-ate lumbar imaging to usual clinical care without immediate imaging for low back pain and found no significant difference in clinical outcome between the two groups [46]. The decision to use any medical test should be based on a risk/benefit assessment. Imaging provides benefit in identify-ing undiagnosed systemic disease and in opera-tive planning for neural compressive lesions requiring intervention. This must be balanced against substantial cost, radiation exposure, the stigmata of labeling individuals as patients with degenerative spine disease (which is inevitably present but almost always asymptomatic) and, in turn, provoking interventions which may have little basis in evidence. It is well established that when we image, we often intervene [47, 48].

Imaging Studies

This section will focus on imaging studies that provide evidence of structural or anatomic abnormalities that can explain the patient's back pain.

The studies include plain X-rays, MRI, plain CT, and CT myelography. Illustrative examples of all three imaging modalities are shown in Figs. 2.2, 2.3, 2.4, and 2.5. Physiologic studies such as electromyography and nerve conduction velocity testing and radionuclide imaging are typically not performed as part of the emergency evaluation of the patient with back pain.

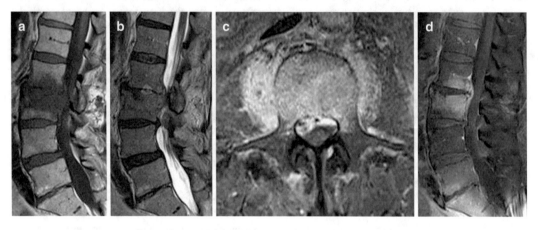

Fig. 2.2 Imaging findings associated with spondylodiscitis. A 65-year-old man with a history of recent abdominal surgery and postoperative sepsis now presents with back pain and right lower limb weakness. Sagittal T1-weighted (**a**) and T2-weighted (**b**) MR images show T1 hypointensity bridging the L2 and L3 vertebral bodies. The central canal is narrowed. Postgadolinium T1-weighted axial (**c**) and sagittal (**d**) images show enhancement in the vertebral bodies, epidural space, and paraspinal tissues consistent with spondylodiscitis. Culture revealed *S. aureus* infection

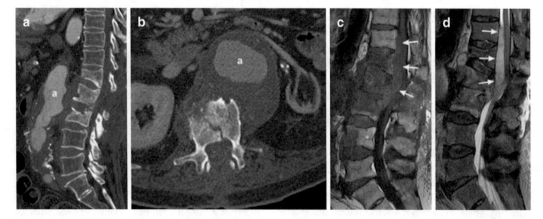

Fig. 2.3 Imaging findings associated with spondylodiscitis. An 85-year-old man presents from another institution with progressive back pain and a history of an aortic graft. A sagittal CT image (**A**) shows multilevel spondylodiscitis with reactive sclerosis, small erosive changes, and pathologic vertebral fractures in direct continuity with a supragraft aortic pseudoaneurysm (a) which is also seen on the axial image (**B**). Sagittal T1-weighted (**C**) and T2-weighted (**D**) MR images also demonstrate spondylodiscitis of L1–L4 and a large ventral epidural abscess (see *arrows*). Surgical exploration confirmed Q fever (*Coxiella burnetii*) mycotic aortic aneurysm, epidural abscess, and spondylodiscitis. The patient succumbed to his disease

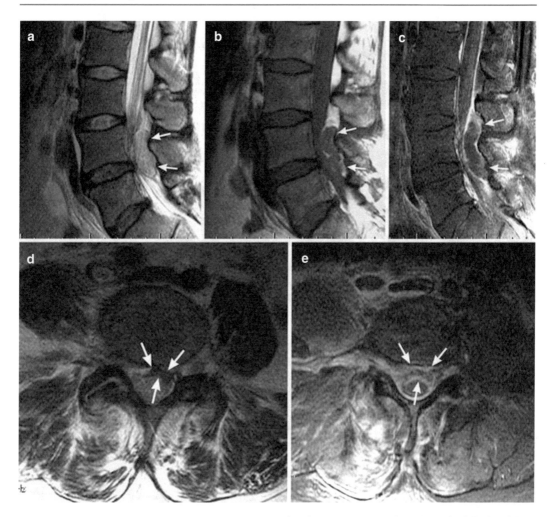

Fig. 2.4 **Epidural abscess.** A 59-year-old woman presents to the emergency department with a 1-week history of increasing back and right lower limb pain. Her right knee reflex is absent. She has a temperature of 38.6 °C. Sagittal T2-weighted (**a**), T1-weighted (**b**), and enhanced T1-weighted (**c**) MR images show a peripherally enhancing dorsal epidural process compressing the thecal sac (see *arrows*). On enhanced axial T2-weighted (**d**) and T1-weighted (**e**) images, the thecal sac is compressed and displaced anteriorly and to the left (see *arrows*) by the posterior mass. Emergent surgical decompression revealed a viridans streptococcal epidural abscess

Plain Radiography

Plain radiography is the imaging technique most commonly available to and used by clinicians to image the lumbar spine. Routine plain lumbosacral spine radiographs are indicated in patients with low back pain in the setting of low-velocity trauma, osteoporosis, chronic steroid use, or when pain has persisted for more than 6–12 weeks despite conservative management [36]. If the clinical presentation suggests, the presence of potential tumor or infection (history of cancer, weight loss, recent infection, fever, IV drug use, or immunosuppression), advanced imaging, and laboratory testing should be obtained instead of plain X-rays.

The standard initial radiographs include two standing views: anteroposterior (AP) and lateral [49, 50]. They enable clinicians to assess lumbar alignment, disc space size, the vertebral bodies, and bone density. The AP view of the lumbar spine also allows for assessment of the sacroiliac

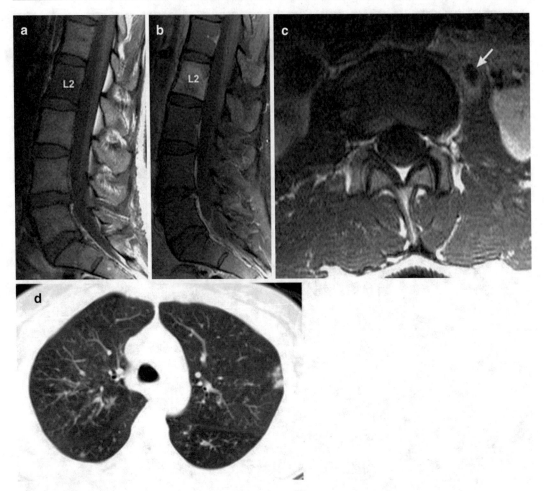

Fig. 2.5 **Spinal tuberculosis**. A 48-year-old woman presents with upper lumbar and abdominal pain. Pre-contrast (**a**) and post-contrast (**b**) sagittal T1-weighted MR images show T1 hypointensity and enhancement confined to the L2 vertebral body, while the discs are unaffected. On the axial postcontrast T1-weighted image (**c**), a small peripherally enhancing tissue collection is seen in the left psoas muscle adjacent to the L2 vertebral body (see *arrow*). Biopsy revealed *Mycobacterium tuberculosis* (TB). Up to 50% of TB spine infections will spare the discs. Chest CT (**d**) demonstrated her pulmonary disease

joints. Additional views, such as spot lateral views of the L5–S1 disc space, oblique views, and flexion and extension views, should be reserved for patients with musculoskeletal spine problems to assess structure and stability.

Advanced Imaging Studies

The three imaging modalities commonly used to help physicians evaluate for anatomic abnormalities are non-contrast CT, MRI, and CT myelogra-

phy. The factors which influence the decision regarding which diagnostic test to use in a patient with acute low back pain include the tissue of greatest interest, claustrophobia, obesity, presence of internal metallic objects including clips and wires, patient and provider preference, availability, and cost of the test [18]. Thoracolumbar axial spine imaging in the setting of blunt trauma is recommended in patients with a high-force mechanism of injury and any of the following: back or posterior midline tenderness, local signs of thoracolumbar injury, abnormal neurological signs, cervical spine fracture, altered or depressed consciousness, a major injury elsewhere in the body which distracts the patient's attention, and evidence of alcohol or drug intoxication [51].

In this section, we will focus on CT and MRI as they are more readily available in all clinical settings (outpatient, inpatient, and emergency department) and most commonly used for the initial evaluation of patients with back pain.

Computed Tomography

Compared to MRI, CT has superior spatial resolution between structures of varying density and enables the clinician to better demonstrate bony pathologies including fractures, bone destruction, spondylolysis, pseudoarthrosis, and facet disease [52, 53]. It is also useful in the postsurgical setting for evaluation of bone graft integrity, surgical fusion, and instrumentation. CT is more widely available and achievable in a short scan time, which is an important factor in the evaluation of patients who suffer from claustrophobia or cannot hold still for the longer intervals required for adequate MR imaging. Also, CT scan can be used as a diagnostic test in patients with contraindications to MRI (e.g., internal metallic objects such as a pacemaker or surgical clips in critical locations).

Technological advances in multidetector CT over the last 15 years have led to less need for MRI in many cases, making it a reasonable alternative in patients with radiculopathy or radicular pain and low clinical likelihood of systemic disease. Thornbury et al. compared MRI with either CT or CT myelography in 95 patients with acute low back and radicular pain due to probable nerve compression from herniated nucleus pulposus. There was no statistically significant difference in the diagnostic accuracy among the three modalities [54]. Another study by van Rijn et al. also found that CT was not inferior to MRI in the detection of disc herniation [55]. However, CT has lower sensitivity than MRI in the detection of spine infection or neoplasm.

Contrast-enhanced or angiographic CT of the chest, abdomen and pelvis ("whole body CT",

trauma CT or "panscan") is used in many trauma centers as the initial imaging test for trauma patients and is often combined with cervical spine CT and non-contrast head CT. These images can be reformatted and used to clear the thoracolumbar spine of significant bony pathology and some soft tissue conditions. Compared to plain radiography, this use of CT has demonstrated superior sensitivity for detecting thoracolumbar spine injury [56, 57].

Magnetic Resonance Imaging

MRI has superior contrast resolution when compared with CT, which allows much better visualization of soft tissues, including the intervertebral discs, ligaments, vertebral bone marrow, and contents of the spinal canal including individual nerve roots and the spinal cord [58]. As such, it is the procedure of choice in patients suspected of cord compression or cord injury or in the presence of red flag symptoms raising concern for infection or malignancy [36]. Additionally, MRI is free of the ionizing radiation used in CT and should be considered the initial imaging modality in patients with persistent or progressive symptoms during or following 6 weeks of conservative management, if the patient is a candidate for intervention or there is diagnostic uncertainty.

In a prospective study of 37 patients with suspected vertebral osteomyelitis, MRI had a higher diagnostic yield (sensitivity 96%, specificity 92%) than plain X-rays or radionuclide bone scanning [59]. MRI can show the extent of infection or tumor burden and help determine if there is a need for surgical intervention [58]. In a patient with a fracture visible on radiographs, MRI provides the best means of characterizing the fracture in terms of its chronicity, benign versus malignant etiology, and whether the patient may be a candidate for vertebral augmentation (vertebroplasty or kyphoplasty). And in the case of radiculopathy, MRI is the best modality to evaluate for intrathecal and extrathecal nerve root impingement, especially when the compressing pathology is also a soft tissue (e.g., herniated nucleus pulposus) [58, 60].

Differential Diagnosis

The differential diagnosis of a patient with low back pain is broad (Table 2.3). In this section, we will cover urgent and emergent conditions which can present with acute lower spine pain as the initial or chief complaint, including infection, tumors, diseases of the aorta, spondylotic conditions (discogenic, spinal stenosis, and spondylolisthesis), and trauma.

Table 2.3 Differential diagnosis of low back pain[a]

Mechanical low back or leg pain (97%)[b]	Nonmechanical spinal conditions (1%)[c]	Visceral disease (2%)
Lumbar strain, sprain (70%)[d]	Neoplasia (0.7%)	Disease of pelvic organs
Degenerative processes of discs and facets, usually age-related (10%)	Multiple myeloma	Prostatitis
Herniated disc (4%)	Metastatic carcinoma	Endometriosis
Spinal stenosis (3%)	Lymphoma and leukemia	Chronic pelvic inflammatory disease
Osteoporotic compression fracture (4%)	Spinal cord tumors	Renal disease
Spondylolisthesis (2%)	Retroperitoneal tumors	Nephrolithiasis
Traumatic fracture (<1%)	Primary vertebral tumors	Pyelonephritis
Congenital disease (<1%)	Infection (0.01%)	Perinephric abscess
Severe kyphosis	Osteomyelitis	Aortic aneurysm
Severe scoliosis	Septic discitis	Gastrointestinal disease
Transitional vertebrae	Paraspinous abscess	Pancreatitis
Spondylolysis[e]	Epidural abscess	Cholecystitis
Internal disc disruption or discogenic low back pain[f]	Herpes zoster	Penetrating ulcer
Presumed instability[g]	Inflammatory arthritis (often associated with HLA-B27) (0.3%) Ankylosing spondylitis Psoriatic spondylitis Reiter syndrome Inflammatory bowel disease Scheuermann disease (osteochondrosis) Paget disease of bone	

From Deyo and Weinstein [17]. Copyright 2002 and reprinted with permission from the Massachusetts Medical Society
[a]Figures in *parentheses* indicate the estimated percentages of patients with these conditions among all adult patients with low back pain in primary care. Diagnoses in *italics* are often associated with neurogenic leg pain. Percentages may vary substantially according to demographic characteristics or referral patterns in a practice. For example, spinal stenosis and osteoporosis will be more common among geriatric patients, spinal infection among injection drug users, etc.
[b]The term "mechanical" is used here to designate an anatomical or functional abnormality without an underlying malignant, neoplastic, or inflammatory disease. Approximately 2% of cases of mechanical low back or leg pain are accounted for by spondylolysis, internal disc disruption or discogenic low back pain, and presumed instability
[c]Scheuermann disease and Paget disease of bone probably account for less than 0.01% of nonmechanical spinal conditions
[d]"Strain" and "sprain" are nonspecific terms with no pathoanatomical confirmation. "Idiopathic low back pain" may be a preferable term
[e]Spondylolysis is as common among asymptomatic persons as among those with low back pain, so its role in causing low back pain remains ambiguous
[f]Internal disc disruption is diagnosed by provocative discography (injection of contrast material into a degenerated disc, with assessment of pain at the time of injection). However, discography often causes pain in asymptomatic adults, and the condition of many patients with positive discograms improves spontaneously. Thus, the clinical importance and appropriate management of this condition remain unclear. "Discogenic low back pain" is used more or less synonymously with "internal disc disruption"
[g]Presumed instability is loosely defined as greater than 10° of angulation or 4 mm of vertebral displacement on lateral flexion and extension radiograms. However, the diagnostic criteria, natural history, and surgical indications remain controversial

Vertebral Infection

Vertebral Osteomyelitis

Vertebral osteomyelitis is one of the etiologies of back pain that can cause significant neurological sequelae if misdiagnosed or left untreated [61]. It is defined as an infection of the bones of the spine. It can be caused by hematogenous spread from any source in the body; by direct inoculation arising from injection, trauma, or spinal surgery; or by contiguous spread from adjacent soft tissue infection [62, 63]. Discitis is an inflammation of the vertebral disc space, usually associated with infection. The presentation, evaluation, and management of vertebral osteomyelitis and discitis are very similar. In fact, they typically occur together (spondylodiscitis) and therefore will be discussed together. Vertebral osteomyelitis and disc space infection account for 1% of all skeletal infections [64], and the incidence seems to be increasing probably due to a greater number of older people, a rise in the prevalence of IV drug abuse, and more spinal injections and surgical procedures [65].

In a systematic review of 14 studies with 1008 patients with vertebral osteomyelitis, Mylona et al. found that back pain was the initial symptom in 86% of patients, followed by fever in 60% of the cases [64]. Neurological symptoms including radiculopathy, limb weakness or paralysis, dysesthesia or sensory loss, and urinary retention were reported in 34% of the cases. Of the studies that reported the vertebral level involved, the lumbar area was affected in 58% of the patients [61]. Usually the pain is well localized, reproducible upon palpation of the spine, and worse at night and with weight-bearing and activity [62, 63]. In a case series of 41 patients with confirmed pyogenic infectious spondylitis, the prevailing clinical symptom was focal back pain aggravated by percussion [66]. Fever may be present [64], although its absence does not exclude the possibility of infection [13]. Other constitutional symptoms such as chills, night sweats, weight loss, and malaise can also occur [67]. Patients should be questioned about possible predisposing factors or events, including underlying illnesses, hospital-

ization, invasive procedures, injection drug use, and travel [63].

The initial evaluation of patients with suspected vertebral osteomyelitis should include CRP, ESR, blood cultures (positive blood cultures can prevent the need for more invasive procedures such as CT-guided or open biopsy [68]), and plain radiographs of the painful portion of the spine. It is important to note that radiographic findings characteristic of vertebral osteomyelitis, such as narrowing of the disc space [69], may not be apparent for up to 4–8 weeks after the onset of infection [59]. If focal spinal tenderness or an elevated CRP or ESR are present, plain films are negative, and the suspicion of spine infection is high, MRI with gadolinium enhancement is recommended for further evaluation [63, 68]. MRI findings include T2 hyperintensity in the disc, T1 hypointensity in adjacent vertebral bodies, and enhancement in the vertebral bodies, disc, epidural space, and paraspinal tissues [59]. CT scanning is primarily useful in providing guidance for percutaneous biopsy, which can rapidly achieve a diagnosis [67, 68].

Tuberculous spondylitis (Pott disease) is the most common spine infection worldwide, and its incidence is increasing in the USA. Compared with pyogenic infection, it is slower and more indolent in onset. MRI findings may be indistinguishable from pyogenic infection, but in up to 50% of cases will spare the disc, presenting as single or multilevel vertebral signal abnormality with paraspinal or epidural extension, often in the form of abscess [70].

The mainstay of treatment for vertebral osteomyelitis or discitis is the prompt administration of antibiotics to reduce the incidence of subsequent adverse outcomes including neurological compromise, vertebral destruction, and abscess formation.

Epidural Abscess

Spinal epidural abscess (SEA) is a suppurative infection of the epidural space, usually arising from hematogenous dissemination, direct inoculation of the spinal canal, or contiguous spread. It is a rare disorder, comprising 0.2–2 cases per 10,000 hospital admissions [71], although its incidence seems to have increased likely due to aging of the population, more spinal injections and surgical interventions, and increased IV drug abuse. A population-based study in Minnesota, from 1990 to 2000, found the incidence of spontaneous epidural abscess to be 0.88 case per 100,000 person-years (95% CI 0.27–1.48) [72]. Risk factors include procedures (e.g., epidural catheter placement [73] and paraspinal, peridural, or spinal injections [74]), diabetes mellitus, alcoholism, HIV infection, trauma, tattooing, acupuncture, contiguous bony or soft tissue infection, bacteremia secondary to distant infection, and IV drug abuse [75, 76].

The presenting symptom is usually severe midline back pain (70%), followed by fever (66%) [13, 71]. In a retrospective study of 31 cases of SEA due to *Staphylococcus aureus*, the lumbar or lumbosacral region was the most frequently involved site (61.3%) [77]. The characteristic triad (fever, back pain, and neurological deficits) was initially present in just 13% of patients with SEA [78]; the absence of any one of the symptoms should not preclude consideration of SEA [13]. Progression of symptoms has been reported to occur in four stages (1) back pain at the affected spinal level; (2) radiculopathic pain radiating from the involved spinal area; (3) decreased motor strength, sensory deficits, and bowel and bladder dysfunction; and (4) paralysis [75, 76].

Early recognition and treatment are critical to avoid permanent disability. When suspected, the initial diagnostic evaluation should include CBC, ESR, and CRP. As previously discussed, contrast-enhanced MRI is the imaging modality of choice for diagnosing spinal infection, such as vertebral osteomyelitis and epidural abscess [58]. MRI can show the full extent of infection (longitudinal and paraspinal) and help determine if there is a need for surgical intervention. Antibiotic treatment alone or following CT-guided needle aspiration can be occasionally curative [76]. However, surgery is the treatment of choice for most symptomatic patients, including all patients with or at risk of severe spinal cord compression. Surgical treatment consists of decompressive laminectomy, drainage, and debridement and culture of infected tissues. Surgery is generally reserved for patients with acceptable operative risk, paralysis that has been present for no longer than 24–48 hours, and without evidence of panspinal infection [75]. Empiric intravenous antibiotic therapy should be started with vancomycin and a third- or fourth-generation cephalosporin until culture results are available. Staphylococcal, streptococcal, and gram-negative bacteria should be covered [76] (Figs. 2.2, 2.3, 2.4, and 2.5).

Tumors

Benign and malignant nonneurogenic tumors of the spine as well as primary neurogenic tumors of the spine can present with low back pain (Table 2.4). While malignant primary and metastatic neoplasms account for less than 1% of low back pain in primary care practice, they are the most common systemic disease affecting the spine [14, 79]. The spine is one of the most common sites of metastasis, with the most frequent primary tumors being breast (17%), lung (16%), prostate (9%), and kidney (7%) [80]. In a retrospective study of 337 patients with a radiographically verified diagnosis of spinal epidural metastases, one out of every five patients presented with spinal epidural metastases as the initial manifestation of malignancy [81].

Malignant tumors can metastasize to the vertebrae and cause pain without neurological symptoms. Back pain is the presenting symptom in 90% of patients with tumors of the spine [82] and is usually constant, progressive, and not relieved by rest. Often, it is worse at night, waking the patient from sleep. It is focal to the level of the lesion and may be associated with lower extremity weakness or symptoms of radiculopathy [62].

If malignancy is suspected, useful laboratory studies include ESR, CRP, CBC, and serum calcium level. Elevated ESR and CRP strongly correlate with systemic neoplasia [62, 70, 79]. It is important to note that ESR and CRP are acute phase reactants and can be elevated in the setting of inflammation or infection as well as cancer. Additionally, blood test results can be normal in the presence of metastatic malig-

Table 2.4 Tumor types

Benign nonneurogenic tumors of spine
Osteoid osteoma
Osteoblastoma
Osteochondroma
Chondroma
Aneurysmal bone cyst
Hemangioma
Giant cell tumor
Eosinophilic granuloma
Malignant nonneurogenic tumors of spine
Chordoma
Chondrosarcoma
Osteosarcoma
Ewing sarcoma
Multiple myeloma
Lymphoma
Metastatic tumors
Extradural
Often in bones of spine
Meningeal
Carcinomatosis and lymphomatosis
Intradural/intramedullary
Metastases within the spinal cord
Neurogenic tumors
Intradural/extramedullary
Nerve sheath tumors (schwannoma, neurofibroma)—
can be extradural
Meningioma
Lipoma of filum terminale
Paraganglioma—can be extradural and extraspinal
Intradural/intramedullary
Astrocytoma
Ependymoma
Hemangioblastoma
Extradural tumor-like conditions
Extramedullary hematopoiesis
Epidural lipomatosis
Sarcoidosis
Paget disease of bone
Vertebral hemangioma
Synovial cyst
Intradural tumor-like conditions
Dural and spinal cord vascular malformations
Syringomyelia not associated with intramedullary
tumor
Sarcoidosis
Arachnoid cyst—can be extradural

From Bartleson and Deen [24], Chap. 1, page 20.
Reproduced with permission of Cambridge University
Press. © 2009 Mayo Foundation for Medical Education
and Research

nancy. In the setting of suspected tumor, ancillary studies can include plain radiography, MRI, CT, and radionuclide imaging. Plain radiographs are less sensitive than other imaging techniques. MRI is more sensitive and specific than other imaging tests for detecting tumors which cause back pain [58, 60]. The management of patients with back pain secondary to benign and malignant tumors will depend on the presence of neurological symptoms, spine stability, and tumor type [13]. Findings of spinal cord or cauda equina compression should prompt consideration of emergent surgical intervention. For patients without neural compression or with compression and a stable course, consultations with an oncologist, radiation oncologist, interventional radiologist, and spine surgeon are recommended.

Signs and symptoms of spinal cord or cauda equina compression by benign or malignant tumors mandate urgent or emergent assessment and treatment. Because of its importance, the following section focuses on spinal cord and cauda equina compression.

Spinal Cord and Cauda Equina Compression

Extrinsic spinal cord and cauda equina compression result in epidural spinal compression syndromes. While rare, spinal cord, conus medullaris, and cauda equina compression need to be considered by the clinician evaluating a patient with acute and chronic low back pain. Up to 90% of cases are due to spinal epidural metastases, but other etiologies include SEA, massive disc herniation, and spinal epidural hematoma. Intradural tumors can also present with back pain and spinal cord or cauda equina compression. In a review of 337 patients with spinal epidural metastases at the Mayo Clinic, the thoracic spinal level was involved in 61%, the lumbosacral level in 29%, and the cervical level in 10% [83]. The conus medullaris forms the distal, bulbous part of the spinal cord. The spinal cord typically terminates at the lower end of the L1 vertebral body in adults, but can end anywhere from the twelfth thoracic vertebra to the interspace between the second and third lumbar vertebrae. The cauda equina consists of a sheaf of bundled lumbosacral nerve roots which run from the bottom of the spinal cord to the end of the vertebral (spinal) canal within the sacrum. It can be clinically difficult to

Table 2.5 Conus medullaris versus cauda equina syndrome

	Conus medullaris	Cauda equina
Vertebral level of injury	Depends on level of termination of spinal cord, usually vertebral level T12–L1; injury is usually to sacral spinal cord (S1–S5)	Between L1 or L2 and the sacrum with injury to multiple lumbosacral nerve roots
Causes	Fracture, primary and secondary tumors, vascular injury, infection, spondylosis (usually disc)	Fractures, primary and secondary tumors, infection, spondylosis (disc or spondylolisthesis), ankylosing spondylitis (rarely)
Pain	Less common and less severe; usually bilateral and affecting perineum and/or thighs	Often and more severe, can be symmetric or asymmetric and typically radicular (sciatica)
Motor findings	Less severe, more symmetric, fasciculations more likely, usually restricted to sacral roots	Less symmetric, can be more severe, fasciculations less common
Reflex loss	Ankle reflex only	Ankle and knee reflexes may be absent
Sensory findings	Bilateral perineal, more likely symmetric, loss of pain and temperature with possible retention of touch	Less symmetric, perineal and lower limb may be affected, all types of sensation can be affected
Bowel and bladder function	Usually early and prominent for both urinary and rectal sphincters	Occurs later and is less severe for both bowel and bladder
Sexual function	Erection and ejaculation more likely to be affected	Less likely to be affected
Onset (depends on cause)	More likely to be acute	More likely to be gradual
EMG findings	Restricted to sacral myotomes, usually bilateral	Multiple lumbosacral levels, usually bilateral root involvement
Prognosis (depends on etiology)	Relatively worse	Relatively better

From Bartleson and Deen [24], Chap. 3, page 55. Reproduced with permission of Cambridge University Press. © 2009 Mayo Foundation for Medical Education and Research

differentiate cauda equina syndrome from conus medullaris compression (Table 2.5).

The first symptom of epidural spinal cord compression due to spinal epidural metastases is usually back pain [84, 85] which precedes neurological symptoms by an average of 7 weeks [86]. Pain gradually increases and may be accompanied by a radicular component which is more common with lumbosacral level involvement. Motor weakness is one of the most common symptoms, affecting 60–85% of patients [85, 86]. If the spinal cord is compressed, the weakness typically follows a corticospinal tract pattern, preferentially involving the flexor muscles in the lower extremities, and if above the thoracic spine, the extensor muscles of the upper limbs. Hyperreflexia below the level of spinal cord compression and extensor plantar responses are typically present. Delayed recognition of epidural spinal cord compression due to spinal epidural metastases reduces the likelihood of a good outcome after treatment [86, 87].

In the lumbar spine, epidural spinal cord compression affects the lumbosacral nerve roots that comprise the cauda equina and typically produces a cauda equina syndrome. Presenting symptoms include low back pain, radicular lower limb pain on one or both sides, motor and/or sensory deficits, and sphincter problems [88]. Common neurological examination findings include positive straight leg raising or other signs of nerve root irritation (unilateral or bilateral), decreased deep tendon reflexes in the lower limbs, and motor and sensory deficits in the distribution of one or more lumbosacral nerve roots. Urinary retention (and resulting overflow incontinence) is the most consistent finding [89–91]. Any history suggestive of urinary retention should prompt a check of postvoid residual volume. The most frequent sensory loss affects the perineal region, buttocks, and posterior thighs and calves. Anal sphincter tone is decreased in up to 80% of patients [89–91].

Expedited imaging is crucial in the evaluation and management of patients with epidural spinal cord compression [78, 84, 92]. All patients with suspected spinal cord or cauda equina compression should undergo urgent MRI; if MRI is not available or the patient cannot undergo MRI, plain CT or CT myelography should be obtained [60]. Recognition of spinal cord or cauda equina compression by cancer should prompt consideration of systemic corticosteroid administration and evaluation by a spine surgeon. Two corticosteroid regimens can be used: a high-dose regimen for patients with paraplegia or rapidly progressive symptoms awaiting definitive therapy and a lower-dose regimen for patients with pain but minimal neurological dysfunction [87]. The high dose of corticosteroid (usually dexamethasone, 10 mg IV followed by 16 mg orally daily in divided doses) has more evidence of benefit and a relatively high rate of serious side effects, such as hyperglycemia, mania, insomnia, and increased risk of infection, while the low dose has fewer side effects but less data to support its use and is primarily for pain control (e.g., 20–40 mg prednisone orally daily or low dose dexamethasone) [87]. Patients with small epidural lesions and normal neurological examinations do not need corticosteroids [87].

Patients with epidural spinal cord compression require a specific diagnosis (tumor and what type, disc, infectious agent, or hematoma). If the patient has a history of a specific tumor with a predilection for spinal metastasis, it can be assumed that the same cancer is responsible for new spinal epidural metastases. For unknown mass lesions, diagnosis is established by imaging-guided needle biopsy or culture or at the time of surgical intervention to remove tumor or drain pus. The definitive treatment of patients with epidural spinal cord compression is usually surgical decompression but can vary depending on the type of tumor and whether or not an SEA needs surgical intervention. Patients with progressive or severe cauda equina or spinal cord compression due to a large herniated disc will typically require emergent or very urgent laminectomy and discectomy, preferably within 24–48 hours of symptom onset [88, 93]. Patients with SEA will require antibiotics and usually will require surgical drainage. The treatment of patients with spinal epidural metastases can be radiotherapy alone or radiotherapy and surgery depending on their initial presentation and the type of tumor [94]. Rarely, patients with spinal epidural metastases might be treated with surgery alone (e.g., a

patient with a single metastasis and gross total surgical resection) or chemotherapy alone (e.g., lymphoma). Surgery is more likely to be recommended if there is spinal instability or the tumor is not radiosensitive (Figs. 2.6, 2.7, and 2.8), and consideration of emergency radiation therapy should be given, in lieu of surgery, to highly radiosensitive expansile tumors often associated with hematological malignancy, especially plasmacytoma.

Vascular Disorders: Thoracic Aortic Dissection and Abdominal Aortic Aneurysms

Thoracic Aortic Dissection

One of the causes of back pain that presents a diagnostic challenge for physicians is thoracic aortic dissection [95]. Acute aortic dissection has an incidence of 3.5 cases per 100,000 people per year; 20% of patients die before reaching hospital, and another 30% die during hospital admission [96]. Thoracic aortic dissections can be divided into those affecting the ascending aorta (Stanford type A and DeBakey types I and II) and those affecting the aorta more distally (Stanford type B and DeBakey type III). Left untreated, 75% of patients with dissection of the ascending aorta die within 2 weeks [97]. Thoracic aortic dissection is more frequent in men between the ages of 50 and 70 years, and the most important predisposing factor is systemic hypertension [98]. Other risk factors include preexisting aortic aneurysm, atherosclerosis, connective tissue disorders (e.g., Marfan syndrome, Ehlers-Danlos syndrome), bicuspid aortic valve, and vascular inflammation (e.g., Takayasu arteritis, giant cell arteritis) [96–98].

The traditional presentation of sudden, ripping or tearing chest pain in a patient with hypertension is not always present [98–101]. While 85–95% of patients with thoracic aortic dissection report chest pain which is usually abrupt in onset and severe, only half describe a ripping or tearing quality [96, 98, 100]. The pain can affect the front or back of the chest, the back, or the abdomen [98]. The location of the pain can vary, depending on the site of tear and its direction of

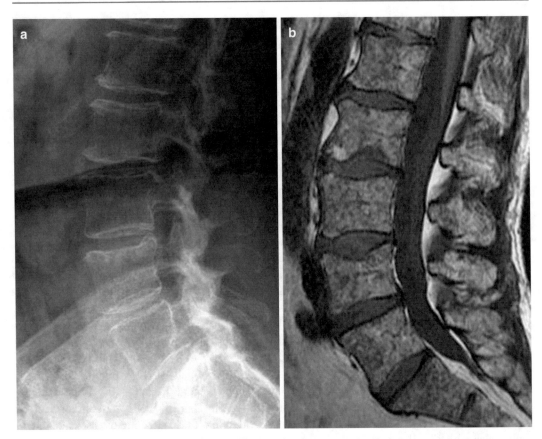

Fig. 2.6 Imaging findings of multiple myeloma affecting the spine. A 70-year-old man presents with low back pain. A lateral radiograph (**a**) shows heterogeneous loss of bone density throughout the lumbar spine. The possibility of multiple myeloma was raised and confirmed on subsequent sagittal T1-weighted MRI (**b**), which demonstrates innumerable tiny marrow-replacing lesions

extension (neck, back, or abdomen). Dissections of the descending aorta are more likely to cause back and abdominal pain than chest pain [100]. Painless presentations are reported in up to 10% of patients [96, 98], especially those with neurological findings such as cerebral, peripheral nerve, or spinal cord ischemia [102, 103]. 10–20% present with syncope, often accompanied by other symptoms [98, 101].

Physical examination findings in a patient with acute thoracic aortic dissection include (1) difference in pulse amplitude between arms, (2) aortic diastolic murmur, and (3) blood pressure differential between arms. A prospective study of 250 patients with clinical suspicion of acute aortic dissection (128 patients with a confirmed diagnosis) found that a difference in systolic blood pressure of more than 20 mmHg between the arms was a significant independent predictor of thoracic aortic dissection [104]. A noticeable pulse amplitude difference and a systolic blood pressure difference of >20 mmHg between arms should raise suspicion for thoracic aortic dissection, but these findings do not establish the diagnosis. A systematic review found that the pooled prevalence for inter-arm blood pressure differences in healthy subjects was 20% for a difference of ≥10 mmHg [105]. The prevalence of asymmetry was greater in patients with high blood pressure and cardiovascular disease.

Emergency diagnostic imaging with CT, transesophageal echocardiogram (TEE), or MRI should follow suspicion of thoracic aortic dissection. Multidetector CT angiography (CTA) is the

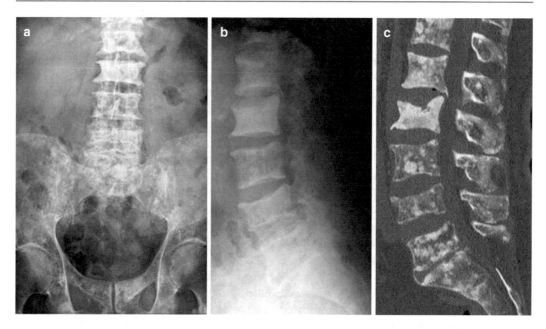

Fig. 2.7 Metastatic prostate cancer affecting the lumbar spine. Frontal (**a**) and lateral (**b**) radiographs in a man with low back pain reveal extensive blastic (bone-forming) metastases due to prostate cancer. The discrete lesions are better seen on a sagittal CT image (**c**), with an age-indeterminate compression fracture of L2

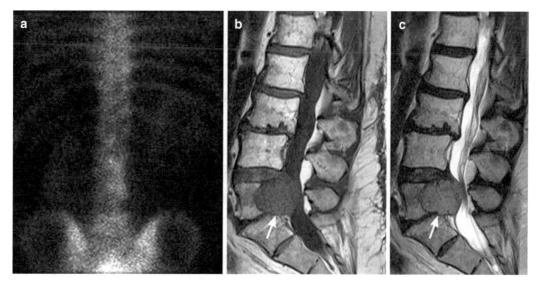

Fig. 2.8 Epidural metastatic tumor compressing the cauda equina. A patient with known colon cancer presents with a cauda equina syndrome despite a recent tumor surveillance radionuclide bone scan (**a**) which fails to show any discrete lesions. Subsequent sagittal T1-weighted (**b**) and T2-weighted (**c**) MR images show a large metastatic lesion occupying the posterior aspect of L5 and extending into the epidural space, effacing the thecal sac (see *arrows*)

initial modality of choice because it provides precise information about the intraluminal and extraluminal structures of the entire aorta and main aortic branches [106]. The diagnostic accuracy of CT for aortic dissection is nearly 100% [107–109]. TEE is a useful bcdside technique to evaluate patients with suspected acute thoracic aortic dissection who are hemodynamically unstable. Pooled sensitivity and specificity with TEE for thoracic aortic dissection have been reported as 98% and 95%, respectively [110]. The main disadvantages to TEE are operator dependence [111] and inability to visualize the distal part of the ascending aorta [112]. A systematic review of TEE, CT, and MRI for the diagnosis of thoracic aortic dissection found that all three techniques provided equally reliable results [110]. MRI is seldom used in the emergent setting as the initial imaging technique due to lack of availability, time delays to obtain images, and restricted patient access and monitoring during the study.

When recognized, the patient with suspected thoracic aortic dissection should be immediately transferred to the closest emergency department [13] and admitted to an intensive care unit. The treatment will be either medical or surgical depending on the localization of the tear [113].

Abdominal Aortic Aneurysm

AAAs are much more common than thoracic [114]. In 2018, AAA was the 19th leading cause of death in the USA with nearly 10,000 fatalities [115]. This is likely to be an underestimate because many sudden or unattended deaths are not correctly attributed to AAA. Risk rupture increases with aneurysm size [114]. Although most AAAs never rupture, the mortality rate is 80% when rupture does occur [116]. The condition is more common in the elderly. It is estimated that the prevalence of AAA in patients over age 65 years ranges between 4% and 8% and increases with every decade [117]. Risk factors include smoking, hyperlipidemia, coronary artery disease, diabetes, connective tissue disorders, and a family history of AAA [13, 117–120].

The clinical presentation of AAA is extremely variable, ranging from no symptoms to flank pain resembling renal colic to retro- or intraperitoneal rupture and shock. Similar to thoracic aortic dissection, the classic clinical presentation for rupturing AAA (the triad of hypotension, abdominal pain, and pulsatile mass) is not the most common, occurring in less than half of patients [121]. Back pain, left lower quadrant abdominal pain, flank pain, syncope, or lower extremity paresthesia can be presenting symptoms. Reports of peripheral nerve injury with weakness of hip flexion and knee extension due to femoral neuropathy have been associated with ruptured AAA [122].

Once the diagnosis of symptomatic AAA is suspected, prompt diagnostic imaging should follow. Ultrasound is the preferred modality to screen, assess, and follow abdominal aneurysms because it is accurate (sensitivity and specificity, 99%), inexpensive, and noninvasive [114, 120, 123]. CT is the preferred imaging technique to delineate the shape and extent of the aneurysm and its relationship with the visceral and renal vasculature. CT angiography can provide more detailed evaluation of the AAA and the renal, mesenteric, and iliac arteries. Disadvantages to CT include radiation exposure, IV contrast administration, and higher cost. Magnetic resonance angiography can also be used [114].

The management of patients with asymptomatic AAA will be medical treatment (e.g., beta-blockers), observation, and elective surgical repair [124]. In patients with ruptured AAA, emergent surgical intervention is needed to prevent death (Figs. 2.9 and 2.10).

Spondylotic Low Back Pain Emergencies

Spondylosis is a general term for usually age-related, wear-and-tear changes affecting the intervertebral discs and vertebrae. Degenerative changes in the facet joints are typically included as are changes in the associated spinal ligaments. Paraspinal muscles may be secondarily affected. Spinal spondylosis is nearly universal with age but is frequently asymptomatic.

Musculoskeletal and mechanical conditions are estimated to account for 97% of adult patients with low back pain in primary care (see Table 2.3). Lumbar spondylosis can present with low back pain, compression of one or more lumbosacral

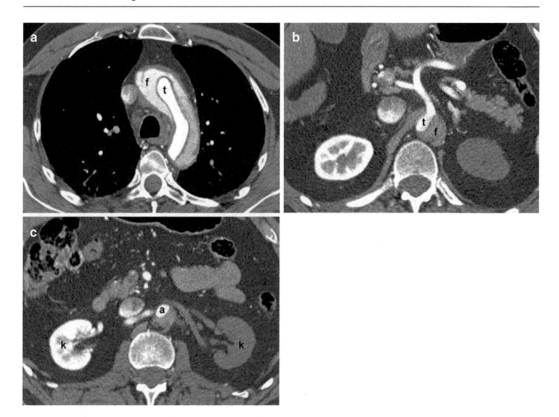

Fig. 2.9 Images of a thoracic aortic dissection. A 60-year-old man presents to the emergency department with the acute onset of severe thoracolumbar back pain. A CTA scan showed Stanford type A and DeBakey type I thoracic aortic dissection which extended from the aortic valve to the aortic bifurcation. Axial CTA image (**A**) at the aortic arch shows differential opacification of the true (t) and false (f) lumina. Axial CTA image at the level of the celiac plexus (**B**) shows a small true lumen (t) filling the celiac plexus, while the false lumen (f) does not opacify. Axial CTA image at the level of the renal arteries (**C**) shows an opacified small true aortic lumen (a). The right renal artery opacifies, and the right kidney (k) enhances, while the left kidney (k) is ischemic

roots, or an acute cauda equina syndrome which requires urgent or emergent attention. Thoracic disc herniations can occur at T11–12 (most common) or T12–L1 and cause low back pain. A herniated lower thoracic disc can present acutely with signs and symptoms of compression of the lower spinal cord and requires urgent or emergent evaluation and treatment. Conus medullaris syndrome and cauda equina syndrome can present with very similar manifestations (see Table 2.5). Spondylotic acute cauda equina syndrome is significantly more common than an acute conus medullaris syndrome, and cauda equina syndrome occurs at the lumbar rather than thoracic level. This section will focus on spondylotic lumbar emergencies.

A large lumbar disc protrusion or extrusion is the most common cause of cauda equina syndrome. Other causes include trauma, tumors, infections, spondylolisthesis, lumbar spinal stenosis, synovial cysts, epidural hematomas, postoperative complications, and arachnoiditis. Lumbar spinal stenosis and synovial cysts, while spondylotic in nature, do not usually present acutely. It is estimated that about 2% of all patients with discogenic low back pain undergo surgery and that disc herniation causing cauda equina syndrome accounts for 1–2% of lumbar disc surgeries [14, 58, 125]. Therefore, the prevalence of discogenic cauda equina syndrome among all patients with low back pain is about 0.04% (1 in 2500 patients).

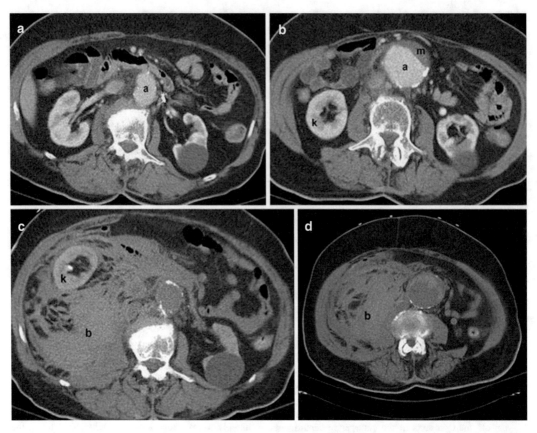

Fig. 2.10 A ruptured AAA. An 80-year-old man presents to the emergency department with new low back and hip pain. He has a known abdominal aortic aneurysm with future plans for an elective repair and is on anticoagulation for atrial fibrillation. Initial contrast-enhanced axial CT images (**A**) and (**B**) show a large abdominal aortic aneurysm (a) containing mural thrombus (m) without evidence of hemorrhage. Five hours later, while still in the emergency department, he developed cardiovascular collapse, and an emergent non-contrast CT was obtained. Axial CT images (**C**) and (**D**) at the same anatomic levels as the previous images show interval massive retroperitoneal bleeding (b) due to aneurysm rupture. Note the shift of his right kidney (k) anteriorly as a result of mass effect from the large retroperitoneal hemorrhage. He survived surgical repair

In one large review, cauda equina syndrome was caused by L4–5 herniation in 46% of cases, L5–S1 herniation in 36.9% of cases, and L2 and L3 herniations in 17.1% of cases [125]. Patients may be predisposed to cauda equina syndrome if they have a congenitally narrow lumbosacral canal or have acquired lumbar spinal stenosis resulting from a combination of degenerative changes affecting the vertebrae (e.g., spondylolisthesis, spurring), intervertebral discs, facet joints, and ligaments. Many, but not all, patients with spondylotic cauda equina syndrome have a past history of low back pain and/or lumbosacral radicular pain. Presenting clinical symptoms can include low back pain, bilateral or unilateral sciatica, perineal/perianal/saddle sensory loss, lower limb motor weakness, lumbosacral root sensory deficits, difficulty with bladder more often than bowel sensation and control, and sexual dysfunction. Neurological findings include weakness and sensory loss in the distribution of multiple lumbosacral nerve roots on one or both sides, positive straight leg raising signs, reduced perianal and perineal sensation, reduced anal sphincter tone and strength, and absent superficial anal and bulbocavernosus reflexes. Three temporal different presentations have been reported: acute, acute or subacute over chronic, and insidiously progressive [91, 126]. A subacute onset is typical of discogenic cauda equina syndrome, but there can be a tendency to "snowball" at the end with rapid progression of neurological impairment.

Not all patients have all clinical features at onset. In one review, only 19% of patients presented with a characteristic combination of bilateral sciatica, lower limb weakness, saddle sensory loss, and sphincter disturbance [127]. Providers and patients and their families should be aware of the worrisome symptoms and signs that can indicate the development of serious compression, which can become a neurological emergency. Men are somewhat more likely than women to develop an acute cauda equina syndrome, and the most common age of onset is between 30 and 60 years.

Cauda equina syndrome due to compression by a large lumbar disc is a spine emergency because recovery of strength and sensation and especially bladder, bowel, and sexual function may depend upon prompt decompression of the nerve roots within the cauda equina [93]. While it is clear that decompressive laminectomy and discectomy are indicated for patients with spondylotic cauda equina syndrome, and that sooner is better than later, the exact urgency of surgical intervention is somewhat controversial and has been the subject of extensive litigation. Early reports emphasized the benefit of rapid decompression; however, Ahn et al. in a meta-analysis reported that there was a significant advantage to treating patients within 48 versus more than 48 hours after the onset of cauda equina syndrome [128] as opposed to shorter intervals. Kohles et al. criticized the methods of this meta-analysis and argued they understated the value of early intervention [129]. Todd analyzed the data and concluded that patients treated less than 24 hours after onset of cauda equine syndrome were more likely to recover bladder function than those treated beyond 48 hours [130]. Gleave and MacFarlane [131] and others [93, 126] subdivide cauda equina syndrome into patients with complete denervation of the bladder and urinary sphincter (those with urinary retention and overflow incontinence) versus patients with incomplete cauda equine syndrome who have reduced urinary sensation, loss of the desire to void, or poor urinary stream, but who do not have urinary retention with overflow incontinence. Many of these authors believe that if the patient has urinary retention with overflow incontinence, implying complete bladder denervation, urgent decompression of the cauda equina confers no benefit [93, 131]. Other authors have reported benefit from early surgery even in the complete cauda equina syndrome group [126]. Other single-series reports did not find significant benefit from early operation [132–135]. In general, better preoperative function predicts even better postoperative function. Despite the lack of clear statistical benefit from operating within 24 hours, cauda equina syndrome due to an acutely herniated large disc should be considered as an emergency and that operating within 24 hours of the onset of sphincter dysfunction is probably optimal and errs on the side of caution, especially in patients with preserved bladder sphincter function. From a practical standpoint, this typically means that a patient who is diagnosed as having an acute or subacute cauda equina syndrome should be referred directly to a medical center with MRI capability and access to emergency consultation with a spine surgeon.

Disc compression of a single lumbosacral nerve root is much more common than cauda equina syndrome. Patients who present with low back pain and severe weakness in the distribution of a single nerve root should be expeditiously evaluated, and many of these patients will be treated with surgery. Laminectomy and discectomy can aid in the recovery of a severely compressed lumbosacral nerve root. However, there is no evidence that outcomes from surgery for a single radiculopathy are better with emergent surgical intervention. Therefore, the patient with a single radiculopathy and a severe motor deficit due to spondylosis should be evaluated and treated urgently but not emergently. The urgency increases if a second nerve root is involved. Apart from cauda equina syndrome or a severe monoradiculopathy, most patients presenting with spondylotic low back pain with or without radicular pain should be treated conservatively. Lumbar spinal stenosis, spondylolisthesis, and synovial cysts rarely present emergently. When they do, it is usually the result of a superimposed disc herniation or trauma.

Current evidence-based guidelines for the evaluation and treatment of acute and chronic low back pain are available (e.g., http://www.icsi.org) [18, 60, 136–141] (Figs. 2.11, 2.12, 2.13, and 2.14).

Traumatic Lower Spine Emergencies

In most instances, the patient with lower spine pain secondary to trauma will be able to describe, sometimes in vivid detail, their injury and current symptoms. However, there are some circumstances where this is not the case, such as (1) minor or no trauma in a patient with osteoporosis; (2) when the patient is confused or unconscious due to a simultaneous head injury or drug or alcohol intoxication; (3) when the patient has dementia, mental retardation, or a significant psychiatric illness; and (4) when the patient has sustained an additional painful injury, such a long bone fracture, which distracts the patient's attention.

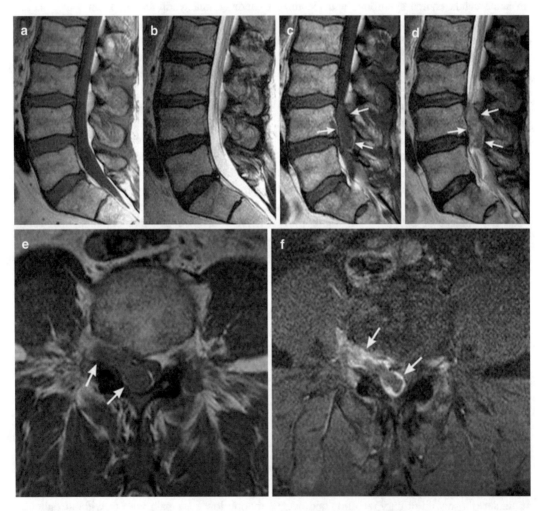

Fig. 2.11 Images of cauda equina compression due to a massive disc extrusion. A 55-year-old man presents with progressive back pain over 6 weeks. T1-weighted (**a**) and T2-weighted (**b**) sagittal MRI images early in his course show only mild disc degeneration with a widely patent central canal. An MRI 6 weeks later, when bilateral lower limb weakness and perineal numbness began, shows a large epidural process effacing the central canal on T1-weighted (**c**) and T2-weighted (**d**) images (see *arrows*). Axial pre-contrast (**e**) and post-contrast (**f**) T1-weighted images show a peripherally enhancing epidural process (see *arrows*) displacing the compressed thecal sac to the left. The radiologist's impression was a probable epidural abscess, but operation showed a massive disc extrusion. Imaging findings are somewhat atypical given the relative preservation of the disc space

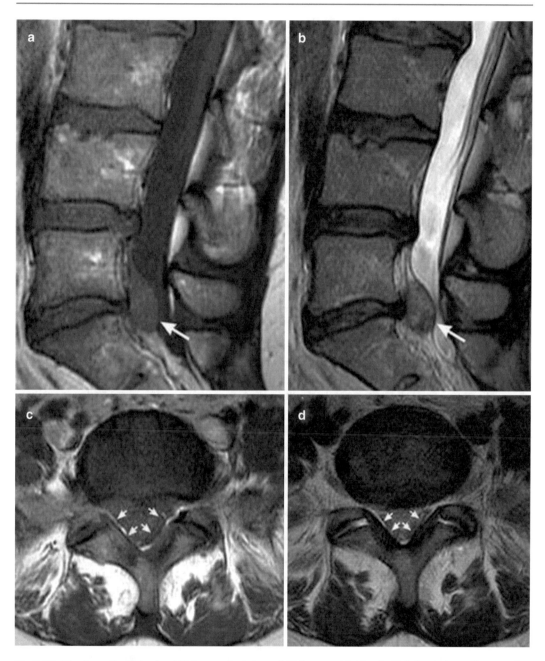

Fig. 2.12 Very large disc extrusion which caused sciatica without neurological deficit. A 44-year-old woman presents with left S1 radicular pain without neurological deficit. Sagittal T1-weighted (**a**) and T2-weighted (**b**) MR images and Axial T1-weighted (**c**) and T2-weighted (**d**) MR images at the level of L5 show a large disc extrusion which severely effaces the thecal sac, which is displaced posteriorly and to the left (see *arrows*). She was treated conservatively, and her sciatica eventually resolved

With or without trauma, vertebral compression fractures are very common. There are an estimated 700,000 new cases of vertebral compression fractures each year in the USA [142]. They are usually due to osteoporosis, but some are due to a pathologic fracture secondary to an osteolytic tumor within the vertebra. Osteoporotic vertebral compression fractures typically affect the lower

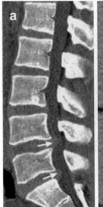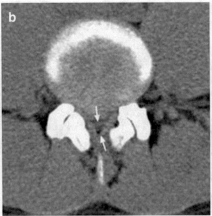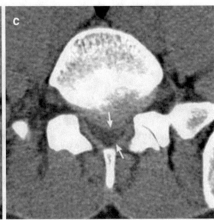

Fig. 2.13 Lumbar spinal canal stenosis. A 38-year-old man presents with progressive lower limb pain and numbness brought on by standing and walking. Sagittal (**a**) and axial CT images at L4 (**b**) and L5 (**c**) show a developmentally narrow spinal canal due to congenitally short pedicles with superimposed disc protrusions at L4 and L5 (see *arrows* in **a**). The thecal sac is severely constricted and has a trefoil shape at the L4 interspace (see *arrows* in **b**) and more room at the level of the L5 vertebral body (see *arrows* in **c**). This patient's lumbar spinal stenosis is currently being treated conservatively

thoracic and lumbar spine. Most patients report some trauma as an inciting cause, but the trigger can be minor such as a fall on the buttocks or lifting an object, and some patients report no injury or inciting event. Plain X-rays, CT, MRI, and even radionuclide bone scanning can help in diagnosis. MRI can help to determine the age of the fracture by showing edema in the affected bone, which typically lasts for at least 3–4 months but can last longer. A minority of patients experience neurological symptoms due to bone fragment displacement into the spinal canal. For these patients, surgical intervention may be necessary. Bone densitometry is often obtained to confirm the presence and gauge the severity of the patient's osteoporosis. Traditionally, patients with vertebral compression fractures are treated with analgesics, bracing, and activity modification. Percutaneous techniques of vertebral augmentation (vertebroplasty and kyphoplasty) have been used to treat painful vertebral compression fractures due to osteoporosis and tumor. Although these injections seem to provide patients with prompt pain relief, two double-blind, placebo-controlled trials failed to show benefit from vertebroplasty [143–145].

Conservative estimates suggest that more than 1 million blunt trauma patients with possible associated spine injuries are seen annually in US emergency departments [146]. The incidence of thoracolumbar fracture following blunt trauma has been reported to be from 2% to 7.5%. Thoracolumbar fractures are associated with neurological injury in 26–40% of patients [51].

Traumatic thoracolumbar spinal fractures are usually due to falls and motor vehicle accidents. Indications for imaging the thoracolumbar spine in patients with trauma include motor vehicle crash at greater than 35 mph; fall from a height greater than 15 ft; automobile hitting a pedestrian with the pedestrian thrown greater than 10 ft; assault with a depressed level of consciousness; known cervical spine injury; and rigid spine disease (e.g., ankylosing spondylitis, diffuse idiopathic skeletal hyperostosis) [146]. Clinical signs associated with thoracolumbar fracture include (1) back pain/midline tenderness (sensitivity 62.1%, specificity 91.5%), (2) palpable midline step (sensitivity 13.8%, specificity 100%), (3) back bruising (sensitivity 6.9%, specificity 98.6%), and (4) abnormal neurological signs (sensitivity 41.4%, specificity 95.8%)

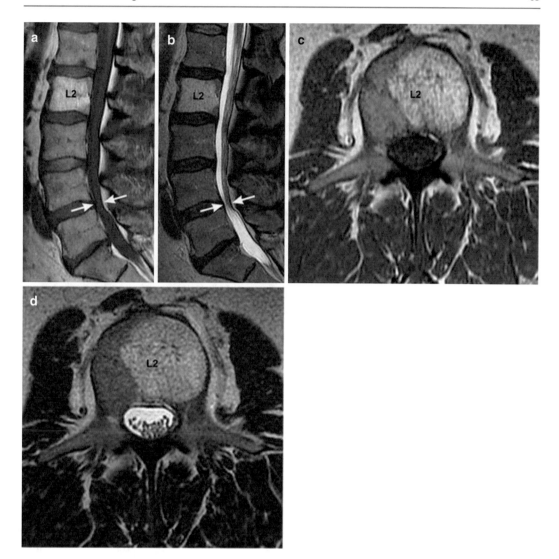

Fig. 2.14 Lumbar spinal canal stenosis. Sagittal and axial T1-weighted (**a**, **c**) and T2-weighted (**b**, **d**) MR images in a patient with low back pain demonstrate hyperintense T1 and T2 signal in the L2 vertebral body. The signal characteristics represent intralesional fat and are essentially pathognomonic for a benign hemangioma, an incidental finding of no clinical consequence. Beware of being distracted from the truly significant finding, which is the congenital central canal stenosis at L4–5 (*arrows* in **a** and **b**)

[51]. The presence of a cervical spine fracture doubles the risk of a thoracolumbar fracture [147]. Major thoracolumbar fracture types include wedge compression, burst, flexion-distraction (or seatbelt), and fracture-dislocation (which are typically highly unstable and usually associated with neurological injury) [148]. The thoracolumbar junction is the most common site for traumatic thoracolumbar fractures [24, 51]. There are several classification systems for thoracolumbar fractures [149]. Penetrating spine trauma, most commonly a gunshot wound, is much less common. In addition to injuring the spine proper, thoracolumbar trauma can also damage the aorta and spinal cord blood supply. Depending on the mechanism and degree of

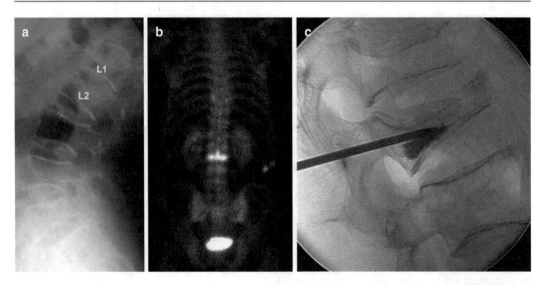

Fig. 2.15 Images of old and recent compression fractures. A 75-year-old man presents with acute upper lumbar pain following minimal trauma. A lateral radiograph (**a**) shows compression of the bodies of L1 and L2. There were no prior films for comparison. A radionuclide bone scan (**b**) shows increased activity at L2 only. L2 is the site of his acute fracture, while the L1 fracture is longstanding and asymptomatic. He was ultimately treated with bone augmentation (vertebroplasty) (**c**)

trauma, many patients will undergo a trauma CT in the emergency room, covering the chest-abdomen-pelvis. Reformatted images of the thoracolumbar spine can be obtained from these trauma studies for adequate assessment of thoracolumbar injury. Further imaging with MRI should be performed in patients who have possible spinal cord injuries secondary to bony compression, disc protrusion, spinal cord ischemia, or hematoma and in patients with suspected ligamentous instability.

Spine fractures are assessed for stability which is judged on a continuum. Patients with a possible spine fracture should be immobilized while they are transported, examined, and imaged. Fractures that are stable and usually without neural compression are typically managed conservatively with external bracing, while unstable injuries or injuries with spinal cord or neural compression may require surgical intervention for decompression and often stabilization with

fusion and segmental instrumentation (e.g., using pedicle screws and rods, or similar constructs in the thoracolumbar spine) (Figs. 2.15, 2.16, and 2.17).

The use of corticosteroids for nonpenetrating acute spinal cord injuries is not recommended in the current guidelines of both major neurosurgical societies, nor by multiple emergency medicine authorities as it is associated with higher rates of medical complications [150]. Multiple studies report a higher incidence of infection, sepsis, complications, increased intensive care unit length of stay, and death with steroid use. The best evidence in support of their use shows only a marginal motor benefit based on a post hoc subgroup analysis from the NASCIS 2 and 3 trials and no change in mortality overall. In the NASCIS 2 trial, at 1 year, there was no significant difference in neurologic function among treatment groups [150–153].

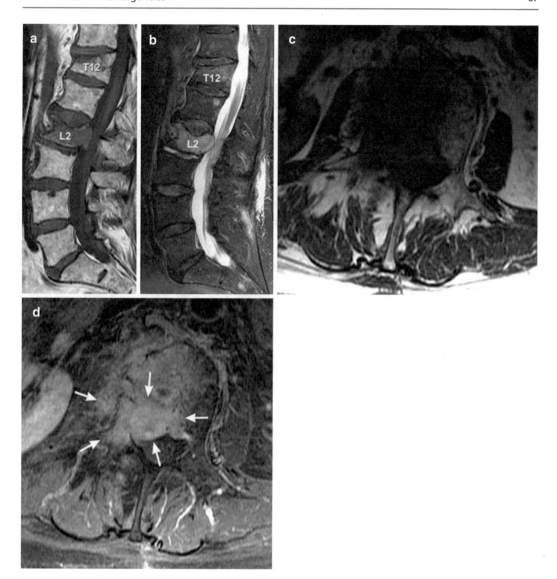

Fig. 2.16 Benign and malignant fractures. A 68-year-old woman presents with new low back pain and right groin and medial thigh pain. Sagittal T1-weighted (**a**) and fat-saturated T2-weighted (**b**) MR images show two compression fractures at T12 and L2. The T12 fracture is benign in appearance, with signal change restricted to the marrow immediately below the fracture endplate. In comparison, at L2, signal abnormality encompasses the entire vertebral body, and the posterior vertebral wall bulges into the spinal canal. Axial pre-contrast (**c**) and post-contrast (**d**) T1-weighted MR images at the L2 level show signal abnormality and enhancement extending from the vertebral body into the right pedicle, with poor delineation of the cortex, and direct extraosseous extension into the epidural and paraspinal soft tissue (see *arrows*). Both sagittal and axial findings at L2 are characteristic of tumor and should raise suspicion for pathologic fracture

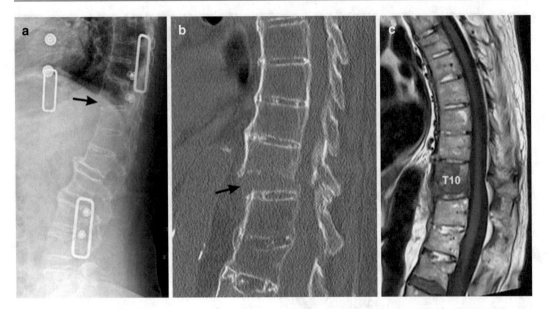

Fig. 2.17 Displaced vertebral fracture in a patient with a rigid spine. A 52-year-old man with known ankylosing spondylitis (AS) presents with low posterior thoracic pain following a low-impact motor vehicle accident. A lateral radiograph (**a**) while the patient is on a backboard demonstrates a displaced fracture through the inferior T10 vertebral body, which is more conspicuous on sagittal CT reconstruction (**b**) (see *arrows*). Diminished signal represents marrow edema throughout the T10 vertebral body on the follow-up sagittal T1-weighted MRI (**c**). Any process rendering the spine unusually stiff (e.g., AS, diffuse idiopathic skeletal hyperostosis [DISH]) predisposes to catastrophic fracture with modest trauma

Conclusions

While most causes of low back pain are benign, some instances represent true medical or surgical emergencies. A search for red flags in the history and on careful general physical and neurological examinations should identify the patient who is likely to harbor a serious condition, such as infection, tumor, aortic dissection or aneurysm, large lumbosacral disc, or traumatic spinal injury. These patients require expeditious investigation and, depending upon the results, possible urgent intervention. MRI is the best imaging study for most of the worrisome causes of low back pain such as infection, tumor, and spondylosis. CT and ultrasound are the preferred imaging modalities for thoracic aortic dissection and AAA, respectively. CT can also help rule out instability in patients with a history of trauma and aid in the diagnosis of other low back emergencies.

References

1. Jonsson E, Nachemson AL. Neck and back pain: the scientific evidence of causes, diagnosis, and treatment. Philadelphia: Lippincott Williams & Wilkins; 2000.
2. Rubin DI. Epidemiology and risk factors for spine pain. Neurol Clin. 2007;25(2):353–71.
3. Hoy D, Bain C, Williams G, March L, Brooks P, Blyth F, et al. A systematic review of the global prevalence of low back pain. Arthritis Rheum. 2012;64(6):2028–37.
4. Milbrett P, Halm M. Characteristics and predictors of frequent utilization of emergency services. J Emerg Nurs. 2009;35(3):191–8; quiz 273.
5. Frymoyer JW. Back pain and sciatica. N Engl J Med. 1988;318(5):291–300.
6. Andersson GB. Epidemiological features of chronic low-back pain. Lancet. 1999;354(9178):581–5.
7. Agency for Healthcare Research and Quality, U.S. Department of Health and Human Services. Medical Expenditures Panel Survey (MEPS), 2008-2011 [Internet] [cited 2020 Aug 5]. Available from: http://meps.ahrq.gov/mepsweb/.

8. Katz JN. Lumbar disc disorders and low-back pain: socioeconomic factors and consequences. J Bone Joint Surg Am. 2006;88(suppl_2):21–4.

9. National Research Council and the Institute of Medicine. Musculoskeletal disorders and the workplace: low back and upper extremities, Chapter 2. In: Panel on musculoskeletal disorders and the workplace commission on behavioral and social sciences and education. Washington, DC: National Academy Press; 2001.

10. Carey TS, Freburger JK, Holmes GM, Castel L, Darter J, Agans R, et al. A long way to go: practice patterns and evidence in chronic low back pain care. Spine. 2009;34(7):718–24.

11. Cassidy JD, Côté P, Carroll LJ, Kristman V. Incidence and course of low back pain episodes in the general population. Spine. 2005;30(24):2817–23.

12. Papageorgiou AC, Croft PR, Thomas E, Ferry S, Jayson MI, Silman AJ. Influence of previous pain experience on the episode incidence of low back pain: results from the South Manchester Back Pain Study. Pain. 1996;66(2–3):181–5.

13. Winters ME, Kluetz P, Zilberstein J. Back pain emergencies. Med Clin North Am. 2006;90(3):505–23.

14. Deyo RA, Rainville J, Kent DL. What can the history and physical examination tell us about low back pain? JAMA. 1992;268(6):760–5.

15. Henschke N, Maher CG, Refshauge KM, Herbert RD, Cumming RG, Bleasel J, et al. Prevalence of and screening for serious spinal pathology in patients presenting to primary care settings with acute low back pain. Arthritis Rheum. 2009;60(10):3072–80.

16. Klineberg E, Mazanec D, Orr D, Demicco R, Bell G, McLain R. Masquerade: medical causes of back pain. Cleve Clin J Med. 2007;74(12):905–13.

17. Deyo RA, Weinstein JN. Low back pain. N Engl J Med. 2001;344(5):363–70.

18. Bigos S, Bowyer O, Braen G, Brown K, Deyo R, Haldeman S, et al. Acute lower back problems in adults. Rockville: Agency for Health Care Policy and Research; 1994.

19. Della-Giustina K, Della-Giustina DA. Emergency department evaluation and treatment of pediatric orthopedic injuries. Emerg Med Clin North Am. 1999;17(4):895–922, vii.

20. Hart LG, Deyo RA, Cherkin DC. Physician office visits for low back pain. Frequency, clinical evaluation, and treatment patterns from a U.S. national survey. Spine. 1995;20(1):11–9.

21. Sapico FL, Montgomerie JZ. Pyogenic vertebral osteomyelitis: report of nine cases and review of the literature. Rev Infect Dis. 1979;1(5):754–76.

22. Baker AS, Ojemann RG, Swartz MN, Richardson EP. Spinal epidural abscess. N Engl J Med. 1975;293(10):463–8.

23. Wiglesworth A, Austin R, Corona M, Schneider D, Liao S, Gibbs L, et al. Bruising as a marker of physical elder abuse. J Am Geriatr Soc. 2009;57(7):1191–6.

24. Bartleson JD, Deen HG. Spine disorders: medical and surgical management. New York/Cambridge: Cambridge University Press; 2009.

25. Arce D, Sass P, Abul-Khoudoud H. Recognizing spinal cord emergencies. Am Fam Physician. 2001;64(4):631–8.

26. Wagner R, Jagoda A. Spinal cord syndromes. Emerg Med Clin North Am. 1997;15(3):699–711.

27. Deyo RA. Early diagnostic evaluation of low back pain. J Gen Intern Med. 1986;1(5):328–38.

28. Kobayashi S, Shizu N, Suzuki Y, Asai T, Yoshizawa H. Changes in nerve root motion and intraradicular blood flow during an intraoperative straight-leg-raising test. Spine. 2003;28(13):1427–34.

29. Breig A, Troup JD. Biomechanical considerations in the straight-leg-raising test. Cadaveric and clinical studies of the effects of medial hip rotation. Spine. 1979;4(3):242–50.

30. Devillé WLJM, van der Windt DAWM, Dzaferagic A, Bezemer PD, Bouter LM. The test of Lasègue: systematic review of the accuracy in diagnosing herniated discs. Spine. 2000;25(9):1140–7.

31. Campbell WW. Clinical signs and symptoms in lumbosacral radiculopathy. In: DeJong's the neurologic examination. Philadelphia: Lippincott Williams & Wilkins; 2012. p. 697.

32. Rabin A, Gerszten PC, Karausky P, Bunker CH, Potter DM, Welch WC. The sensitivity of the seated straight-leg raise test compared with the supine straight-leg raise test in patients presenting with magnetic resonance imaging evidence of lumbar nerve root compression. Arch Phys Med Rehabil. 2007;88(7):840–3.

33. Maitland GD. The slump test: examination and treatment. Aust J Physiother. 1985;31(6):215–9.

34. Majlesi J, Togay H, Unalan H, Toprak S. The sensitivity and specificity of the Slump and the Straight Leg Raising tests in patients with lumbar disc herniation. J Clin Rheumatol. 2008;14(2):87–91.

35. Bourque PR, Dyck PJ. Selective calf weakness suggests intraspinal pathology, not peripheral neuropathy. Arch Neurol. 1990;47(1):79–80.

36. Patel ND, Broderick DF, Burns J, Deshmukh TK, Fries IB, Harvey HB, et al. ACR appropriateness criteria low back pain. J Am Coll Radiol. 2016;13(9):1069–78.

37. Chou R, Qaseem A, Owens DK, Shekelle P. Diagnostic imaging for low back pain: advice for high-value health care from the American College of Physicians. Ann Intern Med. 2011;154(3):181–9.

38. Atlas SJ, Deyo RA. Evaluating and managing acute low back pain in the primary care setting. J Gen Intern Med. 2001;16(2):120–31.

39. Bradley WG. Low back pain. AJNR Am J Neuroradiol. 2007;28(5):990–2.

40. Verhagen AP, Downie A, Popal N, Maher C, Koes BW. Red flags presented in current low back pain guidelines: a review. Eur Spine J. 2016;25(9):2788–802.

41. Downie A, Williams CM, Henschke N, Hancock MJ, Ostelo RWJG, de Vet HCW, et al. Red flags to screen for malignancy and fracture in patients with low back pain: systematic review. BMJ. 2013;347:f7095. Available from: https://www.bmj.com/content/347/bmj.f7095.

42. Boden SD, Davis DO, Dina TS, Patronas NJ, Wiesel SW. Abnormal magnetic-resonance scans of the lumbar spine in asymptomatic subjects: a prospective investigation. J Bone Joint Surg Am. 1990;72(3):403–8.

43. Borenstein DG, O'Mara JW, Boden SD, Lauerman WC, Jacobson A, Platenberg C, et al. The value of magnetic resonance imaging of the lumbar spine to predict low-back pain in asymptomatic subjects: a seven-year follow-up study. J Bone Joint Surg Am. 2001;83(9):1306–11.

44. van Tulder MW, Assendelft WJ, Koes BW, Bouter LM. Spinal radiographic findings and nonspecific low back pain. A systematic review of observational studies. Spine. 1997;22(4):427–34.

45. Brinjikji W, Luetmer PH, Comstock B, Bresnahan BW, Chen LE, Deyo RA, et al. Systematic literature review of imaging features of spinal degeneration in asymptomatic populations. Am J Neuroradiol. 2015;36(4):811–6.

46. Chou R, Fu R, Carrino JA, Deyo RA. Imaging strategies for low-back pain: systematic review and meta-analysis. Lancet. 2009;373(9662):463–72.

47. Jarvik JG, Hollingworth W, Martin B, Emerson SS, Gray DT, Overman S, et al. Rapid magnetic resonance imaging vs radiographs for patients with low back pain: a randomized controlled trial. JAMA. 2003;289(21):2810–8.

48. Lurie JD, Birkmeyer NJ, Weinstein JN. Rates of advanced spinal imaging and spine surgery. Spine. 2003;28(6):616–20.

49. Deyo RA, Bigos SJ, Maravilla KR. Diagnostic imaging procedures for the lumbar spine. Ann Intern Med. 1989;111(11):865–7.

50. Deyo RA, Diehl AK. Lumbar spine films in primary care: current use and effects of selective ordering criteria. J Gen Intern Med. 1986;1(1):20–5.

51. Hsu JM, Joseph T, Ellis AM. Thoracolumbar fracture in blunt trauma patients: guidelines for diagnosis and imaging. Injury. 2003;34(6):426–33.

52. Kelen GD, Noji EK, Doris PE. Guidelines for use of lumbar spine radiography. Ann Emerg Med. 1986;15(3):245–51.

53. Walter J, Falvo T, Martich V, Rosen P, Doris P, Barkin R, et al. Nontraumatic neck and back pain. In: Diagnostic radiology in emergency medicine. St. Louis: Mosby-Year; 1992. p. 475–508.

54. Thornbury JR, Fryback DG, Turski PA, Javid MJ, McDonald JV, Beinlich BR, et al. Disk-caused nerve compression in patients with acute low-back pain: diagnosis with MR, CT myelography, and plain CT. Radiology. 1993;186(3):731–8.

55. van Rijn JC, Klemetso N, Reitsma JB, Bossuyt PM, Hulsmans FJ, Peul WC, et al. Observer variation in the evaluation of lumbar herniated discs and root compression: spiral CT compared with MRI. Br J Radiol. 2006;79(941):372–7.

56. Epstein O, Ludwig S, Gelb D, Poelstra K, O'Brien J. Comparison of computed tomography and plain radiography in assessing traumatic spinal deformity. J Spinal Disord Tech. 2009;22(3):197–201.

57. Inaba K, Munera F, McKenney M, Schulman C, de Moya M, Rivas L, et al. Visceral torso computed tomography for clearance of the thoracolumbar spine in trauma: a review of the literature. J Trauma. 2006;60(4):915–20.

58. Jarvik JG, Deyo RA. Diagnostic evaluation of low back pain with emphasis on imaging. Ann Intern Med. 2002;137(7):586–97.

59. Modic MT, Feiglin DH, Piraino DW, Boumphrey F, Weinstein MA, Duchesneau PM, et al. Vertebral osteomyelitis: assessment using MR. Radiology. 1985;157(1):157–66.

60. Chou R, Qaseem A, Snow V, Casey D, Cross JT, Shekelle P, et al. Diagnosis and treatment of low back pain: a joint clinical practice guideline from the American College of Physicians and the American Pain Society. Ann Intern Med. 2007;147(7):478–91.

61. Jensen AG, Espersen F, Skinhøj P, Frimodt-Møller N. Bacteremic Staphylococcus aureus spondylitis. Arch Intern Med. 1998;158(5):509–17.

62. Siemionow K, Steinmetz M, Bell G, Ilaslan H, McLain RF. Identifying serious causes of back pain: cancer, infection, fracture. Cleve Clin J Med. 2008;75(8):557–66.

63. McDonald M, Peel T. Vertebral osteomyelitis and discitis in adults. In: UpToDate.

64. Mylona E, Samarkos M, Kakalou E, Fanourgiakis P, Skoutelis A. Pyogenic vertebral osteomyelitis: a systematic review of clinical characteristics. Semin Arthritis Rheum. 2009;39(1):10–7.

65. Gasbarrini AL, Bertoldi E, Mazzetti M, Fini L, Terzi S, Gonella F, et al. Clinical features, diagnostic and therapeutic approaches to haematogenous vertebral osteomyelitis. Eur Rev Med Pharmacol Sci. 2005;9(1):53–66.

66. Kapeller P, Fazekas F, Krametter D, Koch M, Roob G, Schmidt R, et al. Pyogenic infectious spondylitis: clinical, laboratory and MRI features. Eur Neurol. 1997;38(2):94–8.

67. An HS, Seldomridge JA. Spinal infections: diagnostic tests and imaging studies. Clin Orthop. 2006;444:27–33.

68. Zimmerli W. Clinical practice. Vertebral osteomyelitis. N Engl J Med. 2010;362(11):1022–9.

69. Szypryt EP, Hardy JG, Hinton CE, Worthington BS, Mulholland RC. A comparison between magnetic resonance imaging and scintigraphic bone imaging in the diagnosis of disc space infection in an animal model. Spine. 1988;13(9):1042–8.

70. Pertuiset E, Beaudreuil J, Lioté F, Horusitzky A, Kemiche F, Richette P, et al. Spinal tuberculosis in adults. A study of 103 cases in a devel-

oped country, 1980–1994. Medicine (Baltimore). 1999;78(5):309–20.

71. Reihsaus E, Waldbaur H, Seeling W. Spinal epidural abscess: a meta-analysis of 915 patients. Neurosurg Rev. 2000;23(4):175–204; discussion 205.

72. Ptaszynski AE, Hooten WM, Huntoon MA. The incidence of spontaneous epidural abscess in Olmsted County from 1990 through 2000: a rare cause of spinal pain. Pain Med. 2007;8(4):338–43.

73. Phillips JMG, Stedeford JC, Hartsilver E, Roberts C. Epidural abscess complicating insertion of epidural catheters. Br J Anaesth. 2002;89(5):778–82.

74. Gaul C, Neundörfer B, Winterholler M. Iatrogenic (para-) spinal abscesses and meningitis following injection therapy for low back pain. Pain. 2005;116(3):407–10.

75. Darouiche RO. Spinal epidural abscess. N Engl J Med. 2006;355(19):2012–20.

76. Sendi P, Bregenzer T, Zimmerli W. Spinal epidural abscess in clinical practice. QJM. 2008;101(1):1–12.

77. Chen W-C, Wang J-L, Wang J-T, Chen Y-C, Chang S-C. Spinal epidural abscess due to Staphylococcus aureus: clinical manifestations and outcomes. J Microbiol Immunol Infect. 2008;41(3):215–21.

78. Davis DP, Wold RM, Patel RJ, Tran AJ, Tokhi RN, Chan TC, et al. The clinical presentation and impact of diagnostic delays on emergency department patients with spinal epidural abscess. J Emerg Med. 2004;26(3):285–91.

79. Deyo RA, Diehl AK. Cancer as a cause of back pain: frequency, clinical presentation, and diagnostic strategies. J Gen Intern Med. 1988;3(3):230–8.

80. Brihaye J, Ectors P, Lemort M, Van Houtte P. The management of spinal epidural metastases. Adv Tech Stand Neurosurg. 1988;16:121–76.

81. Schiff D, O'Neill BP, Suman VJ. Spinal epidural metastasis as the initial manifestation of malignancy: clinical features and diagnostic approach. Neurology. 1997;49(2):452–6.

82. Gilbert RW, Kim JH, Posner JB. Epidural spinal cord compression from metastatic tumor: diagnosis and treatment. Ann Neurol. 1978;3(1):40–51.

83. Schiff D, O'Neill BP, Wang CH, O'Fallon JR. Neuroimaging and treatment implications of patients with multiple epidural spinal metastases. Cancer. 1998;83(8):1593–601.

84. Bach F, Larsen BH, Rohde K, Børgesen SE, Gjerris F, Bøge-Rasmussen T, et al. Metastatic spinal cord compression. Occurrence, symptoms, clinical presentations and prognosis in 398 patients with spinal cord compression. Acta Neurochir. 1990;107(1–2):37–43.

85. Helweg-Larsen S, Sørensen PS. Symptoms and signs in metastatic spinal cord compression: a study of progression from first symptom until diagnosis in 153 patients. Eur J Cancer. 1994;30A(3):396–8.

86. Laufer I, Schiff D, Kelly H, Bilsky M, Post T, Waltham M. Clinical features and diagnosis of neoplastic epidural spinal cord compression. In: UpToDate.

87. Schiff D, Posner JB. Treatment and prognosis of neoplastic epidural spinal cord compression, including cauda equina syndrome. In: UpToDate. 2020.

88. Shapiro S. Medical realities of cauda equina syndrome secondary to lumbar disc herniation. Spine. 2000;25(3):348–51; discussion 352.

89. Kostuik JP, Harrington I, Alexander D, Rand W, Evans D. Cauda equina syndrome and lumbar disc herniation. J Bone Joint Surg Am. 1986;68(3):386–91.

90. O'Laoire SA, Crockard HA, Thomas DG. Prognosis for sphincter recovery after operation for cauda equina compression owing to lumbar disc prolapse. Br Med J (Clin Res Ed). 1981;282(6279):1852.

91. Tay EC, Chacha PB. Midline prolapse of a lumbar intervertebral disc with compression of the cauda equina. J Bone Joint Surg Br. 1979;61(1):43–6.

92. Small SA, Perron AD, Brady WJ. Orthopedic pitfalls: cauda equina syndrome. Am J Emerg Med. 2005;23(2):159–63.

93. Lavy C, James A, Wilson-MacDonald J, Fairbank J. Cauda equina syndrome. BMJ. 2009;338:b936.

94. Loblaw DA, Perry J, Chambers A, Laperriere NJ. Systematic review of the diagnosis and management of malignant extradural spinal cord compression: the Cancer Care Ontario Practice Guidelines Initiative's Neuro-Oncology Disease Site Group. J Clin Oncol. 2005;23(9):2028–37.

95. Sullivan PR, Wolfson AB, Leckey RD, Burke JL. Diagnosis of acute thoracic aortic dissection in the emergency department. Am J Emerg Med. 2000;18(1):46–50.

96. Golledge J, Eagle KA. Acute aortic dissection. Lancet. 2008;372(9632):55–66.

97. Chen K, Varon J, Wenker OC, Judge DK, Fromm RE, Sternbach GL. Acute thoracic aortic dissection: the basics. J Emerg Med. 1997;15(6):859–67.

98. Hagan PG, Nienaber CA, Isselbacher EM, Bruckman D, Karavite DJ, Russman PL, et al. The International Registry of Acute Aortic Dissection (IRAD): new insights into an old disease. JAMA. 2000;283(7):897–903.

99. Rogers RL, McCormack R. Aortic disasters. Emerg Med Clin North Am. 2004;22(4):887–908.

100. Tsai TT, Nienaber CA, Eagle KA. Acute aortic syndromes. Circulation. 2005;112(24):3802–13.

101. Nienaber CA, Eagle KA. Aortic dissection: new frontiers in diagnosis and management: part I: from etiology to diagnostic strategies. Circulation. 2003;108(5):628–35.

102. Gerber O, Heyer EJ, Vieux U. Painless dissections of the aorta presenting as acute neurologic syndromes. Stroke. 1986;17(4):644–7.

103. Greenwood WR, Robinson MD. Painless dissection of the thoracic aorta. Am J Emerg Med. 1986;4(4):330–3.

104. von Kodolitsch Y, Schwartz AG, Nienaber CA. Clinical prediction of acute aortic dissection. Arch Intern Med. 2000;160(19):2977–82.

105. Clark CE, Campbell JL, Evans PH, Millward A. Prevalence and clinical implications of the inter-

arm blood pressure difference: a systematic review. J Hum Hypertens. 2006;20(12):923–31.

106. Salvolini L, Renda P, Fiore D, Scaglione M, Piccoli G, Giovagnoni A. Acute aortic syndromes: role of multi-detector row CT. Eur J Radiol. 2008;65(3):350–8.

107. Sommer T, Fehske W, Holzknecht N, Smekal AV, Keller E, Lutterbey G, et al. Aortic dissection: a comparative study of diagnosis with spiral CT, multiplanar transesophageal echocardiography, and MR imaging. Radiology. 1996;199(2):347–52.

108. Yoshida S, Akiba H, Tamakawa M, Yama N, Hareyama M, Morishita K, et al. Thoracic involvement of type A aortic dissection and intramural hematoma: diagnostic accuracy--comparison of emergency helical CT and surgical findings. Radiology. 2003;228(2):430–5.

109. Zeman RK, Berman PM, Silverman PM, Davros WJ, Cooper C, Kladakis AO, et al. Diagnosis of aortic dissection: value of helical CT with multiplanar reformation and three-dimensional rendering. AJR Am J Roentgenol. 1995;164(6):1375–80.

110. Shiga T, Wajima Z, Apfel CC, Inoue T, Ohe Y. Diagnostic accuracy of transesophageal echocardiography, helical computed tomography, and magnetic resonance imaging for suspected thoracic aortic dissection: systematic review and meta-analysis. Arch Intern Med. 2006;166(13):1350–6.

111. Shiga T, Wajima Z, Inoue T, Ogawa R. Survey of observer variation in transesophageal echocardiography: comparison of anesthesiology and cardiology literature. J Cardiothorac Vasc Anesth. 2003;17(4):430–42.

112. Börner N, Erbel R, Braun B, Henkel B, Meyer J. Diagnosis of aortic dissection by transesophageal echocardiography. Am J Cardiol. 1984;54(8):1157–8.

113. Erbel R, Alfonso F, Boileau C, Dirsch O, Eber B, Haverich A, et al. Diagnosis and management of aortic dissection. Eur Heart J. 2001;22(18):1642–81.

114. Isselbacher EM. Thoracic and abdominal aortic aneurysms. Circulation. 2005;111(6):816–28.

115. U.S. National Center for Injury Prevention and Control, Centers for Disease Control and Prevention. 20 leading causes of death, United States, 2018, all races, both sexes [Internet]. National Center for Health Statistics (NCHS), National Vital Statistics System. 2018 [cited 2020 Aug 5]. Available from: https://webappa.cdc.gov/sasweb/ncipc/leadcause.html.

116. Lederle FA. In the clinic. Abdominal aortic aneurysm. Ann Intern Med. 2009;150(9):ITC5–1.

117. Powell JT, Greenhalgh RM. Clinical practice. Small abdominal aortic aneurysms. N Engl J Med. 2003;348(19):1895–901.

118. Lederle FA, Johnson GR, Wilson SE, Chute EP, Hye RJ, Makaroun MS, et al. The aneurysm detection and management study screening program: validation cohort and final results. Aneurysm Detection and Management Veterans Affairs Cooperative Study Investigators. Arch Intern Med. 2000;160(10):1425–30.

119. Lederle FA, Johnson GR, Wilson SE, Chute EP, Littooy FN, Bandyk D, et al. Prevalence and associations of abdominal aortic aneurysm detected through screening. Aneurysm Detection and Management (ADAM) Veterans Affairs Cooperative Study Group. Ann Intern Med. 1997;126(6):441–9.

120. Lee TY, Korn P, Heller JA, Kilaru S, Beavers FP, Bush HL, et al. The cost-effectiveness of a "quick-screen" program for abdominal aortic aneurysms. Surgery. 2002;132(2):399–407.

121. Steele MA, Dalsing MC. Emergency evaluation of abdominal aortic aneurysms. Indiana Med. 1987;80(9):862–4.

122. Merchant RF, Cafferata HT, DePalma RG. Ruptured aortic aneurysm seen initially as acute femoral neuropathy. Arch Surg. 1982;117(6):811–3.

123. Lindholt JS, Vammen S, Juul S, Henneberg EW, Fasting H. The validity of ultrasonographic scanning as screening method for abdominal aortic aneurysm. Eur J Vasc Endovasc Surg. 1999;17(6):472–5.

124. Upchurch GR, Schaub TA. Abdominal aortic aneurysm. Am Fam Physician. 2006;73(7):1198–204.

125. Spangfort EV. The lumbar disc herniation. A computer-aided analysis of 2,504 operations. Acta Orthop Scand Suppl. 1972;142:1–95.

126. DeLong WB, Polissar N, Neradilek B. Timing of surgery in cauda equina syndrome with urinary retention: meta-analysis of observational studies. J Neurosurg Spine. 2008;8(4):305–20.

127. Jalloh I, Minhas P. Delays in the treatment of cauda equina syndrome due to its variable clinical features in patients presenting to the emergency department. Emerg Med J. 2007;24(1):33–4.

128. Ahn UM, Ahn NU, Buchowski JM, Garrett ES, Sieber AN, Kostuik JP. Cauda equina syndrome secondary to lumbar disc herniation: a meta-analysis of surgical outcomes. Spine. 2000;25(12):1515–22.

129. Kohles SS, Kohles DA, Karp AP, Erlich VM, Polissar NL. Time-dependent surgical outcomes following cauda equina syndrome diagnosis: comments on a meta-analysis. Spine. 2004;29(11):1281–7.

130. Todd NV. Cauda equina syndrome: the timing of surgery probably does influence outcome. Br J Neurosurg. 2005;19(4):301–6; discussion 307.

131. Gleave JRW, Macfarlane R. Cauda equina syndrome: what is the relationship between timing of surgery and outcome? Br J Neurosurg. 2002;16(4):325–8.

132. Hussain SA, Gullan RW, Chitnavis BP. Cauda equina syndrome: outcome and implications for management. Br J Neurosurg. 2003;17(2):164–7.

133. McCarthy MJH, Aylott CEW, Grevitt MP, Hegarty J. Cauda equina syndrome: factors affecting long-term functional and sphincteric outcome. Spine. 2007;32(2):207–16.

134. Qureshi A, Sell P. Cauda equina syndrome treated by surgical decompression: the influence of timing on surgical outcome. Eur Spine J. 2007;16(12):2143–51.

135. Olivero WC, Wang H, Hanigan WC, Henderson JP, Tracy PT, Elwood PW, et al. Cauda equina syndrome (CES) from lumbar disc herniations. J Spinal Disord Tech. 2009;22(3):202–6.

136. Chou R, Atlas SJ, Stanos SP, Rosenquist RW. Nonsurgical interventional therapies for low back pain: a review of the evidence for an American Pain Society clinical practice guideline. Spine. 2009;34(10):1078–93.

137. Chou R, Huffman LH, American Pain Society, American College of Physicians. Medications for acute and chronic low back pain: a review of the evidence for an American Pain Society/American College of Physicians clinical practice guideline. Ann Intern Med. 2007;147(7):505–14.

138. Chou R, Huffman LH, American Pain Society, American College of Physicians. Nonpharmacologic therapies for acute and chronic low back pain: a review of the evidence for an American Pain Society/American College of Physicians clinical practice guideline. Ann Intern Med. 2007;147(7):492–504.

139. Chou R, Loeser JD, Owens DK, Rosenquist RW, Atlas SJ, Baisden J, et al. Interventional therapies, surgery, and interdisciplinary rehabilitation for low back pain: an evidence-based clinical practice guideline from the American Pain Society. Spine. 2009;34(10):1066–77.

140. Chou R, Baisden J, Carragee EJ, Resnick DK, Shaffer WO, Loeser JD. Surgery for low back pain: a review of the evidence for an American Pain Society clinical practice guideline. Spine. 2009;34(10):1094–109.

141. Watters WC, Baisden J, Gilbert TJ, Kreiner S, Resnick DK, Bono CM, et al. Degenerative lumbar spinal stenosis: an evidence-based clinical guideline for the diagnosis and treatment of degenerative lumbar spinal stenosis. Spine J. 2008;8(2):305–10.

142. Kim DH, Vaccaro AR. Osteoporotic compression fractures of the spine; current options and considerations for treatment. Spine J. 2006;6(5):479–87.

143. Buchbinder R, Osborne RH, Ebeling PR, Wark JD, Mitchell P, Wriedt C, et al. A randomized trial of vertebroplasty for painful osteoporotic vertebral fractures. N Engl J Med. 2009;361(6):557–68.

144. Kallmes DF, Comstock BA, Heagerty PJ, Turner JA, Wilson DJ, Diamond TH, et al. A randomized trial of vertebroplasty for osteoporotic spinal fractures. N Engl J Med. 2009;361(6):569–79.

145. Weinstein JN. Balancing science and informed choice in decisions about vertebroplasty. N Engl J Med. 2009;361(6):619–21.

146. Daffner RH, Hackney DB. ACR Appropriateness Criteria on suspected spine trauma. J Am Coll Radiol. 2007;4(11):762–75.

147. Winslow JE, Hensberry R, Bozeman WP, Hill KD, Miller PR. Risk of thoracolumbar fractures doubled in victims of motor vehicle collisions with cervical spine fractures. J Trauma. 2006;61(3):686–7.

148. Frymoyer J, Wiesel S. Chapter 41. In: The adult and pediatric spine. Philadelphia: Lippincott Williams and Wilkins; 2004.

149. Steinmetz MP, Resnick DK. Thoracolumbar fractures: classification and implications for treatment: part I. Contemp Neurosurg. 2006;28(7):1–7.

150. Walters BC, Hadley MN, Hurlbert RJ, Aarabi B, Dhall SS, Gelb DE, et al. Guidelines for the management of acute cervical spine and spinal cord injuries: 2013 update. Neurosurgery. 2013;60(CN_suppl_1):82–91.

151. Bracken MB, Shepard MJ, Collins WF, Holford TR, Young W, Baskin DS, et al. A randomized, controlled trial of methylprednisolone or naloxone in the treatment of acute spinal-cord injury. Results of the Second National Acute Spinal Cord Injury Study. N Engl J Med. 1990;322(20):1405–11.

152. Bracken MB, Shepard MJ, Holford TR, Leo-Summers L, Aldrich EF, Fazl M, et al. Administration of methylprednisolone for 24 or 48 hours or tirilazad mesylate for 48 hours in the treatment of acute spinal cord injury. Results of the Third National Acute Spinal Cord Injury Randomized Controlled Trial. National Acute Spinal Cord Injury Study. JAMA. 1997;277(20):1597–604.

153. Nesathurai S. Steroids and spinal cord injury: revisiting the NASCIS 2 and NASCIS 3 trials. J Trauma. 1998;45(6):1088–93.

Dizziness and Vertigo Presentations in the Emergency Department

3

Kevin A. Kerber

Introduction

Physicians have high levels of uncertainty in the evaluation and management of patients who present with dizziness to the emergency department. In a survey of emergency medicine physicians, "identification of central or serious causes of vertigo" was ranked as the #1 priority for clinical decision support research in adult emergency presentations [1]. Uncertainty also likely contributes to the dramatic increase in the use of imaging studies in emergency department dizziness presentations. In 1995, less than 10% of patients presenting to emergency departments (ED) with dizziness were evaluated with a head computerized tomography (CT) scan, but by 2004, the rate had doubled to greater than 25% [2]. Despite this increase in head CT use, the proportion of ED dizziness visits receiving a central nervous system diagnosis did not increase [2].

Most patients presenting with dizziness can be rapidly assessed and valid estimates can be made regarding diagnostic possibilities—thus informing management decisions. There already exist many effective treatments for dizziness symptoms and specific dizziness disorders. In fact, benign paroxysmal positional vertigo (BPPV) is among the most common causes of dizziness,

and it can be cured by a simple repositioning maneuver (i.e., the Epley maneuver) at the bedside [3, 33]. The goal in the management of dizziness presentations is to get the most effective treatments to the dizziness patients most likely to benefit from them and to do so in an efficient manner. Achieving this goal depends on the bedside assessment and the formulation of the case.

Most of the uncertainty in dizziness presentations occurs when attempting to distinguish "peripheral" (and generally self-limited) from "central" (and potentially life-threatening) causes. The key to distinguishing between these is understanding the three most common peripheral vestibular disorders (i.e., vestibular neuritis, BPPV, and Meniere's disease) (Table 3.1). The most effective way to "rule out" a life-threatening central disorder may be to "rule in" a specific peripheral vestibular disorder. The peripheral vestibular disorders are important because they account for a large proportion of the causes of dizziness, present with highly stereotyped characteristics, and can be effectively treated. The time to consider a central etiology is when the presentation deviates from the stereotyped characteristics of the specific peripheral vestibular disorders and also when the patient is high risk for central disorders, such as stroke.

In this chapter, we highlight the steps in evaluating and managing patients who present with dizziness symptoms in the emergency setting. We focus on the symptom of vertigo and distinguishing peripheral vestibular from central vestibular disorders.

K. A. Kerber (✉)
Department of Neurology, University of Michigan Health System, Ann Arbor, MI, USA
e-mail: kakerber@umich.edu

Table 3.1 The three most common specific peripheral vestibular disorders

	Type of presentation	Symptoms	Exam findings	Red flags for central etiology[a]
Vestibular neuritis	Acute severe prolonged dizziness	Constant vertigo, nausea, and imbalance	Spontaneous unidirectional horizontal nystagmus, positive corresponding head thrust test[b]	Central pattern of nystagmus[c]. Negative head thrust test
Meniere's disease	Recurrent spontaneous attacks	Vertigo, nausea, imbalance lasting hours, unilateral fluctuating hearing loss	Peripheral pattern of nystagmus, unilateral hearing loss	New onset, crescendo attacks lasting minutes, central patterns of nystagmus[c]
Benign paroxysmal positional vertigo	Recurrent positionally triggered attacks	Recurrent positionally triggered attacks of vertigo, duration <1 min	Positional testing Dix–Hallpike test triggers burst of upbeat torsional nystagmus[d]	Central pattern of nystagmus[c], nonresponse to repositioning maneuvers

[a]Red flags for all presentation type include other focal neurological signs or symptoms
[b]With left-sided vestibular neuritis, the spontaneous nystagmus beats to the right side, and the head thrust test reveals a corrective saccade after movements to the left side
[c]Central patterns of nystagmus include spontaneous vertical (up or downbeating) nystagmus, bidirectional gaze-evoked nystagmus, and downbeating nystagmus triggered by positional testing
[d]Benign paroxysmal positional vertigo (BPPV) variant: with horizontal canal BPPV, horizontal nystagmus will be triggered by supine positional testing

Evaluation of Emergency Presentations

The effective clinical evaluation of patients presenting with dizziness in the emergency setting requires an organized approach that allows the physician to gather all of the most relevant information and then to formulate the case in a way that establishes the most likely cause and identifies any relevant "red flags" that could suggest a central disorder.

Step 1: Determine if the Dizziness Is the Principal Symptom as Opposed to a Minor Accompanying Symptom

Dizziness is an incredibly common accompanying symptom. More than 60% of all patients in the emergency department will report having dizziness when specifically asked about it [4]. In most cases, it is a minor accompanying symptom rather than the principal symptom. One of the main problems with dizziness presentations is that the patient's descriptions of dizziness can be very vague, inconsistent, and unreliable [4]. So prior to focusing all attention on the dizziness

symptom, first consider if other symptoms are more prominent. For example, if chest pain is the principal symptom, then an initial focus on cardiac etiologies is probably more effective than a focus on vestibular system etiologies.

Step 2: Define the Characteristics of the Dizziness Symptom

If the dizziness symptom is the principal symptom, then the next step is to more clearly define it. However, defining the dizziness symptom is often not a simple task because it is a subjective experience, and many patients with dizziness have difficulty describing what they are actually experiencing. There can also be problems with being overly reliant on the patient's description of the symptom in informing the potential causes. For example, vertigo (i.e., visualized movement of the environment) is one common type of dizziness symptom, and it should localize to the vestibular system (either the peripheral vestibular system or the central vestibular system). But patients with a variety of non-vestibular disorders (e.g., orthostatic hypotension, cardiac disorders) often report movement of the environment particularly if they are specifically asked about it [5]. An intense visualized room-spinning sensation is probably a more valid indicator of a vestibular system disorder than either an "internal" spinning sensation (i.e., no actual spinning of the environment) or a very mild visualized spinning sensation. Conversely, some patients who have a vestibular disorder will describe the symptom as a nonvertiginous vague type of dizziness, even in the setting of frank nystagmus.

Other types of dizziness symptoms to consider are light-headedness with presyncope, light-headedness (or similar "head" sensation) without presyncope, or imbalance. Some patients will use the label "dizziness" to describe anxiety-like symptoms, general fatigue or weakness, or just not feeling well. It is also important to note that most patient with dizziness will report more than one type of dizziness and are not reliable when asked to select a single type of dizziness [34, 35].

Because of the problem with patient descriptions of dizziness symptoms, the characteristics of the symptom may be equally or even more important than defining the exact symptom itself. Patients have been shown to be more reliable in reporting the timing, duration, and triggers of the dizziness symptom than they are in reporting the type of dizziness [34]. Defining the characteristics of the symptom starts with defining whether the symptom is episodic or constant. If the symptom is episodic, then one should probe regarding triggers of the symptom and the frequency and duration of the episodes. When the symptom is constant, one should determine the onset of the symptom and aggravating and alleviating factors. Determining accompanying symptoms is also a vital step, particularly gathering information about auditory symptoms or focal neurological symptoms.

The information from the history will eventually be a key aspect when formulating the case (see step 5). The details from the history help to categorize the patient into broad classifications of dizziness presentations which are relevant to determining potential etiologies. Helpful classifications of presentations include the following: acute severe prolonged dizziness, recurrent spontaneous dizziness attacks, and recurrent positionally triggered dizziness attacks. The type of presentation is determined based on the details of the history of present illness. Acute severe prolonged dizziness is the sudden onset of a constant symptom that is generally a debilitating symptom. Recurrent spontaneous dizziness attacks are reported by patients who have had at least several attacks that come on without any apparent inciting event. Recurrent positionally triggered dizziness attacks consist of the symptom triggered by certain head movements.

Step 3: Perform a General Neurological Examination

A general neurological examination is important because any relevant motor, sensory, or language deficits will likely warrant a workup for a central disorder regardless of the other characteristics of the dizziness symptom. Most patients presenting with dizziness caused by stroke will have at least subtle signs of a focal central nervous system lesion typically coordination, speech, or sensory defictis [36]. On the other hand, peripheral vestibular disorders and general medical disorders should not cause focal neurological deficits.

For similar reasons, a general medical examination can also be important when trying to exclude a general medical disorder such as a heart arrhythmia or orthostatic hypotension.

Step 4: Perform a Neuro-otologic Assessment

If the source of the symptom is not clear after performing steps 1–3, then the next step is to perform a neuro-otologic assessment. Subtle differences in eye movements or the vestibuloocular reflex can be highly localizing. The key neuro-otologic examination components are the following: an assessment of nystagmus, positional testing when applicable, and the head thrust test when applicable.

Pathological nystagmus occurs as the result of an acute imbalance of the vestibular system which can stem from a lesion (or aberrant stimu-lation) of peripheral or central vestibular struc-tures. Physicians sometimes only note whether nystagmus is present or absent, but it is the pat-tern of nystagmus—not the mere presence—that is important for discriminating a peripheral lesion from a central lesion. The localizing value of the pattern of nystagmus is also dependent on the type of presentation. Some general rules about the localizing value of nystagmus apply (Table 3.2). In patients with acute severe pro-longed vertigo, a unidirectional spontaneous hor-izontal nystagmus is suggestive of a lesion of the vestibular nerve—although a lesion at the cranial nerve 8 root entry zone in the brainstem or the cerebellar hemisphere can less commonly be the cause of unidirectional nystagmus [36]. The lesioned side is the side opposite the direction of the fast phase of nystagmus. Unidirectional spon-taneous nystagmus implies that the nystagmus is present in primary gaze and that the nystagmus never changes direction. For example, if nystag-mus beats to the left side, then it should never transition to beating to the right side. The left-beating nystagmus does increase in velocity when the patient looks to the left side and also decrease (or stop) when the patient looks to the

right side, but it will not transit to a right-beating nystagmus if the lesion is on the vestibular nerve. A central lesion is presumed in acute severe ver-tigo presentations whenever a pattern other than unidirectional horizontal nystagmus is observed. A central nervous system lesion patterns of nys-tagmus in acute severe vertigo presentations include direction-changing gaze-evoked nystag-mus (i.e., patient looks to the right and nystagmus beats to the right; then, patient looks to the left and nystagmus beats to the left) and spontaneous vertical (typically downbeating) nystagmus.

Positional testing is an important component of the bedside examination when the type of pre-sentation is recurrent positional dizziness or when spontaneous or gaze nystagmus is not pres-ent. It is important to note that the patterns of nystagmus that discriminate peripheral from cen-tral etiologies when the presentation type is recurrent positional dizziness are different from the patterns in acute severe dizziness presenta-tions. Generally no spontaneous nystagmus is present in positionally triggered dizziness pre-sentations. In positionally triggered attacks caused by BPPV, the nystagmus can change direction based on changes in head position. In addition, a principally vertical nystagmus is the

Table 3.2 Patterns of nystagmus associated with the type of dizziness presentation

	Spontaneous nystagmus?	Peripheral vestibular patterns of nystagmus	Central vestibular patterns of nystagmus
Acute severe prolonged dizziness	Yes	Unidirectional, horizontal spontaneous[a]	Direction-changing, gaze-evoked[b] Spontaneous vertical or pure torsional
Recurrent spontaneous attacks	Yes/no[c]	Unidirectional, horizontal spontaneous[a]	Direction-changing, gaze-evoked[b] Spontaneous vertical or pure torsional
Recurrent positionally triggered attacks	No	*Dix–Hallpike test*: Burst of upbeat torsional[d] *Supine positional test*: Horizontal nystagmus with direction of nystagmus changing with head movement to opposite side[e]	Downbeating persistent Pure torsional

[a]Pattern can less commonly be caused by central lesions, increasing the importance of assessing risk for central lesion and the results of the head thrust test
[b]Example of direction-changing gaze-evoked nystagmus: left-beating nystagmus with gaze to the left; then, right-beating nystagmus with gaze to the right
[c]May not have nystagmus if evaluation takes place in between attacks
[d]Upon sitting up from Dix–Hallpike test, a burst of downbeating torsional nystagmus will often be triggered. Thus, a direction-changing positionally evoked nystagmus
[e]In rare circumstances, pattern can be caused by a central lesion

characteristic pattern of the most common BPPV variant (i.e., posterior canal BPPV). In posterior canal BPPV, the Dix–Hallpike test (Fig. 3.1) [3, 6] triggers a burst of upbeating and torsional nystag-

mus which lasts less than 1 min. If the patient were to next sit back up from the Dix–Hallpike position, then a burst of downbeating and torsional nystagmus is triggered. The reason for the

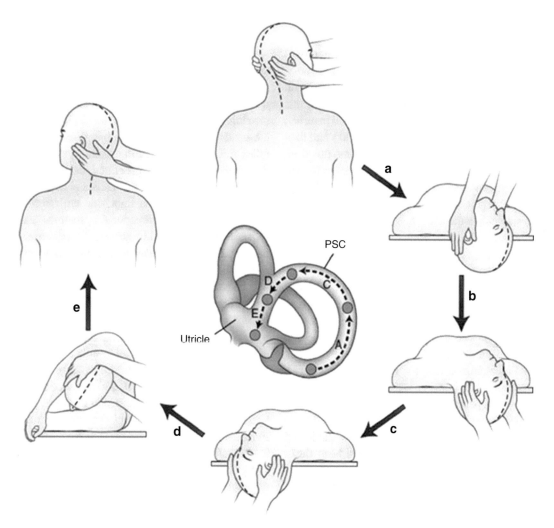

Fig. 3.1 The Dix–Hallpike test for the diagnosis of posterior canal benign paroxysmal positional vertigo affected the right ear, and the Epley maneuver for the treatment of posterior canal benign paroxysmal positional vertigo affecting the right ear. The procedure can be reversed for treating the left ear. The drawing of the labyrinth in the center shows the position of the debris as it moves around the posterior semicircular canal (PSC) and into the utricle (UT). The patient is seated upright, with head facing the examiner, who is standing on the right. (**a**) The patient is then rapidly moved to head-hanging right position (Dix–Hallpike test). This position is maintained until the nystagmus ceases. (**b**) The examiner moves to the head of the table, repositioning hands as shown. (**c**) The head is rotated quickly to the left with right ear upward. This posi- tion is maintained for 30 s. (**d**) The patient rolls onto the left side while the examiner rapidly rotates the head leftward until the nose is directed toward the floor. This position is then held for 30 s. (**e**) The patient is rapidly lifted into the sitting position, now facing left. The entire sequence should be repeated until no nystagmus can be elicited. Following the maneuver, the patient is instructed to avoid head hanging positions to prevent the debris from reentering the posterior canal. (From: Rakel RE. Conn's Current Therapy 1995, p. 839, WB Saunders, 1995. Video clips of the Dix–Hallpike test, Epley maneuver, and other positional test are available from the American Academy of Neurology at http://www.neurology.org/cgi/content/ full/70/22/2067/DC2)

change in direction of the nystagmus after sitting up is that the particles move in the opposite direction after sitting up compared to the head-hanging (i.e., Dix–Hallpike) position. However, if persistent downbeating nystagmus is triggered by the Dix–Hallpike test, then a central nervous system lesion is presumed.

If the Dix–Hallpike positional test does not trigger the nystagmus of BPPV, then supine positional testing is used to test for the less common horizontal canal variant of BPPV [7]. With this test, the patient lies supine and the head is turned first to one side and held for at least 30 s and then to the other side and held for the same duration. A burst of horizontal nystagmus beating toward the ground is characteristic of the horizontal canal variant of BPPV. The side with stronger nystagmus is the abnormal side. More persistent nystagmus beating away from the ground can occur if the debris is stuck within the canal or is attached to the cupula [3, 7].

The head thrust test is an important bedside examination component when the type of dizziness presentation is acute severe dizziness (Fig. 3.2). The head thrust test allows a direct assessment of the vestibular–ocular reflex (VOR), and an abnormal result is highly suggestive of a vestibular nerve lesion when other findings also support a peripheral vestibular lesion [8, 9, 36]. This test is different from the doll's eye test because the doll's eye test uses slow rotation of the head to either side, whereas the head thrust test uses quick movements which isolate the vestibular system function. The corresponding eye movements of the doll's eye test can be generated by either the vestibular system or the smooth pursuit system in a conscious patient. But only the vestibular system generates the reflex movement of the eyes after the quick movement of the head thrust test (the smooth pursuit system only works at low stimulus velocities). To test the VOR using the head thrust test, the examiner stands in front of the patient and holds the patient's head with both hands. The patient is instructed to focus on the examiner's nose, and then the examiner initiates a quick 10–15° movement of the patient's head to one side. When there is a lesion of the VOR on one side, a corrective eye movement (i.e., a corrective "saccade") back to the examiner's nose is seen after the head is moved toward the affected side, and this is considered abnormal. In contrast and serving as an internal control, the eyes will stay on target (i.e., the examiner's nose) after the head thrust test toward the non-lesioned side side which is a normal response. These findings can be appreciated even when spontaneous nystagmus is present. The reason for the corrective saccade with a peripheral vestibular lesion is rooted in the physiology of the vestibular system [10]. When the head is moved quickly in one direction, the reflex (i.e., the VOR) that moves the eyes toward the opposite direction is generated mostly by the side the head moved toward. Thus a patient with vestibular neuritis of the right side will present with a left-beating unidirectional nystagmus, and the head thrust test will be abnormal (i.e., corrective saccade present) with movement toward the right side.

The neuro-otologic examination of the patient with dizziness caused by Meniere's disease is less predictable because most of the symptoms have typically been resolved by the time of the evaluation, the nystagmus can be either toward or away from the affected ear (since it can be a stimulatory or inhibitory lesion), and the head thrust test is typically normal. Regardless, central patterns of nystagmus should be a red flag. Furthermore, a key feature of Meniere's disease is fluctuating hearing loss; however, the auditory symptoms can be mild or unappreciated by the patient during the early phases of the disorder. By mid-to-late stages of the disorder, a persistent unilateral hearing loss will be present.

Step 5: Formulate the Differential Diagnosis

When formulating the case, an initial helpful step is to first determine which classification of dizziness presentation the patient falls under. Likely etiologies can then be determined by further considering the presentation features and the information gathered from the examination.

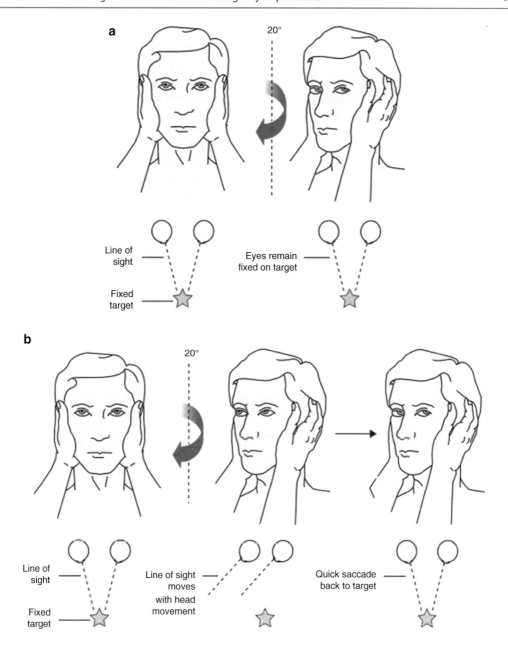

Fig. 3.2 The head thrust test. The head thrust test is a test of vestibular function that can be easily done during the bedside examination. This maneuver tests the vestibuloocular reflex (VOR). The patient sits in front of the examiner and the examiner holds the patient's head steady in the midline. The patient is instructed to maintain gaze on the nose of the examiner. The examiner then quickly turns the patient's head about 10–15 degrees to one side and observes the ability of the patient to keep the eyes locked on the examiner's nose. If the patient's eyes stay locked on the examiner's nose (i.e., no corrective saccade) (*picture* **a**), then the *peripheral vestibular system is assumed to be intact*. Thus, in a patient with acute dizzi- ness, this finding suggests a central nervous system local- ization. If, however, the patient's eyes move with the head (*picture* **b**) and then the patient makes a voluntary eye movement back to the examiner's nose (i.e., corrective saccade), then this *suggests a lesion of the peripheral vestibular system and not the central nervous system*. Thus when a patient presents with the acute vestibular syn- drome, the test result shown in *picture* **a** would suggest a central nervous system lesion, whereas the test result in *picture* **b** would suggest a peripheral vestibular lesion (thus, vestibular neuritis). (From: Edlow JA, et al. Lancet Neurology 2008; 7(10):951–964. Used with kind permis- sion of Elsevier)

Acute Severe Prolonged Vertigo

Vestibular neuritis is a common cause of acute severe prolonged vertigo [11]. It is an acute unilateral vestibulopathy that is presumed to be caused by a viral inflammation of the eighth cranial nerve—although a viral cause can not be specifically identified in individual patients other than those with the Ramsey–Hunt syndrome. Vertigo is accompanied by severe nausea, vomiting, and imbalance. Patients will often describe the need to hold onto objects when walking or may even need to crawl. Typically hearing is not affected, but if it is, then the virus likely involves both auditory and vestibular components, so-called labyrinthitis. As noted earlier, the hallmark examination signs of vestibular neuritis are a spontaneous unidirectional horizontal nystagmus and a positive head thrust test to the side opposite the fasting beating component of the nystagmus. Skew deviation is typically not present. The acronym HINTS (Head Impulse, Nystagmus, Test of Skew) has been used to remind clinicians of the exam components when localizing the lesion in acute dizziness presentations [37, 38]. The findings consistent with an acute unilateral vestibulopathy are unidirectional horizontal nystagmus, an abnormal head impulse test (e.g., corrective saccades) to the side opposite the fast phase of nystagmus, and the absence of a skew deviation.

Patients with vestibular neuritis are typically debilitated for the first day. Then, the natural history of the disorder is a gradual recovery over weeks to months. Vestibular physical therapy programs can help to speed the recovery [12]. In addition, the use of a burst and taper of oral corticosteroids might improve the recovery of the affected vestibular system as measured by the laboratory caloric response [13]. However, systematic reviews of corticosteroids in this condition conclude there is insufficient evidence from these trials to support the administration of corticosteroids to patients with idiopathic acute vestibular dysfunction [39].

In any patient who presents with acute severe vertigo, stroke diagnosis should be considered. Stroke is an obvious concern when the patient reports other focal neurological symptoms or has other focal neurological signs. Though the likelihood of stroke diagnosis drops substantially when the patient presents with isolated vertigo (i.e., no symptoms other than vertigo, nausea, and imbalance) [14], case reports now demonstrate just how closely stroke can mimic vestibular neuritis [15–17]. From epidemiological study designs, the risk of stroke etiology among patients presenting to the ED with dizziness symptoms is about 3% [14]. If the dizziness is an isolated symptom, then the risk of stroke etiology drops to less than 1% [14]. However, the population of this study was patients with any dizziness symptom presentation, not just the acute severe vertigo presentation. This distinction is important because the probability of stroke is higher for acute severe vertigo presentations compared to the other types of dizziness presentations. A recent prospective study in patients with acute severe dizziness with either nystagmus or imbalance found that about 11% (29/272) had a stroke on MRI [36]. Patients with stroke presenting with dizziness will typically have other focal central deficits on exam (e.g., speech changes, coordination problems), truncal ataxia, or central ocular motor findings (e.g., central patterns of nystagmus, normal head impulse test, or skew deviation) [36–38, 40].

Recurrent Spontaneous Attacks of Vertigo

Meniere's disease is the prototypical episodic otological disorder characterized by recurrent vertigo attacks (typically lasting hours). Overall, the prevalence of Meniere's disease in the general population is low [18]. In addition, Meniere's disease patients are probably less likely to present to the ED during acute attacks compared to those with the first ever acute severe vertigo attack. The reason may be that Meniere's disease attacks are typically limited to a couple of hours and patients learn over time that the attacks resolve with rest. To make the diagnosis of Meniere's disease requires the presence of a unilateral hearing loss which is typically a fluctuating symptom early in the course but then later becomes a fixed and progressive feature [41]. Other auditory symptoms are also common, including unilateral tinnitus (typically a low roaring sound rather than a high-pitched sound) or bothersome pressure in one ear. The examination in patients with Meniere's disease can be variable in the acute setting because nystagmus can be caused by either stimulation or inhibition of the affected side. But a central pattern of nystagmus (e.g., spontaneous downbeating nystagmus or bidirectional gaze-evoked nystagmus) would be a reason for a workup for a central disorder. Patients with Meniere's disease do not typically have a positive head thrust test.

Migraine is a common cause of recurrent attacks of vertigo (so-called migrainous vertigo) [42]. Attacks can last from minutes to hours and during attacks patients may exhibit features of both peripheral and central spontaneous and positional vertigo [19]. In between episodes, the exam is normal. The diagnosis rests on identifying other migraine symptoms (headache, aura, photophobia, phonophobia) with at least some attacks [20, 42], but if a patient has recurrent vertigo attacks without hearing loss over time, then the most likely diagnosis remains migraine even if other migraine symptoms are not reported.

Transient ischemic attacks should be considered when brief vertigo attacks (minutes) occur in a patient with vascular risk factors. Usually at least some attacks are accompanied by other neurological symptoms, and they may have a crescendo-like presentation. Sometimes patients who eventually suffer a posterior circulation stroke can have isolated transient vertigo episodes preceding the stroke [21]. As with stroke in general, auditory symptoms can accompany the vertigo symptoms if the anterior inferior cerebellar artery is involved.

Recurrent Positionally Triggered Attacks of Vertigo

BPPV is a very common cause of positionally triggered vertigo [22, 43]—The lifetime prevalence of BPPV is estimated to be about 10% [44]. BPPV can be cured at the bedside with a simple repositioning maneuver [23]. Thus, the ability to identify and treat BPPV is a major step not only for improving patient outcomes but also for reducing unnecessary tests. The key feature of the history is that the episodes are triggered by head movements, not simply worsened by head movements. It is important to know that dizziness of any cause can worsen after certain position changes. But for patients with BPPV, the vertigo attacks are *triggered* by position changes. The patient with constant vertigo who reports that the symptom is better in certain positions and worse with movement should be classified as having acute severe prolonged vertigo rather than recurrent positionally triggered vertigo. The history of the patient with BPPV is vertigo triggered by head tilts (reaching for something on a high shelf), rolling over in bed, or getting in/out of bed. The vertigo attacks last less than 1 min, typically followed by a return to the normal state. Some patients with BPPV report a constant milder dizziness before and even for a time period after treatment for unclear reasons [43].

BPPV is caused by calcium carbonate crystals which are free floating in a semicircular canal, typically the posterior canal. The debris breaks from the otolith membrane for reasons that are not clear. This can occur as the result of head trauma but typically occurs spontaneously (particularly with aging). When the particles enter the posterior canal, they can become trapped and move back and forth with position changes. Since the particles settle quickly after the movement, the symptoms and nystagmus last for only a brief period of time (<1 min). The particles can less commonly enter the horizontal canal and rarely even the anterior canal. The pattern of nystagmus is different depending on which canal is affected [24]. When the particles are in the posterior canal, a burst of upbeat and torsional nystagmus is seen after the patient is placed in the Dix–Hallpike position with the head turned toward the affected side (see Fig. 3.1) [6]. The nystagmus typically lasts only about 20–30 s. When the particles are in the horizontal canal, the nystagmus is horizontal and typically beats toward the ground after turning the head to either side while the patient is supine. The horizontal canal nystagmus lasts longer than the posterior canal nystagmus (as long as a minute) and can persist when the patient returns to the sitting position.

Central disorders can cause positional vertigo attacks, but the attacks typically have features that distinguish them from attacks in BPPV. A downbeating positional nystagmus is the most common pattern of nystagmus indicating a central localization—typically a midline cerebellar lesion. Downbeating positional nystagmus can be caused by the anterior canal variant of BPPV, but this variant is rare. Multiple sclerosis can also cause various types of positional nystagmus as can any other lesion involving central vestibular pathways in the brainstem or cerebellum. Importantly, central lesions do not cause the characteristic vertical torsional nystagmus pattern of posterior canal BPPV. However, central lesions—particularly lesions around the fourth ventricle—may cause a pattern of nystagmus similar to the pattern seen with horizontal canal BPPV [25]. Thus, a central lesion should be considered when a patient with the horizontal canal BPPV pattern of nystagmus has atypical features or is refractory to repositioning.

Other Dizziness Symptoms and Presentations

In the ED setting, the symptom of imbalance is associated with a higher odds of stroke diagnosis compared to the symptom of "dizziness" [14]. In stroke patients with imbalance, the lesion is typically in the midline or superior cerebellum and often the patient requires assistance to ambulate, if ambulation is possible at all [15, 26]. Since the lesions are often in the midline cerebellum, appendicular ataxia may be lacking. Some patients with dizziness in the emergency room will present with a chronic constant dizziness presentation rather than one of the three common presentation types described previously. If the neurological exam is normal in the patient with chronic dizziness, then the chance of a structural neurological disorder is very low. Migraine is the great mimicker of all causes of dizziness [19]. Symptoms in migraine can present as an acute severe attack, positional episodes, recurrent spontaneous attacks, or chronic constant symptoms. An accompanying headache occurs in less than 50% of the presentations, although a personal history of migraine headaches or a strong family history of migraine is common. Consensus diagnostic criteria require migraine symptoms with at least some attacks of vertigo [20, 27, 42]. Unfortunately, the diagnosis of migraine remains a diagnosis of exclusion. Thus, if the symptom is new in onset and does not fit the features of a specific peripheral vestibular disorder, then serious central causes should be considered. However, if the symptoms have been present for at least a couple of months and the neurological exam is nonfocal, then the chance of uncovering a causative structural lesion of the central nervous system is very low.

Panic disorder and anxiety disorder often have dizziness or even vertigo as a symptom. Common accompaniments of these psychiatric disorders are a sense of doom or fear, heart palpitations, shortness of breath, and nonfocal numbness and tingling.

General medical disorders can cause various types of dizziness presentations. Processes that result in transient drops in blood pressure are probably the most common general medical causes of dizziness. Medication side effects or metabolic derangements should also be considered in the differential diagnosis.

Management of Emergency Presentations

The goal in the emergency setting is to stabilize symptoms and identify treatable disorders or monitor those patients at risk for worsening. Proceeding through the above steps will help to identify the most likely causes and red flags. Simply classifying the presentation as a "peripheral" cause or "dizziness not otherwise specified," without proceeding through the above steps, probably leaves too much room for error [28]. BPPV is not only readily identifiable at the time of the clinical presentation, but the most common type (i.e., posterior canal BPPV) can be effectively treated with the Epley maneuver (see Fig. 3.1) [3, 6, 29]. BPPV is unique in clinical medicine because not only can an accurate assessment of the likelihood of the diagnosis be made, but also you can take this one step further and actually prove the diagnosis at the bedside by treating it in a matter of minutes. If the features are atypical for BPPV or the patient does not respond to repositioning maneuvers, then central disorders can be considered (see Table 3.1).

If the patient presents with acute severe dizziness, then the history, baseline vascular risk, and the examination are all important factors [36]. The patient with isolated dizziness has a very low probability of stroke particularly when also low for vascular risk [14]. The probability of stroke drops in patients with isolated dizziness who do not have a central pattern of nystagmus (e.g., the patient has either no nystagmus or the typical peripheral pattern of unidirectional horizontal spontaneous nystagmus) [15, 16, 36]. And the probability of stroke drops even further when the patient has isolated dizziness, low vascular risk, unidirectional horizontal spontaneous nystagmus, and a corresponding positive head thrust test [15, 16, 36].

If a patient presents with recurrent spontaneous episodes of vertigo, the chance of transient ischemic attack as the cause is low if the symptom lasts for hours, the attacks date back more than a couple of months, and prominent unilateral auditory features are reported. These features are highly suggestive of Meniere's disease. On the other hand, if the attacks are new in onset, brief in duration (minutes rather than hours), and not accompanied by prominent unilateral auditory features, then TIA should be a strong consideration.

Vestibular physical therapy is recommended for patients with acute vestibular neuritis [12, 45]. Regarding medication treatments in patients with vestibular neuritis, a Cochrane collaboration meta-analysis of a short course of corticosteroids concluded that there is insufficient

evidence to support their use in presumed vestibular neuritis [39]. Although some studies found improved recovery of the vestibular system measured by caloric testing in treated versus controls, other studies did not [39]. In three trials that measured dizziness disability with the Dizziness Handicap Index (DHI) as the outcome, there was no evidence of benefit to corticosteroids compared with placebo and the trends favored placebo [46–48]. When a short course of corticosteroids is considered, the clinician should also discuss the risks of possible adverse event including infections, blood clots, fractures, hyperglycemia, and hypertension.

Regardless of cause, symptoms can be managed with either oral or intravenous medications (Table 3.3). Few randomized controlled trials have been conducted on the symptomatic treatment of acute dizziness. In one study of 74 patients with acute dizziness, the average effect of 50 mg of intravenous dimenhydrinate was superior to that of 2 mg of intravenous lorazepam [30].

Antinausea medications (e.g., promethazine, prochlorperazine) can be considered when nausea and vomiting are prominent symptoms. One typically begins with less sedating medications. If the effect is not adequate, then more sedating medications are indicated. Patients should be instructed to only use these medicines during the acute phase because use beyond this period is more likely to cause bothersome side effects than any benefit.

Table 3.3 Medication options for symptomatic treatment of dizziness

Medication	Dosing
Less sedating	
Dimenhydrinate	50–100 mg PO/IV every 4–6 h
Meclizine	25–50 mg PO every 4–6 h
Scopolamine	0.4 mg PO every 8 h; 1.5 mg topical disc every 3 days
Diphenhydramine	25–50 mg PO/IV every 4–6 h
More sedating	
Prochlorperazine	10 mg PO every 4–6 h
Promethazine	25 mg PO or suppository every 4–6 h
Lorazepam	0.5–2 mg PO/IV every 6–8 h
Diazepam	2–10 mg PO every 6–8 h

Imaging Studies in Emergency Presentations

The use of neuroimaging studies in ED presentations of dizziness has risen dramatically. As noted earlier, in a population of "vertigo-dizziness" ED presentations, more than 25% of patients had a CT scan in 2004 compared with less than 10% of patients in 1995 [2]. In some subgroups, the percent evaluated with a CT scan was nearly 40% [2]. But the sensitivity of CT scans for identifying stroke in the acute setting is very low (26%) [31], meaning that a negative test does not change the probability of stroke diagnosis in a meaningful way. In addition, CT scans are associated with important downsides, including radiation exposure, increased cost, and increased time in the emergency room. MRI is a much more sensitive test, but can be challenging to obtain in the acute setting, takes more time, and has much greater expense. In addition, the sensitivity of MRI is lowest (thus can miss a stroke) when the test is performed within the first 24 h of symptom onset and when the lesion is small and in the brainstem or cerebellum [16, 31, 32]. The frequency of acute stroke was 11% (95% CI 7–15%; 29/272) in a prospective single center study of patient with acute dizziness and either nystagmus or imbalance (study used active surveillance and research MRIs) [36]. The probability of acute stroke on MRI dropped substantially (<1%; 1 of 109 participants) when vascular risk was low and central ocular motor or general central deficits (e.g., speech, coordination, truncal ataxia) were not present [36].

Conclusion

The evaluation of emergency department dizziness patients is facilitated by an organized approach. An accurate assessment of the most likely diagnosis can be made by categorizing the type of presentation and considering the examination findings. The optimal way to "rule out" a central disorder may be to "rule in" a specific peripheral vestibular disorder (i.e., vestibular neuritis, BPPV, or Meniere's disease). When the key clinical features fit with a specific peripheral vestibular disorder, then the likelihood of a serious central disorder is extremely low. When the presentation is not consistent with a specific peripheral vestibular disorder, then vascular risk factors and findings on the general neurologic assessment should be considered. Dizziness patients who have low vascular risk and no central deficits are unlikely to have an acute stroke as the cause. CT scans are not a valid discriminator of central versus peripheral vertigo presentations in the emergency department.

References (Original List)

1. Eagles D, Stiell IG, Clement CM, et al. International survey of emergency physicians' priorities for clinical decision rules. Acad Emerg Med. 2008;15:177–82.
2. Kerber KA, Meurer WJ, West BT, Fendrick AM. Dizziness presentations in U.S. emergency departments, 1995–2004. Acad Emerg Med. 2008;15:744–50.
3. Fife TD, Iverson DJ, Lempert T, et al. Practice parameter: therapies for benign paroxysmal positional vertigo (an evidence-based review): report of the Quality Standards Subcommittee of the American Academy of Neurology. Neurology. 2008;70:2067–74.
4. Newman-Toker DE, Cannon LM, Stofferahn ME, Rothman RE, Hsieh YH, Zee DS. Imprecision in patient reports of dizziness symptom quality: a cross-sectional study conducted in an acute care setting. Mayo Clin Proc. 2007;82:1329–40.
5. Newman-Toker DE, Dy FJ, Stanton VA, Zee DS, Calkins H, Robinson KA. How often is dizziness from primary cardiovascular disease true vertigo? A systematic review. J Gen Intern Med. 2008;23:2087–94.
6. American Academy of Neurology, online videos. http://www.neurology.org/cgi/content/full/70/22/2067/DC2.
7. Han BI, Oh HJ, Kim JS. Nystagmus while recumbent in horizontal canal benign paroxysmal positional vertigo. Neurology. 2006;66:706–10.
8. Halmagyi GM, Curthoys IS. A clinical sign of canal paresis. Arch Neurol. 1988;45:737–9.
9. Lewis RF, Carey JP. Images in clinical medicine. Abnormal eye movements associated with unilateral loss of vestibular function. N Engl J Med. 2006;355:e26.
10. Baloh RW, Honrubia V. Clinical neurophysiology of the vestibular system. 3rd ed. New York: Oxford University Press; 2001.
11. Baloh RW. Clinical practice. Vestibular neuritis. N Engl J Med. 2003;348:1027–32.
12. Strupp M, Arbusow V, Maag KP, Gall C, Brandt T. Vestibular exercises improve central vestibulospinal compensation after vestibular neuritis. Neurology. 1998;51:838–44.

13. Strupp M, Zingler VC, Arbusow V, et al. Methylprednisolone, valacyclovir, or the combination for vestibular neuritis. N Engl J Med. 2004;351:354–61.
14. Kerber KA, Brown DL, Lisabeth LD, Smith MA, Morgenstern LB. Stroke among patients with dizziness, vertigo, and imbalance in the emergency department: a population-based study. Stroke. 2006;37:2484–7.
15. Lee H, Sohn SI, Cho YW, et al. Cerebellar infarction presenting isolated vertigo: frequency and vascular topographical patterns. Neurology. 2006;67:1178–83.
16. Newman-Toker DE, Kattah JC, Alvernia JE, Wang DZ. Normal head impulse test differentiates acute cerebellar strokes from vestibular neuritis. Neurology. 2008;70:2378–85.
17. Cnyrim CD, Newman-Toker D, Karch C, Brandt T, Strupp M. Bedside differentiation of vestibular neuritis from central "vestibular pseudoneuritis". J Neurol Neurosurg Psychiatry. 2008;79:458–60.
18. Radtke A, von Brevern M, Feldmann M, et al. Screening for Meniere's disease in the general population—the needle in the haystack. Acta Otolaryngol. 2008;128:272–6.
19. von Brevern M, Zeise D, Neuhauser H, Clarke AH, Lempert T. Acute migrainous vertigo: clinical and oculographic findings. Brain. 2005;128:365–74.
20. Neuhauser HK, Lempert T. Diagnostic criteria for migrainous vertigo. Acta Otolaryngol. 2005;125:1247–8.
21. von Campe G, Regli F, Bogousslavsky J. Heralding manifestations of basilar artery occlusion with lethal or severe stroke. J Neurol Neurosurg Psychiatry. 2003;74:1621–6.
22. von Brevern M, Radtke A, Lezius F, et al. Epidemiology of benign paroxysmal positional vertigo: a population based study. J Neurol Neurosurg Psychiatry. 2007;78(7):710–5.
23. Epley JM. The canalith repositioning procedure: for treatment of benign paroxysmal positional vertigo. Otolaryngol Head Neck Surg. 1992;107:399–404.
24. Aw ST, Todd MJ, Aw GE, McGarvie LA, Halmagyi GM. Benign positional nystagmus: a study of its three-dimensional spatio-temporal characteristics. Neurology. 2005;64:1897–905.
25. Johkura K. Central paroxysmal positional vertigo: isolated dizziness caused by small cerebellar hemorrhage. Stroke. 2007;38:e26–e7.
26. Sohn SI, Lee H, Lee SR, Baloh RW. Cerebellar infarction in the territory of the medial branch of the superior cerebellar artery. Neurology. 2006;66:115–7.
27. Neuhauser HK, Radtke A, von Brevern M, et al. Migrainous vertigo: prevalence and impact on quality of life. Neurology. 2006;67:1028–33.
28. Savitz SI, Caplan LR, Edlow JA. Pitfalls in the diagnosis of cerebellar infarction. Acad Emerg Med. 2007;14:63–8.
29. Hilton M, Pinder D. The Epley (canalith repositioning) manoeuvre for benign paroxysmal positional vertigo. Cochrane Database Syst Rev. 2004;(12):CD003162.
30. Marill KA, Walsh MJ, Nelson BK. Intravenous Lorazepam versus dimenhydrinate for treatment of vertigo in the emergency department: a randomized clinical trial. Ann Emerg Med. 2000;36:310–9.
31. Chalela JA, Kidwell CS, Nentwich LM, et al. Magnetic resonance imaging and computed tomography in emergency assessment of patients with suspected acute stroke: a prospective comparison. Lancet. 2007;369:293–8.
32. Oppenheim C, Stanescu R, Dormont D, et al. False-negative diffusion-weighted MR findings in acute ischemic stroke. Am J Neuroradiol. 2000;21:1434–40.

Additional Reference List

33. Bhattacharyya N, Gubbels SP, Schwartz SR, et al. Clinical practice guideline: benign paroxysmal positional Vertigo (update). Otolaryngol Head Neck Surg. 2017;156:S1–S47.
34. Newman-Toker DE, Cannon LM, Stofferahn ME, Rothman RE, Hsieh YH, Zee DS. Imprecision in patient reports of dizziness symptom quality: a cross-sectional study conducted in an acute care setting. Mayo Clin Proc. 2007;82:1329–40.
35. Kerber KA, Callaghan BC, Telian SA, et al. Dizziness symptom type prevalence and overlap: a US Nationally Representative Survey. Am J Med. 2017;130(12):1465–e1.
36. Kerber KA, Meurer WJ, Brown DL, et al. Stroke risk stratification in acute dizziness presentations: a prospective imaging-based study. Neurology. 2015;85:1869–78.
37. Newman-Toker DE, Saber Tehrani AS, Mantokoudis G, et al. Quantitative video-oculography to help diagnose stroke in acute vertigo and dizziness: toward an ECG for the eyes. Stroke. 2013;44:1158–61.
38. Newman-Toker DE, Kerber KA, Hsich YH, et al. HINTS outperforms ABCD2 to screen for stroke in acute continuous vertigo and dizziness. Acad Emerg Med. 2013;20:986–96.
39. Fishman JM, Burgess C, Waddell A. Corticosteroids for the treatment of idiopathic acute vestibular dysfunction (vestibular neuritis). Cochrane Database Syst Rev. 2011;5:CD008607.
40. Carmona S, Martinez C, Zalazar G, et al. The diagnostic accuracy of truncal Ataxia and HINTS as cardinal signs for acute vestibular syndrome. Front Neurol. 2016;7:125.
41. Basura GJ, Adams ME, Monfared A, et al. Clinical practice guideline: Meniere's disease. Otolaryngol Head Neck Surg. 2020;162:S1–S55.
42. Lempert T, Olesen J, Furman J, et al. Vestibular migraine: diagnostic criteria. J Vestib Res. 2012;22:167–72.
43. von Brevern M, Bertholon P, Brandt T, et al. Benign paroxysmal positional vertigo: Diagnostic criteria. J Vestib Res. 2015;25:105–17.

44. von Brevern M, Radtke A, Lezius F, et al. Epidemiology of benign paroxysmal positional vertigo: a population based study. J Neurol Neurosurg Psychiatry. 2007;78:710–5.

45. Hillier SL, Hollohan V. Vestibular rehabilitation for unilateral peripheral vestibular dysfunction. Cochrane Database Syst Rev. 2007;1:CD005397.

46. Goudakos JK, Markou KD, Psillas G, Vital V, Tsaligopoulos M. Corticosteroids and vestibular exercises in vestibular neuritis. Single-blind randomized clinical trial. JAMA Otolaryngol Head Neck Surg. 2014;140:434–40.

47. Ismail EI, Morgan AE, Abdel Rahman AM. Corticosteroids versus vestibular rehabilitation in long-term outcomes in vestibular neuritis. J Vestib Res. 2018;28:417–24.

48. Shupak A, Issa A, Golz A, Margalit K, Braverman I. Prednisone treatment for vestibular neuritis. Otol Neurotol. 2008;29:368–74.

Syncope

4

Mark D. Carlson

Syncope is defined as transient loss of consciousness due to reduced cerebral blood flow associated with postural collapse and rapid spontaneous recovery. It may occur suddenly, without warning, or be preceded by faintness ("presyncope"). Symptoms and signs that precede syncope may include pallor, diaphoresis, a feeling of warmth, nausea, persistent and often progressive generalized weakness, fatigue, cognitive slowing, leg buckling, visual blurring occasionally proceeding to blindness, and the "coat hanger" headache (a triangular headache at the base of the neck due to trapezius ischemia). These may vary in duration and increase in severity until loss of consciousness occurs or may resolve prior to loss of consciousness if the cerebral ischemia is corrected. It is important, but sometimes challenging, to differentiate syncope from seizure. Syncope may be benign when it occurs as the result of normal cardiovascular reflex effects on heart rate and vascular tone and is preceded by symptoms that enable the individual to take actions that prevent injury or serious when it occurs abruptly or is due to a life-threatening arrhythmia. Syncope may occur as a single event or may be recurrent. Studies report syncope prevalence to be as high as 41% and recurrent syncope to be 13.5%. The incidence follows a trimodal distribution, with first episodes common around ages 20, 60, or 80 years and the third peak occurring 5–7 years earlier in males. Recurrent, unexplained syncope, particularly in an individual with structural heart disease, is associated with a high risk of death (40% mortality within 2 years).

Causes

Transiently decreased cerebral blood flow is usually due to one of three general mechanisms: (1) disorders of vascular tone or blood volume, (2) cardiovascular disorders including cardiac arrhythmias, or (3) cerebrovascular disease. Often, the cause of syncope is multifactorial.

Disorders of Vascular Tone or Blood Volume

Disorders of autonomic control of the heart and circulation share common pathophysiologic mechanisms: a cardioinhibitory component (e.g., bradycardia due to increased vagal activity), a vasodepressor component (e.g., inappropriate vasodilatation due to sympathetic withdrawal), or both.

4

4

M. D. Carlson (✉)
Department of Medicine, Case Western Reserve
University School of Medicine, Cleveland, OH, USA

Neurocardiogenic (Vasovagal and Vasodepressor) Syncope

The term *neurocardiogenic* encompasses both vasovagal and vasodepressor forms of syncope. Vasovagal syncope is associated with both sympathetic withdrawal (vasodilatation) and increased parasympathetic activity (bradycardia), whereas vasodepressor syncope is associated with sympathetic withdrawal alone. These types of syncope account for about one-half of syncopal episodes including the common faint that may occur in the absence of disease. Neurocardiogenic syncope is frequently recurrent and is commonly precipitated by a hot or crowded environment, extreme fatigue, severe pain, hunger, alcohol ingestion, prolonged standing, and an emotional or stressful event. The syndrome usually occurs when individuals are in the standing position and rarely occurs when supine. Although often preceded by weakness, nausea, diaphoresis, light-headedness, or blurred vision, in some individuals, syncope may occur abruptly, without warning.

The unconscious patient usually lies motionless with skeletal muscles relaxed, but clonic jerks of the limbs and face may occur. In contrast to a seizure, individuals rarely lose sphincter control. The pulse and blood pressure may be undetectable, and breathing is almost imperceptible. The duration of unconsciousness is rarely longer than a few minutes if the conditions that provoked the episode are reversed. When placed supine, most individuals recover rapidly. Although commonly benign, neurocardiogenic syncope can be associated with prolonged asystole and hypotension, resulting in injury.

In the setting of increased peripheral sympathetic activity and venous pooling, vigorous myocardial contraction of a relatively empty left ventricle activates myocardial mechanoreceptors and vagal afferent nerve fibers that inhibit sympathetic activity and increase parasympathetic activity. The resultant vasodilatation and bradycardia induce hypotension and syncope. Although most investigators have credited the drop in systemic vascular resistance and subsequent vasodilation as the primary cause of vasodepressor syncope, recent articles have focused attention on decreased cardiac output (up to 50%) during presyncope as an important contributor to the syndrome.

Indeed, although the reflexes described above are generally thought to be responsible for neurocardiogenic syncope, other reflexes may also be operative. Patients with transplanted (denervated) hearts have experienced cardiovascular responses identical to those present during neurocardiogenic syncope, which, unless the heart has become reinnervated, should not be possible if the response depends solely on the reflex mechanisms described above. Moreover, neurocardiogenic syncope often occurs in response to stimuli (fear, emotional stress, or pain) that may not be associated with venous pooling in the lower extremities, which suggests a cortical component to the reflex. Thus, a variety of afferent and efferent responses may cause neurocardiogenic syncope. The central nervous system (CNS) mechanisms responsible for neurocardiogenic syncope are uncertain, but a sudden surge in central serotonin levels may contribute to the sympathetic withdrawal. Endogenous opiates (endorphins) and adenosine are also putative participants in the pathogenesis.

Syncope with Normal Heart and ECG and Without Prodrome

Syncope without or with a short prodrome (<5 s) in an individual with a normal heart and electrocardiogram is a recently described phenomenon that is to be differentiated from the typical neurocardiogenic syncope described above. These individuals often present with abrupt asystole due to atrioventricular block, and their plasma adenosine levels are lower than the affinity constant for high – affinity A1 adenosine receptors (<0.7 microM). Theoretically, the A1 adenosine receptors in the sinus and atrioventricular nodes are upregulated which renders them to be very susceptible to cause atrioventricular block or sinus arrest in the setting of even a modest increase in adenosine plasma levels.

Postural (Orthostatic) Hypotension

This occurs in patients who have chronic or episodic instability of vasomotor reflexes. Systemic arterial blood pressure falls on assumption of upright posture due to loss of vasoconstriction reflexes in lower extremity resistance and capacitance vessels. Although the episode differs little from vasodepressor syncope, the effect of posture is critical. Sudden rising from a recumbent position or standing quickly may precipitate episodes. *Orthostatic hypotension may be the cause in up to 30% of elderly individuals who experience syncope; antihypertensive or antidepressant drugs often contribute to syncope in these patients.* Postural syncope may occur in otherwise normal persons with defective postural reflexes. Patients with *idiopathic postural hypotension* may be identified by a characteristic response to upright tilt. Initially, the blood pressure diminishes slightly before stabilizing at a lower level. Thereafter, compensatory reflexes fail and arterial pressure falls precipitously. Orthostatic hypotension, often accompanied by disturbances in sweating, impotence, and sphincter difficulties, also occurs in patients with autonomic nervous system disorders. The most common causes of neurogenic orthostatic hypotension are chronic diseases of the peripheral nervous system that involve postganglionic unmyelinated fibers (e.g., diabetic, nutritional, and amyloid polyneuropathy). Much less common are the multiple system atrophies; CNS disorders in which orthostatic hypotension is associated with (1) parkinsonism but the autonomic dysfunction predominates (Shy–Drager syndrome), (2) olivopontocerebellar atrophy when progressive cerebellar degeneration is a predominant feature, or (3) striatonigral degeneration when parkinsonian features, such as bradykinesia and rigidity, predominate. A rare, acute postganglionic dysautonomia may represent a variant of Guillain–Barre' syndrome. There are several additional causes of postural syncope: (1) after physical deconditioning (such as after prolonged illness with recumbency, particularly in elderly individuals with reduced muscle tone) or after prolonged weightlessness, as in space flight;

(2) after sympathectomy that has abolished vasopressor reflexes; and (3) in patients receiving antihypertensive or vasodilator drugs and those who are hypovolemic because of diuretics, excessive sweating, diarrhea, vomiting, hemorrhage, or adrenal insufficiency.

Carotid Sinus Hypersensitivity

Syncope due to carotid sinus hypersensitivity is precipitated by pressure on the carotid sinus baroreceptors, located just cephalad to the bifurcation of the common carotid artery. Carotid sinus hypersensitivity occurs predominantly in men over 50 years old, typically in the setting of shaving, a tight collar, or turning the head to one side. Activation of carotid sinus baroreceptors gives rise to impulses carried via the nerve of Hering, a branch of the glossopharyngeal nerve, to the medulla oblongata. These afferent impulses activate efferent sympathetic nerve fibers to the heart and blood vessels, cardiac vagal efferent nerve fibers, or both. In patients with carotid sinus hypersensitivity, these responses may cause sinus arrest or atrioventricular (AV) block (a cardioinhibitory response), vasodilatation (a vasodepressor response), or both (a mixed response). The mechanisms responsible for the syndrome are not clear and validated diagnostic criteria do not exist.

Situational Syncope

A variety of activities, including cough, deglutition, micturition, and defecation, are associated with syncope in susceptible individuals. These syndromes are caused, at least in part, by abnormal autonomic control and may involve a cardioinhibitory response, a vasodepressor response, or both. Cough, micturition, and defecation are associated with maneuvers (such as Valsalva and straining) that increase intrathoracic pressure and increase intracranial pressure both of which can contribute to decreased cerebral blood flow. Cough syncope typically occurs during or immediately after prolonged coughing fits in men with chronic bronchitis or chronic obstructive lung disease. Micturition syncope occurs predominantly in middle-aged and older men, particularly those with prostatic hypertrophy and obstruction of the bladder neck; loss of consciousness usually occurs at night during or immediately after voiding. Deglutition syncope and defecation syncope occur in men and women. Deglutition syncope may be associated with esophageal disorders, particularly esophageal spasm. In some individuals, particular foods and carbonated or cold beverages initiate episodes by activating esophageal sensory receptors that trigger reflex sinus bradycardia or AV block. Defecation syncope may occur secondary to a Valsalva maneuver in older individuals with constipation.

Glossopharyngeal Neuralgia

Syncope due to glossopharyngeal neuralgia is preceded by pain in the oropharynx, tonsillar fossa, or tongue. Loss of consciousness is usually associated with asystole rather than vasodilatation. The mechanism is thought to involve activation of afferent impulses in the glossopharyngeal nerve that terminate in the nucleus solitarius of the medulla, and via collaterals that activate the dorsal motor nucleus of the vagus nerve.

Cardiovascular Disorders

Cardiac syncope results from a sudden reduction in cardiac output, caused most commonly by a cardiac arrhythmia but also by structural abnormalities that obstruct blood flow.

Arrhythmias

In healthy individuals, heart rates between 30 and 180 beats/min do not reduce cerebral blood flow, especially when the person is supine. As the heart rate decreases, ventricular filling time and stroke volume increase to maintain normal cardiac output. At rates less than 30 beats/min, stroke volume can no longer increase to compensate

adequately for the decreased heart rate. At rates greater than 180 beats/min, ventricular filling time is often insufficient to maintain adequate stroke volume. Upright posture; cerebrovascular disease; anemia; loss of atrioventricular synchrony; and coronary, myocardial, or valvular disease, all reduce the tolerance to alterations in rate. Bradyarrhythmias may occur as a result of an abnormality of impulse generation (e.g., sinoatrial arrest) or impulse conduction (e.g., AV block). Either may cause syncope if the escape pacemaker rate is insufficient to maintain cardiac output. Syncope due to bradyarrhythmias may occur abruptly, without preceding symptoms, and recur several times daily. Patients with *sick sinus syndrome* may have sinus pauses (>3 s), and those with syncope due to high degree AV block (*Stokes–Adams–Morgagni syndrome*) may have evidence of conduction system disease (e.g., prolonged PR interval, bundle branch block). However, the arrhythmia is often transitory, and the surface electrocardiogram or the continuous electrocardiographic monitor placed later may not reveal the abnormality. The *bradycardia-tachycardia syndrome* is a common form of sinus node dysfunction in which syncope generally occurs as a result of marked sinus pauses, some following termination of an atrial tachyarrhythmia. Drugs are a common cause for bradyarrhythmias, particularly in patients with underlying structural heart disease. Digoxin, adrenergic receptor antagonists, calcium channel blockers, and many antiarrhythmic drugs may suppress sinoatrial node impulse generation or slow AV nodal conduction.

Syncope due to a *tachyarrhythmia* is often preceded by palpitation or light-headedness but may occur abruptly without warning. *Supraventricular tachyarrhythmias* are unlikely to cause syncope in individuals with structurally normal hearts but may do so if they occur in patients with (1) heart disease that also compromises cardiac output, (2) cerebrovascular disease, (3) a disorder of vascular tone or blood volume, or (4) a very rapid ventricular rate. These tachycardias result most commonly from paroxysmal atrial flutter, atrial fibrillation, or reentry involving the AV node or accessory pathways that bypass part or all of the AV conduction system. Patients with the *Wolff–Parkinson–White syndrome* may experience syncope when a very rapid ventricular rate occurs due to reentry across an accessory AV connection. In patients with structural heart disease, ventricular tachycardia is a common cause of syncope, particularly in patients with a prior myocardial infarction. Patients with aortic valvular stenosis and hypertrophic obstructive cardiomyopathy are also at risk for ventricular tachycardia. Individuals with abnormalities of ventricular repolarization (prolongation of the QT interval) are at risk to develop polymorphic ventricular tachycardia (*torsades de pointes*). Those with the inherited form of this syndrome often have a family history of sudden death in young individuals. Genetic markers can identify some patients with familial long QT syndrome, but the clinical utility of these markers remains unproven. Drugs (i.e., certain antiarrhythmics and erythromycin) and electrolyte disorders (i.e., hypokalemia, hypocalcemia, hypomagnesemia) can prolong the QT interval and predispose to torsades de pointes. Antiarrhythmic medications may precipitate ventricular tachycardia, particularly in patients with structural heart disease.

Structural Disorders

In addition to arrhythmias, syncope may also occur with a variety of structural cardiovascular disorders. Episodes are usually precipitated when the cardiac output cannot increase to compensate adequately for peripheral vasodilatation. Peripheral vasodilatation may be appropriate, such as following exercise, or may occur due to inappropriate activation of left ventricular mechanoreceptor reflexes, as occurs in aortic outflow tract obstruction (aortic valvular stenosis or hypertrophic obstructive cardiomyopathy). Obstruction to forward flow is the most common reason that cardiac output cannot increase. Syncope occurs in up to 10% of patients with massive pulmonary embolism and may occur with exertion in patients with severe primary pulmonary hypertension. The cause is an inability of the right ventricle to provide appropriate cardiac output in the presence of obstruction or increased pulmonary vascular resistance. Loss of consciousness is usually accompanied by other symptoms such as chest pain and dyspnea. Atrial myxoma, a prosthetic valve thrombus, and, rarely, mitral stenosis may impair left ventricular filling, decrease cardiac output, and cause syncope. Pericardial tamponade is a rare cause of syncope.

Cerebrovascular Disease

Cerebrovascular disease alone rarely causes syncope but may lower the threshold for syncope in a patient with another cause. In such cases, the vertebrobasilar arteries, which supply brainstem structures responsible for maintaining consciousness, are usually involved. An exception is the unusual patient with tight bilateral carotid stenoses and recurrent syncope, often precipitated by standing or walking. Most patients who experience light-headedness or syncope due to cerebrovascular disease also have symptoms of focal neurologic ischemia, such as arm or leg weakness, diplopia, ataxia, dysarthria, or sensory disturbances. Basilar artery migraine is a rare disorder that can cause syncope in adolescents.

Differential Diagnosis

Anxiety Attacks and the Hyperventilation Syndrome

Anxiety, such as occurs in panic attacks, is frequently interpreted as a feeling of faintness or dizziness resembling presyncope. The symptoms are not accompanied by facial pallor and are not relieved by assuming a recumbent position. The diagnosis is made on the basis of the associated symptoms, such as a feeling of impending doom, air hunger, palpitations, and tingling of the fingers and perioral region. Attacks can often be reproduced by hyperventilation, resulting in hypocapnia, alkalosis, increased cerebrovascular resistance, and decreased cerebral blood flow.

The release of epinephrine also contributes to the symptoms.

Seizures

Unlike syncope, a seizure may be heralded by an aura, which is caused by a focal epileptogenic discharge and hence has localizing significance. The aura is usually followed by a rapid return to normal or by a loss of consciousness. Injury from falling is frequent in a seizure and rare in syncope, since only in generalized seizures are protective reflexes abolished instantaneously. Sustained tonic-clonic movements are characteristic of convulsive seizures but brief clonic, or tonic-clonic, seizure-like activity can accompany fainting episodes. The period of unconsciousness tends to be longer in seizures than in syncope. Urinary incontinence is frequent in seizures and rare in syncope. The return of consciousness is prompt in syncope, slow after a seizure. Mental confusion, headache, and drowsiness are common sequelae of seizures, whereas physical weakness with a clear sensorium characterizes the postsyncopal state. Repeated spells of unconsciousness in a young person at a rate of several per day or month suggest epilepsy rather than syncope.

Hypoglycemia

Severe hypoglycemia is usually due to a serious disease such as a tumor of the islets of Langerhans; due to advanced adrenal, pituitary, or hepatic disease; or to excessive administration of insulin.

Acute Hemorrhage

Hemorrhage, usually within the gastrointestinal tract, is an occasional cause of syncope. In the absence of pain and hematemesis, the cause of the weakness, faintness, or even unconsciousness may remain obscure until the passage of a black stool.

Hysterical Fainting

The attack is usually unattended by an outward display of anxiety. Lack of change in pulse and blood pressure or color of the skin and mucous membranes distinguishes it from the vasodepressor faint.

Approach to the Patient

The diagnosis of syncope is often challenging. The cause may only be apparent at the time of the event, leaving few, if any, clues when the patient is seen later by the physician. The physician should think first of those causes that constitute a therapeutic emergency. Among these are massive internal hemorrhage or myocardial infarction, which may be painless, and cardiac arrhythmias. In elderly persons, a sudden faint, without obvious cause, should arouse the suspicion of complete heart block or a tachyarrhythmia, even though all findings are negative when the patient is seen. Figure 4.1 depicts an algorithmic approach to syncope. A careful history is the most important diagnostic tool, both to suggest the correct cause and to exclude important potential causes. The nature of the events and their time course prior to, during, and after an episode of syncope often provide valuable etiologic clues. Loss of consciousness in particular situations, such as during venipuncture, micturition, or with volume depletion, suggests an abnormality of vascular tone. The position of the patient at the time of the syncopal episode is important; syncope in the supine position is unlikely to be vasovagal and suggests an arrhythmia or a seizure. Syncope due to carotid sinus syndrome may occur when the individual is wearing a shirt with a tight collar, turning the head (turning to look while driving in reverse), or manipulating the neck (as in shaving). The patient's medications must be noted, including nonprescription drugs or health store supplements, with particular attention to recent changes. Heart rate and blood pressure should be evaluated in the supine, sitting, and standing positions. In patients with

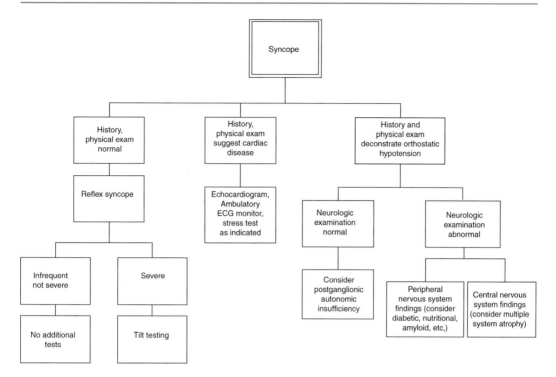

Fig. 4.1 Approach to diagnosing the cause of syncope

unexplained recurrent syncope, an attempt to reproduce an attack may assist in diagnosis.

Anxiety attacks induced by hyperventilation can be reproduced readily by having the patient breathe rapidly and deeply for 2–3 min. Cough syncope may be reproduced by inducing the Valsalva maneuver. Carotid sinus massage should generally be avoided, even in patients with suspected carotid sinus hypersensitivity; it can cause a transient ischemic attack (TIA) or stroke in individuals with carotid atheromas.

Diagnostic Tests

The history and physical examination guide the choice of diagnostic tests. Although unlikely to provide a definitive diagnosis, a surface 12-lead electrocardiogram may provide clues to the cause of syncope *and should be performed in almost all patients.* The presence of conduction abnormalities (PR prolongation and bundle branch block) suggests a bradyarrhythmia, whereas pathologic Q waves or prolongation of the QT interval sug-

gests a ventricular tachyarrhythmia. The approach to heart rhythm monitoring depends on the frequency of the episodes, the likelihood of an arrhythmic cause, and the patient's risk for morbidity or mortality. Inpatients should undergo continuous electrocardiographic monitoring; outpatient monitoring may depend on the frequency of episodes. Holter monitors, which record continuously for 24–48 h, may be useful for patients with frequent episodes. Newer external monitors are able to monitor surface ECG leads for several weeks. In patients with infrequent episodes that are suspected to be due to an arrhythmia, an implantable cardiac monitor, which monitors the heart rhythm continuously for up to 3 years, is useful and cost-effective. Regardless of the monitor type, symptoms should be correlated with the occurrence of arrhythmias. Cardiac event monitors may be useful in patients with infrequent symptoms, particularly in patients with presyncope.

Measurements of serum electrolytes, glucose, and the hematocrit are usually indicated, and cardiac enzymes should be evaluated if myocardial ischemia is suspected. Blood and urine toxicology screens may reveal the presence of alcohol or other drugs. In patients with possible adrenocortical insufficiency, plasma aldosterone and mineralocorticoid levels should be obtained.

Invasive cardiac electrophysiologic testing provides diagnostic and prognostic information regarding sinus node function, AV conduction, and supraventricular and ventricular arrhythmias. Continuous electrocardiographic monitoring is usually more effective for diagnosing sinus node disease. However, invasive electrophysiologic testing is useful for detecting His–Purkinje disease, and in patients who have experienced a myocardial infarction, ventricular arrhythmias may be responsible for syncope.

Upright tilt table testing is indicated for recurrent syncope or a single syncopal episode that caused or could cause injury were it to recur, particularly if the patient is likely to be in a "high-risk" setting (pilot, commercial vehicle driver, etc.). In susceptible patients, upright tilt at an angle between 60° and 80° for 30–60 min induces a vasovagal episode particularly when accompanied with administration of drugs that cause venous pooling or increase adrenergic stimulation (isoproterenol, nitroglycerin, edrophonium, or adenosine). The sensitivity and specificity of tilt table testing are difficult to ascertain because of the lack of validated criteria. Moreover, the reflexes responsible for vasovagal syncope can be elicited in most, if not all, individuals given the necessary stimulus. The reported accuracy of the test ranges from 30% to 80%, depending on the population studied and the techniques used. Whereas the reproducibility of a negative test is 85–100%, the reproducibility of a positive tilt table test is only between 62% and 88%. Importantly, all three recent international guideline and consensus documents recommend that tilt testing be performed only in patients for whom a history, and therefore prodromal symptoms, did not provide a diagnosis.

A variety of other tests may be useful to determine the presence of structural heart disease that may cause syncope. The echocardiogram with Doppler examination detects valvular, myocardial, and pericardial abnormalities. The echocardiogram is the "gold standard" for the diagnosis of hypertrophic cardiomyopathy and atrial myxoma. Cardiac cine magnetic resonance (MR) imaging provides an alternative noninvasive modality that may be useful for patients in whom diagnostic-quality echocardiographic images cannot be obtained. This test is also indicated for patients suspected of having arrhythmogenic right ventricular dysplasia or right ventricular outflow tract ventricular tachycardia. Both are associated with right ventricular structural abnormalities that are better visualized on MR imaging than by echocardiogram. Exercise testing may detect ischemia or exercise-induced arrhythmias. In some patients, cardiac catheterization may be necessary to diagnose the presence or severity of coronary artery disease or valvular abnormalities. Ultrafast computed tomographic scan, ventilation–perfusion scan, or pulmonary angiography is indicated in patients in whom syncope may be due to pulmonary embolus.

In cases of possible cerebrovascular syncope, neuroimaging tests may be indicated, including Doppler ultrasound studies of the carotid and vertebrobasilar systems, MR imaging, MR angiography, and CT angiography of the cerebral vasculature. Electroencephalography is indicated if seizures are suspected.

Decision support algorithms and specialized syncope evaluation units have been used and advocated by some to reduce health service use. However, currently the data are insufficient to demonstrate their efficacy in making patient disposition decisions or that they are financially feasible.

Treatment

The treatment of syncope depends on the underlying cause. With respect to the disorders of autonomic control, certain precautions should be taken regardless of the specific cause of syncope. Patients with frequent episodes, or those who have experienced syncope without warning symptoms, should avoid situations in which sudden loss of consciousness might result in injury (e.g., climbing ladders, swimming alone, operating heavy machinery, driving, etc.). At the onset of symptoms, patients should take steps to avoid injury should they lose consciousness, lowering their head and preferably lying down. Lowering the head by bending at the waist should be avoided because it may further compromise venous return to the heart. Family members or other close contacts should be informed of the problem in order to ensure appropriate therapy and prevent delivery of inappropriate therapy (chest compressions associated with cardiopulmonary resuscitation) that may inflict trauma. Patients who have lost consciousness should be placed in a position that maximizes cerebral blood flow, offers protection from trauma, and secures the airway. Whenever possible, the patient should be placed supine with the head turned to the side to prevent aspiration and the tongue from blocking the airway. Assessment of the pulse and direct cardiac auscultation may assist in determining if the episode is associated with a bradyarrhythmia or tachyarrhythmia. Clothing that fits tightly around the neck or waist should be loosened. Patients should not be given anything by mouth or be permitted to rise until full consciousness has returned.

Patients with vasovagal syncope should be instructed to avoid situations or stimuli that have caused them to lose consciousness and to assume a recumbent position when premonitory symptoms occur. This alone may be sufficient therapy for patients with infrequent and relatively benign episodes of vasovagal syncope, particularly when episodes occur in response to a specific stimulus. Tilt training (standing and leaning against a wall for progressively longer periods each day) has been used with limited success, particularly for those patients who have profound orthostatic intolerance. Episodes associated with intravascular volume depletion may be prevented by salt and fluid loading prior to provocative events.

Prescription drug therapy may be necessary when vasovagal syncope is resistant to these measures, when episodes occur frequently, or when syncope is associated with a significant risk for injury. Adrenergic receptor antagonists (metoprolol, 25–50 mg bid; atenolol, 25–50 mg qd; or nadolol, 10–20 mg bid; all starting doses), the most widely used agents, mitigate the increase in myocardial contractility that stimulates left ventricular mechanoreceptors and also block central serotonin receptors. Serotonin reuptake inhibitors (paroxetine, 20–40 mg qd; or sertraline, 25–50 mg qd) appear to be effective for some patients. A recent meta-analysis indicated that norepinephrine transport inhibitors (sibutramine, reboxetine, and atomoxetine) prevents vasovagal reactions and syncope during head-up tilt testing and is promising for treatment of recurrent syncope. Bupropion SR (150 mg qd), another antidepressant, has also been used with success. Adrenergic receptor antagonists and serotonin reuptake inhibitors are well tolerated and are often used as first-line agents for younger patients. Hydrofludrocortisone (0.1–0.2 mg qd), a mineralocorticoid, promotes sodium retention, volume expansion, and peripheral vasoconstriction by increasing receptor sensitivity to endogenous catecholamines. Hydrofludrocortisone is useful for patients with intravascular volume depletion and those who also have postural hypotension. Proamatine, an alpha agonist, has been used as a first-line agent for some patients. In a randomized controlled trial, proamatine was more effective than placebo in preventing syncope during an upright tilt test. However, in some patients, proamatine and hydrofludrocortisone may increase resting supine systemic blood pressure, a property that may be problematic for those with hypertension.

Disopyramide (150 mg bid), a vagolytic antiarrhythmic drug with negative inotropic properties, and another vagolytic, transdermal scopolamine, have been used to treat vasovagal syncope, as have theophylline and ephedrine. Side effects associated with these drugs have limited their use for this indication. Disopyramide is a type 1A antiarrhythmic drug and should be used with great caution, if at all, in patients who are at risk for ventricular arrhythmias. Although several clinical trials have suggested that pharmacologic therapy for vasovagal syncope is effective, long-term prospective randomized controlled trials have yet to be completed.

Permanent dual-chamber cardiac pacing can be effective for patients with frequent episodes of vasovagal syncope and is indicated for those with prolonged asystole associated with vasovagal episodes. Patients in whom vasodilatation contributes to loss of consciousness may also experience symptomatic benefit from permanent pacing. Pacemakers that can be programmed to transiently pace at a high rate (90–100 beats/min) after a profound drop in the patient's intrinsic heart rate are most effective. Patients with orthostatic hypotension should be instructed to rise slowly and systematically (supine to seated, seated to standing) from the bed or a chair. Movement of the legs prior to rising facilitates venous return from the lower extremities. Whenever possible, medications that aggravate the problem (vasodilators, diuretics, etc.) should be discontinued. Elevation of the head of the bed [20–30 cm (8–12 in)] and use of compression stockings may help. Additional therapeutic modalities include an antigravity or g suit or compression stockings to prevent lower limb blood pooling, salt loading, and a variety of pharmacologic agents including sympathomimetic amines, monoamine oxidase inhibitors, beta blockers, and levodopa.

Glossopharyngeal neuralgia is treated with carbamazepine, which is effective for the syncope as well as for the pain. Patients with carotid sinus syndrome should be instructed to avoid clothing and situations that stimulate carotid sinus baroreceptors. When looking to the side, they should turn their entire body, rather than just their head. Those with intractable syncope due to the cardioinhibitory response to carotid sinus stimulation should undergo permanent pacemaker implantation.

Treatment of the cardiovascular causes of syncope (arrhythmias and structural disorders) is often focused on the underlying cause (myocardial ischemia, valvular disease, etc.). Patients with bradyarrhythmias may benefit from permanent pacing. Those with certain supraventricular arrhythmias may benefit from catheter ablation. An implantable cardioverter defibrillator is indicated for patients with or at high risk for life-threatening ventricular arrhythmias. Surgical replacement is indicated for patients with critical aortic valvular stenosis.

Regardless of the etiology, patients with syncope should be hospitalized with continuous electrocardiographic monitoring when the episode may have resulted from a life-threatening abnormality or if recurrence with significant injury seems likely. Patients who are known to have a normal heart and for whom the history strongly suggests vasovagal or situational syncope may be treated as outpatients if the episodes are neither frequent nor severe.

Further Reading

Brignole M. Mechanism of syncope without prodromes with normal heart and normal electrocardiogram. Heart Rhythm. 2017;14:234–9.

Lei LY. Pharmacological norepinephrine transporter inhibition for the prevention of vasovagal syncope in young and adult subjects. A systematic review and meta-analysis. Heart Rhythm. 2020;17:1151–8.

Shen WK. 2017 ACC/AHA/HRS guideline for the evaluation and management of patients with syncope. Heart Rhythm. 2017;14:e155–217.

Sutton R. Pacing in vasovagal syncope: physiology, pacemaker sensors, and recent clinical trials – precise patient selection and measurable benefit. Heart Rhythm. 2020;17:821–8.

Wieling W. Cardiac output and vasodilation in the vasovagal response: an analysis of the classic papers. Heart Rhythm. 2016;13:798–805.

Acute Visual Loss

5

Jane H. Lock, Cédric Lamirel, Nancy J. Newman, and Valérie Biousse

Introduction

Acute visual changes often precipitate emergency consultation. Although ocular causes are usually identified by eye care specialists, many patients appear in the emergency department or a neurologist's office when the ocular examination is normal or when it suggests a neurologic disorder. Indeed, many causes of monocular or binocular acute visual loss may reveal or precede a neurologic process. In this situation, a quick and simple clinical examination in the emergency department allows the neurologist to localize the lesion and determine whether urgent neurologic workup or further ophthalmologic consultation is necessary [1, 2].

The original version of this chapter was revised. A correction to this chapter can be found at https://doi.org/10.1007/978-3-030-75778-6_19

J. H. Lock
Neuro-Ophthalmology Unit, Emory University School of Medicine, Atlanta, GA, USA

Department of Ophthalmology, Royal Perth Hospital, Perth, WA, Australia

Department of Ophthalmology, Sir Charles Gairdner Hospital, Nedlands, WA, Australia
e-mail: jane.lock@health.wa.gov.au

C. Lamirel
Service d'ophtalmologie, Fondation Ophtalmologique Adolphe Rothschild, Paris, France
e-mail: clamirel@fo-rothschild.fr

N. J. Newman · V. Biousse (✉)
Neuro-Ophthalmology Unit, Emory University School of Medicine, Atlanta, GA, USA
e-mail: ophtnjn@emory.edu; vbiousse@emory.edu

The Neuro-ophthalmologic Examination in the Emergency Department

Evaluation of visual function, pupils, extraocular movements and the ocular fundus are all part of a routine neurologic examination. They are particularly important when the neurologic disorder involves the intracranial visual pathways or is classically associated with neuro-ophthalmologic manifestations. Ophthalmic findings can provide helpful clues regarding the mechanism of disease and guide acute management decisions in a patient with visual complaints. The only tools needed are a near visual acuity card (or a smartphone), a bright red object, a bright light for external and pupil examination and a direct ophthalmoscope.

Visual Acuity

Visual acuity can easily be measured in the emergency department or in the neurologist's office. Each eye must be tested separately and patients should wear their refractive correction (glasses or contact lens) during the examination. A standardized vision chart (usually a Snellen chart) at the designated distance from the patient will give the most accurate assessment. If unavailable, then a near vision card or a vision chart displayed on a smartphone will suffice, provided that patients older than 45 years wear reading glasses or are

K. L. Roos (ed.), *Emergency Neurology*, https://doi.org/10.1007/978-3-030-75778-6_5

provided with +3.00 sphere lenses to account for presbyopia. If visual acuity improves when looking through a pinhole (easily fashioned by perforating small holes in a piece of cardboard), then the problem is refractive and is not neurologic in origin. Pinhole testing is also useful to estimate distance visual acuity when patients do not have their glasses. If the vision loss is so profound that the patient cannot see anything on the vision chart or near card, visual acuity can be quantified as "count fingers," "hand motion," "light perception," or "no light perception."

Color Vision

Color vision testing can help localize the lesion to the optic nerve or detect subtle optic neuropathies when visual acuity is normal. Altered color vision may be the only sign of an early optic neuropathy. The red desaturation test is a simple bedside assessment for patients complaining of unilateral vision loss, which involves asking the patient to estimate the amount of "redness" seen by each eye when viewing a bright red object. Unilateral optic neuropathies will produce red desaturation (dimmer or darker red) in the affected eye.

More formal and quantitative bedside color vision testing includes Ishihara or Hardy-Rand-Rittler pseudoisochromatic color plates and the City University Test. While Ishihara plates are the most widely available, the latter two tests are better for detecting acquired color vision deficiency in optic neuropathies [3].

Visual Fields

Visual fields are usually assessed in the emergency department by confrontation methods and can be of great value in localizing the lesion. As for visual acuity, visual fields are tested monocularly, with special attention directed to the horizontal and vertical axes of the visual field. One eye is occluded and the patient is instructed to fixate on the examiner's eye or nose. The examiner presents fingers in each quadrant within the central 30° and the patient is asked to count the fingers [1]. The patient must perform the task equally well in all four quadrants. Visual field deficits that respect the horizontal midline are most suggestive of optic nerve disease, whereas visual field deficits that respect the vertical meridian are indicative of intracranial pathology. The peripheral visual field may be tested with finger movements as it is more sensitive to motion than form. If the visual field defect is within the central 10°, then an Amsler grid is a more effective bedside test.

Standardized visual field testing, such as Goldmann (kinetic) or Humphrey (automated static) perimetry, reveals more subtle abnormalities and can quantify the defects to facilitate monitoring of disease progression. These tests are easily performed in an ophthalmologist's office once the patient is stable and able to cooperate.

Examination of the Pupils

Pupillary examination in light and dark provides valuable information about the afferent and efferent visual pathways. Dim lighting is essential for an accurate examination, which may be challenging in the emergency department or ICU.

Firstly, one should assess for pupil size and asymmetry. Unless the patient has a history of an ocular disorder (such as surgery or uveitis), anisocoria reflects an efferent problem which may either be impaired dilation (the smaller pupil does not dilate well) or impaired constriction (the larger pupil does not constrict well). Poor dilation reflects a lesion of the sympathetic pathways, e.g., Horner syndrome, whereas poor constriction reflects a lesion of the parasympathetic pathways, e.g., third nerve palsy, tonic pupil and pharmacologic mydriasis. Horner syndrome with acute visual loss may be the first sign of a carotid dissection, while an acute third nerve palsy with vision loss is highly suggestive of pituitary apoplexy with cavernous sinus and chiasmal compression.

Pupillary responses to light should then be examined. The search for a relative afferent pupillary defect (RAPD) by the swinging flash-light test is of great importance, particularly when visual loss is unilateral or asymmetric. Presence of a RAPD in the setting of a normal appearing retina is diagnostic of a unilateral or asymmetric optic neuropathy. Exceptions include extensive retinal diseases such as retinal vascular occlusions and large retinal detachments, which are easily seen on funduscopic examination. Corneal abnormalities, cataracts and macular disorders do *not* cause a RAPD.

Eye Movements

Diplopia and ocular motility are discussed in detail in Chap. 6. Some patients describe subtle diplopia as "blurred vision" that resolves with covering either eye. True monocular or binocular visual loss in association with abnormal eye movements can help localize the lesion (e.g., to the orbital apex or to the sellar region).

Ocular Examination and Funduscopic Examination

The ocular examination itself is usually the domain of the ophthalmologist, but careful pen-light examination can reveal obvious abnormalities of the anterior segment (cornea, iris and lens), which may be capable of causing decreased vision or obstructing an adequate view of the fundus. Ocular media opacities that are sufficient to cause severe visual loss usually result in a poor fundal view: "If you can't see in, the patient can't see out." When media opacity is suspected, visual acuity should be tested without and with pinhole as a refractive change may underlie the visual disturbance.

Conjunctival injection may be indicative of anterior segment disease. Ocular redness or pain associated with vision loss should prompt immediate ophthalmologic consultation. Corneal ulcers, uveitis and angle-closure glaucoma are examples of ophthalmic emergencies presenting with acute painful vision loss (Fig. 5.1).

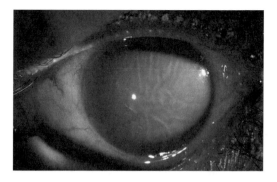

Fig. 5.1 Acute angle-closure glaucoma in the left eye with acute painful vision loss. The eye is red and the cornea is cloudy and edematous. The pupil is mid-dilated and non-reactive to light. On palpation, the eye feels hard

Examination of the ocular fundus is essential in all patients complaining of visual loss. Pharmacologic dilation of the pupils with short-acting drops, such as a parasympathetic antagonist (tropicamide) and a sympathetic agonist (phenylephrine), allows the best view of the optic nerve, macula and retinal vessels. Phenylephrine should be avoided in patients with severe systemic hypertension or malignant hypertension. Pupillary dilation occurs within 30 minutes and usually resolves within 6 hours. Both pupils should be dilated to facilitate comparison and time of eye drop instillation should be noted in the medical chart. Nonmydriatic ocular fundus cameras provide an alternative method of assessing the ocular fundus, providing real-time high quality digital photographs of the posterior pole of the eye without pupillary dilation [4, 5].

Identification of optic disc edema, optic disc pallor, retinal whitening, retinal hemorrhages, arterial attenuation, venous dilation, retinal emboli and vitreous hemorrhages can be extremely useful in neurologic emergencies. It allows the neurologist to manage these patients appropriately, even before requesting an ophthalmic consultation. Optic nerve pallor takes about 6 weeks to develop, regardless of the mechanism of optic nerve injury. Therefore, the presence of optic nerve pallor in a patient with acute vision loss suggests a chronic underlying process. For example, a patient with a previously undiagnosed pituitary mass may only notice vision loss at the time of pituitary apoplexy. On the other hand, patients with long-standing optic atrophy may erroneously blame their acute visual deterioration on recent trauma.

Where Is the Lesion?

In most cases, vision loss results from ocular disorders and an ophthalmologist should be consulted first in the emergency department when a patient presents with acute visual changes. Ocular redness, eye pain or abnormal fundus appearance usually localizes the lesion to the eye. In the rare instances that the ocular examination does not explain the visual symptoms, optic neuropathy or an intracranial process is then suspected. Sometimes the ophthalmologist or emergency physician identifies a sign suggestive of a neurologic disorder, such as optic nerve head edema, bitemporal or homonymous visual field changes, an efferent pupillary disorder or abnormal extraocular movements. A neurologic consultation should also be requested when the patient is diagnosed with acute retinal ischemia (transient or permanent) or retinal emboli, as these conditions may herald an imminent cerebral infarction and warrant urgent neurovascular evaluation [6–8].

Ocular Causes of Acute Vision Loss: What the Neurologist Should Know

Painful Red Eye with Vision Loss

Acute vision loss with ocular pain, photophobia, epiphora and eye redness suggests anterior segment disease and is usually unilateral. Trauma, corneal infections, anterior uveitis and acute angle-closure glaucoma are classic causes of acute visual loss with pain that warrant immediate examination by an ophthalmologist.

Patients with corneal ulcers or trauma may struggle to open their eye due to reflex blepharospasm. Instillation of topical anesthesia may facilitate eye opening such that one can at least perform a cursory macroscopic examination

looking for white lesions on the cornea, a hypopyon or hyphema.

Uveitis is difficult to diagnose without a slit lamp examination, unless there is an obvious hypopyon. Most patients complain of photophobia, floaters and mild pain.

Acute angle-closure glaucoma is suspected when vision loss is preceded by severe eye pain, headaches and nausea. The patient may complain of seeing halos in addition to blurred vision. Typical signs include corneal clouding that may obstruct a clear view of the iris and a mid-dilated pupil that is poorly reactive to light (Fig. 5.1). Palpation of both eyes allows the neurologist to ascertain that the affected eye feels much firmer than the unaffected eye.

Vision Loss with an Abnormal Retina

A few neurologic emergencies may present with acute visual loss and retinal changes. Intravitreal and preretinal hemorrhages cause painless vision loss. The anterior segment looks normal, there is no RAPD and the fundal view is hazy. A dull or dark red reflex can be appreciated through a direct ophthalmoscope held at arm's length from the patient. Comparison with the red reflex of the unaffected eye may help confirm that it is abnormal. Vitreous hemorrhage is common in diabetic patients but may rarely occur in patients with acute intracranial hypertension, especially from subarachnoid hemorrhage (Terson syndrome) (Fig. 5.2) [9].

Retinal diseases such as central retinal artery occlusion (CRAO) (Fig. 5.3) and large retinal detachments can produce acute painless monocular vision loss with a RAPD. The RAPD is indicative of the involvement of retinal ganglion cells, whose axonal projections become the optic nerve. This exemplifies why dilated funduscopy is necessary before localizing the lesion to the optic nerve in all patients with vision loss and a RAPD.

CRAO produces sudden, painless, severe and permanent monocular vision loss resulting from acute inner retinal ischemia, which includes the ganglion cells and their axons. Fundoscopy shows marked attenuation of the retinal arteries and edema of the ischemic inner retinal layers that is most prominent at the macula. There is relatively less obscuration of the choroidal vasculature at the fovea, where the inner retinal layers are at their thinnest. This creates the classic "cherry-red spot" (Fig. 5.3) with whitening of the macula surrounding a red fovea. This sign may not always be apparent immediately after the insult, but tends to evolve over a day or two.

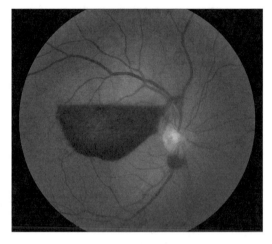

Fig. 5.2 Terson syndrome in the right eye of a patient with subarachnoid hemorrhage. There is a large preretinal hemorrhage as well as two small peripapillary hemorrhages

Acute CRAO is effectively an infarction of the anterior cerebral circulation and therefore necessitates immediate stroke workup to prevent further ischemic events [6–8]. In patients older than 50 years, giant cell arteritis must also be considered as an underlying etiology [10, 11].

Acute treatments for CRAO are limited and stroke neurologists may be consulted for consideration of thrombolysis within the first few hours of visual loss. Currently the risks are thought to outweigh the benefits of intra-arterial thrombolysis for CRAO [12]. Meanwhile, the safety and efficacy of intravenous thrombolysis continues to be investigated [13].

Central retinal vein occlusion (Fig. 5.4) can also cause painless monocular vision loss, but is not usually associated with neurologic disorders. Rarely, severe and ischemic forms of central retinal vein occlusions can exhibit a RAPD. Fundoscopy reveals a "blood and thunder" appearance with dilated veins, intraretinal hemorrhages and cotton wool spots.

Numerous macular disorders may produce central visual loss, but typically without a RAPD. Exacerbation of age-related macular degeneration with acute bleeding of a choroidal neovascular membrane is a common cause of acute central visual loss or distortion in the elderly. Often there is a preceding history of

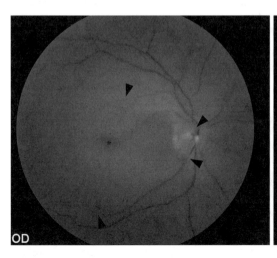

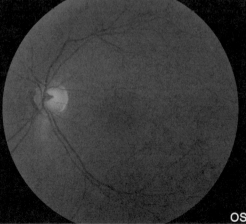

Fig. 5.3 Acute central retinal artery occlusion in the right eye (OD). Note the attenuated central retinal artery with segmental narrowing in the right eye (*arrows*) compared with the left eye. The ischemic retina is edematous and appears whitish compared to the left eye and there is a *cherry-red spot* at the fovea (*)

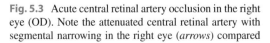

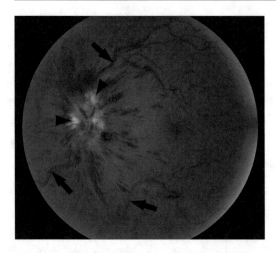

Fig. 5.4 Acute central retinal vein occlusion in the left eye. There are numerous flame retinal hemorrhages and cotton wool spots (*arrow heads*), the veins are dilated (*arrows*) and there is optic disc edema

gradual visual decline. The peripheral vision tends to be spared. A grossly disorganized macula or a macular hemorrhage may be seen on fundoscopy.

Central serous retinopathy is a cause of acute painless unilateral central vision loss with no RAPD and a normal-appearing optic nerve, most often occurring in young men. Careful examination of the macula shows a "blister" in the macular region that can be difficult to detect on fundoscopy, but is easily seen on optical coherence tomography (OCT) of the macula.

Optic Neuropathies

Optic neuropathies typically manifest with decreased visual acuity, altered color vision and abnormal visual fields. A RAPD is always present when the optic neuropathy is unilateral or asymmetric. Acutely, the optic disc may appear normal (posterior optic neuropathy) or may be swollen (anterior optic neuropathy) (Fig. 5.5). Optic disc pallor ensues 4–6 weeks later, regardless of the mechanism. Optic neuropathies with acute or subacute vision loss are often evaluated in the emergency department. These are best classified by mechanism and their clinical characteristics facilitate diagnosis (Table 5.1).

Dedicated optic nerve imaging is often helpful, particularly to demonstrate optic nerve inflammation, infiltration or compression (Fig. 5.5). However, it is important to emphasize that most brain scans (CT or MRI) do not allow proper evaluation of the optic nerves. A CT of the orbits with contrast, thin cuts and coronal reconstructions is helpful when emergent MRI cannot be obtained, or in the setting of trauma. MRI of the orbits with contrast and fat suppression is the most sensitive test with which to image the optic nerves in the orbits, at the level of the orbital apex and intracranially (see Fig. 5.5b). It is particularly important when an optic nerve sheath meningioma or an orbital apex syndrome is suspected.

Inflammatory Optic Neuropathy (Optic Neuritis)

Isolated optic neuritis is often the first manifestation of multiple sclerosis (MS) and is one of the classic clinically isolated syndromes. However, inflammation of the optic nerve may also occur in association with numerous infectious and non-infectious inflammatory disorders.

Patients with optic neuritis present with acute or subacute painful monocular visual loss. Central vision typically deteriorates over hours or days. In mild optic neuritis, color vision change can be the first or the only visual complaint. Pain on eye movement is a frequent early complaint accompanying the visual loss. On examination, there is decreased visual acuity, decreased color vision and central visual field loss. A RAPD will be present if the optic neuritis is unilateral or asymmetric. In isolated optic neuritis associated with demyelinating disease, two-thirds of patients have a normal optic disc appearance acutely and one-third of patients have moderate optic nerve head swelling (so-called "anterior" optic neuritis or "papillitis") (see Fig. 5.5) [14]. Optic neuritis with a normal-appearing optic disc acutely is called "retrobulbar" or "posterior" optic neuritis. In all cases, optic nerve head pallor develops 4–6 weeks later.

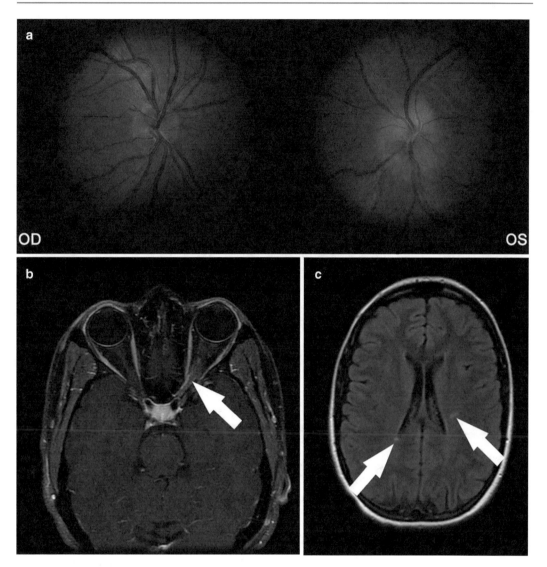

Fig. 5.5 Left anterior optic neuritis. (**a**) Fundus photograph of both eyes showing mild optic nerve head edema in the left eye (OS) compared with the right eye (OD). (**b**) Axial T1-weighted MRI of the orbits with contrast and fat suppression demonstrating enhancement of the left optic nerve (*arrow*). (**c**) Axial FLAIR MRI of the brain showing two periventricular ovoid lesions suggestive of demyelinating disease

Evaluation of the patient with optic neuritis varies based on the clinical presentation and the suspected diagnosis. A brain MRI is usually obtained in patients with isolated optic neuritis to look for demyelinating disease (see Fig. 5.5). Blood tests and specific serologies may be obtained depending on the patient's clinical characteristics. Syphilis, cat scratch disease, sarcoidosis, neuromyelitis optica spectrum disorder and myelin oligodendrocyte glycoprotein (MOG) antibody-associated disease are important alternate causes of optic neuritis. A lumbar puncture may also be useful in this setting, especially assessing for oligoclonal bands. In most cases, optic neuritis remains idiopathic or is associated with multiple sclerosis.

In patients with typical isolated optic neuritis, the risk of multiple sclerosis is best predicted by a brain MRI: patients without lesions have an estimated risk of 25% at 15 years, whereas those

Table 5.1 Most common causes of acute optic neuropathies

Mechanism	Optic neuropathies that often present with acute visual loss
Inflammatory (optic neuritis)	Clinically isolated syndrome or associated with multiple sclerosis Not associated with multiple sclerosis: Neuromyelitis optica spectrum disorder Myelin oligodendrocyte glycoprotein antibody-associated disease Infectious diseases (syphilis, cat scratch) Systemic inflammatory and autoimmune diseases (sarcoidosis)
Vascular	Ischemic optic neuropathy: Arteritic–Giant cell arteritis Nonarteritic anterior ischemic optic neuropathy
Compressive/infiltrative	Acute compression of the intracranial portion of the optic nerve or of the chiasm: Pituitary mass (pituitary apoplexy) Craniopharyngioma Internal carotid artery aneurysm Any intracranial mass close to the anterior visual pathways
Toxic/nutritional	Methanol poisoning
Hereditary	Leber hereditary optic neuropathy
Traumatic	Direct or indirect mechanism
Raised intracranial pressure	Papilledema
Malignant hypertension	Stage IV hypertensive retinopathy

with at least one typical demyelinating lesion have an estimated risk of 72% at 15 years (see Fig. 5.5) [15]. Among the patients with no lesions on MRI, any of the following features is associated with virtually no risk of multiple sclerosis: male gender, absence of pain, severe optic nerve edema, peripapillary hemorrhages or macular changes suggesting neuroretinitis [15]. This emphasizes the importance of a funduscopic examination by an ophthalmologist in all cases of presumed optic neuritis.

The visual prognosis of isolated optic neuritis is usually good even without treatment [16–18]. High-dose intravenous methylprednisolone (1 g/day for 3 days followed by oral prednisone 1 mg/kg/day for 11 days) only accelerates visual recovery, but does not alter long-term visual outcome or the long-term risk of subsequent MS [18–20]. The Optic Neuritis Treatment Trial showed that 1 mg/kg/day of oral prednisone for 2 weeks did not improve visual outcome and doubled the risk of recurrent optic neuritis [20, 21]. Therefore, low-dose oral prednisone is currently not recommended for patients with isolated optic neuritis and intravenous steroids should be discussed on a case-by-case basis.

A subgroup of patients with optic neuritis are found to have aquaporin 4 antibodies, leading to the diagnosis of neuromyelitis optica spectrum disorder (NMOSD), even in the absence of transverse myelitis [22, 23]. These patients often present with severe optic neuritis characterized by poor recovery, bilateral involvement and a higher risk of recurrence. They usually require more aggressive initial intravenous steroid therapy with escalation to plasma exchange if there is little improvement, followed by a more prolonged course of oral steroid taper. Hence, early consideration of this diagnosis is imperative for minimizing long-term morbidity. The majority of patients with NMOSD will continue on long-term immunomodulatory therapy because of the high risk of unpredictable and devastating relapses [23].

A recently described disorder that frequently manifests as optic neuritis is MOG antibody-associated disease. Features suggestive of MOG antibody associated optic neuritis include bilaterality, recurrent disease, anterior optic nerve involvement with optic disc edema and peripapillary folds and longitudinally enhancing optic nerves with optic sheath involvement seen on MRI [23]. Our understanding of MOG antibody associated disease continues to evolve rapidly; hence, treatment paradigms are also shifting. Essentially, early consideration of MOG antibody associated disease may instigate a more prolonged steroid taper and discussion of possible long-term immunomodulation, in an effort to stave off recurrences.

Neuroretinitis characterizes patients with an anterior optic neuritis associated with retinal exudates, usually in the shape of a star at the macula. In most cases, neuroretinitis is due to an infection such as cat scratch disease or syphilis, or is caused by a noninfectious inflammatory disorder such as sarcoidosis. Neuroretinitis is not associated with a risk of developing MS [24, 25]. Treatment of neuroretinitis or infectious optic neuritis depends on the underlying disease.

Ischemic Optic Neuropathy

Ischemic optic neuropathies are classified into anterior ischemic optic neuropathy (AION), in which case there is always optic nerve head swelling acutely (Fig. 5.6), and posterior ischemic optic neuropathy (PION), in which the posterior part of the optic nerve is ischemic with normal-appearing optic disc acutely. AION is much more common, accounting for 90% of ischemic optic neuropathies [26], and PION remains a diagnosis of exclusion. Ischemic optic neuropathies are further classified as "nonarteritic" and "arteritic"; the latter is most often associated with giant cell arteritis. Ischemic optic neuropathies present with painless, acute or subacute vision loss with visual field defects, and a RAPD. Four to six weeks later, the optic nerve becomes pale.

Nonarteritic AION (NAION) is the most common form of acute optic neuropathy in older patients, affecting 2.3–10.2 individuals per 100,000 persons 50 years or older [27, 28]. The main risk factor is a small crowded optic disc with no cup, the so-called disc at risk (see Fig. 5.6), but other disc anomalies such as optic disc drusen and papilledema can also predispose to NAION [29, 30]. Most patients with NAION are at least 50 years of age and have at least one cardiovascular risk factor. NAION is a small vessel disease involving the short posterior ciliary arteries. It is not embolic and is neither associated with an increased risk of cerebrovascular disease nor with carotid occlusive disease. The pathophysiology involves local arteriolosclerosis of the small vessels, in addition to the "disc at risk." Therefore, atheromatous vascular risk factors should be identified and aggressively treated; however, searching for a carotid or cardiac source of emboli is usually not necessary in patients with isolated NAION [26].

There is currently no proven treatment for ischemic optic neuropathies, and the only emergency in evaluating a patient with AION or PION is to rule out giant cell arteritis [26]. Indeed, giant cell arteritis should be considered in all patients older than 50 years with AION or PION, and blood tests looking for raised inflammatory markers should be obtained urgently. High-dose steroids are commenced in patients in whom there is high clinical suspicion of giant cell arteritis and a temporal artery biopsy should be subsequently obtained in these patients [31]. Administration of high doses of intravenous steroids at the initiation of treatment for giant cell arteritis may decrease the duration of treatment and the total dose of steroids used, as might the use of tocilizumab [32].

Fig. 5.6 Anterior ischemic optic neuropathy in the right eye. There is optic nerve head edema, worse superiorly, and a small superior peripapillary hemorrhage. The patient had an inferior altitudinal visual field defect

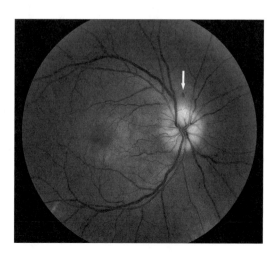

Traumatic Optic Neuropathy

Monocular visual loss after head trauma can result from direct or indirect traumatic optic neuropathy. Direct traumatic optic neuropathy is a consequence of mechanical stresses applied directly to the optic nerve such as compression, laceration or avulsion due to penetrating orbital trauma or optic canal fracture [33]. Indirect traumatic optic neuropathy results from transference of force from head trauma to the bony structures that convey the optic nerve [33]. Affected patients frequently have associated brain and systemic injuries, and recognition of vision loss is often delayed if there is no external sign of ocular injury. A RAPD may be the only evidence of traumatic optic neuropathy in a sedated or unconscious patient and should be systematically checked in all head trauma patients [1]. Visual loss may be isolated and the optic disc may appear normal or swollen in the acute phase. There may also be associated signs of globe rupture or signs of orbital trauma with proptosis, ophthalmoplegia and elevated intraocular pressure. Orbital non-contrast CT is essential to rule out an orbital fracture or an orbital hematoma, which may require immediate treatment. An ophthalmologist must perform an urgent detailed examination when there is suspected ocular or orbital trauma.

Direct traumatic optic neuropathies may require surgical intervention, whereas indirect traumatic optic neuropathies are usually observed. There is evidence that steroids are not effective in this subgroup of patients and are potentially harmful, particularly in the setting of associated brain and systemic injuries [33, 34].

Compressive Optic Neuropathy

Patients with compressive optic neuropathies classically develop gradual progressive unilateral or bilateral vision loss. However, many of these patients are unaware due to the insidious onset and present emergently when their central vision acutely worsens or keeps them from reading and driving. These patients already have optic nerve pallor at presentation. Rarely, sudden vision loss can result from compressive optic neuropathy. This may be due to an orbital apex lesion, typically metastases or fungal lesions or a lesion involving the intracranial optic nerve and chiasm, most commonly due to pituitary tumors, pituitary apoplexy, ophthalmic artery aneurysms and craniopharyngiomas. Associated signs such as an orbital syndrome and ocular motor cranial nerve palsies help localize the lesion to the orbital apex or the intracranial portion of the optic nerve, respectively. Emergent evaluation with dedicated MRI of the brain and orbits with contrast and fat suppression is indicated. MRA or CTA should be obtained when an aneurysm is suspected or when the MRI is normal.

Acute Bilateral Optic Neuropathies

Rarely, simultaneous bilateral optic neuropathies may cause acute binocular vision loss. These patients are usually severely visually disabled and often present to the emergency department. Because both optic nerves are affected, a RAPD may not be apparent. When the optic nerves appear normal (e.g., acute bilateral posterior optic neuropathies), the diagnosis may be difficult and relies on pupil examination (sluggish pupillary response to light) and visual field testing.

Bilateral inflammatory optic neuritis, with or without disc edema, suggests an infectious or non-infectious inflammatory disorder and should prompt a more extensive evaluation than isolated unilateral optic neuritis. A lumbar puncture is usually performed, looking for a meningeal process. Sarcoidosis, NMOSD and MOG antibody-associated disease are classic causes.

Bilateral simultaneous ischemic optic neuropathies in patients older than 50 are highly suggestive of giant cell arteritis [35]; therefore erythrocyte sedimentation rate and C-reactive protein should be systematically obtained in the emergency department.

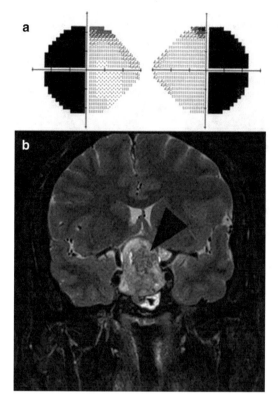

Fig. 5.7 Acute binocular visual loss with bitemporal hemianopia from pituitary apoplexy. The patient also had headaches and diplopia due to a left third nerve palsy. (**a**) Humphrey visual fields showing a bitemporal hemianopia. (**b**) Coronal T2-weighted MRI demonstrating a large pituitary mass (*arrowhead*) with chiasmal compression and cavernous sinus compression

Pituitary apoplexy with sudden chiasmal and optic nerve compression is another classic cause of acute bilateral optic neuropathies (Fig. 5.7). Most patients also experience headaches, sometimes with abnormal extraocular movements and altered mental status.

Hypertensive retinopathy with bilateral optic nerve head edema can also produce acute or subacute bilateral visual loss (Fig. 5.8).

In cases of papilledema that are associated with visual loss, the onset tends to slowly progressive, rather than acute. However, fulminant idiopathic intracranial hypertension or acute causes of raised intracranial pressure such as cerebral venous thrombosis can cause severe

bilateral papilledema and rapidly progressive bilateral visual loss (Fig. 5.9) [36].

Leber hereditary optic neuropathy often presents with acute or subacute bilateral optic neuropathies and profound painless vision loss [37]. Brain and orbit MRIs are typically normal without optic nerve enhancement. The diagnosis should be suspected in any patient with bilateral or rapidly sequential painless optic neuropathies, especially in a young man with a family history of visual loss in maternal relatives and absence of visual recovery. Testing for mitochondrial DNA mutations can be easily performed on a peripheral blood sample.

Nutritional and toxic optic neuropathies are typically bilateral and slowly progressive. Acute vision loss can occur after ingestion of methanol (homemade alcohol or antifreeze). The optic nerves usually appear swollen in the acute phase and patients typically have associated neurologic signs with confusion and altered mental status [38]. The visual prognosis is poor.

Bilateral Optic Disc Edema

Bilateral optic disc edema may be the result of bilateral anterior optic neuritis, bilateral anterior ischemic optic neuropathies, raised intracranial pressure (papilledema) or systemic hypertension (stage IV hypertensive retinopathy). Patients with bilateral anterior optic neuropathies have visual acuity loss, decreased color vision and abnormal visual fields.

When there is bilateral disc edema and central visual acuity is normal, papilledema from raised intracranial pressure should be suspected. All causes of raised intracranial pressure can produce papilledema, which is associated with progressive visual field constriction, secondary optic atrophy and irreversible visual loss if treatment is delayed. Indeed, visual loss is the main complication of idiopathic intracranial hypertension and is often encountered in patients with cerebral venous thrombosis (see Fig. 5.9), intracranial mass lesions or unrecognized hydrocephalus,

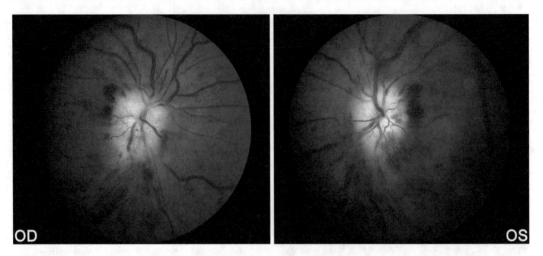

Fig. 5.8 Hypertensive retinopathy with bilateral optic disc edema and retinal hemorrhages. The retinal arteries are attenuated. Blood pressure was 210/130 mmHg. This is consistent with stage IV hypertensive retinopathy

emphasizing the importance of systematic performance of fundoscopy on all patients with chronic headaches (Fig. 5.10).

Malignant systemic hypertension (or hypertensive crisis) is often associated with bilateral optic nerve head edema (see Fig. 5.8). Usually, there are accompanying retinal and vascular changes suggestive of hypertensive retinopathy, such as attenuation of retinal arteries, retinal hemorrhages and retinal exudates (hypertensive retinopathy stage IV).

Binocular Vision Loss from Chiasmal Lesions

Acute binocular visual loss may result from simultaneous damage to the intracranial portions of the optic nerves, often in association with chiasmal compression. Pituitary tumors, sphenoid wing meningiomas and craniopharyngiomas are the most common causes of the chiasmal syndrome. Pituitary apoplexy is a classic cause of acute chiasmal syndrome often associated with headaches, whereas other intracranial processes usually present with more insidious, progressive visual loss. Detection of a bitemporal visual field defect (the hallmark of the chiasmal syndrome) requires immediate brain imaging in patients with acute visual changes (see Fig. 5.7). Internal carotid artery aneurysms can also produce compressive chiasmal syndromes.

Binocular Vision Loss from Retrochiasmal Lesions

A lesion of the retrochiasmal visual pathways (optic tract, lateral geniculate body, optic radiations or occipital cortex) classically produces a contralateral homonymous hemianopia (Fig. 5.11) [1]. Visual acuity should be normal in each eye, unless there is superimposed damage to the anterior visual pathways. In cases of bilateral injury (most often bilateral occipital lobe lesions), visual acuity may be decreased, but the amount of visual acuity loss is symmetric in both eyes. Any central nervous system disorder involving both occipital lobes may produce bilateral visual loss from so-called cerebral

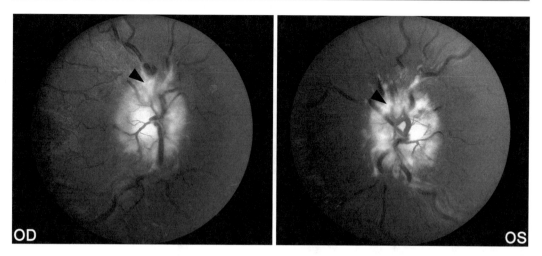

Fig. 5.9 Bilateral severe optic disc edema consistent with papilledema (from raised intracranial pressure). The optic discs are elevated with numerous cotton wool spots (*arrows*) and severe dilation of the veins. The patient had thrombosis of the superior sagittal sinus with elevated CSF opening pressure

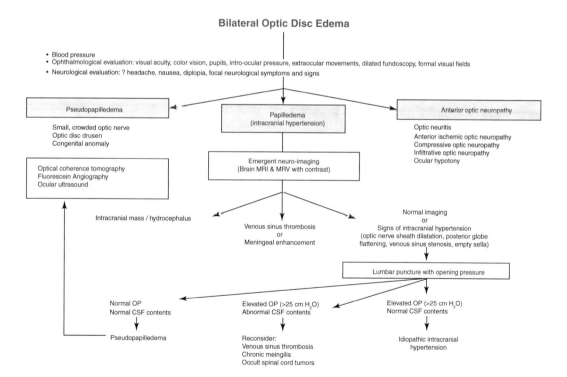

Fig. 5.10 Flowchart detailing the diagnosis of disc edema

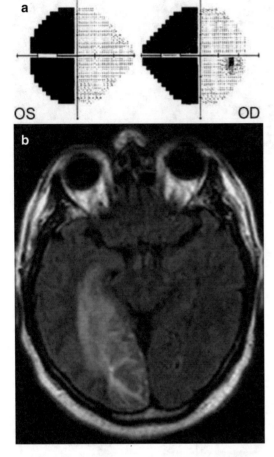

OS   OD

Fig. 5.11 Left homonymous hemianopia secondary to a right occipital infarction. (**a**) Humphrey visual fields showing a complete left homonymous hemianopia. (**b**) Axial FLAIR MRI of the brain showed a right occipital infarction in the territory of the right posterior cerebral artery

Table 5.2 Common neurologic causes of acute binocular visual loss (producing either a homonymous visual field defect or binocular "cerebral" visual loss)

Cerebral causes of acute visual loss
• Vascular
Occipital infarction or hemorrhage
Optic radiations or optic tract infarction or hemorrhage
Superior sagittal venous sinus thrombosis with occipital venous infarction
Arteriovenous malformation involving the visual pathways
• Intracranial mass
Any mass involving the intracranial visual pathways
• Occipital seizures
• Hypoglycemia
• Multiple sclerosis
• Leukoencephalopathies
• Creutzfeldt–Jakob disease
• Posterior reversible encephalopathy syndrome (PRES)
• Hypertensive encephalopathy
• Trauma
• Carbon monoxide intoxication

radiations. The most common cause of an isolated homonymous hemianopia is a stroke (most often a posterior cerebral artery distribution infarction) (see Fig. 5.11) [39].

Transient Visual Loss

The most important step in evaluating a patient with transient visual loss is establishing whether the visual loss is monocular (a disorder of the eye or the optic nerve) or binocular (a disorder affecting the chiasm or retrochiasmal visual pathways) (Table 5.3).

Deciding whether an episode of transient visual loss occurred in one eye or both is not always easy. Very few patients realize that binocular hemifield loss (homonymous visual field defects) affects both eyes. They usually localize their visual disturbance to the eye that lost its temporal field. Clues suggestive of binocular transient visual loss include reading impairment (monocular visual loss does not impair reading unless the unaffected eye had prior vision impairment) and visual loss confined to a lateral hemifield, i.e., to the right or left of the vertical midline

blindness (Table 5.2). A complete homonymous hemianopia (see Fig. 5.11) has no other specific localizing value than the contralateral retrochiasmal visual pathways, but associated symptoms and signs are very helpful in localizing the lesion along the intracranial visual pathways. Optic tract lesions produce a contralateral RAPD, whereas parietal lesions are associated with abnormal optokinetic nystagmus. Congruous incomplete homonymous hemianopias (when the two abnormal fields are similar in both eyes) are most suggestive of an occipital lesion, whereas incongruous homonymous hemianopias suggest a lesion along the more anterior optic

Table 5.3 Causes of transient visual loss

Monocular transient visual loss

Ocular (non-vascular) causes

Ocular surface disease (e.g., dry eyes)

Corneal edema

Intermittent angle-closure glaucoma

Anterior chamber inflammation/hyphema

Phacodonesis

Vitreous hemorrhage or vitreous floaters

Incomplete retinal detachment (moving curtain)

Abnormal optic nerve head (papilledema, optic disc drusen)

Previous optic neuritis (Uhthoff's)

Orbital vascular malformation

Vascular causes

Retinal arterial transient ischemic attack

Choroidal ischemia (giant cell arteritis)

Impending central retinal vein occlusion

Ocular ischemic syndrome

Ischemic optic neuropathy (giant cell arteritis)

Binocular transient visual loss

Ocular causes

Ocular surface disease (e.g., dry eyes)

Corneal edema, corneal dystrophy

Refractive error (accommodative spasm, hyperglycemia)

Pigment dispersion syndrome

Bilateral optic neuropathies

Abnormal optic nerve head (papilledema, optic disc drusen)

Chiasmal or Retrochiasmal causes

Chiasmal compression

Migrainous visual aura

Occipital seizures

Occipital transient ischemic attack

Posterior reversible encephalopathy syndrome

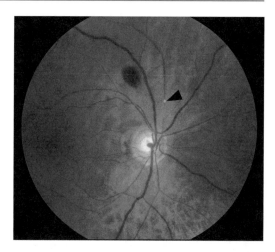

Fig. 5.12 Branch retinal arterial embolus in a patient with an episode of transient loss of vision in the right eye. Fundus photograph of the right eye showing a retinal cholesterol embolus (*arrow head*) from a carotid artery atheroma. There is a large intraretinal hemorrhage superiorly related to retinal ischemia

(monocular visual loss does not usually manifest with this pattern of field defect).

A detailed ocular examination is essential to detect clues to the underlying mechanism, e.g., narrow anterior chamber, elevated intraocular pressure, abnormal pupil, retinal emboli (Fig. 5.12), retinal ischemia, optic nerve edema or residual visual field defect.

Monocular Transient Visual Loss

Neurologists are often called to evaluate patients with transient monocular visual loss (TMVL). However, it is important to keep in mind that numerous ocular conditions can also produce TMVL and need to be ruled out by a detailed ocular examination before assuming that the mechanism of TMVL is vascular (see Table 5.3).

Ocular Causes of Monocular Transient Visual Loss

Most ocular disorders can produce fluctuations in vision and may be described as "TMVL" by patients. Ocular disorders usually produce transient blurry vision rather than complete blackout of vision as in vascular TMVL. Blurry vision worsened by reading (during which blink rate is reduced) and improved with blinking or eye rubbing is highly suggestive of dry eyes, abnormal tear film and other ocular surface disorders. Acute increase in intraocular pressure can produce transient visual changes, including blurred vision, halos around lights and associated eye pain. Transient ocular hypertension can be due to spontaneously resolving angle-closure glaucoma or pigment dispersion syndrome after exercise in young myopic patients. In patients with diabetes mellitus, acute hyperglycemia can cause transient refractive or macular changes that manifest as blurred vision, lasting hours to days. Abnormally crowded optic discs, such as papilledema, drusen and congenitally small or tilted optic discs, can produce recurrent episodes of TMVL lasting a few seconds (transient visual obscurations), often precipitated by postural changes. Orbital tumors may present as episodes of monocular TMVL precipitated by eye movements in a specific gaze direction.

Mechanisms of Vascular Transient Monocular Visual Loss

Vascular TMVL may result from a retinal transient ischemic attack (TIA) in the carotid circulation and should be managed emergently, similar to hemispheric TIAs, in order to reduce the risk of permanent visual loss, stroke or cardiovascular death (Table 5.4) [10, 40]. Vascular TMVL may result from emboli in the ophthalmic artery or in the central retinal artery, from ocular hypoperfusion or more rarely from central retinal artery spasm [10, 40]. Vascular TMVL resulting from optic nerve ischemia is rare and is highly suggestive of giant cell arteritis, in which case the optic nerve is usually swollen. Rarely, TMVL may

Table 5.4 Differential diagnosis of transient monocular visual loss (TMVL)

Vascular
Orbital ischemia (ophthalmic artery)
Retinal ischemia (central retinal artery and its branches, central retinal vein)
Optic nerve ischemia (short posterior ciliary arteries/ophthalmic artery)
Choroidal ischemia (posterior ciliary arteries)
Ocular diseases
Anterior segment disorders (dry eyes, hyphema, intermittent angle-closure glaucoma)
Optic nerve disorders
Papilledema (transient visual obscurations)
Optic disc drusen (transient visual obscurations)
Congenitally anomalous optic disc (transient visual obscurations)
Optic nerve compression (gaze-evoked TMVL)
Uhthoff phenomenon (demyelination)

inaugurate a central retinal vein occlusion, with dilated veins on funduscopic examination.

The description of the visual loss, its duration and the ocular examination are helpful in determining the mechanism of TMVL. Findings of retinal arterial emboli suggest a carotid, aortic arch or cardiac source of emboli (see Fig. 5.12). Retinal hemorrhages and dilation of the veins suggest chronic ocular hypoperfusion or ocular ischemic syndrome. Optic disc edema suggests optic nerve ischemia and should prompt immediate treatment and workup for giant cell arteritis (see Fig. 5.6). Association of TMVL and an ipsilateral painful Horner syndrome is highly suggestive of internal carotid artery dissection. Often, however, the ocular examination is normal, and the patient is evaluated for all causes of retinal TIAs. All patients over the age of 50 years require emergent workup for giant cell arteritis.

Binocular Transient Visual Loss

Binocular transient visual loss usually results from intracranial processes involving the chiasmal and retrochiasmal visual pathways. Less commonly, it can be related to bilateral ocular disorders or to transient visual obscurations associated with papilledema (see Table 5.3). Migrainous visual aura, occipital seizures and occipital TIAs are the most classic causes of binocular transient visual loss and can usually be discriminated based on the patient's description (Table 5.5).

Migrainous Visual Aura

Migrainous visual aura is the most common cause of transient binocular visual loss and is usually easily diagnosed based on the patient's description. Patients describe a scintillating scotoma expanding over several minutes into a visual field, surrounded by jagged, luminous, shimmering edges [1]. The scotoma can lead to a

Table 5.5 Characteristics of the three most common causes of binocular transient visual loss

	Migrainous visual aura	Occipital seizures	Occipital transient ischemic attack
Visual symptoms	Positive Very rich, moving Often black and white, scintillating, shimmering, jagged edges	Positive Simple visual phenomena (phosphenes, bubbles) Colored	Negative (hemianopia or blindness)
Progression of symptoms	Typical migrainous march, with progression of symptoms over time	Usually not progressive	Sudden onset and disappearance
Duration of visual symptoms	Typically 20–30 minutes less than an hour	Usually brief (seconds) Often repeated	A few minutes
Associated symptoms	Migrainous headache typically follows the aura Visual aura may be followed by other migrainous aura (mostly sensory)	Often none May be associated with other seizures	Brow headache possible at the time of visual symptoms Vertebrobasilar ischemia: Vertigo, dizziness Imbalance Diplopia Bilateral extremity weakness

complete hemianopia and disappears gradually. Episodes usually last no longer than 30 minutes and may be followed by a headache, orbital pain, photophobia, phonophobia or nausea [41]. Migrainous visual aura without headache (acephalgic migraine) is common.

Occipital Seizures

Occipital seizures typically produce brief binocular positive visual phenomena often described as flashing lights, bubbles or bright colors seen in one hemifield or diffusely throughout their entire field of vision [1, 41]. Episodes last a few seconds, but they are usually repetitive and are relatively stereotyped in the same patient.

Occipital Transient Ischemic Attack

Episodes of transient, complete binocular visual loss may represent a TIA in the distribution of the basilar artery or the posterior cerebral arteries. A unilateral occipital TIA manifests as a transient homonymous hemianopia, whereas a bilateral occipital TIA manifests as transient "cortical blindness." As opposed to migraine, hemianopic

events of ischemic origin are typically sudden in onset and last only a few minutes [1]. There may be associated headache, especially over the brow contralateral to the visual field loss; but the pain is usually coincident with the visual loss, rather than following the visual loss as in migraine [1]. Other symptoms of vertebrobasilar ischemia are often present, such as vertigo, dizziness, imbalance, diplopia or bilateral extremity weakness.

Posterior Reversible Encephalopathy Syndrome

Posterior reversible encephalopathy syndrome (PRES) classically produces acute bilateral visual loss lasting hours or days, usually associated with headaches and altered mental status. Malignant systemic hypertension, medications such as cyclosporine or tacrolimus and various metabolic disorders are classic causes of PRES. Brain MRI shows T2 hyperintense lesions involving most often the white matter of both occipital lobes (Fig. 5.13). Treatment of the underlying disorder usually results in dramatic improvement of visual function within days, followed by complete resolution of the MRI changes within weeks [42].

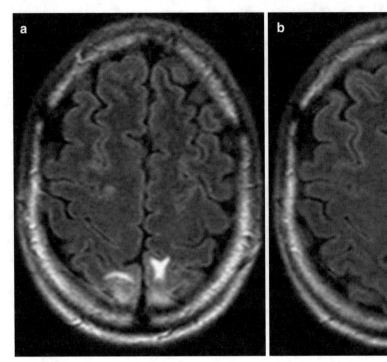

Fig. 5.13 Posterior reversible encephalopathy syndrome (*PRES*) secondary to hypertensive crisis. The patient presented with headaches and binocular visual loss. (**a**) Axial FLAIR MRI showing white matter hyperintense lesions involving both parieto-occipital lobes. (**b**) Six weeks after treatment of hypertension, the MRI has normalized (the vision had returned to normal within 24 hours of blood pressure reduction)

Conclusion

Visual loss is a common symptom in neurologic emergencies. Simple bedside examination including ocular funduscopy is crucial for localizing the lesion and identifying ocular changes such as retinal emboli or optic nerve head edema, facilitating accurate diagnosis and timely management in the acute setting.

References

1. Biousse V, Newman NJ. Neuro-ophthalmology illustrated. 3rd ed. New York: Thieme; 2020.
2. Purvin V, Kawasaki A. Neuro-ophthalmic emergencies for the neurologist. Neurologist. 2005;11(4):195–233.
3. Simunovic MP. Acquired color vision deficiency. Surv Ophthalmol. 2016;61(2):132–55.
4. Biousse V, Bruce BB, Newman NJ. Ophthalmoscopy in the 21st century: the 2017 H. Houston Merritt lecture. Neurology. 2018;90(4):167–75.
5. Irani NK, Bidot S, Peragallo JH, Esper GJ, Newman NJ, Biousse V. Feasibility of a nonmydriatic ocular fundus camera in an outpatient neurology clinic. Neurologist. 2020;25(2):19–23.
6. Fallico M, Lotery AJ, Longo A, Avitabile T, Bonfiglio V, Russo A, et al. Risk of acute stroke in patients with retinal artery occlusion: a systematic review and meta-analysis. Eye (Lond). 2019;
7. Biousse V, Nahab F, Newman NJ. Management of acute retinal ischemia: follow the guidelines! Ophthalmology. 2018;125(10):1597–607.
8. Lavin P, Patrylo M, Hollar M, Espaillat KB, Kirshner H, Schrag M. Stroke risk and risk factors in patients with central retinal artery occlusion. Am J Ophthalmol. 2018;196:96–100.
9. Biousse V, Mendicino ME, Simon DJ, Newman NJ. The ophthalmology of intracranial vascular abnormalities. Am J Ophthalmol. 1998;125(4):527–44.
10. Vodopivec I, Cestari DM, Rizzo JF 3rd. Management of transient monocular vision loss and retinal artery occlusions. Semin Ophthalmol. 2017;32(1):125–33.
11. Chen JJ, Leavitt JA, Fang C, Crowson CS, Matteson EL, Warrington KJ. Evaluating the incidence of arteritic ischemic optic neuropathy and other causes of vision loss from giant cell arteritis. Ophthalmology. 2016;123(9):1999–2003.

12. Schumacher M, Schmidt D, Jurklies B, Gall C, Wanke I, Schmoor C, et al. Central retinal artery occlusion: local intra-arterial fibrinolysis versus conservative treatment, a multicenter randomized trial. Ophthalmology. 2010;117(7):1367–75 e1.

13. Nantes University Hospital. A phase III randomized, blind, double dummy, multicenter study assessing the efficacy and safety of iv thrombolysis (alteplase) in patients with acute central retinal artery occlusion (THEIA) 2018 [updated August 3, 2018]; Available from: https://ClinicalTrials.gov/show/NCT03197194.

14. Optic Neuritis Study Group. The clinical profile of optic neuritis. Experience of the Optic Neuritis Treatment Trial. Optic Neuritis Study Group. Arch Ophthalmol. 1991;109(12):1673–8.

15. Optic Neuritis Study Group. Multiple sclerosis risk after optic neuritis: final optic neuritis treatment trial follow-up. Arch Neurol. 2008;65(6):727–32.

16. Optic Neuritis Study Group. Visual function 5 years after optic neuritis: experience of the Optic Neuritis Treatment Trial. The Optic Neuritis Study Group. Arch Ophthalmol. 1997;115(12):1545–52.

17. Beck RW, Gal RL, Bhatti MT, Brodsky MC, Buckley EG, Chrousos GA, et al. Visual function more than 10 years after optic neuritis: experience of the Optic Neuritis Treatment Trial. Am J Ophthalmol. 2004;137(1):77–83.

18. Optic Neuritis Study Group. Visual function 15 years after optic neuritis: a final follow-up report from the Optic Neuritis Treatment Trial. Ophthalmology. 2008;115(6):1079–82 e5.

19. Optic Neuritis Study Group. The 5-year risk of MS after optic neuritis. Experience of the Optic Neuritis Treatment Trial. Neurology. 1997;49(5):1404–13.

20. Beck RW, Cleary PA, Anderson MM Jr, Keltner JL, Shults WT, Kaufman DI, et al. A randomized, controlled trial of corticosteroids in the treatment of acute optic neuritis. N Engl J Med. 1992;326(9):581–8.

21. Beck RW, Cleary PA. Optic Neuritis Treatment Trial. One-year follow-up results. Arch Ophthalmol. 1993;111(6):773–5.

22. Wingerchuk DM, Banwell B, Bennett JL, Cabre P, Carroll W, Chitnis T, et al. International consensus diagnostic criteria for neuromyelitis optica spectrum disorders. Neurology. 2015;85(2):177–89.

23. Abel A, McClelland C, Lee MS. Critical review: typical and atypical optic neuritis. Surv Ophthalmol. 2019;64:770–9.

24. Parmley VC, Schiffman JS, Maitland CG, Miller NR, Dreyer RF, Hoyt WF. Does neuroretinitis rule out multiple sclerosis? Arch Neurol. 1987;44(10):1045–8.

25. Purvin V, Sundaram S, Kawasaki A. Neuroretinitis: review of the literature and new observations. J Neuroophthalmol. 2011;31(1):58–68.

26. Biousse V, Newman NJ. Ischemic optic neuropathies. N Engl J Med. 2015;372(25):2428–36.

27. Johnson LN, Arnold AC. Incidence of nonarteritic and arteritic anterior ischemic optic neuropathy. Population-based study in the state of Missouri and Los Angeles County, California. J Neuroophthalmol. 1994;14(1):38–44.

28. Hattenhauer MG, Leavitt JA, Hodge DO, Grill R, Gray DT. Incidence of nonarteritic anterior ischemic optic neuropathy. Am J Ophthalmol. 1997;123(1):103–7.

29. Purvin V, King R, Kawasaki A, Yee R. Anterior ischemic optic neuropathy in eyes with optic disc drusen. Arch Ophthalmol. 2004;122(1):48–53.

30. Burde RM. Optic disk risk factors for nonarteritic anterior ischemic optic neuropathy. Am J Ophthalmol. 1993;116(6):759–64.

31. Hellmich B, Agueda A, Monti S, Buttgereit F, de Boysson H, Brouwer E, et al. 2018 update of the EULAR recommendations for the management of large vessel vasculitis. Ann Rheum Dis. 2020;79:19–30.

32. Stone JH, Tuckwell K, Dimonaco S, Klearman M, Aringer M, Blockmans D, et al. Trial of tocilizumab in giant-cell arteritis. N Engl J Med. 2017;377(4):317–28.

33. Chaon BC, Lee MS. Is there treatment for traumatic optic neuropathy? Curr Opin Ophthalmol. 2015;26(6):445–9.

34. Yu-Wai-Man P, Griffiths PG. Steroids for traumatic optic neuropathy. Cochrane Database Syst Rev. 2013;(6):CD006032.

35. De Smit E, O'Sullivan E, Mackey DA, Hewitt AW. Giant cell arteritis: ophthalmic manifestations of a systemic disease. Graefes Arch Clin Exp Ophthalmol. 2016;254(12):2291–306.

36. Bidot S, Bruce BB. Update on the diagnosis and treatment of idiopathic intracranial hypertension. Semin Neurol. 2015;35(5):527–38.

37. Fraser JA, Biousse V, Newman NJ. The neuro-ophthalmology of mitochondrial disease. Surv Ophthalmol. 2010;55(4):299–334.

38. Grzybowski A, Zulsdorff M, Wilhelm H, Tonagel F. Toxic optic neuropathies: an updated review. Acta Ophthalmol. 2015;93(5):402–10.

39. Pula JH, Yuen CA. Eyes and stroke: the visual aspects of cerebrovascular disease. Stroke Vasc Neurol. 2017;2(4):210–20.

40. Biousse V, Trobe JD. Transient monocular visual loss. Am J Ophthalmol. 2005;140(4):717–21.

41. Lawlor M, Perry R, Hunt BJ, Plant GT. Strokes and vision: the management of ischemic arterial disease affecting the retina and occipital lobe. Surv Ophthalmol. 2015;60(4):296–309.

42. Tetsuka S, Ogawa T. Posterior reversible encephalopathy syndrome: a review with emphasis on neuroimaging characteristics. J Neurol Sci. 2019;404:72–9.

Diplopia, Third Nerve Palsies, and Sixth Nerve Palsies

6

Janet C. Rucker and Rachel Calix

Introduction

Ocular motor deficits are common clinical manifestations of neurological emergencies and may be the distinctive clinical feature facilitating accurate lesion localization. Two of the most common ocular motor deficits, third nerve (oculomotor, CN III) palsies and sixth nerve (abducens, CN VI) palsies, are the focus of this chapter. Ocular misalignment from dysfunction of these nerves causes binocular diplopia that resolves with monocular covering of either eye.

Comprehensive coverage of the myriad causes of third and sixth nerve palsies is not the goal of this chapter and can be found in other sources [1, 2]. Rather, the focus is on the relationship between these cranial nerve palsies and true neurological emergencies (Table 6.1) with high risk of mortality or morbidity. As with most neurological signs, accurate localization is achieved by consideration of the sign and "the company it keeps." A patient with a third or sixth nerve palsy should be questioned regarding headache, eye pain, vision loss in one eye, facial numbness or tingling, stiff neck, fever, confusion, changes in

Table 6.1 Neurologic emergencies that cause third and sixth nerve palsies

Alterations in intracranial pressure (ICP)
High intracranial pressure—intracranial space occupying lesion, venous sinus thrombosis
Low intracranial pressure—spontaneous intracranial hypotension
Intracranial saccular aneurysms (especially posterior communicating artery aneurysms causing third nerve palsies)
Fungal sinusitis with extension to the orbital apex or cavernous sinus
Suppurative thrombophlebitis of the internal jugular vein
Herpes zoster ophthalmicus
Cavernous sinus thrombosis
Giant cell arteritis
Meningitis (infectious, neoplastic)
Pituitary apoplexy
Stroke (ischemic and hemorrhagic)
Wernicke encephalopathy

level of consciousness, and other systemic or neurological symptoms. Brief attention in this chapter is given to third and sixth nerve palsies in combination with other signs, such as hemiparesis, hemisensory changes, ataxia, and Horner syndrome. However, the true diagnostic challenge in third and sixth nerve palsies is identification of the emergencies when they occur in neurological isolation. Cranial mononeuropathies have several benign and spontaneously resolving etiologies. Thus, clinical prowess is required to diagnose and exclude neurologic emergencies.

J. C. Rucker (✉)
Departments of Neurology and Ophthalmology, New York University Langone Medical Center, New York, NY, USA
e-mail: janet.rucker@nyulangone.org

R. Calix
Department of Neurology, New York University Langone Medical Center, New York, NY, USA

© The Author(s), under exclusive license to Springer Nature Switzerland AG 2021
K. L. Roos (ed.), *Emergency Neurology*, https://doi.org/10.1007/978-3-030-75778-6_6

Epidemiology

Epidemiologic studies on the etiologic incidence of third and sixth nerve palsies vary in analytical approach and study design and, thus, present variable etiologic distributions. Factors that significantly influence these distributions include study population (socioeconomic status, age distribution), study location (inpatient-based versus outpatient tertiary care center versus outpatient population-based studies), inclusion of unilateral versus bilateral ocular motor cranial nerve palsies, and inclusion of neurologically isolated ocular motor nerve palsies versus those associated with other neurological signs. For example, studies including primarily inpatients at tertiary care centers present much higher etiologic percentages of neurologic emergencies than outpatient-based studies, and studies including neurologically non-isolated cranial nerve palsies (such as those with coexisting papilledema) present higher percentages of neoplasm than studies including only neurologically isolated cranial mononeuropathies. In general, these epidemiologic studies are helpful in providing perspective with regard to common causative third and sixth nerve palsy lesions; however, they provide little guidance in assisting the clinician with prompt recognition of neurologic emergencies.

Third Nerve

Third nerve palsies represent approximately 30% of ocular motor cranial nerve palsies, being less common than sixth nerve palsies and more common than fourth nerve palsies [3, 4]. In large ret- rospective series of third nerve palsies with defined etiologic causes, vascular causes [most often referring to microvascular ischemic cranial mononeuropathy (not a neurologic emergency unless due to giant cell arteritis, see "Diagnosis" section below)] was among the most common identified etiologies in most series (Table 6.2), representing up to 42% of cases [3–8]. However, aneurysmal and neoplastic causes were also common, representing up to 30% and 18%, respectively, of cases, and a large percentage of patients in each series had an undetermined etiology. Thirty-four to 61% of posterior communicating artery aneurysms (PComA) are associated with third nerve paresis [9]. In the 1966 series by Rucker, metastatic neoplasms were responsible for 40% of neoplastic cases, with primary intracranial tumors representing the rest [3]. Pituitary adenomas were causative in 28% of neoplastic cases. Additional neurologic emergencies were often classified as "other," including infectious meningitis, subdural hematoma, pituitary apoplexy, and giant cell arteritis [3]. Although each of these "other" diagnoses represented less than 2% of third nerve palsies, they are true emergencies and must be differentiated from benign causes of cranial nerve dysfunction.

The presence or absence of pupillary involvement has historically been considered critical to defining the differential diagnosis of the etiology of a third nerve palsy (see "Clinical Features" and "Diagnosis" sections); however, the etiologic series in Table 6.2 represent all third nerve palsies, regardless of pupillary function.

Bilateral third nerve palsies (Figs. 6.1 and 6.2) are much less common than unilateral third nerve palsies. The series in Table 6.2 included both uni-

Table 6.2 Causes of third nerve palsies

	Trauma	Neoplasm	Vascular [a]	Aneurysm	Undetermined	Other
Rucker 1958 $n = 335$	15[b]	11	19	19	28	8
Rucker 1966 $n = 274$	12	18	17	18	20	15
Rush 1981 $n = 290$[c]	16	12	21	14	23	14
Park 2008 $n = 48$	19	6	35	11	19	11
Chen 2019 $n = 121$	6	5	36	30	15	18
Fang 2017 $n = 145$	12	11	42	6	4	25

[a]Specifically, microvascular ischemia
[b]All numbers given in percentage of the total n and rounded to nearest whole number
[c]First study following widespread use of head CT imaging

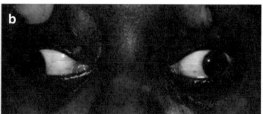

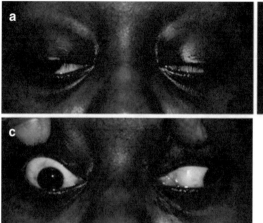

Fig. 6.1 Bilateral third nerve palsies in a 34-year-old woman status-post resection of a midbrain cavernous malformation following midbrain hemorrhage. Pupils were dilated to 8 mm bilaterally and were nonreactive to light; upgaze was almost completely absent in both eyes, and there was minimal depression of each eye. (**a**) Primary position with bilateral ptosis and a large outward devia-tion of the eyes (exotropia). (**b**) Attempted right gaze reveals full abduction of the right eye (normal sixth nerve function) but completely absent adduction of the left eye. (**c**) Attempted left gaze reveals full abduction of the left eye (normal sixth nerve function) but completely absent adduction of the right eye

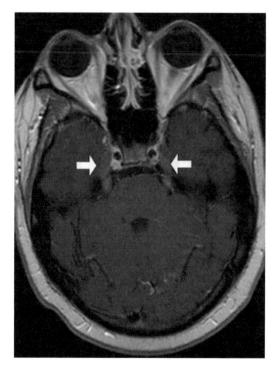

Fig. 6.2 Axial gadolinium-enhanced T1-weighted brain MRI reveals enhancement along the course of both fifth (CN V, trigeminal) nerves (*white arrows*) in a patient with systemic lymphoma. On examination, the patient had bilateral loss of facial sensation and bilateral third nerve palsies from involvement of both cavernous sinuses

lateral and bilateral cases in the etiologic distributions. In the largest case series specifically addressing the frequency of bilateral involvement of a single cranial nerve, bilateral third nerve palsies represented only 5% of 578 cases of simultaneous involvement of a single nerve among all 12 cranial nerves [10]. Vascular causes, including subarachnoid and brainstem hemorrhage and brainstem infarction, were the most common etiologies. Bilateral posterior communicating artery aneurysm (PComA) causing bilateral third nerve palsies are very rare, but can occur [11].

Sixth Nerve

Sixth nerve palsies are more common than third or fourth nerve palsies, representing up to 40–50% of ocular motor cranial nerve palsies [3, 4]. In large retrospective series of sixth nerve palsies with defined etiologic causes in patients of all ages, wider variability is seen than in the third nerve palsy series. Of sixth nerve palsies in adults, approximately 30% are due to microvascular ischemia (not a neurologic emergency unless due to giant cell arteritis, see "Diagnosis" section), 30% due to neoplasm (Table 6.3) and, in

Table 6.3 Causes of sixth nerve palsies

	Trauma	Neoplasm	Vascular[a]	Aneurysm	Undetermined	Other
Rucker1958 n = 545	16[b]	21	11	6	30	16
Shrader 1960 n = 104	3	7	36	0	24	30
Rucker 1966 n = 515	11	31	8	3	22	25
Robertson 1970 n = 133 (children)	20	39	<1[c]	2	9	29
Keane 1976 Bilateral VI, n = 125	10	22	0	0	2	66
Keane 1976 n = 143	14	18	2	1	4	61
Rush 1981 n = 419	17	14	18	3	30	18
Moster 1984 n = 49 (age <50)	6	16	29	0	22	27
Lee 1999 n = 75 (children)	12	45	0	0	5	37
Patel 2004 n = 137	12	5	35	2	26	20
Park 2008 n = 108	19	5	28	4	24	20

[a]Specifically, microvascular ischemia (with exception of Robertson study in children, see notation[c])
[b]All numbers given in percentage of the total n and rounded to nearest whole number
[c]Vascular in this case refers to an arteriovenous malformation

most series, between 20% and 30% have an undetermined etiology [3–6, 12–15]. In series dedicated to children, neoplasms were the most common cause of sixth nerve dysfunction and, in many cases, were accompanied by papilledema and nystagmus [16, 17]. In the 1966 series by Rucker, metastatic neoplasms were responsible for 40% of neoplastic cases, with nasopharyngeal carcinoma being the most common [3]. Primary intracranial tumors represented the rest. Pontine gliomas (the majority in children) were the most common primary brain tumor and pituitary adenomas were causative in only 5% of neoplastic cases. Neurologic emergencies were included among the large number of cases classified as "other," including intracranial hypertension, Wernicke encephalopathy, infectious meningitis, subdural hematoma, and giant cell arteritis. As with third nerve palsies, each of these represented a small percentage of cases, but they are of extreme importance as neurologic emergencies [3, 13].

Bilateral sixth nerve palsies (Fig. 6.3) are much less common than unilateral sixth nerve palsies, but are more common than bilateral third nerve palsies. The series in Table 6.3 included both unilateral and bilateral cases without distinction in the etiologic distributions, with exception of the series by Keane, in which etiologies were compared between bilateral sixth nerve palsies (125 cases) and unilateral sixth nerve palsies

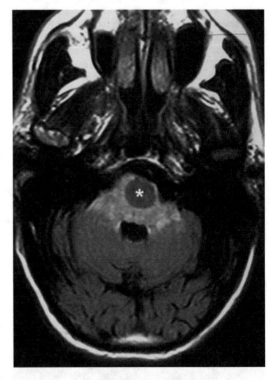

Fig. 6.3 Axial T1-weighted brain MRI through the pons reveals a metastatic lesion (white asterisk) with surrounding edema. The patient presented with binocular, horizontal diplopia due to bilateral sixth nerve palsies

(143 cases) [13]. In the acute inpatient setting of this series, the majority of both bilateral and unilateral sixth nerve palsies fell into the "other" category, with subarachnoid hemorrhage, infection,

stroke, and raised intracranial pressure as common etiologies. In the case series specifically addressing the frequency of bilateral involvement of a single cranial nerve, bilateral sixth nerve palsies represented 40% of 578 cases of simultaneous involvement of single nerve among all 12 cranial nerves. Trauma was the most common etiology [10].

Pathophysiology and Anatomy

Third Nerve

Paired third nerve nuclei lie at the level of the superior colliculus ventral to the periaqueductal gray matter. Each nucleus contains inferior rectus, medial rectus, and inferior oblique subnuclei providing ipsilateral innervation; a superior rectus subnucleus providing contralateral innervation; and an Edinger–Westphal nucleus supplying ipsilateral preganglionic parasympathetic output to the iris sphincter and ciliary muscles. A single midline caudal central subnucleus provides innervation to both levator palpebrae superioris muscles.

The third nerve fascicle originates ventrally from each nucleus, passes through or near to the red nucleus, and emerges from the ventral midbrain as rootlets in the interpeduncular fossa. The rootlets converge into a nerve trunk that passes through the subarachnoid space and between the superior cerebellar and posterior cerebral arteries. The third nerve travels parallel to the posterior communicating artery (PCom) and is very near to the anterior PCom at its junction with the intracranial internal carotid. In the cavernous sinus, the third nerve is within the lateral dural wall, lateral to the pituitary gland and sella. In the anterior cavernous sinus, it physically separates into superior and inferior divisions, although patterns of pupil and muscle involvement in more posterior lesions suggest that functional division occurs in the midbrain [18–21]. The inferior division innervates the inferior and medial recti, the inferior oblique, and the iris sphincter and ciliary

muscles. The superior division innervates the superior rectus and the levator palpebrae superioris. Inferior and superior divisions enter the orbit through the superior orbital fissure. Parasympathetic fibers synapse in the ciliary ganglion in the orbit prior to innervating the iris sphincter and ciliary body.

The most important third nerve neurological emergency occurs as the third nerve passes through the subarachnoid space in close approximation to the PCom at its junction with the internal carotid artery. This is the location of PComA that cause third nerve dysfunction via direct aneurysmal compression of the ipsilateral nerve (Fig. 6.4). Other less common third nerve emergencies include ischemic or hemorrhagic stroke at the level of the midbrain fascicle, unilateral or bilateral third nerve compression in the cavernous sinus from pituitary apoplexy, and giant cell arteritis which may cause ischemia of the third nerve anywhere along its course.

Sixth Nerve

Paired sixth nerve nuclei in the medial dorsal pons in the fourth ventricular floor lie in close proximity to the facial nerve fascicles. Each nucleus contains abducens motoneurons that form the ipsilateral sixth nerve and interneurons that decussate at the nuclear level and ascend in the medial longitudinal fasciculus to the contralateral medial rectus subnucleus of the third nerve nucleus. These interneurons facilitate conjugate horizontal gaze in the direction ipsilateral to the interneuron nuclear origin. From the ventral surface of the nucleus, the sixth nerve fascicle passes through the pons, emerges from the caudoventral pons, and passes through the subarachnoid space. It then ascends near the clivus, pierces the dura, and passes under the petroclinoid (Gruber's) ligament into Dorello's canal. In the cavernous sinus, the sixth nerve is free within the sinus body lateral and adjacent to the internal carotid artery. It enters the orbit through the superior orbital fissure to innervate the lateral rectus muscle.

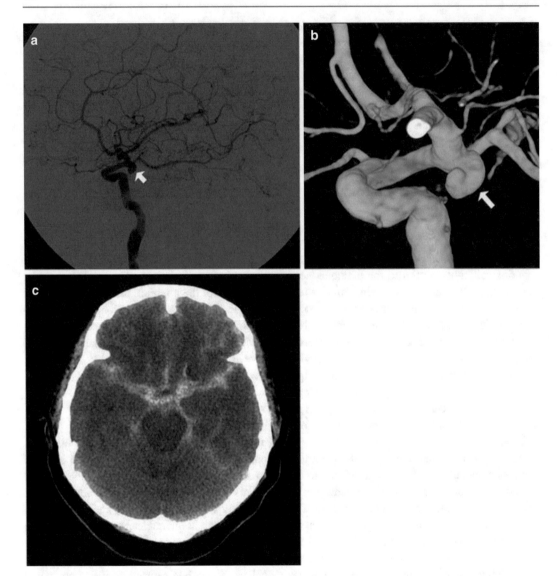

Fig. 6.4 Conventional cerebral angiogram (left internal carotid artery catheterization) reveals a 6–7-mm aneurysm on standard images (**a**) and 3D reconstructed images (**b**) at the junction of the left internal carotid artery and a fetal origin posterior communicating artery. The 55-year-old patient presented with a left third nerve palsy, syncope, severe headache, and confusion. Head CT reveals subarachnoid hemorrhage (**c**). (Images courtesy of Deborah Carson and Dr. Aman Patel)

Sixth nerve palsies due to neurological emergencies tend to occur at the level of the sixth nerve fascicle within the pons or as the nerve passes into Dorello's canal. Pontine ischemic or hemorrhagic infarction and Wernicke encephalopathy affect the former, whereas alterations in intracranial pressure affect the latter.

Clinical Features

Third Nerve

General Clinical Appearance

A third nerve palsy may result in paresis of any third nerve innervated muscle: inferior, superior,

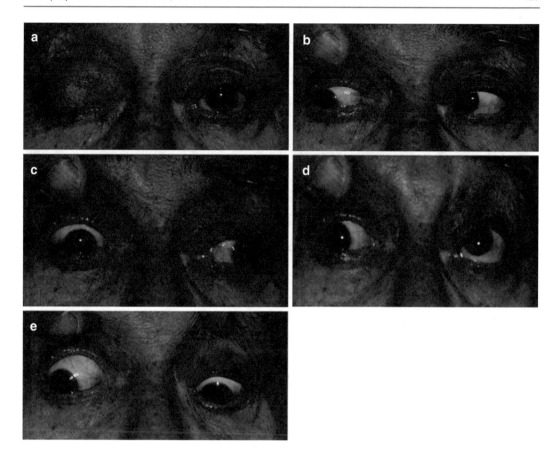

Fig. 6.5 Partial right third nerve palsy from a right intra-cavernous carotid artery aneurysm. The pupil was partially affected with the right pupil larger than the left and slightly less reactive to light. (**a**) Complete right ptosis. (**b**) Right gaze with normal abduction of the right eye. (**c**) Left gaze with impaired adduction of the right eye. (**d**) Upgaze with absent elevation of the right eye, which is also shown to be exotropic. (**e**) Downgaze with fairly intact depression of the right eye

or medial recti; inferior oblique; levator palpebrae superioris; or pupillary iris sphincter (Figs. 6.1, 6.5, and 6.6). The structures may be individually affected, affected in any partial combination with or without pupillary involvement, or all may be simultaneously affected. When all innervated structures are simultaneously fully paralyzed, the classic appearance of a complete third nerve palsy results in an eye that is "down and out" (in other words, hypotropic and exodeviated) and completely ptotic with a dilated nonreactive pupil. Eye depression (from inferior rectus involvement), elevation (from superior rectus and inferior oblique involvement), and adduction (from medial rectus involvement) are all eliminated in a complete third nerve palsy. Complete

superior divisional third nerve palsies cause ptosis and impaired elevation (especially in an abducted eye position) of the ipsilateral eye, whereas complete inferior divisional third nerve palsies cause impaired elevation, depression, and adduction with pupillary involvement of the ipsilateral eye. Historically, great emphasis was placed on the presence or absence of pupillary involvement in a third nerve palsy as a guide to determine likely etiology; however neither this, nor demographic features or the presence or absence of pain, can be used to fully rule out emergent etiologies [22].

The presence or absence of aberrant regeneration should be specifically sought in the clinical examination of any third nerve palsy. Retraction

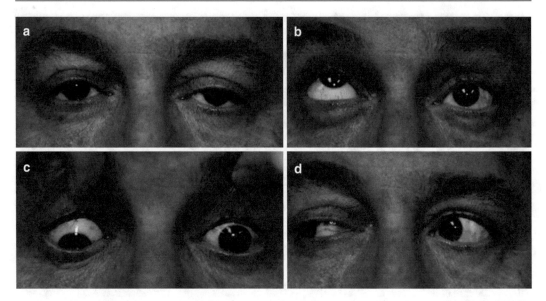

Fig. 6.6 Partial left third nerve palsy due to a left cavernous sinus meningioma. Left sixth nerve function was intact (not shown). Prior to pharmacologic dilation, there was pupillary involvement (not shown) with 2-mm anisocoria and a large, poorly reactive left pupil. In all photos, pupils are pharmacologically dilated. (**a**) Left ptosis and a small exotropia in primary position. (**b**) Minimal elevation of left eye in attempted upgaze. (**c**) Minimal depression of the left eye in attempted downgaze. (**d**) Mild impairment of adduction of the left eye in attempted right gaze. Note the widening of the palpebral fissure upon adduction, consistent with aberrant regeneration

of the upper lid (pseudo von Graefe phenomenon) or miosis during adduction or depression of the eye, or adduction occurring with downgaze provide evidence of aberrant regeneration, or anomalous axonal reinnervation [23, 24]. This is almost always due to third nerve dysfunction caused by a compressive or traumatic etiology (see Fig. 6.6) and is thought to be due either to misdirection of regenerating axons or to ephaptic transmission caused by disruption of endoneurial integrity. This does not occur in microvascular ischemic third nerve palsy and should raise concern for an alternative etiology [25].

Full neurological examination should be performed to determine if the third nerve is affected in isolation. In order to determine that the sixth and fourth nerves are not affected, abduction of the affected eye (sixth nerve function) and intorsion of the abducted eye upon attempted downgaze (fourth nerve function) should be intact.

PCom Aneurysm

PComA (at the junction of the PCom and internal carotid artery) is the etiology of any pupi-linvolving or partial third nerve palsy (even if not involving the pupil) [3, 9, 21] until definitively proven otherwise. The pupil is particularly prone to involvement from PComA because parasympathetic fibers to the iris pupillary sphincter muscle are in a peripheral and superomedial location in the third nerve as it passes near the PCom [26, 27]; however, 33% of PCom aneurysmal partial third nerve palsies have normal pupillary function at initial presentation, although the majority will develop pupillary involvement within 1 week [9]. Complete third nerve dysfunction is found immediately upon presentation in up to 36% of PComA [9, 28]. By 24 h and 1 week after presentation, 46% and 66% of third nerve palsies are complete, respectively. Fourteen percent remain partial and incomplete [28].

It is worth emphasizing that the term pupil-sparing complete third nerve palsy refers only to the situation in which the function of all third nerve-innervated structures except the pupil is 100% absent. It is a common misconception that recognition of pupil-sparing in any third nerve palsy makes PComA less probable. This is absolutely untrue and clinical application of this misconception may result in subarachnoid hemorrhage and death from rupture of an untreated aneurysm [22]. A fair degree of confidence in a non-aneurysmal third nerve palsy etiology can only be attained when pupil-sparing occurs in the setting of an otherwise complete third nerve palsy. The necessity of imaging in this setting to rule out an aneurysm is controversial [29]; however, it is generally accepted in this era of access to non-invasive imaging that *all* third nerve palsies warrant urgent intracranial vascular imaging in order to avoid errors in examination interpretation and missed diagnoses [22, 30, 31]. The onset of a third nerve palsy after mild to moderate head trauma also warrants intracranial vascular imaging for an underlying aneurysm.

Spontaneous improvement in third nerve function may occur prior to aneurysm treatment and should not dissuade from full diagnostic evaluation for underlying PComA as the cause of a third nerve palsy [32]. Aberrant regeneration in the setting of third nerve dysfunction from a PComA usually develops following the acute third nerve palsy. Primary aberrant regeneration in the absence of an acute third nerve palsy is often due to a meningioma in the cavernous sinus or an intracavernous carotid artery aneurysm; however, it is also reported in the setting of PComA [33–35].

Third nerve dysfunction may occur in isolation due to an unruptured aneurysm, or it may accompany subarachnoid hemorrhage (Figs. 6.4, 6.7, and 6.8) with other neurologic symptoms and signs. Pain is present in over 60% of patients with an ipsilateral third nerve palsy due to PComA, even in the absence of subarachnoid hemorrhage, and may precede development of ptosis or diplopia by up to 2 weeks [28, 36]. The location of the pain is generally ipsilateral and periocular or retrobulbar and is thought to be due

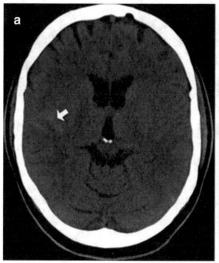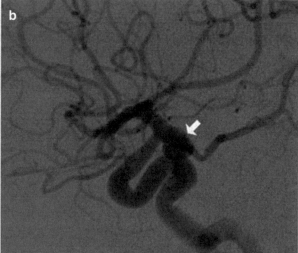

Fig. 6.7 (**a**) Head CT scan reveals focal subarachnoid hemorrhage in the right sylvian fissure (*white arrow*). Conventional cerebral angiogram demonstrates a 6.5×6×5.4-mm aneurysm at the junction of the right internal carotid artery and a fetal origin right posterior cerebral artery pretreatment (**b**, *white arrow*) and following endovascular coil embolization (**c**, *white arrow*). (Images courtesy of Deborah Carson and Dr. Aman Patel)

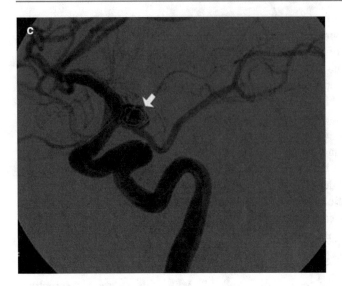

Fig. 6.7 (continued)

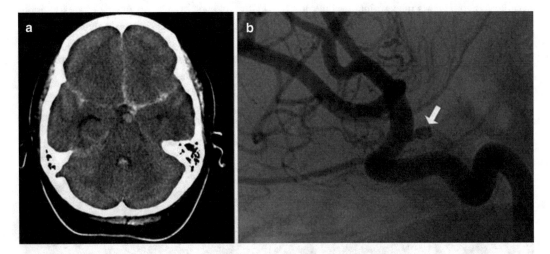

Fig. 6.8 (**a**) Head CT scan reveals subarachnoid hemorrhage. Conventional angiogram demonstrates a $3 \times 2 \times 2.8$-mm aneurysm at the junction of the left internal carotid and posterior communicating arteries pretreatment (**b**, *white arrow*) and following endovascular coil emboliza-

tion (**c**, *black arrow*). Compare the more extensive hemorrhage caused by this small aneurysm with the small amount of hemorrhage caused by the larger aneurysm in Fig. 6.7. (Images courtesy of Deborah Carson and Dr. Aman Patel)

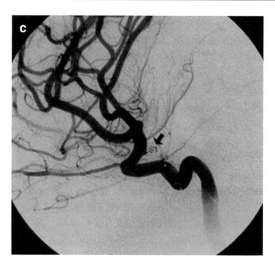

Fig. 6.8 (continued)

to involvement of sensory afferent fibers from the ophthalmic division of the fifth nerve that travel in the periphery of the third nerve [37]. Pain in this location accompanying a third nerve palsy, however, is not specific to PComA. It is also common with microvascular third nerve palsies [8, 38]. The absence of pain also does not exclude PComA as the cause of a third nerve palsy.

While PComA are, by far, the most common aneurysmal cause of third nerve palsies, any saccular or cerebrospinal fluid cisternal aneurysm is a neurologic emergency, and third nerve palsy occurs occasionally from aneurysms in other locations, such as the basilar tip or anterior choroidal artery [36, 39, 40]. Superior division third nerve palsies lacking pupillary involvement may occur with such aneurysms [21]. Basilar aneurysm is a reported cause of a pupil-sparing otherwise complete third nerve palsy. The reports on these non-PCom aneurysms underscore the limited utility of the pupillary exam in ruling out emergency causes of third nerve dysfunction [41]. Rarely, subarachnoid hemorrhage and third nerve palsy occur in the absence of an identified aneurysm. In this setting, an aneurysm may or may not be found upon repeat diagnostic evaluation [42, 43].

Brainstem Stroke

Ischemic and hemorrhagic midbrain stroke may cause unilateral or bilateral third nerve palsies due to involvement of the third nerve fascicle [44, 45]. Inferior and superior divisional partial third nerve palsies (see above subsection "General Clinical Appearance" in this section) are reported, as are paresis of a single muscle and isolated mydriasis and ptosis in the absence of ocular motility deficits [19, 46–48]. Although isolated third nerve dysfunction has been reported with midbrain strokes, it is rare and accompanying neurological signs are typically present. Named brainstem syndromes occur most often from stroke. Current syndromic descriptions vary somewhat from the original descriptions [49, 50]. All include an ipsilesional third nerve palsy in combination with other findings: contralesional ataxia (Claude syndrome, superior cerebellar peduncle involvement), ipsilesional ataxia (Nothnagel syndrome, superior cerebellar peduncle or pedunculopontine nucleus involvement), contralesional hemiparesis (Weber syndrome, cerebral peduncle involvement) (Fig. 6.9), or contralesional chorea or tremor (Benedikt syndrome, red nucleus involvement). Details regarding the clinical appearance of the third nerve palsy in these syndromes are few, but in Claude syndrome, pupil-sparing partial third nerve dysfunction with predominant medial rectus involvement may be most common [51].

Third nerve palsies may also occur in combination with vertical supranuclear gaze palsies, as the midbrain is the location of the rostral interstitial medial longitudinal fasciculus and interstitial nucleus of Cajal, structures responsible for vertical gaze control. Third nerve dysfunction occurs in 35% of infarctions restricted to the midbrain [44, 52]. Aberrant regeneration following an intra-axial cause of third nerve palsy is exceedingly rare, but reported [53]. Demyelinating lesions, including neuromyelitis optica, and brainstem encephalitides may also affect the third nerve brainstem fascicle or nuclei in isola-

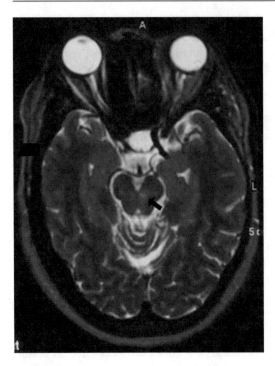

Fig. 6.9 T2-weighted axial brain MRI reveals increased T2 signal in the left ventral midbrain in a patient with ischemic Weber syndrome with right hemiparesis and a left third nerve palsy

tion [4, 54–57], or theoretically, with any of the above combination of neurological signs.

Uncal Herniation

In the subarachnoid space, the third nerve passes in close proximity to the medial temporal lobe. Herniation of the temporal lobe uncus secondary to increased intracranial pressure may cause compression of the third nerve. This most commonly manifests clinically as sudden enlargement and poor reactivity of the pupil ipsilateral to the herniating uncus and is termed the "Hutchison's pupil [58]." Uncal herniation may also present with third nerve compression due to a contralateral supratentorial lesion [59].

Meningitis

Third nerve involvement in the interpeduncular fossa and subarachnoid space may occur secondary to infectious or neoplastic meningitis [60]. Usually, the third nerve palsy will be persistent, but rarely may be transient and episodic. In the

latter scenario, it may be due to an accompanying infectious vasculitis with transient ischemia to the nerve or to raised intracranial pressure [61, 62]. The patient will often have accompanying signs suggesting meningitis, such as fever, nuchal rigidity, papilledema, or Kernig's and Brudzinski's signs.

Pituitary Apoplexy

Pituitary apoplexy is due to hemorrhage and necrosis within a preexisting pituitary adenoma. It may occur spontaneously or following a medical procedure, such as cardiac surgery (Fig. 6.10). Given the anatomic location of the third nerves within the dural walls of the cavernous sinuses directly lateral to the pituitary gland and sella, sudden lateral expansion of a pituitary adenoma from apoplexy often leads to unilateral or bilateral third nerve palsies [63]. They may occur as an isolated sign [64, 65] (often associated with severe headache), but often are also accompanied

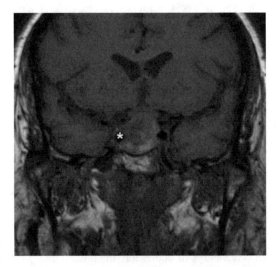

Fig. 6.10 Coronal T1-weighted noncontrasted brain MRI showing a pituitary adenoma in a 62-year-old patient who developed a right third nerve palsy, right optic neuropathy, and a bitemporal hemianopia with severe headache acutely following cardiac stent placement. Note the heterogenous signal characteristics within the adenoma, suggestive of hemorrhage and/or necrosis within a preexisting tumor. Also note the predominant lateral expansion of the mass toward the right (*asterisk* is placed within the right internal carotid flow void within the cavernous sinus), which explains the predominant right-sided presentation

by other ocular motor nerve involvement and severe vision loss due to intracranial optic nerve and chiasmal compression via upward expansion of the pituitary mass [66]. This condition is a true medical emergency not only because of the possibility of permanent vision loss if the optic apparatus is not quickly decompressed but also because of its propensity to lead to Addisonian crisis.

Infectious Orbital and Cavernous Sinus Disease

Infectious sinus disease from aspergillosis, mucormycosis, or bacterial pathogens may spread to the orbital apex or cavernous sinus and cause third nerve dysfunction, often accompanied by dysfunction of neighboring structures. Septic cavernous sinus thrombosis may also occur [67–70]. In the orbital apex, structures include the optic nerve, first division of the fifth nerve (trigeminal, CN V), fourth nerve (trochlear, CN IV), and sixth nerve (abducens, CN VI). In the cavernous sinus, structures include the first and second divisions of the fifth nerve, fourth nerve, and sixth nerve. With orbital apex involvement, proptosis and conjunctival injection and swelling may also be present. This diagnosis should be particularly suspected in patients with diabetes and in those who are immunosuppressed.

Suppurative thrombophlebitis of the internal jugular vein is a rare but potentially fatal complication of anaerobic septicemias and can progress to internal jugular venous thrombosis with retrograde propogation into the cavernous sinus [71, 72]. Lemierre's syndrome is a septicemia traditionally due to acute oropharyngeal infection progressing to thrombophlebitis of the internal jugular vein; however, infection in many adjacent structures (ear, mastoid, or dental) can present similarly in various age groups. Non-neuro-ophthalmologic complications of this syndrome include septic pulmonary emboli, empyema, intra-abdominal abscesses, and soft tissue lesions. Rarely, aseptic cavernous sinus thrombosis may occur, which is usually seen in the context of hypercoaguable states, trauma, or

mechanical compression of the venous system [70, 73].

Herpes zoster infection can present with ocular motor dysfunction including third nerve palsy via meningitis or tracking of infection to the cavernous sinus. (See section on "Clinical Appearance of Sixth Nerve Palsy" for more details on ophthalmoplegia in herpes zoster ophthalmicus.)

Giant Cell Arteritis

Ocular motor presentations of giant cell arteritis are uncommon but are important to identify due to the high risk of bilateral blindness from ischemic optic neuropathies if left undiagnosed. Third nerve palsies may be pupil-involving or pupil-sparing and are reported both in isolation and with simultaneous ischemic optic neuropathy [74–76]. Any patient over the age of 70 with an acute-onset third nerve palsy should be questioned about typical giant cell arteritis symptoms of fatigue, jaw claudication, and scalp tenderness and should have a sedimentation rate and C-reactive protein checked, followed by steroid treatment and temporal artery biopsy if there is clinical suspicion.

Sixth Nerve

General Clinical Appearance

A fascicular sixth nerve palsy results in impaired ipsilateral abduction of the eye and deviation of the eyes towards one another (esotropia). Binocular horizontal diplopia and the esotropia are worse with gaze in the direction of impaired abduction. This is in contrast to a nuclear sixth nerve palsy which results in conjugate horizontal gaze palsy towards the side of the lesion.

Brainstem Stroke

Ischemic and hemorrhagic pontine stroke may cause unilateral or bilateral sixth nerve palsies due to involvement of the sixth nerve fascicle. Although isolated sixth nerve dysfunction is reported [77, 78], accompanying neurological signs are often present. The following named brainstem syndromes occur most commonly with stroke. All include an ipsilesional sixth nerve palsy in combination with other signs: contralesional ataxia and ipsilesional facial weakness, Horner syndrome, deafness, and loss of facial sensation and taste (Foville syndrome); contralesional hemiparesis and ipsilesional facial weakness (Millard-Gubler syndrome); or contralateral hemiparesis (Raymond syndrome). Demyelinating lesions and brainstem encephalitities may also affect the sixth nerve fascicle in isolation or, theoretically, with any of the above combinations of signs [79].

Wernicke Encephalopathy

The classic triad of Wernicke encephalopathy is confusion, ophthalmoplegia, and ataxia. Horizontal gaze dysfunction, including sixth nerve palsy, is a common clinical finding. Nystagmus is the only ocular motor feature that occurs with a higher frequency than sixth nerve palsy, and the majority of patients exhibit both nystagmus and unilateral or bilateral sixth nerve palsies [80]. The accompanying nystagmus is generally gaze-evoked nystagmus, but may also be upbeat nystagmus. Characteristic MRI findings include increased T2 signal in the dorsal midbrain and medial thalami surrounding the third ventricle (Fig. 6.11). Improvement in sixth nerve dysfunction often begins within hours to days of treatment with thiamine.

Meningitis and Alterations in Intracranial Pressure

Sixth nerve involvement in the subarachnoid space may occur secondary to infectious, inflammatory, and neoplastic meningitis, either from direct involvement of the nerve or secondary to raised intracranial pressure. The sixth nerves are particularly prone to dysfunction from alterations in intracranial pressure, including raised intracranial pressure from cerebral vein thrombosis (Fig. 6.12) or idiopathic intracranial hypertension, as well as to low intracranial pressure from spontaneous intracranial hypotension [81]. It was historically suggested that the sixth nerve was affected by alterations in intracranial pressure

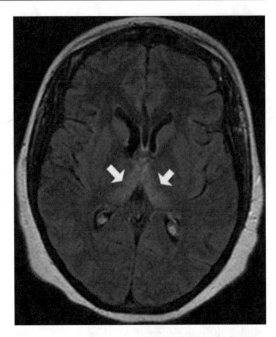

Fig. 6.11 Axial T2-weighted FLAIR brain MRI in a patient with Wernicke encephalopathy demonstrating increased T2 signal in the medial thalami surrounding the third ventricle

because of its long intracranial course; however it is shorter than the fourth nerve (trochlear nerve, CN IV), which is not prone to such injury. Rather, it is likely the tethering of the sixth nerve to the dura at its point of entry to Dorello's canal (see above section on "Pathophysiology and Anatomy of the Sixth Nerve") that leads to stretching and distortion of the nerve with alterations in intracranial pressure [82]. Within the subarachnoid space, the sixth nerve is also in close approximation with the clivus and the basilar and vertebral arteries and may be affected by neoplastic clivus disease, compression by an aneurysm, or inferior petrosal vein thrombosis [83, 84].

Pituitary Apoplexy

Sixth nerve dysfunction is more commonly due to pituitary apoplexy than is third nerve dysfunction in some series (see above section on "Clinical Appearance of Third Nerve Palsy") [63, 66]. When it occurs, it may be unilateral and isolated, although bilateral sixth nerve palsies and multiple cranial nerve palsies are also well-described

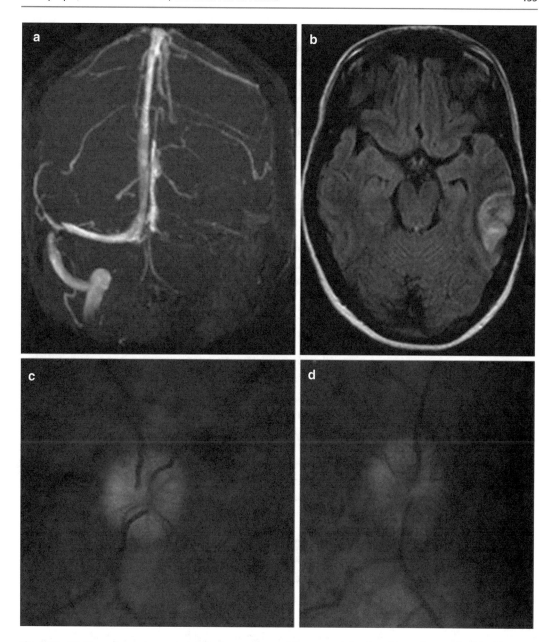

Fig. 6.12 (**a**) Magnetic resonance venogram demonstrating acute venous sinus thrombosis with lack of signal in the left transverse and sigmoid sinuses. (**b**) Axial T2-weighted FLAIR brain MRI reveals a left temporal lobe venous infarction. The patient presented with severe headaches, binocular horizontal diplopia due to bilateral sixth nerve palsies, and bilateral papilledema (**c**, right eye; **d**, left eye)

in pituitary apoplexy [66]. A single case of an isolated sixth nerve palsy as the presentation of pituitary apoplexy resulting in death has been reported [85]. Early pituitary surgery (≤14 days) has been associated with higher rate of ocular motor dysfunction resolution [66].

Infectious Orbital and Cavernous Sinus Disease

A sixth nerve palsy may result from orbital apex or cavernous sinus extension of fungal or bacterial sinus disease with or without accompanying septic cavernous sinus thrombosis (see above section on "Clinical Appearance of Third Nerve Palsy" for more details about fungal and bacterial sinus disease). Herpes zoster ophthalmicus has many ocular manifestations which affect nearly every structure of the eye. Ocular motor dysfunction occurs in 5–31% of patients and rarely can present with complete unilateral ophthalmoplegia [86, 87]. Ocular motor nerve dysfunction can be unilateral or bilateral, isolated, or in combination with other cranial nerve palsies depending on structures involved [88, 89].

Giant Cell Arteritis

Sixth nerve palsies are reported in giant cell arteritis [31, 90] (see above section on "Clinical Appearance of Third Nerve Palsy" for more details about giant cell arteritis).

Diagnosis

Third Nerve

Emergent neuroimaging to evaluate for PComA is critical in all third nerve palsies, with the sole exception of a pupil-sparing third nerve palsy that is otherwise complete, meaning complete ptosis and the complete absence of function of inferior, superior, and medial recti and the inferior oblique.

Pupil-sparing in this setting must also be complete, with no pupillary enlargement and a reaction to light that is equal in amplitude to the pupillary light reaction in the unaffected eye. The argument can be made, however, that every patient with a third nerve palsy should undergo neuroimaging regardless of pupillary status in order to avoid errors in exam interpretation and misdiagnosis [22, 31].

Non-invasive diagnostic tests for aneurysm detection include magnetic resonance angiography (MRA) and CT angiography (CTA) (Fig. 6.13). Neither of these techniques is 100% sensitive and interpretation requires skill, time, and experience, so conventional angiography should be performed when clinical suspicion for an aneurysm is high, even if noninvasive imaging techniques are normal [91, 92]. Aneurysms large enough to cause third nerve palsies are usually at least 4–5 mm, but are often less than 10 mm [36]. The sensitivity of MRA for aneurysms 5 mm or greater is in the 95–97% range but drops to roughly 50% for aneurysms less than 5 mm; for CTA, the sensitivity for aneurysms 5 mm or greater is at least 95%, but drops to less than 90% for aneurysms less than 3 mm [92]. CT angiography, even if performed with a brain CT scan, will fail to detect most non-aneurysmal causes of third nerve palsy. If aneurysm is effectively excluded by CTA and/or conventional angiogra-

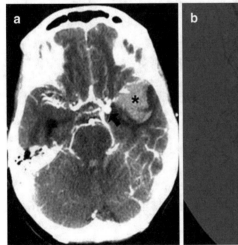 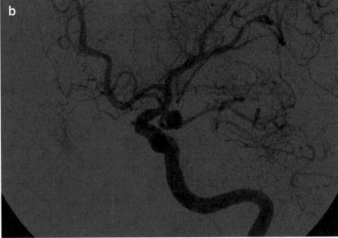

Fig. 6.13 (**a**) CT angiogram demonstrating a left temporal intraparenchymal hemorrhage (*asterisk*) and a 5× 7-mm left posterior communicating artery aneurysm. (**b**) Conventional angiogram demonstrates the aneurysm pretreatment. (Images courtesy of Deborah Carson and Dr. Aman Patel)

phy, gadolinium-enhanced brain MRI may still be necessary to seek an alternative etiology.

Microvascular

Although microvascular third nerve palsies are not neurological emergencies, they are among the most frequent causes of third nerve palsies. Although the diagnosis is not an emergent one, microvascular third nerve palsies have been shown to be associated with higher future stroke risk, especially within the first year, even after adjusting for demographics and confounding vascular risk factors [93, 94]. An isolated, painful, pupil-sparing third nerve palsy in an older patient with vascular risk factors is likely to be due to microvascular ischemia to the nerve; however, as discussed in the above section on "Clinical Features" of third nerve palsy due to PComA, a large percentage of third nerve palsies from PComA progress over several days to weeks, so one can only be relatively confident in a microvascular diagnosis if third nerve dysfunction in a pupil-sparing third nerve palsy is otherwise complete. As stated above, emergent vascular neuroimaging to evaluate for PComA should be strongly considered for all third nerve palsies.

Relative pupil involvement with an average of 0.8 mm of anisocoria may be seen in up to one-third of patients with microvascular third nerve ischemia; however, the pupil generally remains reactive [95]. Relative pupil involvement is also commonly seen with compressive mass lesions [96]. Rarely, up to 2 mm of anisocoria is seen with microvascular ischemia [97]. Spontaneous resolution of a microvascular cranial mononeuropathy occurs over 8–12 weeks. As up to 13% of patients with microvascular third cranial nerve palsies will be found to have an alternative diagnosis with MRI with gadolinium, MRA head, and sedimentation rate and C-reactive protein testing, all of these should be strongly considered at the time of diagnosis of an isolated third nerve palsy [31]. In the absence of complete, spontaneous resolution, diagnostic testing to include brain MRI with gadolinium is

essential and lumbar puncture to exclude an alternative etiology should be considered. Development of aberrant regeneration following a presumed microvascular etiology should also immediately prompt neuroimaging, as aberrant regeneration does not generally occur in this setting [25].

Head Trauma

A third nerve palsy caused by closed mechanical head trauma may or may not be a neurological emergency. A third nerve palsy due to raised intracranial pressure with uncal herniation from intracranial (epidural, subdural, or intraparenchymal) hemorrhage is a neurological emergency. Direct traumatic mechanical injury to the third nerve may not be. When third nerve dysfunction is found in the setting of mild to moderate head injury, a previously asymptomatic underlying lesion, such as PComA or skull-based intracranial tumor [98, 99], should be sought unless the head trauma was extremely severe, usually with loss of consciousness and basilar skull fracture [100, 101]. Onset of a third nerve palsy following trivial head injury suggests that the nerve is stretched over or compressed by an underlying lesion, although cases lacking identification of an underlying lesion are reported [102–105].

Sixth Nerve

The need for emergent neuroimaging in acute isolated sixth nerve palsy is controversial, especially in patients over the age of 50 with vascular risk factors [97, 106].

Microvascular

Although microvascular sixth nerve palsies are not neurological emergencies and may not warrant immediate neuroimaging, they are among the most frequent cause of sixth nerve palsies and must be distinguished from other emergent causes of sixth nerve dysfunction. An isolated, painful sixth nerve palsy in an older patient with vascular risk factors is likely to be due to micro-vascular ischemia. Compared with third nerve palsies where a PComA must not be missed, the decision if and when to perform neuroimaging in the scenario of a probable microvascular isolated sixth nerve palsy is generally considered less emergent; however, up to 19% of patients with microvascular ischemic sixth nerve palsies will be found on neuroimaging to have alternative etiologies [31], and immediate neuroimaging is preferred. Spontaneous resolution of a microvascular cranial mononeuropathy occurs over 8–12 weeks. In the absence of complete, spontaneous resolution, neuroimaging is critical.

Head Trauma

A sixth nerve palsy caused by closed mechanical head trauma may or may not be a neurological emergency. A sixth nerve palsy due to raised intracranial pressure from traumatic intracerebral (epidural, subdural, or intraparenchymal) hemorrhage is a neurological emergency. Direct traumatic mechanical injury to the sixth nerve is not. Such mechanical injury may occasionally be caused by even minor head trauma without loss of consciousness [101].

Treatment and Prognosis

Third Nerve

Treatment for a third nerve palsy consists of treatment of the underlying etiology (aneurysm, stroke, meningitis, sinusitis, etc.), as well as treatment directed at alleviating binocular diplopia. When complete ptosis is present, the affected eye is essentially patched. Ptosis often resolves before ocular motor deficits and diplopia. Treatment may consist of patching one eye, placement of temporary Fresnel press-on prisms on the patient's glasses, and ultimately strabismus surgery if the deficits fail to improve and demonstrate stability for several months. Complete or partial recovery occurs in approximately 84% of all third nerve palsies [4, 6].

With regard to intracranial aneurysms, the annual rupture rate of aneurysms less than 10 mm is less than 0.9–1.1% and 2.8–6.7% for aneurysms greater than 10 mm [107–110]. A higher rate is associated with prior subarachnoid hemorrhage, symptomatic presentation, posterior aneurysm location, and larger aneurysm size; however, even small, unruptured aneurysms presenting with third nerve palsy may rupture and lead to death before treatment occurs [36, 39, 107, 108]. The true rupture risk for small aneurysms is ill-defined, but has been shown to be as low as 0.33% [111, 112]. Treatment options include surgical clipping and neurointerventional endovascular coiling (Fig. 6.14). In a review of retrospective studies, the rate of third nerve recovery in patients treated with surgical clipping was 78%, compared to 44% in patients treated with endovascular coiling [36, 107, 108]. Higher rates of recovery occurred when managed with surgical clipping as compared to endovascular coiling in most, but not all, studies in this review. However, surgical intervention carries significant peri-procedural morbidity, and treatment decisions must consider patient status, aneurysmal morphology, and treating physician experience [108]. The presence of complete third nerve dysfunction at presentation is a poor prognostic sign, with 82.5% of patients with partial third nerve palsy reaching complete recovery compared to 38.7% of patients with complete third nerve palsy at presentation. Shorter preoperative interval also confers improved prognosis in patients with and without pre-operative subarachnoid hemorrhage [113].

Sixth Nerve

Treatment for a sixth nerve palsy consists of treatment of the underlying etiology (stroke, meningitis, sinusitis, raised intracranial pressure, etc.), as well as treatment directed at alleviating binocular diplopia. This may consist of patching one eye, placement of temporary Fresnel press-on prisms on the patient's glasses, and ultimately strabismus surgery if the deficits fail to improve and demonstrate stability for several months. Complete or partial recovery occurs in approximately 50% of all sixth nerve palsies [4].

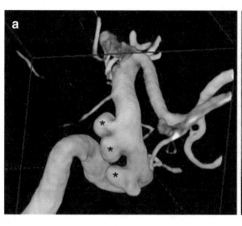
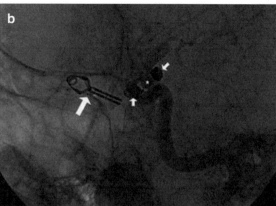

Fig. 6.14 (**a**) Three-dimensional conventional angiographic reconstructed image demonstrating three untreated aneurysms along the supraclinoid left internal carotid artery (*three black asterisks*). The most proximal is a superior hypophyseal artery aneurysm. The distal two are in the region of the posterior communicating artery. (**b**) Posttreatment angiogram demonstrating different treatment approaches. The proximal and distal left-sided aneurysms were treated with endovascular coil embolization (*two small white arrows*). The middle aneurysm (*white asterisk*) was ultimately treated by stent placement across its base due to catheter inaccessibility for coiling. The surgical clip used to treat a previously diagnosed right internal carotid artery aneurysm is also visible (*large white arrow*). (Images courtesy of Deborah Carson and Dr. Aman Patel)

Conclusion

Third and sixth nerve palsies, whether isolated or with accompanying neurological symptoms and signs, may represent true neurologic emergencies with a high risk of morbidity and mortality. A systematic and careful approach to each patient and a low threshold for neuroimaging are required to avoid common diagnostic pitfalls and misconceptions.

References

1. Miller NR, et al. Walsh & Hoyt's Clinical Neuro-Ophthalmology. 6th ed, . N.R. Miller, et al. Philadelphia: Lippincott Williams & Wilkins; 2005.
2. Leigh RJ, Zee DS. The neurology of eye movements, Contemporary neurology series. 5th ed. Oxford ; New York: Oxford University Press. xx; 2015. 1109 pages.
3. Rucker CW. The causes of paralysis of the third, fourth and sixth cranial nerves. Am J Ophthalmol. 1966;61(5 Pt 2):1293–8.
4. Rush JA, Younge BR. Paralysis of cranial nerves III, IV, and VI. Cause and prognosis in 1,000 cases. Arch Ophthalmol. 1981;99(1):76–9.
5. Rucker CW. Paralysis of the third, fourth and sixth cranial nerves. Am J Ophthalmol. 1958;46(6):787–94.
6. Park UC, et al. Clinical features and natural history of acquired third, fourth, and sixth cranial nerve palsy. Eye. 2008;22(5):691–6.
7. Chen H, et al. The aetiologies of unilateral oculomotor nerve palsy: a clinical analysis on 121 patients. Somatosens Mot Res. 2019;36(2):102–8.
8. Fang C, et al. Incidence and Etiologies of acquired third nerve palsy using a population-based method. JAMA Ophthalmol. 2017;135(1):23–8.
9. Kissel JT, et al. Pupil-sparing oculomotor palsies with internal carotid-posterior communicating artery aneurysms. Ann Neurol. 1983;13(2):149–54.
10. Keane JR. Bilateral involvement of a single cranial nerve: analysis of 578 cases. Neurology. 2005;65(6):950–2.
11. Gomez-Figueroa E, et al. Bilateral third nerve palsy in Mirror aneurysms of the posterior communicating arteries. Eur J Case Rep Intern Med. 2018;5(8):000912.
12. Shrader EC, Schlezinger NS. Neuro-ophthalmologic evaluation of abducens nerve paralysis. Arch Ophthalmol. 1960;63:84–91.
13. Keane JR. Bilateral sixth nerve palsy. Analysis of 125 cases. Arch Neurol. 1976;33(10):681–3.
14. Moster ML, et al. Isolated sixth nerve palsies in younger adults. Arch Ophthalmol. 1984;102:1328–30.
15. Patel SV, et al. Incidence, associations, and evaluation of sixth nerve palsy using a population-based method. Ophthalmology. 2004;111(2):369–75.
16. Robertson DM, Hines JD, Rucker CW. Acquired sixth nerve paresis in children. Arch Ophthalmol. 1970;83:574–9.

17. Lee MS, et al. Sixth nerve palsies in children. Pediatr Neurol. 1999;20(1):49–52.
18. Saeki N, Yamaura A, Sunami K. Bilateral ptosis with pupil sparing because of a discrete midbrain lesion: magnetic resonance imaging evidence of topographic arrangement within the oculomotor nerve. J Neuroophthalmol. 2000;20(2):130–4.
19. Ksiazek SM, et al. Divisional oculomotor nerve paresis caused by intrinsic brainstem disease. Ann Neurol. 1989;26:714–8.
20. Bhatti MT, et al. Superior divisional third cranial nerve paresis: clinical and anatomical observations of 2 unique cases. Arch Neurol. 2006;63:771–6.
21. Guy JR, Day AL. Intracranial aneurysms with superior division paresis of the oculomotor nerve. Ophthalmology. 1989;96(7):1071–6.
22. Newman NJ, Biousse V. Third nerve palsies-less frequent but just as concerning. JAMA Ophthalmol. 2017;135(1):29–30.
23. Sibony PA, Evinger C, Lessell S. Retrograde horseradish peroxidase transport after oculomotor nerve injury. Invest Ophthalmol Vis Sci. 1986;27(6):975–80.
24. Fernandez E, et al. Oculomotor nerve regeneration in rats. Functional, histological, and neuroanatomical studies. J Neurosurg. 1987;67(3):428–37.
25. Sibony PA, Lessell S, Gittinger JW Jr. Acquired oculomotor synkinesis. Surv Ophthalmol. 1984;28(5):382–90.
26. Kerr FWL, Hollowell OW. Location of pupillomotor and accommodation fibres in the oculomotor nerve: experimental observations on paralytic mydriasis. J Neurol Neurosurg Psychiatry. 1964;27:473–81.
27. Sunderland S. Mechanism responsible for changes in the pupil unaccompanied by disturbances of extra-ocular muscle function. Br J Ophthalmol. 1952;36:638–44.
28. Soni SR. Aneurysms of the posterior communicating artery and oculomotor paresis. J Neurol Neurosurg Psychiatry. 1974;37(4):475–84.
29. Miller NR. When should emergent imaging be performed? JAMA Ophthalmol. 2017;135(7):820.
30. Trobe JD. Searching for brain aneurysm in third cranial nerve palsy. J Neuroophthalmol. 2009;29(3):171–3.
31. Tamhankar MA, et al. Isolated third, fourth, and sixth cranial nerve palsies from presumed microvascular versus other causes: a prospective study. Ophthalmology. 2013;120(11):2264–9.
32. Arle JE, et al. Pupil-sparing third nerve palsy with preoperative improvement from a posterior communicating artery aneurysm. Surg Neurol. 2002;57:423–7.
33. Carrasco JR, Savino PJ, Bilyk JR. Primary aberrant oculomotor nerve regeneration from a posterior communicating artery aneurysm. Arch Ophthalmol. 2002;120(5):663–5.
34. Cox TA, Wurster JB, Godfrey WA. Primary aberrant oculomotor regeneration due to intracranial aneurysm. Arch Neurol. 1979;36(9):570–1.
35. Grunwald L, Sund NJ, Volpe NJ. Pupillary sparing and aberrant regeneration in chronic third nerve palsy secondary to a posterior communicating artery aneurysm. Br J Ophthalmol. 2008;92(5):715–6.
36. Yanaka K, et al. Small unruptured cerebral aneurysms presenting with oculomotor nerve palsy. Neurosurgery. 2003;52(3):553–7; discussion 556–7.
37. Lanzino G, et al. Orbital pain and unruptured carotid-posterior communicating artery aneurysms: the role of sensory fibers of the third cranial nerve. Acta Neurochir. 1993;120:7–11.
38. Wilker SC, et al. Pain in ischemic ocular motor cranial nerve palsies. Br J Ophthalmol. 2009;93(12):1657–9.
39. Friedman JA, et al. Small cerebral aneurysms presenting with symptoms other than rupture. Neurology. 2001;57(7):1212–6.
40. Ajtai B, Lincoff N. Pupil-sparing, painless compression of the oculomotor nerve by expanding basilar artery aneurysm: a case of pseudomyasthenia. Arch Neurol. 2004;61:1448–50.
41. Lustbader JM, Miller NR. Painless, pupil-sparing but otherwise complete oculomotor nerve paresis caused by basilar artery aneurysm. Case report. Arch Ophthalmol. 1988;106(5):583–4.
42. Marquardt G, et al. Long term follow up after perimesencephalic subarachnoid hemorrhage. J Neurol Neurosurg Psychiatry. 2000;69:127–30.
43. Kamat AA, Tizzard S, Mathew B. Painful third nerve palsy in a patient with perimesencephalic subarachnoid haemorrhage. Br J Neurosurg. 2005;19(3):247–50.
44. Kim JS, Kim J. Pure midbrain infarction: clinical, radiologic, and pathophysiologic findings. Neurology. 2005;64(7):1227–32.
45. Mizushima H, Seki T. Midbrain hemorrhage presenting with oculomotor nerve palsy: case report. Surg Neurol. 2002;58(6):417–20.
46. Chen L, Maclaurin W, Gerraty RP. Isolated unilateral ptosis and mydriasis from ventral midbrain infarction. J Neurol. 2009;256(7):1164–5.
47. Ksiazek SM, et al. Fascicular arrangement in partial oculomotor paresis. Am J Ophthalmol. 1994;118(1):97–103.
48. Castro O, Johnson LN, Mamourian AC. Isolated inferior oblique paresis from brain-stem infarction. Perspective on oculomotor fascicular organization in the ventral midbrain tegmentum. Arch Neurol. 1990;47(2):235–7.
49. Liu GT, et al. Midbrain syndromes of Benedikt, Claude, and Nothnagel: setting the record straight. Neurology. 1992;42(9):1820–2.
50. Hathout GM, Bhidayasiri R. Midbrain ataxia: an introduction to the mesencephalic locomotor region and the pedunculopontine nucleus. AJR Am J Roentgenol. 2005;184(3):953–6.
51. Seo SW, et al. Localization of Claude's syndrome. Neurology. 2001;57(12):2304–7.

52. Ogawa K, et al. Clinical study of eleven patients with midbrain infarction-induced oculomotor nerve palsy. J Stroke Cerebrovasc Dis. 2016;25(7):1631–8.
53. Messe SR, et al. Oculomotor synkinesis following a midbrain stroke. Neurology. 2001;57(6):1106–7.
54. Bentley PI, Kimber T, Schapira AH. Painful third nerve palsy in MS. Neurology. 2002;58(10):1532.
55. de Seze J, et al. Unusual ocular motor findings in multiple sclerosis. J Neurol Sci. 2006;243(1–2):91–5.
56. Kremer L, et al. Brainstem manifestations in neuromyelitis optica: a multicenter study of 258 patients. Mult Scler. 2014;20(7):843–7.
57. Yasuda K, et al. Bilateral oculomotor nerve palsy in a case of anti-aquaporin-4 antibody-positive neuromyelitis optica spectrum disorder. J Clin Neurosci. 2019;66:271–2.
58. Koehler PJ, Wijdicks EF. Fixed and dilated: the history of a classic pupil abnormality. J Neurosurg. 2015;122(2):453–63.
59. Chung KH, Chandran KN. Paradoxical fixed dilation of the contralateral pupil as a false-localizing sign in intraparenchymal frontal hemorrhage. Clin Neurol Neurosurg. 2007;109(5):455–7.
60. Li X, et al. Clinical characteristics of tuberculous meningitis combined with cranial nerve palsy. Clin Neurol Neurosurg. 2019;184:105443.
61. Azran MS, et al. Episodic third nerve palsy with cryptococcal meningitis. Neurology. 2005;64(4):759–60.
62. Keane JR. Intermittent third nerve palsy with cryptococcal meningitis. J Clin Neuroophthalmol. 1993;13(2):124–6.
63. Kim SH, Lee KC, Kim SH. Cranial nerve palsies accompanying pituitary tumour. J Clin Neurosci. 2007;14:1158–62.
64. Chen Z, Murray AW, Quinlan JJ. Pituitary apoplexy presenting as unilateral third cranial nerve palsy after coronary artery bypass surgery. Anesth Analg. 2004;98(1):46–8, table of contents.
65. Saul RF, Hilliker JK. Third nerve palsy: the presenting sign of a pituitary adenoma in five patients and the only neurological sign in four patients. J Clin Neuroophthalmol. 1985;5(3):185–93.
66. Hage R, et al. Third, fourth, and sixth cranial nerve palsies in pituitary apoplexy. World Neurosurg. 2016;94:447–52.
67. Fujikawa T, Sogabe Y. Septic cavernous sinus thrombosis: potentially fatal conjunctival hyperemia. Intensive Care Med. 2019;45(5):692–3.
68. Wang YH, et al. A review of eight cases of cavernous sinus thrombosis secondary to sphenoid sinusitis, including a12-year-old girl at the present department. Infect Dis (Lond). 2017;49(9):641–6.
69. Frank GS, et al. Ophthalmic manifestations and outcomes after cavernous sinus thrombosis in children. J AAPOS. 2015;19(4):358–62.
70. Lai PF, Cusimano MD. The spectrum of cavernous sinus and orbital venous thrombosis: a case and a review. Skull Base Surg. 1996;6(1):53–9.
71. Riordan T, Wilson M. Lemierre's syndrome: more than a historical curiosa. Postgrad Med J. 2004;80(944):328–34.
72. Golpe R, Marin B, Alonso M. Lemierre's syndrome (necrobacillosis). Postgrad Med J. 1999;75(881):141–4.
73. Dinkin M, Patsalides A, Ertel M. Diagnosis and management of cerebral venous diseases in neuro-ophthalmology: ongoing controversies. Asia Pac J Ophthalmol (Phila). 2019;8(1):73–85.
74. Lazaridis C, Torabi A, Cannon S. Bilateral third nerve palsy and temporal arteritis. Arch Neurol. 2005;62(11):1766–8.
75. Oncel C, Bir F, Bir LS. Simultaneous ischemic optic neuropathy and third cranial nerve palsy in giant cell arteritis. J Neuroophthalmol. 2007;27(4):315–6.
76. Thurtell MJ, Longmuir RA. Third nerve palsy as the initial manifestation of giant cell arteritis. J Neuroophthalmol. 2014;34(3):243–5.
77. Paik JW, Kang SY, Sohn YH. Isolated abducens nerve palsy due to anterolateral pontine infarction. Eur Neurol. 2004;52(4):254–6.
78. Fukutake T, Hirayama K. Isolated abducens nerve palsy from pontine infarction in a diabetic patient. Neurology. 1992;42(11):2226.
79. Barr D, et al. Isolated sixth nerve palsy: an uncommon presenting sign of multiple sclerosis. J Neurol. 2000;247(9):701–4.
80. Victor M, Adams R, Collins GH. The Wernicke-Korsakoff Syndrome and Related Neurological Disorders Due to Alcoholism and Malnutrition, Contemporary Neurology Series. 2nd ed. Philadelphia: F. A. Davis Company; 1989.
81. Porta-Etessam J, et al. Orthostatic headache and bilateral abducens palsy secondary to spontaneous intracranial hypotension. J Headache Pain. 2011;12(1):109–11.
82. Hanson RA, et al. Abducens length and vulnerability? Neurology. 2004;62(1):33–6.
83. Pallini R, et al. Clivus metastases: report of seven patients and literature review. Acta Neurochir. 2009;151(4):291–6; discussion 296.
84. Mittal SO, Siddiqui J, Katirji B. Abducens nerve palsy due to inferior petrosal sinus thrombosis. J Clin Neurosci. 2017;40:69–71.
85. Warwar RE, et al. Sudden death from pituitary apoplexy in a patient presenting with an isolated sixth cranial nerve palsy. J Neuroophthalmol. 2006;26(2):95–7.
86. Sanjay S, et al. Complete unilateral ophthalmoplegia in herpes zoster ophthalmicus. J Neuroophthalmol. 2009;29(4):325–37.
87. Kedar S, Jayagopal LN, Berger JR. Neurological and ophthalmological manifestations of varicella zoster virus. J Neuroophthalmol. 2019;39(2):220–31.
88. Marsh RJ, Dulley B, Kelly V. External ocular motor palsies in ophthalmic zoster: a review. Br J Ophthalmol. 1977;61(11):677–82.

89. Temnogorod J, et al. Acute orbital syndrome in herpes zoster ophthalmicus: clinical features of 7 cases. Ophthalmic Plast Reconstr Surg. 2017;33(3):173–7.

90. Lunagariya A, et al. Temporal arteritis presenting as an isolated bilateral abducens nerve palsy: a rare case of a 65-year-old male. Cureus. 2018;10(5):e2667.

91. Elmalem VI, et al. Underdiagnosis of posterior communicating artery aneurysm in noninvasive brain vascular studies. J Neuroophthalmol. 2011;31(2):103–9.

92. Chaudhary N, et al. Imaging of intracranial aneurysms causing isolated third cranial nerve palsy. J Neuroophthalmol. 2009;29(3):238–44.

93. Park SJ, et al. Ocular motor cranial nerve palsy and increased risk of stroke in the general population. PLoS One. 2018;13(10):e0205428.

94. Rim TH, et al. Stroke risk among adult patients with third, fourth or sixth cranial nerve palsy: a Nationwide cohort study. Acta Ophthalmol. 2017;95(7):e656–61.

95. Jacobson DM. Pupil involvement in patients with diabetes-associated oculomotor nerve palsy. Arch Ophthalmol. 1998;116(6):723–7.

96. Jacobson DM. Relative pupil-sparing third nerve palsy: etiology and clinical variables predictive of a mass. Neurology. 2001;56(6):797–8.

97. Chou KL, et al. Acute ocular motor mononeuropathies: prospective study of the roles of neuroimaging and clinical assessment. J Neurol Sci. 2004;219(1–2):35–9.

98. Eyster EF, Hoyt WF, Wilson CB. Oculomotor palsy from minor head trauma. An initial sign of basal intracranial tumor. JAMA. 1972;220(8):1083–6.

99. Walter KA, Newman NJ, Lessell S. Oculomotor palsy from minor head trauma: initial sign of intracranial aneurysm. Neurology. 1994;44(1):148–50.

100. Jefferson A. Ocular complications of head injuries. Trans Ophthalmol Soc U K. 1961;81:595–612.

101. Dhaliwal A, et al. Third, fourth, and sixth cranial nerve palsies following closed head injury. J Neuroophthalmol. 2006;26(1):4–10.

102. Muthu P, Pritty P. Mild head injury with isolated third nerve palsy. Emerg Med J. 2001;18(4):310–1.

103. Levy RL, Geist CE, Miller NR. Isolated oculomotor palsy following minor head trauma. Neurology. 2005;65(1):169.

104. Chen CC, et al. Isolated oculomotor nerve palsy from minor head trauma. Br J Sports Med. 2005;39(8):e34.

105. Tajsic T, et al. Isolated oculomotor nerve palsy in patients with mild head injury. Br J Neurosurg. 2017;31(1):94–5.

106. Bendszus M, et al. MRI in isolated sixth nerve palsies. Neuroradiology. 2001;43(9):742–5.

107. Brennan JW, Schwartz ML. Unruptured intracranial aneurysms: appraisal of the literature and suggested recommendations for surgery, using evidence-based medicine criteria. Neurosurgery. 2000;47(6):1359–71; discussion 1371–2.

108. Micieli JA, et al. Intracranial aneurysms of neuroophthalmologic relevance. J Neuroophthalmol. 2017;37(4):421–39.

109. Vlak MH, et al. Prevalence of unruptured intracranial aneurysms, with emphasis on sex, age, comorbidity, country, and time period: a systematic review and meta-analysis. Lancet Neurol. 2011;10(7):626–36.

110. Wermer MJ, et al. Risk of rupture of unruptured intracranial aneurysms in relation to patient and aneurysm characteristics: an updated meta-analysis. Stroke. 2007;38(4):1404–10.

111. Lee AG, Hayman LA, Brazis PW. The evaluation of isolated third nerve palsy revisited: an update on the evolving role of magnetic resonance, computed tomography, and catheter angiography. Surv Ophthalmol. 2002;47(2):137–57.

112. Murayama Y, et al. Risk analysis of Unruptured intracranial aneurysms: prospective 10-year cohort study. Stroke. 2016;47(2):365–71.

113. Zhong W, et al. Posterior communicating aneurysm with oculomotor nerve palsy: predictors of nerve recovery. J Clin Neurosci. 2019;59:62–7.

Facial Nerve Palsy

7

Jennifer Siriwardane

Introduction

The facial nerve, cranial nerve VII, innervates the muscles of facial expression and supplies innervation for lacrimation, salivation, taste on the anterior two-thirds of the tongue, dampening of sound, as well as sensation for the auricle. Bell's palsy is the term for facial nerve paralysis of unknown cause, and it is named after Sir Charles Bell who first identified the syndrome and the function of the facial nerve [1]. The facial nerve has an extended course which involves an intracranial and extracranial path, with some areas of difficulty along its course, particularly the temporal bone and at its entrance to the bony facial canal. In addition to the psychological toll of facial nerve paralysis, there is risk of corneal abrasion due to inability to blink, along with alterations of speech and smiling, and inadequate facial animation.

Epidemiology

Bell's palsy is more common in those aged 15–45 years old; those with diabetes, upper respiratory disease, or immune compromise; and during pregnancy. It has an estimated incidence of 11.5–53.3 per 100,000 person-years [2]. In a retrospective study which looked at 1989 patients referred for facial nerve palsy, Bell's palsy was the diagnosis in 38%, acoustic neuroma resection in 10%, malignancy in 7%, iatrogenic injury in 7%, varicella zoster virus infection in 7%, Lyme disease in 4%, and other etiologies in 17% [3]. Women made up a majority of cases at 62% and the mean age was 44.5 years [3].

In a study of 1701 patients with Bell's palsy, 71% eventually achieved normal facial nerve function, with a majority of patients having a complete recovery by 2 months [4]. Complete recovery is less likely if there has been no or minimal improvement after 3 months from symptom onset. Prognosis is better for those with incomplete Bell's palsy as compared to those with complete Bell's palsy [4].

The occurrence of bilateral facial nerve palsy is rare; an estimated 0.3–2.0% of facial nerve palsies are bilateral [5]. Of those with facial diplegia, 20% are idiopathic. The causes of facial diplegia include Guillain-Barre syndrome, sarcoidosis, multiple sclerosis, HIV, Lyme disease, diabetes, acute leukemia, and porphyria [6].

Facial Nerve Anatomy

An understanding of the anatomy of the facial nerve's course is immensely helpful in understanding the pathogenesis of facial nerve palsy (Fig. 7.1). The facial nerve has a motor division

J. Siriwardane (✉)
Department of Neurology, Indiana University School of Medicine, Indianapolis, IN, USA
e-mail: jemasiri@iupui.edu

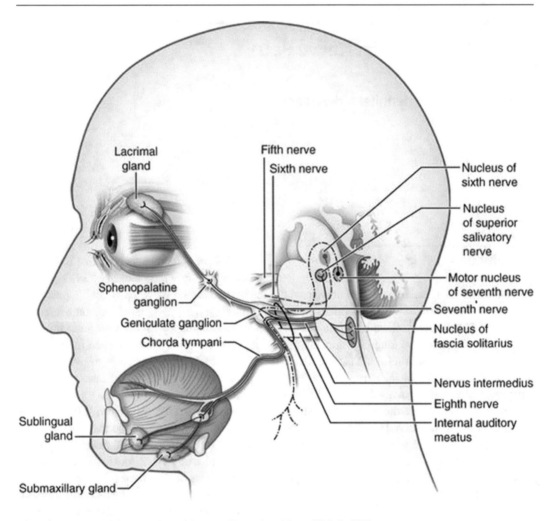

Fig. 7.1 Anatomy of the seventh cranial nerve. (Reproduced from Gilchrist [51])

and a sensory division. Within the sensory root of the facial nerve are sensory fibers which end in the spinal nucleus of cranial nerve V and preganglionic parasympathetic fibers and taste axons [7]. The facial nucleus is in the lateral pons, and the motor fibers exit the brainstem ventrolaterally at the pontomedullary junction. The sensory division of the facial nerve is separate from the motor division between the brainstem and the internal acoustic canal, but the two divisions join to enter the internal auditory meatus and course through the auditory canal of the petrous temporal bone. Cranial nerve VIII also travels through the auditory canal with cranial nerve VII. The facial nerve path through the temporal bone can be separated into four parts: the meatus, labyrinthine, tym-

panic, and mastoid parts. The meatus is the narrowest portion of the facial canal and is implicated as the site of facial nerve compression in Bell's palsy as it is quite narrow at 0.68 mm, with little room for the facial nerve to swell from any potential inflammation [8]. The labyrinthine segment is named for its proximity to the superior semicircular canal. This segment ends at the geniculate ganglion, which contains sensory neurons for taste of the anterior two-thirds of the tongue and general somatic sensation for the region near the external auditory meatus. The greater petrosal nerve branches out from the geniculate ganglion, and this eventually supplies lacrimation through parasympathetic fibers. In the tympanic segment, the stapedius nerve branches off to supply the stapedius muscle, which works to dampen sound by stabilizing the stapes bone. The stapedius muscle is interesting as it is the smallest muscle in the human body, and the stapes is the smallest bone in the human body. The mastoid segment descends to the stylomastoid foramen to proceed extracranially. The chorda tympani branches off the facial nerve in the mastoid segment, and this ultimately supplies parasympathetic fibers to the sublingual and submandibular glands, along with relaying taste from the anterior two-thirds of the tongue [9]. Most saliva production (about 70 percent) originates from the submandibular salivary glands [10]. The facial nerve then travels through the parotid gland and branches into the five major branchial motor branches which control the muscles of facial expression: the temporal, zygomatic, buccal, mandibular, and cervical branches [9].

The facial nerve has four main functional subdivisions: special visceral efferent, general visceral efferent, special afferent, and general somatic afferent subdivisions. The special visceral efferent subdivision, also known as the branchial branch, supplies motor innervation to the muscles of facial expression, the stylohyoid, stapedius, and the posterior belly of the digastric muscle. The general visceral efferent subdivision supplies parasympathetic innervation to the submandibular, sublingual, and lacrimal glands. The special sensory afferent subdivision of facial nerve supplies taste from the anterior two-thirds of the tongue. General somatic afferents provide sensory information from the tympanic membrane, external auditory canal, and the auricle [11].

Pathophysiology and Pathogenesis

As Bell's palsy is the term for acute facial nerve paralysis when no other medical etiology of facial weakness is determined, it is therefore a diagnosis of exclusion. There are a vast number of etiologies for facial nerve paralysis (Table 7.1). The two broad main categories are an acquired

Table 7.1 Causes of unilateral seventh cranial neuropathy

Relatively common	*HIV*
Bell's palsy (idiopathic)	Osteomyelitis of skull base
Herpes simplex virus	Otogenic infections
Ramsay Hunt syndrome (varicella zoster)	Parotitis/abscess
Lyme	Mastoiditis
Zoster sine herpete	Sinusitis
Trauma	Leprosy
Diabetes mellitus	Mycoplasma
Pregnancy	Influenza
Guillain-Barré syndrome	HTLV-1
Sarcoid	*Miscellaneous*
Neoplastic meningitis	Benign intracranial hypertension
Pontine infarct	Melkersson-Rosenthal
Pontine hemorrhage	Amyloidosis
Multiple sclerosis	Wegener's granulomatosis
Brainstem tumor	Polyarteritis
Facial neuropathy from forceps/birth trauma	Sjogren's syndrome
Acoustic neuroma	Hereditary neuropathy with pressure palsies (HNPP)
Relatively less common	Familial Bell's
Pontine brainstem encephalitis	CIDP
Brainstem abscess	Charcot-Marie-Tooth
Congenital/postnatal	Histiocytosis X
Mobius syndrome	Interferon therapy
Hemicranial microsomia	Sclerosteosis
Congenital lower lip paralysis	Ethylene glycol intoxication
Kawasaki disease	Wernicke-Korsakov syndrome
Albers-Schoenberg (osteopetrosis)	Stevens-Johnson syndrome
Infantile hypercalcemia	
Cardiofacial syndrome	
Tumor	
Meningioma	
Cholesteatoma	
Metastatic	
Neurinoma	
Parotid tumor	
Infectious	
Bacterial meningitis	
Fungal meningitis	
Tuberculous meningitis	
Syphilis	

Reproduced from Gilchrist [51]

deficit of the facial nerve, such as infection or injury to the nerve, or congenital malformations [12]. True developmental anomalies are rare and include Moebius syndrome and neonatal asymmetric crying facies. Moebius syndrome is a rare neurologic condition, with an incidence of about one in 50,000 in which children have trouble with muscles of facial expression and eye movement, along with micrognathia and microstomia [13].

Acquired facial nerve paralysis is much more common than congenital. The most common infectious causes of facial nerve paralysis are herpes simplex virus and varicella zoster virus. Infectious causes can lead to inflammation which compresses the nerve in the small enclosures of the facial canal. Both viruses are acquired in childhood and can reactivate from their latent state in the trigeminal or geniculate ganglia causing inflammation and paralysis [14]. McCormick first suggested that herpes simplex virus was a cause of acute facial nerve paralysis in 1972, hypothesizing that the virus remained in nerve cell endings and axons [15]. Using PCR testing on autopsy specimens, herpes simplex virus was present in 94 percent of trigeminal ganglia and 88 percent of geniculate ganglia [16]. There is increased incidence of facial paralysis in diabetic patients, and it has been suggested based on an animal study that reactivation of HSV-1 in the geniculate ganglion may be responsible for the increased incidence in diabetic patients [17].

Ramsay Hunt syndrome is peripheral facial neuropathy with an accompanying vesicular rash of the ear (herpes zoster oticus) or mouth. The cause of Ramsey Hunt syndrome is varicella zoster virus. Patients presenting with Ramsay Hunt syndrome may also complain of tinnitus, hearing loss, nausea, and vertigo, and they tend to have a severe facial paralysis with poor recovery [18]. Hunt described the proximity of the vestibulocochlear nerve to the geniculate ganglion in the confines of the bony facial canal [19], and this explains the symptoms of tinnitus, hearing loss, nausea, and vertigo seen in Ramsay Hunt syndrome.

Borrelia burgdorferi, the tick-born spirochete that causes Lyme disease, can cause a unilateral or bilateral facial nerve paralysis. Lyme disease should be considered in those presenting with facial palsy as well tick exposure, arthralgia, or the classic bull's eye skin rash of erythema nodosa associated with Lyme disease. It is reported that 10 percent of patients with Lyme disease have facial nerve palsy [20], and a study from the UK found that younger patients with Lyme disease were more likely to develop facial paralysis, possibly due to a younger population of hikers and campers [21]. Facial nerve paralysis due to Lyme disease has a good prognosis, with 95 percent of patients having a complete recovery if diagnosed early [22].

Facial nerve palsy in pregnancy is hypothesized to be due to relative immunosuppression that allows for reactivation of herpes virus, or increased extracellular volume, hypertension, or changes in hormone levels [23]. Retrospective data has shown that pregnant women may have a worse prognosis of facial nerve paralysis, as pregnant women are more likely to have a complete facial nerve paralysis [24].

Central processes are also responsible for facial palsy and include ischemia, tumor, stroke, and multiple sclerosis, among others. Facial palsy sometimes is the first sign of multiple sclerosis, but will typically present with other brainstem signs [25]. Bilateral and unilateral facial paralysis has been described in neurosarcoidosis, which can also present with myelopathy, optic neuropathy, cerebral mass lesions, and polyneuropathy. The treatment is 1 milligram per kilogram per day of prednisone or, in severe cases, intravenous methylprednisolone [26].

Clinical Presentation

The onset of acute facial nerve paralysis is typically less than 72 h [2]. Patients often present with inability to close the eye, drooping of the corner of the mouth, and loss of the nasolabial fold. There is a facial asymmetry on examination of the face: the facial creases and the nasolabial fold disappear; the affected side also may have a drooping mouth, eyelid widening, and lagophthalmos, all of which are static signs. Dynamic signs include the inability to whistle, puff the checks, frown, and close the eyelid [27]. Paralysis of all muscles of facial expression on one side is consistent with a lower motor neuron pathology, while an upper motor neuron pathology, such as a stroke, spares the frontalis muscle of the forehead.

Many experience a Bell's phenomenon, which is the rolling of the eye upwards upon trying to close the eyelid. Patients may complain of food and beverage spilling out of their mouth, and some complain of subjective numbness of the paralyzed area [28]. A postulated mechanism for this numbness is herpetic viral spread along an anatomical course involving the trigeminal nerve [29].

Along with facial muscle weakness, patients can experience impaired salivation and lacrimation due to compromise of the parasympathetic fibers of the seventh cranial nerve. Hearing loss is not a typical sign, although hyperacusis does occur as the seventh cranial nerve supplies innervation to the stapedius muscle. Damage to the chorda tympani nerve can result in dysgeusia.

Bell's palsy is a complication of pregnancy with an incidence in pregnant women of 45.1 per 100,000 births, while nonpregnant women of the same age group is 17.4 in 100,000. Of 42 cases of Bell's palsy in pregnancy, 31 of those cases occurred in the third trimester [30]. It is important to distinguish an upper motor neuron facial nerve palsy, such as a stroke, from a lower motor neuron facial nerve palsy in a pregnant woman with facial weakness as the management is distinctly different.

As a general rule, a complete facial paralysis on initial presentation carries a poorer prognosis for recovery as compared to partial facial paralysis. The presence of complete facial paralysis, hypertension, and non-ear pain all are associated with incomplete recovery [28]. A cohort study of 368 patients with Bell's palsy found that normal stapedius reflex testing and no pathological spontaneous activity in EMG were significant prognostic factors of recovery, and prednisolone therapy initiated after 96 h had a decreased recovery rate then when it was started earlier in the course. In the same study, the median onset of

treatment was 1.5 days, and the median recovery time was 2.6 months [31].

In the process of recovery, regenerating fibers can reach the wrong target, leading to phenomena such as crocodile tears, in which a person exhibits lacrimation instead of salivation at the sight of food [10]. Abnormal recovery of motor fibers can lead to synkinesis, which is an abnormal involuntary movement that occurs during voluntary movement of another muscle. For example, a patient may try to volitionally close the eye, but instead, the muscles of the mouth contract.

The presence of bilateral facial nerve palsy, which is far more rare than unilateral facial nerve palsy, should broaden the differential diagnosis to include Lyme disease, Guillain-Barré syndrome, HIV, sarcoidosis, multiple sclerosis, diabetes, or leukemia [6].

Diagnosis

The diagnosis of acute facial nerve palsy does not typically require a plethora of testing and can be made with bedside examination. The ear should be examined to assess for herpes zoster oticus, which presents as vesicles on the external auditory canal, concha, or helix, although the absence of visible lesions does not exclude Ramsay Hunt syndrome [32]. Imaging is not absolutely required, and clinicians can rely mostly on history and physical to establish the diagnosis readily. The most important question to answer in an acute setting is whether the facial weakness is due to a central or peripheral cause. An upper motor neuron pattern of weakness, or a central cause of weakness, spares the forehead of weakness; this pattern of facial weakness should alarm clinicians for a stroke or other central causes.

Upper motor neuron facial weakness will not have accompanied hyperacusis or dysgeusia, and stroke or other upper motor neuron dysfunction will likely present with other deficits beyond the face. The muscles that supply the forehead receive bilateral supranuclear innervation, while the facial muscles of the middle and lower face receive unilateral innervation from contralateral upper motor neurons [33]. A lower motor neuron pattern of weakness causes paralysis of an entire side of the face, including the forehead. This weakness is ipsilateral to the facial nerve paralysis.

Imaging is not necessary if there is high suspicion for isolated facial nerve paralysis. However, if facial weakness if suspected to be secondary to another cause, then imaging can be helpful in evaluating for pontine lesions or an internal acoustic canal mass. Bilateral facial paralysis or the involvement of multiple cranial nerves should also prompt imaging and examination of cerebrospinal fluid evaluation, as this can be the presentation of multiple sclerosis, neurosarcoidosis, or cancer with central nervous system involvement.

Testing for Lyme disease is warranted if there is suspicion that the patient has been exposed to a tick, especially in areas where the disease is more prevalent. The first is an enzyme immunoassay (EIA) or immunofluorescence assay of antibodies to the spirochete *Borrelia burgdorferi*. A positive result may indicate past or current infection, or it may be a false positive. If the result of this first step is positive or equivocal, then obtain a Western blot (immunoblot) assay for IgM and IgG; this test is more specific for Lyme disease than the EIA. The Western blot for IgM is particularly helpful when symptoms have been present for less than 4 weeks [34]. After 1 month into the course of the disease, there should be an IgG response and so an isolated IgM antibody is most likely a false positive [35]. False positives may occur with testing of IgM, the largest antibody, as there can be cross-reactivity with other pathogens [36]. The sensitivity of this two-step testing method is 70–100 percent with above 95 percent specificity [37].

EMG can be considered in those with complete facial nerve paralysis, as those with greater than 90 percent axonal loss of facial nerve can be considered for facial nerve decompression [38]. However, strong evidence for the efficacy of surgical decompression of the facial nerve is lacking, as there are limited randomized controlled trials with low power [39]. Risks of the surgery include persistent vertigo [39] and unilateral sensorineural hearing loss, with one study reporting deafness in 15 percent of patients who underwent surgical decompression [40].

MRI can be considered in those with multiple cranial nerve dysfunction or other neurologic signs. Gadolinium enhancement of the facial nerve can be seen on MRI in some patients with facial nerve paralysis, but the presence of this enhancement does not indicate a worse prognosis [41].

Management and Treatment

The main pearls of management of acute facial nerve palsy are corticosteroids with the use of eye lubricants to prevent corneal abrasion [1]. Antiviral therapy may also be beneficial (see below).

Steroids in the treatment of acute facial nerve palsy have proven to be an effective treatment. Earlier studies, including a 2004 meta-analysis of four randomized controlled trials, showed no benefit of facial nerve paralysis treatment with corticosteroids [42]. A 2009 meta-analysis of 18 randomized controlled trials, which involved 2786 patients, concluded that corticosteroids were associated with greater benefit (reduced risk of unsatisfactory recovery) than antivirals alone, and there was added benefit if corticosteroids and antivirals were used together [43].

A randomized, double-blind, placebo-controlled, multicenter trial was conducted with the primary outcome of time to complete recovery of facial function. Patients were randomized to placebo, prednisolone 60 milligrams per day for 5 days then reduced by 10 milligrams per day plus placebo, 1000 milligrams valacyclovir three times a day for 7 days plus placebo, or prednisolone for 10 days plus valacyclovir for 7 days. Time to recovery was shorter in patients who received prednisolone compared to those who did not (hazard ratio 1.40, 95 percent CI 1.18–1.64; $p < 0.0001$). There was no difference in time to recovery in those treated with valacyclovir and those who did not receive valacyclovir [44].

Additional treatment with antivirals appears to have a very modest effect on recovery, with a reported 7 percent increase in probability of facial functional recovery. A large review of 14 trials showed that corticosteroid monotherapy was probably more effective than monotherapy with antivirals, and antivirals with corticosteroids were more effective than placebo or no treatment [45]. The antiviral of choice is valacyclovir 1 gram three times per day for 7 days. Prednisone is administered at a dose of 60 milligrams per day for 10 days. Complications of prednisone can include dyspepsia, duodenal ulcer activation, uncontrolled diabetes, and acute psychosis; however, these complications occur in less than 4 percent of patients who received prednisone [46].

Early medical attention is preferred as there is no benefit of medications administered after 4 days of onset of symptoms [1]. Patients should be prescribed eye lubrication to be used hourly throughout the day, and those with corneal abrasions should be referred to ophthalmology.

For those with Lyme disease as the identified cause of facial paralysis, doxycycline is the recommended antibiotic. Doxycycline is given in a dose of 100 milligrams orally twice daily for 10–21 days. Alternatively, other antibiotic regimens include cefuroxime 500 milligrams orally twice daily or amoxicillin 500 milligrams orally three times daily for 14–21 days [47].

For pregnant women who present with acute facial nerve paralysis, the risks and benefits should be evaluated in the clinical context. Although recovery tends to be worse in pregnant women with facial paralysis, there is extra risk with use of steroids in the presence of concurrent hyperglycemia and hypertension. Steroids are FDA pregnancy category C and are probably safe during lactation. In the absence of clear viral infection, antiviral therapy, which is category B and considered safe in breast-feeding, can probably be held in pregnant women with facial nerve paralysis as the benefit is modest [24].

There lack sufficient data and consensus as to the benefit of decompressive surgery as a therapy for facial paralysis, along with a lack of uniformity of who should get surgery and when during the disease surgery is most efficacious [48]. A small non-randomized, non-blinded study did show benefit of surgical treatment with decompression in patients with severe facial paralysis.

Patients who were offered surgery had total facial paralysis with greater than 90 percent decrease in motor amplitude compared to the unaffected side and no voluntary motor unit potentials on needle EMG exam [49]. However, the benefit of surgical decompression has been a controversial topic [50].

Conclusion

Facial neuropathy manifests as unilateral facial weakness, and an unknown cause of facial nerve paralysis is a Bell's palsy. Clinicians should make the distinction between acute stroke and facial nerve paralysis. In facial nerve paralysis, there is weakness of the entire unilateral side of the face, while stroke produces an upper motor neuron pattern of weakness which spares the forehead muscles. Patients with facial nerve palsy commonly have a drooping mouth and inability to close the eye and may have alterations in lacrimation, taste, salivation, and hearing. Common causes of facial nerve palsy include infectious etiologies, such as herpes zoster oticus (Ramsay Hunt syndrome) or herpes simplex virus. Treatment should be initiated within 3 days of onset, and this consists of at least a 5-day course of corticosteroids at a suggested dose of 60 milligrams per day of prednisone. There is some additional benefit in treating with valacyclovir. Diagnostic workup should be tailored to each clinical scenario, and generally imaging and cerebrospinal fluid analysis should be reserved for those presenting with multiple cranial nerve deficits or other neurologic signs.

References

1. Tiemstra JD, Khatkhate N. Bell's palsy: diagnosis and management. Am Fam Physician. 2007;76(7):997–1002.
2. Baugh RF, Basura GJ, Ishii LE, Schwartz SR, Drumheller CM, Burkholder R, et al. Clinical practice guideline: Bell's palsy. Otolaryngol Head Neck Surg. 2013;149(3 Suppl):S1–27.
3. Hohman MH, Hadlock TA. Etiology, diagnosis, and management of facial palsy: 2000 patients at a facial nerve center. Laryngoscope. 2014;124(7):E283–93.

4. Peitersen E. Bell's palsy: the spontaneous course of 2,500 peripheral facial nerve palsies of different etiologies. Acta Otolaryngol Suppl. 2002;549:4–30.
5. Jung J, Park DC, Jung SY, Park MJ, Kim SH, Yeo SG. Bilateral facial palsy. Acta Otolaryngol. 2019;139(10):934–8.
6. Kumar P, Charaniya R, Bahl A, Ghosh A, Dixit J. Facial diplegia with paresthesia: an uncommon variant of guillain-barre syndrome. J Clin Diagn Res. 2016;10(7):Od01–2.
7. DeMyer W. Neuroanatomy. 2nd ed. Baltimore: Williams & Wilkins; 1998. p. xi, 463 p.
8. Kochhar A, Larian B, Azizzadeh B. Facial nerve and parotid gland anatomy. Otolaryngol Clin N Am. 2016;49(2):273–84.
9. Gilchrist JM. Seventh cranial neuropathy. Semin Neurol. 2009;29(1):5–13.
10. Blumenfeld H. Neuroanatomy through clinical cases. 2nd ed. Sunderland: Sinauer Associates; 2010. ©2010; 2010.
11. Chu EA, Byrne PJ. Treatment considerations in facial paralysis. Facial Plast Surg. 2008;24(2):164–9.
12. Owusu JA, Stewart CM, Boahene K. Facial nerve paralysis. Med Clin North Am. 2018;102(6):1135–43.
13. Domeshek LF, Zuker RM, Borschel GH. Management of bilateral facial palsy. Otolaryngol Clin N Am. 2018;51(6):1213–26.
14. Schirm J, Mulkens PS. Bell's palsy and herpes simplex virus. APMIS. 1997;105(11):815–23.
15. McCormick DP. Herpes simplex virus as a cause of Bell's palsy. 1972. Rev Med Virol. 2000;10(5):285–9.
16. Takasu T, Furuta Y, Sato KC, Fukuda S, Inuyama Y, Nagashima K. Detection of latent herpes simplex virus DNA and RNA in human geniculate ganglia by the polymerase chain reaction. Acta Otolaryngol. 1992;112(6):1004–11.
17. Esaki S, Yamano K, Katsumi S, Minakata T, Murakami S. Facial nerve palsy after reactivation of herpes simplex virus type 1 in diabetic mice. Laryngoscope. 2015;125(4):E143–8.
18. Sweeney CJ, Gilden DH. Ramsay hunt syndrome. J Neurol Neurosurg Psychiatry. 2001;71(2):149–54.
19. Hunt JR. On herpetic inflammation of the geniculate ganglion: a new syndrome and its complications. J Nerv Mental Dis. 1907;34(2):73–96.
20. Masterson L, Vallis M, Quinlivan R, Prinsley P. Assessment and management of facial nerve palsy. BMJ. 2015;351:h3725.
21. Cooper L, Branagan-Harris M, Tuson R, Nduka C. Lyme disease and Bell's palsy: an epidemiological study of diagnosis and risk in England. Br J Gen Pract. 2017;67(658):e329–e35.
22. Duncan CJ, Carle G, Seaton RA. Tick bite and early Lyme borreliosis. BMJ. 2012;344:e3124.
23. Evangelista V, Gooding MS, Pereira L. Bell's palsy in pregnancy. Obstet Gynecol Surv. 2019;74(11):674–8.
24. Massey EW, Guidon AC. Peripheral neuropathies in pregnancy. Continuum (Minneap Minn). 2014;20(1 Neurology of Pregnancy):100–14.
25. Fukazawa T, Moriwaka F, Hamada K, Hamada T, Tashiro K. Facial palsy in multiple sclerosis. J Neurol. 1997;244(10):631–3.
26. Jain V, Deshmukh A, Gollomp S. Bilateral facial paralysis: case presentation and discussion of differential diagnosis. J Gen Intern Med. 2006;21(7):C7–C10.
27. Ciorba A, Corazzi V, Conz V, Bianchini C, Aimoni C. Facial nerve paralysis in children. World J Clin Cases. 2015;3(12):973–9.
28. Katusic SK, Beard CM, Wiederholt WC, Bergstralh EJ, Kurland LT. Incidence, clinical features, and prognosis in Bell's palsy, Rochester, Minnesota, 1968–1982. Ann Neurol. 1986;20(5):622–7.
29. Vanopdenbosch LJ, Verhoeven K, Casselman JW. Bell's palsy with ipsilateral numbness. J Neurol Neurosurg Psychiatry. 2005;76(7):1017–8.
30. Hilsinger RL Jr, Adour KK, Doty HE. Idiopathic facial paralysis, pregnancy, and the menstrual cycle. Ann Otol Rhinol Laryngol. 1975;84(4 Pt 1):433–42.
31. Urban E, Volk GF, Geissler K, Thielker J, Dittberner A, Klingner C, et al. Prognostic factors for the outcome of Bells' palsy: a cohort register-based study. Clin Otolaryngol. 2020;45(5):754–61.
32. Wagner G, Klinge H, Sachse MM. Ramsay hunt syndrome. J Dtsch Dermatol Ges. 2012;10(4):238–44.
33. Sanders RD. The trigeminal (V) and facial (VII) cranial nerves: head and face sensation and movement. Psychiatry (Edgmont). 2010;7(1):13–6.
34. Marques AR. Laboratory diagnosis of Lyme disease: advances and challenges. Infect Dis Clin N Am. 2015;29(2):295–307.
35. Halperin JJ. Neurologic manifestations of lyme disease. Curr Infect Dis Rep. 2011;13(4):360–6.
36. Lager M, Dessau RB, Wilhelmsson P, Nyman D, Jensen GF, Matussek A, et al. Serological diagnostics of Lyme borreliosis: comparison of assays in twelve clinical laboratories in Northern Europe. Eur J Clin Microbiol Infect Dis. 2019;38(10):1933–45.
37. Branda JA, Linskey K, Kim YA, Steere AC, Ferraro MJ. Two-tiered antibody testing for Lyme disease with use of 2 enzyme immunoassays, a whole-cell sonicate enzyme immunoassay followed by a VlsE C6 peptide enzyme immunoassay. Clin Infect Dis. 2011;53(6):541–7.
38. Zandian A, Osiro S, Hudson R, Ali IM, Matusz P, Tubbs SR, et al. The neurologist's dilemma: a comprehensive clinical review of Bell's palsy, with emphasis on current management trends. Med Sci Monit. 2014;20:83–90.
39. McAllister K, Walker D, Donnan PT, Swan I. Surgical interventions for the early management of Bell's palsy. Cochrane Database Syst Rev. 2011;(2):CD007468.
40. Brown JS. Bell's palsy: a 5 year review of 174 consecutive cases: an attempted double blind study. Laryngoscope. 1982;92(12):1369–73.
41. Engstrom M, Abdsaleh S, Ahlstrom H, Johansson L, Stalberg E, Jonsson L. Serial gadolinium-enhanced magnetic resonance imaging and assessment of facial

nerve function in Bell's palsy. Otolaryngol Head Neck Surg. 1997;117(5):559–66.

42. Salinas RA, Alvarez G, Ferreira J. Corticosteroids for Bell's palsy (idiopathic facial paralysis). Cochrane Database Syst Rev. 2004;(4):CD001942.

43. de Almeida JR, Al Khabori M, Guyatt GH, Witterick IJ, Lin VY, Nedzelski JM, et al. Combined corticosteroid and antiviral treatment for Bell palsy: a systematic review and meta-analysis. JAMA. 2009;302(9):985–93.

44. Engstrom M, Berg T, Stjernquist-Desatnik A, Axelsson S, Pitkaranta A, Hultcrantz M, et al. Prednisolone and valaciclovir in Bell's palsy: a randomised, double-blind, placebo-controlled, multicentre trial. Lancet Neurol. 2008;7(11):993–1000.

45. Gagyor I, Madhok VB, Daly F, Sullivan F. Antiviral treatment for Bell's palsy (idiopathic facial paralysis). Cochrane Database Syst Rev. 2019;9:CD001869.

46. Adour KK, Wingerd J, Bell DN, Manning JJ, Hurley JP. Prednisone treatment for idiopathic facial paralysis (Bell's palsy). N Engl J Med. 1972;287(25):1268–72.

47. Hu LT. Lyme disease. Ann Intern Med. 2016;164(9):Itc65–itc80.

48. Adour KK. Decompression for Bell's palsy: why I don't do it. Eur Arch Otorhinolaryngol. 2002;259(1):40–7.

49. Gantz BJ, Rubinstein JT, Gidley P, Woodworth GG. Surgical management of Bell's palsy. Laryngoscope. 1999;109(8):1177–88.

50. Bodenez C, Bernat I, Willer JC, Barre P, Lamas G, Tankere F. Facial nerve decompression for idiopathic Bell's palsy: report of 13 cases and literature review. J Laryngol Otol. 2010;124(3):272–8.

51. Gilchrist JM. Facial nerve palsy. New York: Springer Nature; 2012.

Evaluation and Management of Acute Ischemic Stroke

8

Richard V. Scheer

Introduction

The American Heart Association (AHA) defines ischemic stroke as brain, spinal cord, or retinal cell death attributable to ischemia, based on neuropathological, neuroimaging, and/or clinical evidence of permanent injury [1]. This modern definition of stroke was adopted by the AHA in 2013 in an effort to better define stroke in the context of our current understanding of the nature, causes, and clinical and imaging characteristics of stroke. The need for this updated, more modern definition of stroke reflects the major advancements which have taken place in the field in the last 40 years. The goal of this chapter is to provide an up-to-date overview of current ischemic stroke epidemiology, pathophysiology, and acute treatment techniques. The scope of this chapter is limited to acute ischemic stroke not caused by intracerebral hemorrhage (ICH), subarachnoid hemorrhage (SAH), or cerebral venous sinus thrombosis (CVST)—in-depth information about these entities can be found elsewhere in this textbook.

Epidemiology

In 2003 stroke was the third leading cause of death in the United States. By 2013, however, it had fallen to fifth behind heart disease, cancer, chronic lower respiratory diseases, and unintentional injury [2]. More specifically, from 2003 to 2013, the number of stroke deaths declined by more than 18% due to both a decline in overall incidence and lower individual fatality rates [3]. This success parallels improvements across all aspects of stroke care which occurred over the same time period—from primary prevention and risk factor modification (including interventions to recognize and treat hypertension, diabetes, hyperlipidemia, and smoking) to stroke education (including improved stroke symptom awareness and early recognition) and improvements in acute stroke interventions (including intravenous thrombolysis and mechanical thrombectomy).

Despite these encouraging trends, approximately 795,000 people experience a stroke annually. Of these, 87% are ischemic and 610,000 are first-time ischemic strokes. Additionally, stroke remains the leading cause of serious long-term disability in the United States. The highest death rates from stroke are in the southeastern United States.

Moreover, significant racial, gender, and geographic disparities in stroke persist. Compared to whites, a higher incidence of stroke has been reported in African-Americans; Hispanics and Mexican Americans; and American Indians and

R. V. Scheer (✉)
Indiana University School of Medicine, Indianapolis, IN, USA
e-mail: rvscheer@iupui.edu

Alaska Natives. Annually, females have approximately 55,000 more strokes than males and have a higher lifetime risk of stroke [4].

Thus, despite encouraging trends, significant work to improve stroke outcomes remains.

Etiology and Classification

Well-established, independent, and modifiable risk factors for acute ischemic stroke include physical inactivity, dyslipidemia, hypertension, obesity, diabetes mellitus, cigarette smoking, atrial fibrillation, and poor diet (including low intake of fruits and vegetables and high intake of sodium). Non-modifiable risk factors include age, race/ethnicity, and numerous genetic factors. Interactions between these risk factors may also play an important role in the overall risk of stroke [5].

Together these risk factors lead to a variety of pathologies within the cardiovascular system including but not limited to atherosclerosis, small artery lipohyalinosis and fibrinoid necrosis, coronary artery disease, and myocardial injury. The presence of these pathologies can be informative to the mechanism of stroke occurrence, to the risk for recurrence, and to the optimal secondary prevention strategy. As such, a system which classifies stroke subtypes based on the underlying mechanism of stroke (i.e., by cause) can be very useful to the clinician. The TOAST classification system [6] is the most widely utilized of these systems and classifies stroke into five different subtypes based on the underlying mechanism. The categories are summarized in Table 8.1 and include large artery atherosclerosis, cardioembo-

Table 8.1 TOAST criteria

Subtypes of ischemic stroke
Large artery atherosclerosis
Cardioembolic
Small vessel disease
Stroke of other determined etiologies
Stroke of undetermined etiology
(a) Two or more possible causes identified
(b) Negative evaluation
(c) Incomplete evaluation

Reproduced from Adams et al. [6]. With permission from Wolters Kluwer Health, Inc

lism, small vessel occlusion, stroke of other determined etiologies, and stroke of undetermined etiology.

Atherosclerosis is the most common pathology underlying large artery-related strokes. Plaques may cause luminal narrowing and reduction in distal blood flow or may ulcerate or rupture leading to distal embolization of plaque material or thrombus. Other pathologies of large arteries which may lead to stroke include dissection, arteritis, and other vasculopathies, such as moyamoya disease.

The most common cause of cardioembolism is atrial fibrillation. Other causes include paradoxical emboli via a patent foramen ovale, left ventricular thrombus formation from reduced ejection fraction or post-myocardial infarction wall motion abnormalities, valvular abnormalities, and endocarditis. Aortic arch pathologies may also lead to embolization and stroke.

Small vessel occlusion occurs secondary to lipohyalinosis and fibrinoid necrosis (most common) or atherosclerosis (less common) within small capillaries of the brain. Strokes associated with this pathology are typically lacunar in nature (see section on Clinical Presentation, Lacunar Stroke Syndromes).

Pathophysiology

The brain's metabolic rate is high, and it depends on continuous blood flow to supply the oxygen and glucose necessary to produce such high levels of energy. Fortunately, by regulating cerebral blood flow (mainly through vasoconstriction and vasodilation) and fractional extraction of oxygen, the brain is able to maintain normal energy production and function across a wide range of physiologic conditions. However, if cerebral perfusion is reduced beyond the capacity of these compensatory mechanisms, a cascade of cellular and molecular events may quickly lead to cell death. Among these, glutamate excitotoxicity is thought to play a central role in ischemia-induced cellular death. As ischemic conditions lead to decreased energy production, neuronal cells depolarize, leading to a massive release of glutamate via voltage gated calcium channel depolarization. The resultant excessive activation of NMDA and AMPA receptors leads to increased inflow and release of intracellular calcium which, in turn, activates cell death pathways, such as apoptosis and necrosis. It is estimated that under ischemic conditions, this and many other biochemical processes lead to the death of approximately 1.9 million neurons per minute.

The ability of brain cells to tolerate ischemia depends on the cell type (e.g., gray matter vs. white matter) and both the magnitude and duration of the ischemia. During an acute ischemic stroke, the ischemic area of involved brain tissue is often comprised of two distinct areas termed the core and the penumbra. Within the core, which is often at or very near the site of vessel occlusion, the magnitude of ischemia is so great that cells in this region are irreversibly injured within minutes of the onset of ischemia. Because of autoregulation and collateral circulation, however, a second region (often more distal to the site of vessel occlusion) with less profound ischemia exists. Within this penumbral region, cells are dysfunctional and clinical symptoms arise from their dysfunction, but they are not immediately irreversibly damaged (although if the ischemia persists long enough, irreversible injury will eventually occur). The duration in which cells of the ischemic penumbra can remain viable is variable and again depends largely on the magnitude of ischemia to this area. However, during this period, if blood flow is restored, cells of the ischemic penumbra may recover and resume normal cellular function. Thus, it is the goal of reperfusion therapy to restore blood flow to the area of ischemic penumbra and thereby minimize the amount of brain tissue which is irreversibly injured.

Clinical Presentation

The cardinal feature of acute ischemic stroke is the acute and rapid onset of focal neurological deficits. The specific deficits depend largely on the size and location of the stroke and the area of the brain that is affected. However, more than 95% of stroke presentations will have at least one of the following features: imbalance, vision/eye changes, facial palsy/droopiness, asymmetric arm weakness, and speech or language abnormalities [7]. Based on this, the American Heart Association has adopted the mnemonic BE-FAST for public stroke education. The mnemonic stands for balance, eyes, face, arm, speech, and time (as in time to call 9-1-1) and represents an easy way for the public to remember and recognize stroke symptoms as well as to remember to quickly access and utilize emergency medical services for these symptoms (see below).

A number of specific stroke syndromes have also been well described. These consist of both syndromes accompanying occlusion of large arteries and syndromes seen in subcortical or lacunar strokes. A knowledge and understanding of these syndromes can aid in immediate localization of a stroke, as well as be predictive of the underlying pathophysiology. For example, the presence of deficits localizing to specific cortical regions such as aphasia, hemi-neglect, forced gaze deviation, and/or visual field deficits (anopsia) may predict the presence of a large vessel occlusion and should cue the physician to assess for mechanical thrombectomy eligibility.

Large Artery Syndromes

Occlusion of the middle cerebral artery (MCA) (Fig. 8.1) is characterized by contralateral hemiparesis and hemisensory loss (typically with greater involvement of the arm and face than the leg), forced-gaze deviation with the direction of deviation towards the side of the occluded vessel, and aphasia or hemi-neglect depending on whether the dominant or nondominant hemisphere, respectively, is involved (Table 8.2 and Fig. 8.2). The degree of the above mentioned deficits is variable, with more distal occlusions typically resulting in milder or a less complete set of symptoms than an occlusion at the MCA origin [8].

Occlusion of the anterior cerebral artery (ACA) (Fig. 8.3) is characterized by weakness

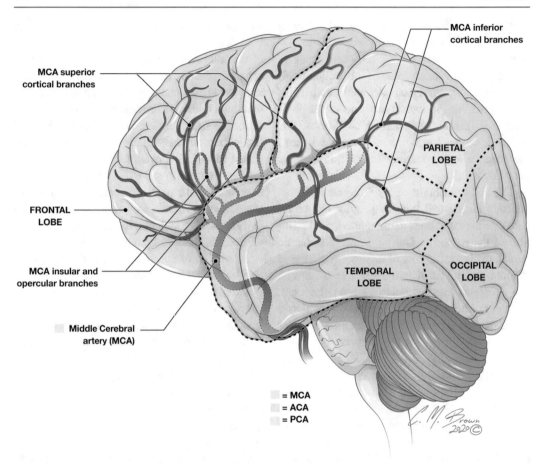

Fig. 8.1 Middle cerebral artery and the regions of the brain supplied by the middle cerebral artery. (Illustration by Christopher M. Brown, BFA, MS. (C. M. Brown © 2020))

Table 8.2 Middle cerebral artery syndrome

Middle cerebral artery syndrome	
Contralateral weakness (arm>leg)	Primary motor cortex (pre-central gyrus)
Contralateral sensory loss	Primary sensory cortex (post-central gyrus)
Forced eye deviation	Frontal eye fields
Aphasia (dominant)	Language areas (i.e., Broca's area, Wernicke's area)
Visuospatial neglect (nondominant)	Parietal association cortex

and anesthesia of the contralateral leg. Here leg involvement is typically more extensive than involvement of the arm and face. Additional features of ACA strokes can include akinetic mutism (abulia) and other behavioral disturbances and disconnection syndromes due to involvement of the anteromedial frontal lobes, cingulate gyrus, and corpus callosum (Table 8.3) [9].

Occlusion of the posterior cerebral artery (PCA) (Fig. 8.4) is characterized by contralateral anopia, usually a homonymous hemianopia due to the involvement of the visual radiations and primary visual cortex, both of which receive some or all of its blood supply from the PCA. The thalamus is also perfused via arteries which branch from the proximal portion of the PCA. As a result, a variety of thalamic-related behavioral and cognitive disturbances as well as contralateral hemisensory disturbances can be seen with PCA infarctions when thalamic structures are involved (Table 8.4) [10].

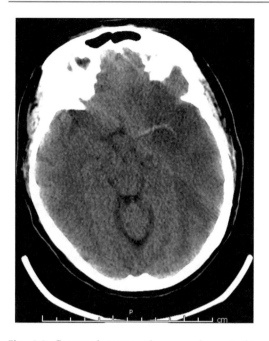

Fig. 8.2 Computed tomography scan demonstrating hyperdensity within the left middle cerebral artery due to thrombosis and hypodensity of the left middle cerebral artery territory secondary to infarction. This patient presented with a left middle cerebral artery syndrome characterized by right hemiparesis and aphasia

Brainstem Stroke Syndromes

Hallmark features of brainstem stroke include the so-called crossed deficits, in which motor or sensory symptoms are seen on one side of the face and the opposite side of the body. This typically occurs due to involvement of an ipsilateral cranial nerve or nerve nucleus and the corresponding descending fibers (corticospinal tract for motor deficits, spinothalamic tracts for sensory deficits, etc.) above their decussation (resulting in contralateral body symptoms). Similarly, vision disturbances such as diplopia are frequently seen in brainstem stroke syndromes due to involvement of cranial nerves III, IV, and VI and the resultant abnormalities of extra-ocular motility. Also common is vertigo and imbalance due to involvement of motor and cerebellar pathways within the brainstem. In addition to these hallmark features, a number of specific stroke syndromes have been described. Selected syndromes are described in more detail below.

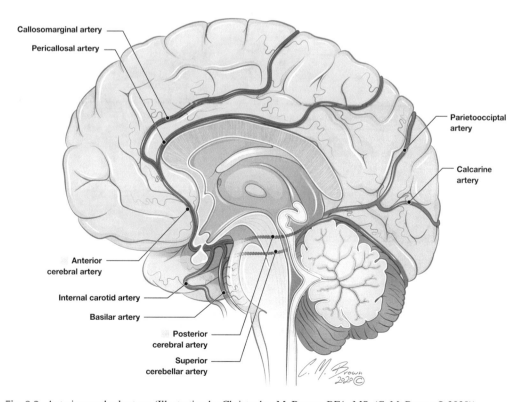

Fig. 8.3 Anterior cerebral artery. (Illustration by Christopher M. Brown, BFA, MS. (C. M. Brown © 2020))

Table 8.3 Anterior cerebral artery syndrome

Anterior cerebral artery syndrome	
Contralateral weakness (leg>arm)	Primary motor cortex (pre-central gyrus)
Contralateral sensory loss	Primary sensory cortex (post-central gyrus)
Abulia	Inferomedial frontal lobe

Table 8.4 Posterior cerebral artery syndrome

Posterior cerebral artery syndrome	
Contralateral anopia	Primary visual cortex (occipital lobe)
Contralateral sensory loss	Thalamus
Cognitive and behavioral disturbance	Thalamus

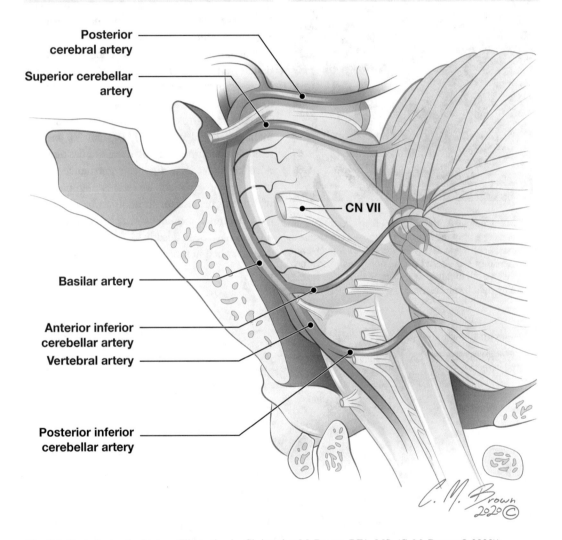

Fig. 8.4 Posterior cerebral artery. (Illustration by Christopher M. Brown, BFA, MS. (C. M. Brown © 2020))

Midbrain Infarction (Weber Syndrome, Claude Syndrome)

The cranial portion of the midbrain is supplied predominantly by the PCA (Fig. 8.3). Small midline perforators supply the ventral paramedian portion of the midbrain, while long and short circumferential arteries supply much of the lateral and posterior midbrain. Weber syndrome is char-

acterized by an ipsilateral third nerve palsy and contralateral hemiparesis. It is classically caused by a lesion within the proximal PCA (P1 segment) resulting in ischemia to the ventromedial midbrain where the exiting cranial nerve III fibers and descending corticospinal tract fibers (above their decussation) are involved (Fig. 8.5). When nearby cerebellar fibers are involved, contralat-

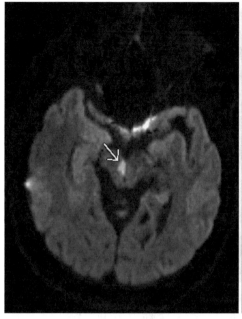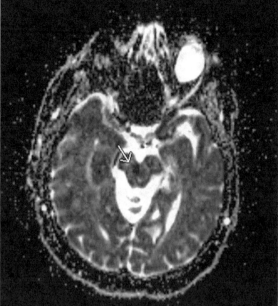

Fig. 8.5 Diffusion weighted (left) and apparent diffusion coefficient (right) MR images showing an acute infarction in the medial midbrain (arrows). This patient presented with an ipsilateral (right) cranial nerve 3 palsy and contralateral (left) hemiparesis

Table 8.5 Midbrain stroke symptoms and the involved structures

Midbrain Infarction	
Ipsilateral 3rd nerve palsy	CN 3 exiting fibers
Contralateral hemiparesis	Crus cerebri (corticospinal tract)
Contralateral ataxia, involuntary movement	Cerebellar pathways, red nucleus

eral ataxia may accompany the third nerve palsy (Claude syndrome) (see Table 8.5).

Lateral Medullary Infarction (Wallenberg Syndrome)

The posterior lateral medulla is densely populated with cranial nerve nuclei and ascending and descending fibers for multiple somatic and visceral functions. This area receives blood supply predominantly from the posterior inferior cerebellar artery (PICA) (Fig. 8.3) and associated perforating branches as the artery wraps around the dorsolateral surface of the medulla. Pathology within a vertebral artery or the PICA itself can, therefore, result in infarction of the lateral

medulla. Infarction in this area produces the Wallenberg syndrome which is characterized by loss of pain and temperature sensation on the ipsilateral face and contralateral body. Severe dysphagia, hypophonia, hypogeusia, and ipsilateral Horner's syndrome are also variably seen in Wallenberg syndrome (Fig. 8.6). The structures associated with each of these deficits are provided in Table 8.6.

Lacunar Stroke Syndromes

Lacunar strokes are small, subcortical infarcts which occur within areas of the brain supplied by small penetrating arteries (Fig. 8.7). Specifically, lacunar infarcts occur within the regions supplied by the lenticulostriate arteries (basal ganglia, internal capsule), thalamoperforating arteries (thalamus, ventral midbrain), and pontine perforators (pons). These small arteries are unique in the sense that they are small penetrating arteries which arise directly off of large arteries without

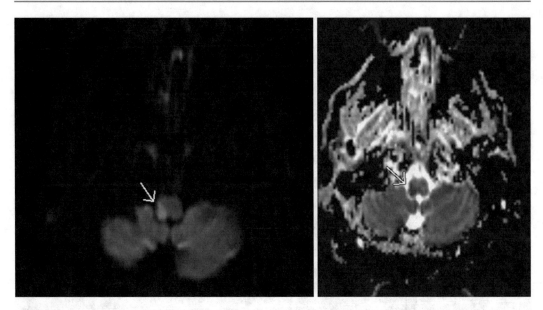

Fig. 8.6 Diffusion weighted (left) and apparent diffusion coefficient (right) MR images showing an acute infarction in the lateral medulla (arrows). This patient presented with loss of pain and temperature sensation on the ipsilateral (right) face and contralateral (left) body, severe dysphagia, partial ptosis, and right pupillary miosis

Table 8.6 Lateral medullary stroke symptoms and the involved structures

Lateral medullary infarction	
Loss of pain and temperature sensation—ipsilateral face	Spinal trigeminal nucleus and tract
Loss of pain and temperature sensation—contralateral body	Spinothalamic tract
Dysphagia	Nucleus ambiguus
Hypophonia	Nucleus ambiguus
Hypogeusia	Nucleus and tractus solitarius
Ipsilateral Horner's syndrome	Descending sympathetic fibers

intervening arteries and arterioles which sequentially decrease in diameter (as is seen on surface vessels). Because of this anatomy, these vessels are particularly susceptible to injury from hypertension, diabetes, and other traditional vascular risk factors. As a result, the underlying pathology leading to stroke in these vessels is more often thickening and disruption due to lipohyalinosis and fibrinoid necrosis rather than the atherosclerosis and thrombotic occlusion seen in larger arteries of the brain [11]. A summary of the specific lacunar stroke syndromes discussed below can be found in Table 8.7.

Pure Motor, Pure Sensory, and Motor-Sensory Syndromes

Most commonly lacunar strokes present with isolated deficits in one modality—motor or sensory—without other accompanying features (such as visual field disturbance, language disturbance, vertigo, diplopia, etc.). The pure motor syndrome is classically due to lacunar infarction in the region of the internal capsule but is also well described with lacunes occurring in the corona radiata and brainstem. Similarly, the pure sensory syndrome may be seen with lacunar infarctions of the thalamus (most common), corona radiata, internal capsule, and brainstem. In addition to the "pure" variants, a combination of isolated motor and sensory symptoms can be seen with lacunes of the same regions [12].

Dysarthria Clumsy Hand

The dysarthria clumsy hand syndrome is characterized by dysarthria (usually with accompanying contralateral facial weakness) and profound ataxia of the contralateral upper extremity significantly out of proportion to any degree of weakness in that limb. The syndrome is classically attributed to a lesion in the anterior limb of

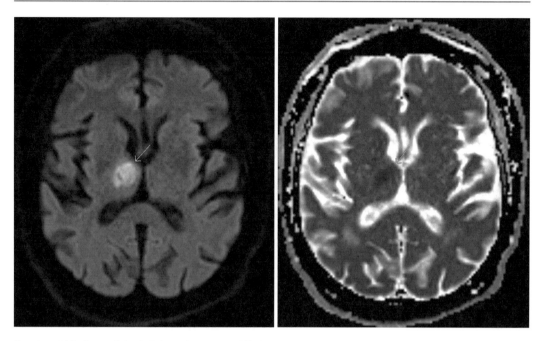

Fig. 8.7 Diffusion weighted (left) and apparent diffusion coefficient (right) MR images showing an acute lacunar infarction of the right thalamus (arrows)

Table 8.7 Lacunar stroke syndromes, the involved structures, and vascular supply

Lacunar syndromes			
Syndrome	Symptom	Structure	Vascular supply
Pure motor	Contralateral hemiparesis	Corticospinal tract Corona radiata Internal capsule Ventral pons	Small MCA (lenticulostriate) or basilar penetrating arteries
Pure sensory	Contralateral sensory loss	Spinothalamic tract, Medial lemniscus ventral posterolateral VPL nucleus of thalamus	Lenticulostriate MCA arteries PCA penetrating arteries
Sensorimotor	Contralateral weakness Contralateral sensory loss	Corticospinal tract Spinothalamic tract Medial Lemniscus Ventral posterolateral nucleus of thalamus	Lenticulostriate MCA arteries
Dysarthria-clumsy hand	Slurred speech Contralateral hand weakness	Pons	Penetrating basilar arteries
Ataxia hemiparesis	Contralateral limb ataxia Mild contralateral weakness	Posterior limb internal capsule Pons	MCA or basilar penetrating arteries

the internal capsule but has also been described in lacunes of other locations. Many authors describe the dysarthria clumsy hand syndrome as a variant of ataxia hemiparesis [12].

Ataxia Hemiparesis

Ataxia hemiparesis is characterized by mild to moderate contralateral weakness, more so of the lower extremity than of the face and arm, with associated profound ataxia of gait. This ataxia is significantly out of proportion to the imbalance and ataxia that would be expected from the weakness alone. Classically, it is ascribed to a lesion of the brainstem, but its occurrence with lesions in the internal capsule, corona radiata, and basal ganglia and cerebellum is also described [12].

Acute Treatment

Prehospital Care

Awareness and recognition of stroke symptoms and activation of emergency medical services are critical for receiving timely stroke treatments. According to the 2014 National Health Interview Survey, 68.3% of participants were able to correctly identify all five stroke symptoms (numbness of face, arm, leg, side; confusion/trouble speaking; sudden trouble seeing; trouble walking; sudden severe headache), which is an improvement since 2005 (54.1%). However, data suggest considerably lower awareness of stroke symptoms among African-Americans and Hispanics, placing them at an increased risk for treatment delay and worsened outcomes. The use of emergency medical services is associated with decreased onset-to-door times, door-to-imaging times, and door-to-needle times and an increase in the use of tissue plasminogen activator among eligible patients. Despite 95% of survey participants answering that they would contact emergency medical services at the onset of stroke symptoms, real-world data from Get With the Guidelines (GWTGs) showed that more than one third of stroke patients do not utilize emergency medical services (hospital arrival by EMS was 63.7%) [13–17].

One emerging and promising method to combat delayed and low utilization of emergency medical services is the use of mobile stroke units (MSUs)—essentially ambulances outfitted with the ability to perform appropriate neuroimaging and deliver thrombolytic therapy in the field, prior to transporting a stroke patient to the nearest stroke center. In April 2020 results of the Berlin Pre-Hospital or Usual care Delivery (B_ PROUD) trial were reported at the American Stroke Association International Stroke Conference in Los Angeles, California. This prospective, quasi-randomized trial with blinded outcome assessment compared functional outcomes at 90 days for patients 18 years of age or older, with acute ischemic stroke who requested medical dispatch for stroke-like symptoms that started ≤4 h prior. Patients were randomized to receive care via a MSU or traditional EMS service (standard ambulance, transport and care in an emergency department). One thousand five-hundred and forty-three patients were enrolled. At 3 months, the odds of death and disability was significantly reduced with care delivered via MSU versus standard care (aOR 0.74, 95% CI 0.60–0.90, $p = 0.003$). In addition, use of a MSU increased thrombolysis rates (60% vs. 48%) and dispatch-to-treatment times (50 min, IQR 43–64 vs. 70 min IQR 59–85, $p \leq 0.001$). Additional studies of MSUs, including the BEST-MSU study in the United States, are ongoing.

Reperfusion Therapy

The core-penumbra hypothesis, as discussed in detail above, guides the selection and use of reperfusion therapies. All reperfusion strategies share the common goal of restoration of blood flow to ischemic tissue (i.e., the ischemic penumbra), thereby avoiding permanent infarction and, in turn, reducing the extent of a stroke and the related disability. Over the last 25 years, a number of reperfusion strategies have successfully demonstrated benefit in clinical trials and are now considered standard of care for stroke; these include intravenous thrombolysis and mechanical thrombectomy.

Proper patient selection has been a key driver of success for these therapies. Whereas both intravenous thrombolysis and mechanical thrombectomy had early trials which were negative, further trials and ongoing prospective databases have demonstrated the overwhelming benefit of these treatments in the properly selected populations of patients. As such, the selection criteria which guide the use of these therapies remain a highly important part of reperfusion therapy in the emergency department and at the bedside. For this reason, the selection criteria for each therapy are highlighted throughout this section's text and in figures throughout this chapter.

Modern stroke trials have mainly utilized the modified Rankin Scale (mRS) as the outcome measure of choice. The components of this ordinal scale are illustrated in Table 8.8.

Alteplase

In 1995 the National Institutes of Neurological Disorders and Stroke (NINDS) rt-PA Stroke Study Group published the results of a 624-patient prospective randomized clinical trial utilizing recombinant tissue plasminogen activator (Activase [alteplase], Genentech, San Francisco) (tPA) for the treatment of acute ischemic stroke in patients presenting within 3 h from last known normal. Participants were randomized to receive placebo or tPA at a dose of 0.9 mg/kg (90 mg maximum, with 10% delivered as a bolus over 1 min, and the remaining 90% delivered as a continuous infusion over 60 min). Current inclusion and exclusion criteria for the administration of rtPA endorsed by the AHA/ASA are listed in Table 8.9 and remain largely unchanged from those utilized in the NINDS tPA trial. The outcome mea-

sure for this trial was disability at 90 days after stroke onset, as measured by four validated disability measures: the Barthel Index, the Modified Rankin Scale (mRS), the National Institutes of Health Stroke Scale (NIHSS), and the Glasgow Outcome Scale. Treatment with tPA resulted in an increase in the percentage of patients achieving a better mRS score. Symptomatic intracranial hemorrhage (sICH) occurred in 7% of patient's treated with rtPA and 1% of patients treated with placebo. Despite this, there was no increase in mortality from tPA (17% rtPA group vs. 21 percent placebo group, $p = 0.30$).

Tenecteplase

Tenecteplase is a genetically modified variant of alteplase which has been engineered for increased

Table 8.8 The modified Rankin Scale

Grade	Description
0	No symptoms at all
1	No significant disability despite symptoms: able to carry out all usual duties and activities
2	Slight disability: unable to carry out all previous activities but able to look after own affairs without assistance
3	Moderate disability: requiring some help, but able to walk without assistance
4	Moderately severe disability: unable to walk without assistance, and unable to attend to own bodily needs without assistance
5	Severe disability: bedridden, incontinent, and requiring constant nursing care and attention

Table 8.9 Inclusions, exclusions, and contraindications for the administration of tPA in acute ischemic stroke

0–3 h	3–4.5 h
Inclusions	
Presentation consistent with stroke	Presentation consistent with stroke
Non-contrasted CT head without hemorrhage or frank hypodensity	Non-contrasted CT head without hemorrhage or frank hypodensity
Onset or LKN within 0–3 h	Onset or LKN within 3–4.5 h

Absolute contraindications and exclusions
Mild, non-disabling stroke
Extensive CT hypoattenuation/frank hypodensity
History of intracranial hemorrhage
History of recent (within 3 months) ischemic stroke
Recent (within 3 months), severe head trauma
Recent (within 3 months) intracranial or intraspinal surgery
Blood pressure >185/110 mmHg
Presence of coagulopathy
 Platelets <100,000
 INR >1.7, PT >15s
 aPTT >40s
 Recent (within 24 h) full treatment dose heparin or LMWH administration
 Recent (within 48 h) DTI or Factor Xa inhibitor administration
BG <50 mg/dL or >400 mg/dL
Known or suspected infective endocarditis
Known or suspected aortic arch dissection
Known or suspected intra-axial, intracranial neoplasm
Relative contraindications, exclusions, and considerations

(continued)

Table 8.9 (continued)

0–3 h	3–4.5 h
Recent (within 21 days) GI bleed or known GI malignancy	All 0–3-h criteria
Recent (within 21 days) GU bleeding; menorrhagia causing significant anemia or hypotension	Severe stroke (NIHSS >25)
Recent (within 14 days) major trauma not involving the head	
Recent (within 14 days) major surgery	
Recent (within 7 days) arterial puncture (particularly if puncture was at a non-compressible site)	
Intracranial arterial dissection	
Known or suspected large (>10 mm), unsecured intracranial aneurysm	
Known or suspected large, untreated intracranial vascular malformation	
Known high burden (>10) cerebral microbleeds felt to be associated with cerebral amyloid angiopathy	
Recent (within 3 months) left anterior STEMI	

LKN last known normal, *LMWH* low molecular weight heparin, *DTI* direct thrombin inhibitor, *NIHSS* National Institutes of Health Stroke Scale

fibrin specificity, a longer half-life (allowing delivery as a single bolus), and increased resistance to inactivation by plasminogen activator inhibitor 1 (PAI-1).

The Tenecteplase versus Alteplase before Endovascular Therapy for Ischemic Stroke (EXTEND-IA TNK) trial, a multicenter, prospective, randomized, open-label, blinded outcome trial, randomized patients with acute ischemic stroke, within 4.5 h from onset, and large vessel occlusion of the intracranial carotid artery, middle cerebral artery, or basilar artery to receive tenecteplase 0.25 mg/kg (max 25 mg) or alteplase 0.9 mg/kg (max 90 mg) followed by mechanical thrombectomy. The primary outcome of reperfusion of greater than 50% of the involved ischemic territory (as assessed by digital subtraction angiography (DSA) or computed tomography perfusion (CTP)) or absence of retrievable thrombus at the time of thrombectomy occurred

in 22% of those treated with tenecteplase versus 10% of those treated with alteplase (incidence ratio 2.2, 95% CI 1.1–4.4; $p = 0.002$ for noninferiority and $p = 0.03$ for superiority). Moreover, there was a significant difference in median 90-day mRS scores in the tenecteplase group (median mRS 2, IQR 0–3) versus the alteplase group (median mRS 3, IQR 1–5) (common OR 1.7, 95%CI 1.0–2.8; $p = 0.04$), though no significant difference in the achievement of functional independence (mRS 0–2) was seen (64% tenecteplase vs. 51% alteplase; aOR 1.8, 95% CI 1.0–3.4; $p = 0.006$).

In 2017, the largest phase III clinical trial comparing tenecteplase to alteplase was published. The Norwegian Tenecteplase Stroke Trial (NOR-TEST) trial was a multicenter, prospective, randomized, open-label, blinded end-point, phase 3, study in which patients ≥18 years of age with a clinically suspected acute ischemic stroke with onset in the 4.5 h prior to presentation and who were otherwise eligible to receive thrombolytic therapy were randomized to receive either tenecteplase 0.4 mg/kg (max 40 mg) or alteplase 0.9 mg/kg (max 90 mg) plus usual care. One thousand one hundred patients were randomized (549 to tenecteplase and 551 to alteplase). The mean NIHSS score for both groups was 4, with the majority of participants having mild (NIHSS 0–7) stroke symptoms at randomization (78% receiving tenecteplase, and 73% receiving alteplase). In the intention-to-treat analysis, 354 (64%) patients in the tenecteplase group and 345 (63%) patients in the alteplase group achieved the primary outcome of mRS score 0–1 at 90 days (OR 1.08, 95% CI 0.84–1.38; $p = 0.52$). Symptomatic intracranial hemorrhage occurred in 15 (3%) and 13 (2%) of patients in these groups, respectively (OR 1.16, 95% CI 0.51–2.68; $p = 0.70$). Thus, patients treated with tenecteplase showed similar rates of functional independence at 90 days compared to those treated with alteplase, and the safety of tenecteplase with regard to ICH was similar to alteplase.

Because of differences between these two trials—namely, the dose of tenecteplase used (0.25 mg/kg and 0.4 mg/kg in EXTEND-IA TNK and NOR-TEST, respectively) and stroke severity in the treated cohort (median NIHSS 17 vs. 4, respectively)—EXTEND-IA TNK part 2 randomized clinical trial was designed to examine the optimal dose of tenecteplase. Part 2 included a more severely affected cohort of patients, those with acute ischemic stroke due to occlusion of the intracranial carotid, middle cerebral, or basilar artery (large vessel occlusion [LVO]). In this phase III, multicenter, randomized, open-label, blinded end-point assessment trial, patients ≥18 years of age with acute ischemic stroke due to LVO and symptom onset within 4.5 h prior to randomization were treated with either tenecteplase 0.4 mg/kg (max 40 mg) or tenecteplase 0.25 mg/kg (max 25 mg). Three hundred patients were randomized (150 in each group). The median NIHSS was 17 and 16 in the 0.4 mg/kg and 0.25 mg/kg groups, respectively. The primary outcome of reperfusion of greater than 50% of the involved ischemic territory (as assessed by DSA or CTP) or absence of retrievable thrombus at the time of thrombectomy occurred in 19.3% of patients at both doses. Additionally, there was no difference in outcomes, as measured by the mRS at 90 days, in either group (mRS 0–2 occurred in 59% of the 0.4 mg/kg group and 56% of the 0.25 mg/kg group; aRR 1.08, 95% CI 0.90–1.29; $p = 0.4$), and there was a nonsignificant trend towards lower rates of sICH (4.7% vs. 1.3%, RR 3.5, 95% CI 0.74–16.62; $p = 0.12$).

Mechanical Thrombectomy

Mechanical thrombectomy is indicated for patients with a large vessel occlusion presenting within 6 h of last known normal, and for select patients presenting within 24 h of last known normal. Large vessel occlusion is generally defined as a causative occlusion of the internal carotid artery or the first segment of the middle cerebral artery (M1). In some of the individual studies discussed below, the second middle cerebral artery segment (M2) and the first and second anterior cerebral artery segments (A1 and A2, respectively) were also considered large vessel occlusions. However, the number of patients with these lesions enrolled in the trials was small, and the overall benefit of mechanical thrombectomy in this population remains uncer-

tain. Similarly, the use of mechanical thrombectomy for the treatment of causative occlusions in the posterior circulation (vertebral arteries, basilar artery) has not been well studied, and the benefit remains uncertain. In these situations, mechanical thrombectomy may be reasonable, but consultation with a vascular expert such as a vascular neurologist is recommended, and treatment decisions should be made on a case-by-case basis [18].

0–6 Hours

In 2015, six randomized trials of mechanical thrombectomy (MR. CLEAN [19], SWIFT-PRIME [20], EXTEND-IA [21], ESCAPE [22], REVASCAT [23], and THRACE) were published. These trials overwhelmingly demonstrated the benefit of mechanical thrombectomy for the treatment of large vessel occlusion 0–6 h from last known normal. Inclusion criteria among the trials were slightly different. However, the least restrictive (most inclusive) of these trials, MR CLEAN, showed significant benefit. MR CLEAN was a multicenter randomized controlled trial conducted in the Netherlands. The trial's major inclusion and exclusion criteria are presented in Table 8.10. Eligible patients were 18 years of age or older and presented with an acute ischemic stroke caused by an occlusion of the M1, M2, A1, or A2 segments as confirmed by CT angiography, MR angiography, or digital subtraction angiography. The mechanical thrombectomy procedure had to be possible within 6 h of LKN. The primary outcome was the score on the modified Rankin Scale at 90 days. Five hundred patients were enrolled in the study. At 90 days, 32.6% of patients in the mechanical thrombectomy group and 19.1% of patients in the control group (usual medical care) were functionally independent (defined as a mRS score of 2 or less) (aRR 13.5, 95% CI 5.9–21.2), with an adjusted odds ratio of 2.16 (95% CI 1.39–3.38). The number needed to treat for this trial was 7.4.

A subsequent meta-analysis of five of the trials (MR. CLEAN [19], SWIFT-PRIME [20],

Table 8.10 Inclusion criteria for mechanical thrombectomy in the 0–6-h window

Age	≥18
Location of LVO	ICA, M1, M2[b], A1, A2[b], tandem
NIHSS	≥6[a]
ASPECTS	≥6[a]
mRS	0-1[a]

mRS modified Rankin Scale; *ASPECTS* Alberta Stroke Program Early CT Score; *LVO* large vessel occlusion; *ICA* internal carotid artery; *M1 and M2* middle cerebral artery, first and second segments, respectively; *A1 and A2* anterior cerebral artery, first and second segments, respectively
[a]Although the benefit is uncertain, mechanical thrombectomy may be useful in patients with a pre-stroke mRS score >1, ASPECTS <6, or NIHSS score <6 [18]
[b]Pooled analyses of patient-level clinic trial data have shown a trend (non-statistically significant) towards favorable outcome for mechanical thrombectomy over standard care in M2 occlusions [18]

EXTEND-IA [21], ESCAPE [22], and REVASCAT [23]) using patient-level data confirmed the beneficial effect of MT in the 0–6 h window. Of 1287 patients analyzed (634 assigned to MT, 653 assigned to control), mRS of 0–2 was achieved by 46% of patients in the MT group and 26.5% in the control group (aRR 19.5%) for an adjusted odds ratio of 2.7 (95% CI 2.07–3.55, $p < 0.0001$; NNT 5.1). In this meta-analysis, a subgroup analysis of M2 occlusions showed a trend favoring MT, but did not reach statistical significance (adjusted cOR 1.28, 95% CI 0.51–3.21) [24]. Other meta-analyses have reached similar conclusions [25].

It is recommended that patients who are also eligible for tPA or tenecteplase should receive these treatments prior to mechanical thrombectomy. Furthermore, after the administration of these treatments, observation for improvement prior to performing MT is not recommended as delays in recanalization are associated with worse outcomes [25].

6–24 Hours and Perfusion Imaging

Perfusion imaging measures blood flow to different regions of the brain. Specifically, rapid, sequential imaging allows for a bolus of contrast to be tracked as it passes through the brain tissue, thereby generating data from which the three main parameters of cerebral perfusion—cerebral blood flow (CBF), cerebral blood volume (CBV), and mean transit time (MTT)—can be calculated. Cerebral blood flow is the amount of blood flowing through a given volume of brain over a given amount of time (typically 100 g of brain over 1 min; mL g^{-1} min^{-1}). In a healthy, resting, adult brain, typical CBF for gray matter is 80 mL 100 g^{-1} min^{-1} and 20 mL 100 g^{-1} min^{-1} in white matter. Cerebral blood volume is the amount of blood in a given volume of brain at any given time (100 g of brain; mL 100 g^{-1}). The average value in a healthy, resting, adult brain is 3.7 mL 100 g^{-1}. The mean transit time is the time it takes for blood to traverse a given volume of brain tissue, typically measured in seconds. In the normal human brain, MTT is 4.7 s. These parameters are related by the equation MTT = CBV/CBF.

For a given large vessel occlusion, a great degree of patient-to-patient heterogeneity exists in the size and extent of the resulting core and penumbra regions. Moreover, the time it takes for the penumbral (ischemic) region to progress to irreversible infarction (core) is variable. This variability depends largely on the degree of collateral circulation and ability of the brain vasculature to autoregulate. As a result of this variability, early work in reperfusion-related outcomes demonstrated that patients with smaller core sizes and larger penumbral regions at the time of reperfusion had better outcomes [26, 27].

The culmination of this research occurred in 2018 when two large clinical trials demonstrated the benefits of endovascular therapy within 16 h and 24 h, respectively, of symptom onset. In the Clinical Mismatch in the Triage of Wake Up and Late Presenting Strokes Undergoing Neurointervention with Trevo (DAWN) trial, eligible patients were 18 years of age or older presenting between 6 and 24 h of last known normal with an occlusion of the intracranial ICA, M1 segment, or both and had a clinical imaging mismatch. Clinical imaging mismatch was defined as a mismatch between the severity of clinical deficits and the infarct (core) volume on perfusion imaging. Three groups of clinical imaging mismatch were defined based on age and clinical stroke severity: Group A were 80 years of age or older, had a score of 10 or higher on the NIHSS, and had an infarct volume of <21 ml; Group B were <80 years of age, had an NIHSS of 10 or higher, and had an infarct volume of <31 ml; and Group C were <80 years of age, had an NIHSS of ≥20, and had an infarct volume of 31–50 ml. Quantitative measurement of infarct core volume was obtained using automated perfusion analysis software (RAPID, IschemaView) (Fig. 8.8). Patients meeting these criteria were randomly assigned to thrombectomy plus usual care or usual care alone. The primary outcome was the rate of functional independence, defined as a score of ≤2, on the mRS at 90 days. Two hundred and six patients were enrolled (107 MT, 99 usual care alone). The trial was terminated early due to a prespecified interim analysis showing overwhelming benefit in the mechanical thrombectomy group. At 90 days, the rate of functional independence was 49% in the mechanical thrombectomy group and 13% in the control group (aRR 36%, 95% CI 21–44%, posterior probability of superiority >0.999). The rate of sICH did not differ between the two groups (6% vs. 3%, $p = 0.5$) nor did 90-day mortality (19% vs. 18%, $p = 1.00$) [28].

In the Endovascular Therapy Following Imaging Evaluation of Ischemic Stroke 3 (DEFUSE 3) trial, patients 18 year of age or older with stroke due to occlusion of the intra-cranial ICA or M1 segment whose symptoms started within 6–16 h of enrollment underwent perfusion imaging. Patients who had a favorable perfusion profile, defined as core of <70 mL, tissue at risk of at least 15 mL, and a core/infarcted tissue volume to ischemic tissue volume ratio of ≥1.8 were randomized to mechanical thrombectomy plus standard medical care or standard medical care alone. The primary outcome was the shift in mRS score at 90 days. The trial was terminated early due to overwhelming efficacy. A favorable shift in mRS score at 90 days was seen (OR 2.77, 95% CI 1.63–4.70; $p < 0.001$), and functional independence (mRS of ≤2) was achieved in 45% of patients in the mechanical thrombectomy group as compared to 17% in the standard medical care group (risk ratio 2.67, 95% CI 1.6–4.48, $p < 0.001$). Ninety-day mortality (mRS shift from 6 [death] to lower scores) was significantly improved with mechanical thrombectomy (14% vs. 26%, $p = 0.05$). There was no difference in sICH (7% vs. 4%, $p = 0.75$) or other adverse events between the groups [29].

The inclusion criteria for the DEFUSE 3 trial were less restrictive than those of DAWN, allowing patients with larger cores size, a lower NIHSS, and a higher premorbid mRS to be enrolled. Conversely, DAWN enrolled patients up to 24 h from last known normal, whereas DEFUSE 3 criteria only went to 16 h—excluding

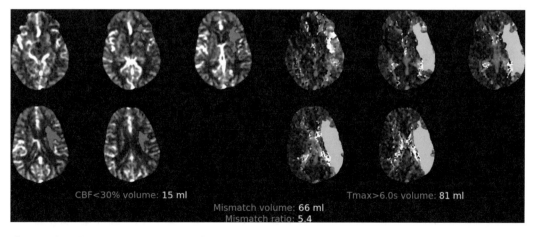

CBF<30% volume: **15 ml**   Tmax>6.0s volume: **81 ml**

Mismatch volume: **66 ml**
Mismatch ratio: **5.4**

Fig. 8.8 Quantitative measurement of infarct core volume as obtained by automated perfusion analysis software (RAPID, IschemaView)

some otherwise eligible patients presenting between 16 and 24 h. Retrospective analysis of patients presenting to a single DAWN trial-participating center during the trial enrollment period demonstrated that of 103 patients who met eligibility criteria for both trials, 15 (14.6%) would have been excluded if only DEFUSE 3 criteria were applied, and 28 (27.2%) would have been excluded if only the DAWN criteria were applied—confirming the higher inclusivity of DEFUSE 3 criteria. Approximately 13%, or nearly all of those excluded by DEFUSE 3 criteria, were due to presentation beyond 16 h [30]. Thus, the greatest inclusion of patients would come from application of DEFUSE 3 criteria to patients up to 24 h. In order to ensure that benefit was retained under the broader inclusion criteria, a retrospective, patient level data, review was undertaken in which the DAWN criteria were applied to DEFUSE 3 patients. Of patients enrolled in DEFUSE 3 who otherwise would have been excluded in DAWN (due to core too large, premorbid mRS too high, or NIHSS too low), the benefit of mechanical thrombectomy was significantly retained in the core too large group (OR 20.9), and a trend towards benefit remained in those with NIHSS too low. There was an inadequate number of patients with mRS = 2 to address the retention of benefit in this subgroup [31].

As a result of the above data, guidelines from the AHA/ASA currently recommend mechanical thrombectomy for patients presenting in the 6–16 h window who meet criteria for either DAWN or DEFUSE 3 and for patients presenting within 16–24 h who meet DAWN eligibility criteria [18]. Many stroke centers across the United States, however, have made the decision, outside of the above recommendations, to apply the DEFUSE 3 criteria up to 24 h for patient selection. The safety and benefit of this practice have been argued due to the similarities in the patients actually enrolled in both trials. For example, the median NIHSS for the thrombectomy groups in DAWN and DEFUSE 3 was 17 and 16, respectively, while the median core infarct volume was 7.6 mL (IQR 2.0–18.0) and 9.4 mL (IQR 2.3–25.6), respectively.

Early Supportive Care

Blood Pressure

The blood pressure target which optimizes favorable outcomes in patients with acute ischemic stroke is uncertain. A U-shaped relationship between initial BP and mortality has been suggested [32]. Additionally, some studies have demonstrated a deleterious effect on outcomes with lower BPs, but this finding is not consistent. Indeed, the optimal BP target is likely a highly individual factor based on stroke symptoms, location, subtype, and the patient's underlying comorbidities. In general, it is recommended that mild to moderate hypertension (typically defined as blood pressures up to 220/120 mmHg) go untreated in the early period (first 24–72 h) of an acute ischemic stroke. Blood pressure lowering is generally recommended with more severe hypertension (>220/120 mmHg) and when comorbidities requiring it are present. Following the administration of alteplase, a BP goal of <180/105 is recommended to minimize the risk of intracranial hemorrhage [33]. The optimal blood pressure target following mechanical thrombectomy remains uncertain and is a matter of ongoing research. Preliminary data suggest an association between higher post-mechanical thrombectomy blood pressures and worse functional outcomes [34, 35].

Early Dual-Antiplatelet Therapy in Minor Stroke or High-Risk TIA

In the Clopidogrel with Aspirin in Acute Minor Stroke of Transient Ischemic Attack (CHANCE) [36] trial, patients 40 years of age or older presenting within 24 h of onset with a minor ischemic stroke (defined as an NIHSS of ≤3) or high-risk TIA (defined as ABCD2 score ≥4) were randomly assigned to receive aspirin alone or aspirin plus a 300 mg loading dose of clopidogrel followed by clopidogrel 75 mg daily for a total of 21 days, followed by clopidogrel monotherapy. The trial enrolled 5170 patients (2584 clopidogrel + aspirin, 2586 aspirin alone) with a median age of 62 years. The index event was a high-risk TIA in 1445 (27.9%) of the enrolled patients. The primary outcome of recurrent stroke (ischemic or hemorrhagic) at 90 days occurred in 212 (8.2%) patients assigned to aspirin + clopidogrel and 303 (11.7%) patients assigned to aspirin alone (HR 0.68, 95% CI 0.57–0.81; $p < 0.001$). Moderate or severe bleeding, hemorrhagic stroke, and death did not differ between the two groups.

In the Clopidogrel and Aspirin in Acute Ischemic Stroke and High-Risk TIA (POINT) [37] trial, patients 18 years of age or older presenting within 12 h of onset with minor ischemic stroke (defined as NIHSS ≤3) or high-risk TIA (defined as ABCD2 score ≥4) were randomly assigned to receive aspirin alone or aspirin plus a 600 mg loading dose of clopidogrel followed by clopidogrel 75 mg for a total of 90 days. The trial was stopped early due to exceeding both a prespecified safety boundary for major hemorrhage in the aspirin + clopidogrel group and an efficacy boundary. A total of 4883 patients were enrolled (2432 clopidogrel + aspirin, 2449 aspirin alone) with a median age of 65 years. The index event was a high-risk TIA in 2108 (43%) of the enrolled patients. At the time of stoppage, 4557 (93.4%) of patients had completed the 90-day trial visit or had died (i.e., complete data was available). Recurrent stroke occurred in 116 (4.8%) of the aspirin + clopidogrel group and 156 (6.4%) of the aspirin only group (HR 0.74, 95% CI 0.58–0.94, $p = 0.01$). Major hemorrhage occurred in 23 (0.9%) of the aspirin + clopidogrel group and 10 (0.4%) in the aspirin only group (HR 2.32, 95% CI 1.10–4.87; $p = 0.02$). However, in a secondary analysis, the benefit of clopidogrel plus aspirin was concentrated in the first few weeks of treatment ($p = 0.04$ for days 0–7 and $p = 0.02$ for days 0–30), while the risk of hemorrhage with clopidogrel plus aspirin was greater during the period from 8 to 90 days than during the first 7 days ($p = 0.04$ for days 8 to 90 and $p = 0.34$ for days 0–7). Therefore, similar to the CHANCE trial, the use of dual-antiplatelet therapy for a short duration following minor stroke or high-risk TIA appears to be efficacious without increasing the risk of major hemorrhage. The optimal duration of dual-antiplatelet therapy remains uncertain, but based on the trial data above, most would opt for 21 days.

References

1. Sacco RL, Kasner SE, Broderick JP, Caplan LR, Connors JJ, Culebras A, et al. An updated definition of stroke for the 21st century. Stroke. 2013;44(7):2064–89.
2. Yang Q, Tong X, Schieb L, et al. Vital signs: recent trends in stroke death rates — United States, 2000–2015. MMWR Morb Mortal Wkly Rep. 2017;66:933–9.
3. Mozaffarian D, Benjamin EJ, Go AS, Arnett DK, Blaha MJ, Cushman M, et al. Heart disease and stroke statistics-2016 update. Circulation. 2016;133(4):e38–e360.
4. Benjamin Emelia J, Muntner P, Alonso A, Bittencourt Marcio S, Callaway Clifton W, Carson April P, et al. Heart disease and stroke statistics—2019 update: a report from the American Heart Association. Circulation. 2019;139(10):e56–e528.
5. Meschia J, Bushnell C, Boden-Albala B, Braun L, Bravata D, Chaturvedi S, et al. Guidelines for the primary prevention of stroke. A statement for healthcare professionals from the American Heart Association/American Stroke Association. Stroke. 2014;45:3754–832.
6. Adams H, Bendixen B, Kappelle L, Biller J, Love BB, Gordon DL, Marsh EE. Classification of subtype of acute ischemic stroke. Definitions for use in a multicenter clinical trial. TOAST. Trial of Org 10172 in acute stroke treatment. Stroke. 1993;24:35–41.
7. Aroor S, Singh R, Goldstein L. BE-FAST (Balance, Eyes, Face, Arm, Speech, Time). Reducing the proportion of strokes missed using the FAST mnemonic. Stroke. 2017;48:479–81.
8. Sharma VK, Wong LKS. Middle cerebral artery disease. In: Grotta JC, Albers GW, Broderick JP, Kasner SE, Lo EH, Mendelow AD, et al., editors. Stroke pathophysiology, diagnosis, and management. 6th ed. New York: Elsevier; 2016.
9. Brust JCM, Chamorro A. Anterior cerebral artery disease. In: Grotta JC, Albers GW, Broderick JP, Kasner SE, Lo EH, Mendelow AD, et al., editors. Stroke pathophysiology, diagnosis, and management. 6th ed. New York: Elsevier; 2016.
10. Kim JS. Posterior cerebral artery disease. In: Grotta JC, Albers GW, Broderick JP, Kasner SE, Lo EH, Mendelow AD, et al., editors. Stroke pathophysiology, diagnosis, and management. 6th ed. New York: Elsevier; 2016.
11. Caplan LR. Lacunar infarction and small vessel disease: pathology and pathophysiology. J Stroke. 2015;17(1):2–6.
12. Norrving B. Lacunar syndromes, lacunar infarcts, and cerebral small-vessel disease. In: Grotta JC, Albers GW, Broderick JP, Kasner SE, Lo EH, Mendelow AD, et al., editors. Stroke pathophysiology, diagnosis, and management. 6th ed. New York: Elsevier; 2016.
13. Cruz-Flores S, Rabinstein A, Biller J, Elkind MS, Griffith P, Gorelick PB, et al. Racial-ethnic disparities in stroke care: the American experience: a statement

for healthcare professionals from the American Heart Association/American Stroke Association. Stroke. 2011;42(7):2091–116.

14. Ekundayo OJ, Saver JL, Fonarow GC, Schwamm LH, Xian Y, Zhao X, et al. Patterns of emergency medical services use and its association with timely stroke treatment. Circ Cardiovasc Qual Outcomes. 2013;6(3):262–9.

15. Fang JKN, Ayala C, Dai S, Merritt R, Denny CH. Awareness of stroke warning symptoms – 13 states and the District of Columbia, 2005. MMWR. 2008;57(18):481–5.

16. Ojike N, Ravenell J, Seixas A, Masters-Israilov A, Rogers A, Jean-Louis G, et al. Racial disparity in stroke awareness in the US: an analysis of the 2014 National Health Interview Survey. J Neurol Neurophysiol. 2016;7(2):365.

17. Patel A, Fang J, Gillespie C, Odom E, King SC, Luncheon C, et al. Awareness of stroke signs and symptoms and calling 9-1-1 among US adults: National Health Interview Survey, 2009 and 2014. Prev Chron Dis. 2019;16:E78.

18. Powers WJ, Rabinstein AA, Ackerson T, Adeoye OM, Bambakidis NC, Becker K, et al. Guidelines for the early management of patients with acute ischemic stroke: 2019 update to the 2018 guidelines for the early management of acute ischemic stroke: a guideline for healthcare professionals from the American Heart Association/American Stroke Association. Stroke. 2019;50(12):e344–418.

19. Berkhemer OA, Fransen PSS, Beumer D, Van Den Berg LA, Lingsma HF, Yoo AJ, et al. A randomized trial of intraarterial treatment for acute ischemic stroke. N Engl J Med. 2015;372(1):11–20.

20. Saver JL, Goyal M, Bonafe A, Diener H-C, Levy EI, Pereira VM, et al. Stent-retriever thrombectomy after intravenous t-PA vs. t-PA alone in stroke. N Engl J Med. 2015;372(24):2285–95.

21. Campbell BCV, Mitchell PJ, Kleinig TJ, Dewey HM, Churilov L, Yassi N, et al. Endovascular therapy for ischemic stroke with perfusion-imaging selection. N Engl J Med. 2015;372(11):1009–18.

22. Goyal M, Demchuk AM, Menon BK, Eesa M, Rempel JL, Thornton J, et al. Randomized assessment of rapid endovascular treatment of ischemic stroke. N Engl J Med. 2015;372(11):1019–30.

23. Jovin TG, Chamorro A, Cobo E, De Miquel MA, Molina CA, Rovira A, et al. Thrombectomy within 8 hours after symptom onset in ischemic stroke. N Engl J Med. 2015;372(24):2296–306.

24. Goyal M, Menon BK, van Zwam WH, Dippel DW, Mitchell PJ, Demchuk AM, Dávalos A, Majoie CB, van der Lugt A, De Miquel MA, Donnan GA. Endovascular thrombectomy after large-vessel ischaemic stroke: a meta-analysis of individual patient data from five randomised trials. Lancet. 2016;387(10029):1723–31.

25. Bush CK, Kurimella D, Cross LJS, Conner KR, Martin-Schild S, He J, et al. Endovascular treatment with stent-retriever devices for acute ischemic stroke: a metaanalysis of randomized controlled trials. PLoS One. 2016;11:e0147287.

26. Albers GW, Thijs V, Wechsler L, Kemp S, Schlaug G, Skalbrin E, et al. Magnetic resonance imaging profiles predict clinical response to early reperfusion: the diffusion and perfusion imaging evaluation for understanding stroke evolution (DEFUSE) study. Ann Neurol. 2006;60(5):508–17.

27. Lansberg MG, Straka M, Kemp S, Mlynash M, Wechsler L, Jovin TG, et al. MRI profile and response to endovascular reperfusion after stroke (DEFUSE 2): a prospective cohort study. Lancet Neruol. 2006;11(10):860–7.

28. Nogueira RG, Jadhav AP, Haussen DC, Bonafe A, Budzik RF, Bhuva P, et al. Thrombectomy 6 to 24 hours after stroke with a mismatch between deficit and infarct. N Engl J Med. 2017;378(1):11–21.

29. Albers GW, Marks MP, Kemp S, Christensen S, Tsai JP, Ortega-Gutierrez S, et al. Thrombectomy for stroke at 6 to 16 hours with selection by perfusion imaging. N Engl J Med. 2018;378(8):708–18.

30. Jadhav AP, Desai S, Kenmuir C, Rocha M, Starr M, Molyneaux B, et al. Eligibility for endovascular trial enrollment in the 6- to 24-hour time window: analysis of a single comprehensive stroke center. Stroke. 2018;49:1015–7.

31. Leslie-Mazwi TM, Hamilton S, Mlynash M, Patel AB, Schwamm LH, Lansberg MG, et al. DEFUSE 3 non-DAWN patients. Stroke. 2019;50(3):618–25.

32. Vemmos K, Tsivgoulis G, Spengos K, Zakopoulos N, Synetos A, Manios E, et al. U-shaped relationship between mortality and admission blood pressure in patients with acute stroke. J Intern Med. 2004;255:257–65.

33. Demaerschalk BM, Kleindorfer DO, Adeoye OM, Demchuk AM, Fugate J, Grotta JC, et al. Scientific rationale for the inclusion and exclusion criteria for intravenous alteplase in acute ischemic stroke. A statement for healthcare professionals from the American Heart Association/American Stroke Association. Stroke. 2016;47:581–641.

34. Goyal N, Tsivgoulis G, Pandhi A, Chang J, Dillard K, et al. Blood pressure levels post mechanical thrombectomy and outcomes in large vessel occlusion strokes. Neurology. 2017;89:1–8.

35. Mistry E, Mistry A, Nakawah M, Khattar N, Fortuny E, et al. Systolic blood pressure within 24 hours after mechanical thrombectomy for acute ischemic stroke correlates with outcome. J Am Heart Assoc. 2017;6(5):e006167.

36. Wang Y, Wang Y, Zhao X, Liu L, Wang D, Wang C, et al. Clopidogrel with aspirin in acute minor stroke or transient ischemic attack. N Engl J Med. 2013;369:11–9.

37. Johnston S, Easton J, Farrant M, Barsan W, Conwit R, Elm J, et al. Clopidogrel and aspirin in acute ischemic stroke and high-risk TIA. N Engl J Med. 2018;379:215–25.

Intracerebral Hemorrhage

David Dornbos III, Kendrick Johnson,
Pratik V. Patel, and Lucas Elijovich

Introduction

Distinct from subarachnoid hemorrhage (SAH) and isolated intraventricular hemorrhage (IVH), intracerebral hemorrhage (ICH) is defined as bleeding into the brain parenchyma. Despite improved control of hypertension and a decrease in ICH secondary to hypertension, the incidence of overall ICH has not appreciably changed with time due to an increase in lobar ICH due to amyloid angiopathy in an aging population [1]. Due to an incidence that steadily increases with advancing age [1], the overall incidence of ICH is expected to continue to increase with the growing elderly population [2]. As such, intimate knowledge of this disease process is critical for a wide range of medical practitioners from the emergency room to the intensive care

unit (ICU). Neurologists, intensivists, and neurosurgeons must work closely together to make critical decisions regarding the prognostication, medical management, utility of emergency interventions, and potential surgical interventions. Predominantly a disease process best treated with medical management, further clinical trials are underway to assess the utility of novel, cutting-edge surgical interventions as well.

Epidemiology

Intracerebral hemorrhage is a common neurological emergency, accounting for 10–20% of the nearly 800,000 strokes per year in the United States [1, 2]. The overall incidence of ICH in the United States is approximately 12–15 cases per 100,000 [3]. Spontaneous primary ICH occurs secondary to rupture of small intraparenchymal arterioles, physiologically distinct from subarachnoid hemorrhage secondary to rupture of an intracranial aneurysm. Primary ICH typically occurs secondary to long-standing hypertension or amyloid angiopathy (Table 9.1). The long-standing effects of hypertension on small arterioles account for two-thirds of all ICH [4], although the prevalence of cerebral amyloid angiopathy (CAA) has been steadily increasing with the aging population. Further, the risk of recurrent hemorrhage in patients with amyloid angiopathy is increased threefold with the pres-

D. Dornbos III · K. Johnson
Department of Neurosurgery, Semmes-Murphey Clinic and University of Tennessee Health and Science Center, Memphis, TN, USA
e-mail: kdjohnson@semmes-murphey.com

P. V. Patel
Department of Anesthesiology and Pain Medicine, Harborview Medical Center, University of Washington School of Medicine, Seattle, WA, USA
e-mail: pratikv@uw.edu

L. Elijovich (✉)
Department of Neurology and Neurosurgery, Semmes-Murphey Clinic, University of Tennessee Health Sciences Center, Memphis, TN, USA
e-mail: lelijovich@semmes-murphey.com

Table 9.1 Etiology of spontaneous intracerebral hemorrhage

Primary ICH	Secondary ICH
Hypertension	Vascular malformations
Cerebral amyloid angiopathy	Arteriovenous malformation
Sympathomimetic drugs	Cavernous malformation
Cocaine	Aneurysm
Methamphetamine	Dural arteriovenous fistula
Coagulopathy	Moyamoya disease/syndrome
	Ischemic stroke with hemorrhagic conversion
	Cerebral venous sinus thrombosis
	Tumor
	Cerebral vasculitis

ence of the E2 and E4 alleles of the apolipoprotein E gene [5]. Additionally, primary ICH may also be seen in the setting of coagulopathy or sympathomimetic drugs, such as cocaine or methamphetamines.

Secondary ICH is observed with spontaneous ICH in the setting of an underlying predisposing disorder. This pathology is frequently observed in the setting of an underlying structural lesion, such as a tumor (primary or metastatic) or vascular malformation (cavernous malformation, arteriovenous malformation, or dural arteriovenous fistula). Cerebral vasculitis, moyamoya disease, cerebral venous sinus thrombosis, and hemorrhagic conversion following ischemic stroke may also lead to secondary causes of spontaneous ICH. Ultimately, the underlying etiology of ICH is determined from the clinical presentation, risk factors, imaging hemorrhage characteristics (particularly the location), and tissue pathology (if available).

The basal ganglia are the most frequent location for hypertensive ICH, observed in over 70% of cases [1]. Other common locations for hypertensive ICH include the thalamus, cerebellum, pontine tegmentum, and deep lobar white matter. CAA-associated ICH is typically located in the peripheral lobar white matter near the gray-white junction, a distinction that helps identify the underlying etiology in primary ICH (Fig. 9.1).

Risk Factors

The underlying risk factors responsible for primary ICH are relatively well established. Hypertension, increasing age, ethnicity, high alcohol intake, and lower low-density lipoprotein C (LDL-C) are all known to contribute to ICH risk. Hypertension generates a fivefold increase in the risk of subsequent ICH, a risk that increases in a dramatic fashion with increasing hypertensive severity [6–8]. Excessive alcohol intake is also an independent risk factor for ICH, extending a higher degree of risk with increasing alcohol consumption [9, 10]. Interestingly, numerous studies have identified that increasing levels of LDL-C and triglycerides impart a protective effect regarding ICH risk [7, 11, 12]. Of note, the SPARCL trial demonstrated that high-dose atorvastatin therapy following ischemic stroke was associated with an increased risk of subsequent ICH [13, 14].

Nonmodifiable risk factors, including ethnicity, age, and gender, also play a significant role as they pertain to primary ICH risk. Socioeconomic factors (lack of access to healthcare and poorly controlled hypertension) are certainly responsible for the increased ICH risk experienced by non-white individuals in part; however, this does not fully explain the disparity between African-Americans and whites with African-Americans experiencing a near twofold elevated risk of ICH [7, 15]. Furthermore, Hispanic and Asian individuals also experience an increased risk of ICH, although this is likely due to associated pathologies (cavernous malformations, moyamoya disease) and elevated risk of secondary ICH [16, 17]. Age is the most profound risk factor for primary ICH with a nearly twofold increase in ICH risk per decade of life [6, 7]. Men also have an increased risk of ICH compared with females [18].

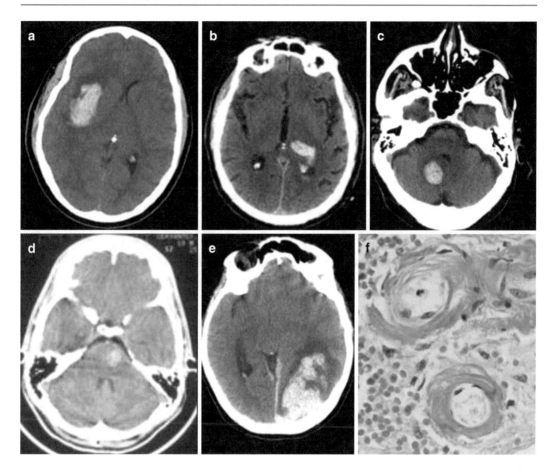

Fig. 9.1 Typical locations for hypertensive intracerebral hemorrhage. (**a**) Putaminal. (**b**) Thalamic. (**c**) Cerebellar white matter. (**d**) Pontine tegmentum. (**e**) Lobar white matter. (**f**) Hematoxylin and eosin photomicrograph demonstrating lipohyalinosis of small penetrating arteries that weaken the arterial wall and are the source of typical hypertensive ICH. (Photomicrographs provided courtesy of UCSF Neuropathology, Han Lee, MD PhD & Andrew W. Bollen, MD, DVM)

Prognosis

While ICH accounts for only 10–20% of strokes in the United States, this pathology is responsible for a disproportionately large amount of the overall morbidity, mortality, and socioeconomic burden of stroke. Short-term mortality is nearly 40%, and less than one-third of patients will be functionally independent following ICH. These outcomes have not changed appreciably despite decades of research [18]. This is a direct reflection of the absence of any effective proven treatments for ICH despite decades of investigation and numerous clinical trials. This lack of scientific progress and historically poor outcomes have resulted in significant heterogeneity in care and therapeutic nihilism manifested by early limitations in aggressive care that lead to self-fulfilling prophecy of poor outcomes [19–22]. In addition to the high degree of morbidity and mortality posed by this disease entity, the socioeconomic impact of ICH is exceedingly high, with hospital stays costing nearly $24,000 in the United States [19], imposing a nearly 6 billion dollar burden on the healthcare industry [20].

Pathophysiology

The underlying pathologic process that leads to rupture of small arterioles (<100 micron diameter) in hypertensive ICH has been termed lipohyalinosis. This process is characterized by subintimal fibroblast proliferation, deposition of lipid-filled macrophages, and replacement of smooth muscle cells with collagen in the tunica media of larger vessels (Fig. 9.1) [21]. This results in reduced blood vessel elasticity and increased susceptibility to spontaneous rupture.

The loss of neurological function that occurs following ICH has classically been ascribed to the tissue destruction caused by the initial hemorrhage as blood transects white matter tracts and destroys neurons. More recently, the importance of this form of mechanical tissue damage has been accompanied by a growing interest in mechanisms of secondary brain injury and potential therapeutic targets for these novel injury pathways. This has been spurred by the observation that many patients deteriorate clinically, even in the absence of early hematoma expansion or rehemorrhage. Importantly, this secondary clinical deterioration coincides with the time frame in which edema develops and clot absorption and hematoma breakdown occur.

Plasma proteins that are abundant in vasogenic edema and are increased by clot resorption have harmful effects on the brain. Further, patients with a higher ratio of edema to hematoma volume have been shown to have poorer clinical outcomes as well [22]. Thrombin, hemoglobin, and their breakdown products demonstrate neurotoxicity via glutamate-mediated excitotoxicity, acute perihematoma edema, and disruption of the blood-brain barrier [23]. Additionally, interleukin-1 and matrix metalloproteinases (MMPs) are upregulated in neurons and astrocytes within the perihematoma region, and perihematoma edema has been shown to be reduced in experimental models of ICH with both

MMP–9 knockout mice and following administration of IL-1 receptor antagonists [24, 25]. In addition to these deleterious changes, the toxic effects of iron and a range of inflammatory mediators have led to the concept of neurohemoinflammation as a descriptor for a variety of different pathways, which result in secondary brain injury after ICH. These small molecules and their biochemical signaling pathways, and even the potential use of iron-chelating agents such as deferoxamine, represent promising potential targets for future acute ICH therapy [26–29]. The results of a modified phase 2 randomized controlled trial (i-DEF) demonstrated safety of deferoxamine in acute ICH but did not demonstrate the pre-specified clinical efficacy endpoint in improving good outcomes at 3 months to warrant a phase 3 trial based upon the trial design [29].

Concern for perihematoma ischemia has been another area of active investigation regarding mechanisms of ICH-related secondary brain injury. Cerebral blood flow studies using single photon emission computed tomography (SPECT) and MRI perfusion and diffusion have attempted to demonstrate a perihematoma penumbra at risk for additional injury and neuronal loss due to hypoperfusion [30–32]. The significance of these findings has been called into question by more subsequent computed tomography (CT) perfusion studies that have failed to show a penumbra, by positron emission tomography (PET) studies that have found that these penumbral regions may, in fact, be appropriately perfused in the setting of reduced metabolic activity, and by animal studies which suggest a zone of hypoperfusion without impaired oxygen metabolism [33–35].

Historically, ICH was considered a monophasic event with an initial hemorrhage, growing to its maximal size within moments, with rehemorrhage or hematoma expansion as rare events suggestive of coagulopathy or underlying vascular anomaly. More recently, however, numerous studies have demonstrated that hematoma expansion is common early after acute ICH, even in the absence of an underlying lesion or coagulopathy. In a single-center prospective study, substantial hematoma growth (>33% enlargement of the baseline hematoma volume) occurred within the first day in 38% of patients who underwent initial CT within 3 hours of the ictus. Over a quarter of patients demonstrated enlargement within 1 hour after initial CT scan [36]. Retrospective studies have found similar rates of rebleeding, ranging from 18% to 36%, with substantially lower rates of delayed rebleeding beyond 6 hours from ictus, ranging from 2% to 10% [37–39]. Given that hematoma expansion is an important independent determinant of overall outcome, early aggressive blood pressure (BP) control to limit hematoma growth remains of utmost importance in initial patient management [40].

Clinical Presentation and Diagnosis

The clinical presentation of ICH is characterized by the sudden onset of focal neurological dysfunction, generally accompanied by severe headache. Prior to the advent of modern imaging, the presence of headache with the ictus was often cited as the defining characteristic of hemorrhagic stroke. However, headache at onset does not reliably distinguish ICH as it also occurs in up to 30% of patients with ischemic stroke [41]. Patients with large hemispheric ICH resulting in mass effect or those with significant IVH obstructing cerebrospinal fluid drainage may have profoundly elevated intracranial pressure (ICP) and often present with nausea and vomiting, in addition to headache and focal neurological deficits, which may rapidly progress to herniation and coma. The distinct presentation of coma with pinpoint pupils should immediately alert the practitioner to the possibility of a pontine tegmental hemorrhage.

Various baseline clinical and neuroimaging characteristics are predictive of outcome in ICH. These include hematoma volume, Glasgow Coma Scale Score, IVH, advanced age, and infratentorial ICH location [42–46]. There are several ICH scoring tools, which can provide practitioners a basis for grading the severity of illness and communicating among each other. The two most commonly used scores are the ICH (Table 9.2) and FUNC (Table 9.3) scores. The

Table 9.2 Intracerebral hemorrhage score

Predictor	Component score	ICH score	30-day mortality
Glasgow Coma Scale		0	0%
3–4	2	1	13%
5–12	1	2	26%
13–15	0	3	72%
Age (years)		4	97%
≥80	1	5	100%
<80	0		
ICH volume (cc)			
≥30	1		
<30	0		
Infratentorial location			
Yes	1		
No	0		
Intraventricular hemorrhage			
Yes	1		
No	0		

Table 9.3 FUNC score and outcomes

Predictor	Component score	FUNC score	Functional independence at 90 days
Glasgow Coma Scale		0	0%
≥9	2	1	0%
≤8	0	2	0%
Age		3	0%
<70	2	4	0%
70–79	1	5	4–10%
≥80	0	6	0–11%
ICH volume (cc)		7	18–22%
<30	4	8	39–47%
30–60	2	9	60–69%
>60	0	10	50–75%
ICH location		11	75–86%
Lobar	2		
Deep	1		
Infratentorial	0		
Pre-ICH cognitive impairment			
No	1		
Yes	0		

FUNC score builds upon the ICH score and includes pre-ICH cognitive impairment, drops IVH, and has been shown to better predict functional independence at 90 days post-hemorrhage [47]. It also has the advantage of accounting for the effect of withdrawal of care on outcome. It is essential to understand that both of these scores were developed to better understand factors that influence outcomes, but are not intended as the sole basis of prognostication. In addition, these scores have been largely validated during the early period of recovery (first 90 days); however, ICH recovery occurs over a longer period with significant recovery occurring up to 1 year post-ictus. ICH is a heterogenous disease with patients that are critically ill, often with multi-organ failure. Synthesis of the entire clinical scenario incorporating many factors not included in these scores is essential to both plan care and to guide families in terms of prognosis. A prospective study of patients with ICH clearly demonstrates that NICU staff (MDs and RNs) more accurately predicts outcome than ICH scores alone [48].

The widespread use of CT scanning has made the diagnosis of ICH relatively straightforward and remains the most widely used neuroimaging technique. Acute stroke MRI protocols utilizing susceptibility-weighted imaging that exploit the paramagnetic properties of hemoglobin can also accurately identify ICH with very high sensitivity and specificity as compared with CT (Fig. 9.2) [49]. Intracranial vascular imaging with conventional angiography is recommended for identifying vascular malformations, particularly in younger patients (age < 45), atypical hemorrhage location for hypertensive etiology, or if the patient has no history of hypertension [50]. Vascular imaging is also recommended in cases where the hemorrhage appears to originate from the ventricle, as the yield of angiography is quite high in this population [51]. Multi-slice computed tomography angiography (CTA) has been proposed as a surrogate for conventional angiography [52], although the sensitivity is insufficient to advocate foregoing conventional angiography. CTA with early and delayed image acquisition may be helpful in cases of acute ICH to identify patients with active contrast extravasation, as this is an important predictor of hematoma expansion and worse outcome [53–56]. This could also the-

oretically help target interventions toward patients most likely to experience ongoing hematoma expansion, although studies using the spot sign to enrich the population for intervention have not demonstrated benefit [57].

Management of Intracerebral Hemorrhage

Blood Pressure

Elevated BP is extremely common in the setting of acute ICH. Blood pressure management in this setting, however, remains controversial due to concerns over balancing the competing interests of limiting hematoma expansion or rebleeding while simultaneously avoiding the theoretical risk of secondary ischemic injury through hypoperfusion of the perihematoma brain parenchyma.

Previous studies have conflicted over whether elevated BP predisposes to hematoma expansion after acute ICH [58–60]. However, more recent studies have suggested that perihematoma ischemia is unlikely to be a major contributor to ICH-related brain injury in most cases [34, 35, 61]. Two large randomized controlled trials were undertaken to shed further light on this clinical conundrum. The Second Intensive Blood Pressure Reduction in Acute Cerebral Haemorrhage Trial (INTERACT-2) randomized patients within 6 hours of ICH onset into groups targeting either SBP <140 or <180 mm Hg, with this blood pressure parameter tightly followed for 7 days [62]. While no difference was observed between the groups regarding death and disability at 90 days, functional outcomes were improved in the more intensive blood pressure regimen (<140 mm Hg). Based on the INTERACT-2 findings, the AHA guidelines in 2015 recommended treating acute hypertension in these patients to target SBP <140 mm Hg [63].

A subsequent randomized clinical trial (The Second Intensive Blood Pressure Reduction in Acute Cerebral Haemorrhage Trial; ATACH-2) evaluated patients treated with the same SBP targets, although initiating treatment within

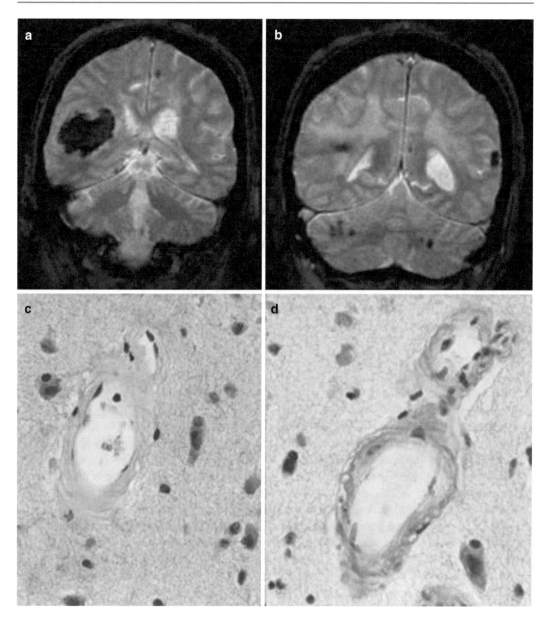

Fig. 9.2 Histopathology and neuroimaging of cerebral amyloid angiopathy (CAA). (**a, b**) MRI T2 susceptibility-weighted image demonstrates a parietal-occipital lobar hemorrhage with several asymptomatic microhemorrhages scattered throughout the cerebral and cerebellar hemispheres. (**c**) Hematoxylin and eosin photomicrograph of a cerebral arteriole demonstrating medial thickening secondary to amyloid deposition. (**d**) Congo-red staining of B-amyloid deposition in the media diagnostic of CAA. (Photomicrographs provided courtesy of UCSF Neuropathology, Han Lee, MD PhD & Andrew W. Bollen, MD, DVM)

4.5 hours of onset and maintaining this threshold for only 24 hours [64]. This study found no difference between the two groups in death and disability at 90 days or in functional outcomes, but did identify a higher rate of renal adverse events within 7 days in patients treated with the higher intensity regimen. Further analysis of these two trials identified that the BP reduction in ATACH-2 was more profound and rapid (average SBP 120–130 mm Hg in first 24 hours) compared to that observed in INTERACT-2 (average SBP 135–145 mm Hg), a possible explanation for the difference in outcomes between the two trials [65]. Importantly, patients experiencing SBP <130 mm Hg and patients with greater BP lability in the INTERACT-2 trial were found to have worse clinical outcomes [66, 67]. In fact, a post hoc analysis of the ATACH-2 trial revealed that intensive and rapid blood pressure reduction in patients presenting with SBP >220 mm Hg was associated with a higher rate of neurologic deterioration within 24 hours without any benefit in reducing hematoma expansion [68]. Given that combined data from these trials did not identify broad benefit for tight SBP targets and that rapid and aggressive BP reduction can be harmful, recent guidelines from the American College of Cardiology/American Heart Association Task Force recommend against immediate SBP reduction to SBP <140 mm Hg in patients that present within 6 hours of onset and have SBP between 150 and 220 mm Hg [69].

While the data still certainly supports blood pressure control and reduction, caution should be emphasized exercised to avoid excessive and rapid blood pressure lowering and Individualized blood pressure goals based upon individual patient characteristics such as presumed etiology of hemorrhage (hypertension vs underlying vascular anomaly), history of chronic hypertension and baseline blood pressure, and known or suspected major vessel arterial stenosis where a significant decline in blood pressure could cause secondary organ damage are recommended [70]. For patients presenting with SBP between 150 and 220 mm Hg and without contraindication to acute BP treatment, acute lowering of SBP to 140 mm Hg is safe, although care should be taken to avoid overcorrection, and use of a continuous intravenous infusion and frequent monitoring of BP and neurological examination are recommended [63]. When SBP >220 mm Hg, it is reasonable to use continuous intravenous drug infusion and close BP monitoring to lower SBP [69]. In these patients in particular, if there is evidence of or suspicion for elevated ICP, it is important to consider monitoring ICP and reducing BP with continuous intravenous medications to keep the cerebral perfusion

pressure (CPP) between 60 and 80 mm Hg. In situations where SBP exceeds 220 mm Hg without suspicion of elevated ICP, a modest reduction in SBP to <160 mm Hg should be considered. The choice of BP-lowering agent should be individualized based on factors such as heart rate and medical comorbidities (e.g., renal or heart failure); however, our standard preference is to use agents that preferentially affect cardiac output or act as arterial vasodilators, such as bolus doses of intravenous labetalol or continuous IV infusion of nicardipine or clevidipine. We try to avoid medications that might cause significant venodilation such as hydralazine or nitroprusside.

Coagulopathy

While not the leading cause of ICH, anticoagulation is responsible for approximately 10–15% of spontaneous ICH, accounting for significant morbidity and mortality [71]. The routine use of anticoagulation for any indication carries an annual 2% risk of ICH [72]. Historically, warfarin (half-life 36 hours) was used with the greatest frequency, although non-vitamin K oral anticoagulants (NOACs) have become increasingly more prevalent given their ease of use and maintenance. The risk of warfarin-related ICH increases with increasing international normalized ratio (INR) [73, 74] and is associated with an even higher rate of mortality than ICH in the absence of coagulopathy [75]. In these patients, the obvious goal is to immediately reverse the coagulopathy. This has historically been done using vitamin K and fresh frozen plasma (FFP); however, this approach is suboptimal and often leads to excessively slow correction or failure to adequately correct the coagulopathy [76].

Current guidelines recommend the use of 5–10 mg of vitamin K, usually administered intravenously by slow push, and concurrent treatment with a more rapidly acting reversal agent [77, 78]. Full warfarin correction usually necessitates the administration of large volumes of FFP, and the logistics surrounding crossmatching, thawing, and infusion rates makes this generally a slower option for correction. In the setting of potentially life-threatening ICH, interest has turned to the use of concentrated factor preparations such as prothrombin complex concentrate (PCC) [79–81]. PCC comes in two variations, including either the three-factor (factors II, IX, and X) or four-factor (factors II, VII, IX, and X) formulations, and dosing is titrated based on the presenting INR [82]. Despite the time savings afforded by PCC compared to FFP, no difference in hematoma growth has been observed in patients whose INR was corrected within 2 hours, strongly suggesting that the timing of coagulopathy reversal is what makes the difference, rather than a specific agent [83]. Numerous current guidelines for warfarin reversal in the setting of life-threatening hemorrhage now emphasize the use of a rapid reversal agent, such as PCC, in combination with vitamin K [77, 84, 85].

Non-vitamin K Oral Anticoagulants

New-generation oral anticoagulants, including factor Xa inhibitors (rivaroxaban, edoxaban, and apixaban) and direct thrombin inhibitors (dabigatran), are in frequent use for the treatment of venous thromboembolism, atrial fibrillation, and numerous other indications [82]. The primary benefit of these medications in comparison to warfarin is that they do not require close monitoring of effect level and they offer a much more regimented dosing schedule. While this offers a significant quality of life benefit, reversal agents are not as readily available in the setting of life-threatening or significant ICH.

The direct factor Xa inhibitors selectively bind to and inhibit factor Xa without the need for the enzymatic activity of antithrombin, decreasing the downstream conversion of prothrombin to thrombin. Rivaroxaban (half-life 5–9 hours) is a synthetic direct factor Xa inhibitor, typically reserved for prophylactic deep venous thrombosis (DVT) treatment and atrial fibrillation [86]. The drug demonstrates high bioavailability at 80–100% and is highly protein bound (92–95%). Apixaban (half-life 12 hours) is another oral factor Xa inhibitor, predominantly used in stroke prevention secondary to atrial fibrillation and for

the treatment and prevention of DVT [87, 88]. In comparison to rivaroxaban, apixaban demonstrates prolonged absorption, is 87% protein bound, and is only partially renally excreted. Finally, edoxaban (half-life 10–14 hours) demonstrates 62% bioavailability [89]. Edoxaban is indicated for stroke risk reduction in the setting of non-valvular atrial fibrillation and for both treatment and prevention of DVT.

While the high bioavailability and protein-bound nature of this drug class make it an attractive option for anticoagulation, they also lend limited options when seeking drug removal in the event of ICH. The rapid and near complete absorption from the gastrointestinal system renders gastric lavage or charcoal administration relatively ineffective. Furthermore, the high protein binding renders hemodialysis ineffective as well [90]. In the setting of spontaneous ICH, prothrombin Complex Concentrate (PCC) is the primary treatment of choice for effective antithrombotic reversal [91]. PCC is given as a 50 IU/kg bolus, which effectively reverses the effects of factor Xa inhibitors within minutes [92]. More recently, andexanet alpha has been approved for reversal of direct factor Xa inhibitors [93]. This antidote is a recombinant modified human factor Xa decoy protein that exhibits its prothrombotic effect by mimicking factor Xa and binding direct factor Xa inhibitors [92, 93]. Studies evaluating its clinical use have found it to be effective in reversing the antithrombotic effects of this drug class within minutes of administration [93, 94]. Andexanet alpha is indicated for any life-threatening or uncontrolled bleeding in the setting of factor Xa inhibitors, although the cost of the antidote is prohibitive at many centers.

Dabigatran (half-life 8 hours), the lone direct thrombin inhibitor, is able to competitively inhibit thrombin directly and prevent thrombus formation. One potential advantage that dabigatran holds is that it can inhibit fibrin-bound thrombin and thrombin-mediated platelet activation and aggregation [95]. Indicated for the prevention of stroke in the setting of non-valvular atrial fibrillation, for the prevention and treatment of PE, and in the setting of heparin-induced thrombocytopenia, dabigatran is only 3–7% bioavailable with normal to marginal renal function. These favorable biochemical properties lend themselves to more strategies for drug reversal. The lipophilic nature of dabigatran facilitates removal via gastric charcoal, although this must be done within 2–3 hours after administration. Also, given that the majority of the drug is freely circulating, this facilitates removal via hemodialysis [96]. Importantly, an antibody fragment, idarucizumab, has been synthesized as a specific antidote for dabigatran in the setting of severe or life-threatening hemorrhage. Idarucizumab binds dabigatran with 350x more affinity than it does with thrombin [97]. Numerous studies have shown that this antidote can inhibit the effects of dabigatran within minutes of administration [96–98]. When not available, a 50 IU/kg bolus of PCC may also be attempted [82].

Antiplatelet Agents

The role of prior antiplatelet therapy on hematoma expansion and outcome for patients presenting with ICH is unclear, although there is mounting evidence that the use of antiplatelet agents increases the degree of ICH, IVH, and neurologic morbidity and mortality risk in patients that present with ICH [99–102]. Unfortunately, there does not exist an antidote or universal strategy for reversal of this medication class. For this reason, there is wide heterogeneity in clinical practice, ranging from practitioners who advocate platelet transfusion in patients with ICH while taking antiplatelet agents, to those who advocate the use of laboratory tests for platelet function, to those who choose not to treat.

While COX inhibitors (aspirin) and P2Y12 inhibitors (clopidogrel, ticagrelor, prasugrel, and cangrelor) are most frequently encountered in clinical practice, dipyridamole (thromboxane inhibitor), cilostazol (phosphodiesterase inhibitor), and vorapaxar (protease-activated receptor 1 inhibitor) are additional antiplatelet agents of which practitioners should be aware in this patient population. Working through different mechanisms, all of these agents effectively inhibit

platelet activation and aggregation. Reversal strategies for antiplatelet agents are similar across the drug class. While platelet transfusion with or without desmopressin is often used in patients presenting with significant spontaneous ICH, the only randomized clinical trial assessing the utility of platelet transfusion for ICH was the Platelet transfusion versus standard care after acute stroke due to spontaneous cerebral haemorrhage associated with antiplatelet therapy (PATCH) trial [103]. The study randomized patients on baseline antiplatelet therapy who presented within 6 hours of spontaneous supratentorial ICH ictus to receive either platelet transfusion or standard therapy, finding no difference in ICH growth between the two groups. Patients treated with platelet transfusion in this trial demonstrated higher rates of death and dependency and a nonsignificant trend toward increased in-hospital serious adverse events compared to those that received standard therapy.

Despite the negative findings in the PATCH trial and other studies [103–106], a number of studies have shown benefit from platelet transfusion in patients presenting with spontaneous ICH, and this reversal strategy is often employed in routine clinical practice [107–109]. Platelet transfusion typically utilizes 1 pool ($>3 \times 10^9$ platelets/L) to offset the antiplatelet agent, although 2 pools are typically given for P2Y12 inhibitors [82]. Desmopressin (0.3 mg/kg) is often given as well to augment platelet reactivity through the release of von Willebrand factor multimers from platelet alpha-granules and Weibel-Palade bodies of endothelial cells, although no clinical trials have established efficacy for this regimen [110].

Intensive Care Management: Intracranial Pressure

Patients with moderate or large ICH or intraventricular hemorrhage often have increased ICP or hydrocephalus that warrants consideration of treatment. The AHA/ASA guidelines advocate a graded stepwise approach with initial routine use of less invasive measures prior to instituting more invasive measures. These less invasive measures include elevation of the head of the bed to 30 degrees, maintenance of the neck in a neutral position to facilitate jugular venous drainage, and adequate analgesia and sedation. More invasive measures include cerebrospinal fluid (CSF) drainage via an external ventricular drain (EVD) placed directly into the ventricles or surgical decompression. An EVD allows continuous measurement of ICP as well as drainage of CSF to treat elevated ICP, but does carry a small risk of hemorrhage or infection.

Osmotic agents such as mannitol and hypertonic saline may be used to decrease ICP, but overuse of mannitol may cause hypovolemia, renal failure, and cerebral vasoconstriction. Neuromuscular blockade may also be considered in patients with refractory elevated ICP, but is likely associated with an increased risk of infection and critical illness neuromuscular disease. Although hyperventilation may rapidly reduce elevated ICP by causing cerebral arterial vasoconstriction, this effect is generally transient (few hours) and reduces cerebral blood flow, which might potentially engender secondary brain injury. Thus, we tend to reserve hyperventilation for use as a temporizing measure in preparation for more definitive medical or surgical treatments. Finally, barbiturate coma may be considered in patients that have failed other therapies, but is associated with a significant risk of hypotension and requires continuous electroencephalographic monitoring to titrate effective dosing. Induced hypothermia to 32 °C to 34 °C may also be attempted for a brief period, but is associated with a high rate of complications. The use of barbiturate coma and induced hypothermia has not been systematically investigated in ICH, and they are considered as salvage last-tier medical therapies.

Intensive Care Management: Fever, Glucose, and Deep Venous Thrombosis Prophylaxis

Fever is a common occurrence in patients with ICH, and increased fever duration is associated with poor outcomes [111]. Thus, fever should be aggressively treated even as appropriate testing for systemic infection is being undertaken. Hyperglycemia on admission is predictive of 14-day and 28-day mortality in patients with ICH [112, 113]. Intensive insulin treatment of hyperglycemia during critical illness has been shown to decrease systemic morbidity and mortality and to decrease the incidence of critical illness polyneuropathy [114]. Thus, it is reasonable to vigilantly avoid hyperglycemia in patients with ICH and to institute aggressive approaches to achieve normoglycemia. Even so, randomized trials in this patient population have not been performed, and concerns have been raised about the possibility of hypoglycemic episodes and their particularly detrimental effects in patients with brain injury [115]. Deep venous thrombosis (DVT) and pulmonary embolism are frequently encountered in patients presenting with ICH, with DVT being diagnosed in 2% of patients during their acute hospitalization [116]. The combination of compression stockings plus intermittent pneumatic compression has been shown to decrease the rate of asymptomatic DVT from 15.9% to 4.7% in patients recovering from ICH [117]. The initiation of low-dose subcutaneous heparin (unfractionated heparin 5000 units three times per day) for DVT prophylaxis can be started as early as the second day following presentation with ICH [118]. This regimen has a proven statistically significant decrease in the incidence of pulmonary embolism with no increase in intracranial rehemorrhage.

Traditional Open Surgery

Surgical intervention via decompressive hemicraniectomy with or without hematoma evacuation for spontaneous intraparenchymal hemorrhage is typically reserved for patients with clinical deterioration and significant mass effect, imminent brain herniation, or signs of elevated intracranial pressure. In the absence of significant mass effect and/or clinical deterioration, clinical decision-making regarding surgery for primary ICH remains quite controversial and is heavily influenced by the biases of the practitioners and consultants caring for individual patients [119]. Initial studies were composed of single institution case series with mixed results and no clear indicator as to the clinical utility of surgical evacuation aside from theoretical benefits.

Open surgical intervention has not yet demonstrated clear superiority to medical management in the International Surgical Trial in Intracerebral Hemorrhage (STICH) series [120, 121]. STICH I was an international multicenter trial evaluating patients presenting within 72 hours of onset of a spontaneous supratentorial ICH with clinical equipoise regarding the utility of surgery [120]. Patients were randomized to either early surgical intervention (within 24 hours of randomization) or medical management. The primary outcome measure was death and disability (extended Glasgow Outcome Score at 6 months), different outcome metrics were used depending on expected prognosis from the initial hemorrhage, and outcomes were assessed using questionnaires sent to the patients or their families [122]. A quarter of patients initially randomized to medical management (26%) ultimately underwent surgery for hematoma evacuation, predominantly due to neurological deterioration [123]. Using intention-to-treat analysis, there was no statistically significant difference in either mortality or functional outcome, and as such, early surgery was neither beneficial nor harmful. While STICH I cannot be used to conclude that surgical evacuation has no role in supratentorial ICH, it did demonstrate that early surgery is not a panacea for all patients. Importantly, pre-specified subgroup analyses identified that patients with hematomas <1 cm from the cortical surface who underwent a craniotomy had a nonsignificant trend toward benefit with early surgery.

Based upon the results of the subgroup analysis in STICH I, a second international multicenter randomized trial (STICH II) was undertaken to evaluate the role of surgical intervention for spontaneous supratentorial lobar ICH [121]. Patients were randomized to either early surgical intervention (within 12 hours of randomization) or medical management. Similar to STICH I, the primary outcome measure was a prognosis-based dichotomized outcome on the extended Glasgow Outcome Scale at 6 months, and outcomes were assessed using questionnaires sent to the patients or their families. Substantial crossover was again experienced with 21% of patients initially randomized to medical management ultimately requiring surgical intervention. Nonetheless, the STICH II trial revealed similar outcomes between patients managed with early surgery compared to medical management alone, observing unfavorable outcomes in 59% and 62%, respectively. Despite these findings, further subset analyses and meta-analyses incorporating these results have suggested that a small, but clinically relevant survival advantage may exist for patients with spontaneous lobar ICH in the absence of intraventricular hemorrhage [121].

Reduction or elimination of hematoma volume remains an appealing treatment option given the deleterious effects of perilesional edema and the physiologic and biochemical impacts of the hematoma on adjacent parenchyma. Despite these theoretical benefits of hematoma evacuation, however, trials evaluating open surgical management of spontaneous ICH have only established a clinical benefit for surgical treatment of cerebellar hemorrhage (Class I, Level B, evidence) for patients with a large hematoma (>3 cm), obstructive hydrocephalus, or clinical deterioration [63]. Aside from this indication, open surgical management of spontaneous ICH is largely reserved for large hematomas causing mass effect or uncontrolled ICP crises.

Minimally Invasive Surgery

While open surgical evacuation of ICH has shown little utility, minimally invasive surgical (MIS) options hold the potential to safely reduce hematoma volume with minimal disruption of healthy parenchymal tissue. Minimally invasive surgical hematoma evacuation has been shown to be safe and efficacious with numerous surgical approaches, including minimally invasive parafascicular surgery (MIPS), stereotactic intracerebral hemorrhage underwater blood aspiration (SCUBA), or catheter-based techniques [124–

127]. In comparison to open surgical techniques, these MIS options have demonstrated encouraging preliminary results in terms of clinical outcomes and decreased mortality [128–130].

Several randomized clinical trials have evaluated the utility of MIS evacuation of spontaneous ICH in comparison to standard medical therapy. The Intraoperative Stereotactic Computed Tomography-Guided Endoscopic Surgery (ICES) trial randomized patients presenting with primary ICH within 48 hours of ictus into MIS evacuation via SCUBA technique or standard therapy [124]. Patients undergoing MIS evacuation demonstrated significant ICH volume reduction. While underpowered, the ICES study demonstrated a trend toward improved neurologic outcomes in patients treated with MIS evacuation (42.9% vs. 23.7%), although this failed to reach statistical significance. A similar study, the Minimally Invasive Surgery plus rt-PA for Intracerebral Hemorrhage Evacuation (MISTIE-II) trial, also sought to assess the efficacy of catheter-based MIS hematoma evacuation in primary ICH [131]. This trial randomized patients to standard therapy and treatment with catheter-based aspiration followed by rt-PA infusion, finding a significant reduction in hematoma volume without a significant increase in adverse events.

Based on these findings, MISTIE-III was undertaken to evaluate the effect of the MISTIE catheter-based technique for hematoma evacuation in comparison to standard therapy [132]. Patients randomized to MIS evacuation demonstrated equivalent rates of good functional outcome (mRS 0–3) at 1 year compared to standard therapy (45% vs. 41%) with a trend toward improved 30-day mortality (9% vs. 15%). Despite the equivocal results, subgroup and post hoc analyses identified a potential benefit of MIS techniques. Within the MISTIE-III trial, less than two-thirds of patients undergoing MIS evacuation demonstrated the targeted post-treatment hematoma volume of <15 mL [132]. Subsequent analysis suggested that patients with postsurgical hematoma volumes of <15 mL had better functional outcomes and patients with postsurgical hematoma volumes of <30 mL experienced a mortality benefit compared to patients treated

with medical management [133]. Further studies have demonstrated that MIS evacuation of ICH, when achieving adequate volume reduction, produces favorable long-term results [130, 134]. Ongoing clinical trials (MIND, INVEST-FEASIBILITY, and ENRICH) are currently evaluating the impact of other MIS techniques on clinical outcomes in ICH [130, 134–136].

Conclusion

Despite enhanced understanding of the underlying etiology and pathophysiology of ICH, it remains a substantial source of neurologic morbidity and mortality. While improved understanding of optimal medical management has developed over the past decade, significant controversy still remains, and further research is needed to define optimal treatment strategies. The advent of new-generation anticoagulants and antiplatelet agents also poses new challenges in treating this patient population, and a firm understanding of reversal strategies in the setting of ICH is of utmost importance for practitioners. Further, while trials evaluating surgical intervention have been underwhelming thus far, recent studies have identified a subset of patients and new surgical strategies that may provide clinical benefit for patients suffering from spontaneous ICH.

References

1. Sacco S, Marini C, Toni D, et al. Incidence and 10-year survival of intracerebral hemorrhage in a population-based registry. Stroke. 2009;40(2):394–9. https://doi.org/10.1161/STROKEAHA.108.523209 [published Online First: 2008/11/29].
2. Qureshi AI, Tuhrim S, Broderick JP, et al. Spontaneous intracerebral hemorrhage. N Engl J Med. 2001;344(19):1450–60. https://doi.org/10.1056/NEJM200105103441907 [published Online First: 2001/05/11].
3. Gebel JM, Broderick JP. Intracerebral hemorrhage. Neurol Clin. 2000;18(2):419–38. https://doi.org/10.1016/s0733-8619(05)70200-0 [published Online First: 2000/04/11].
4. McCormick WF, Rosenfield DB. Massive brain hemorrhage: a review of 144 cases and an exami-

nation of their causes. Stroke. 1973;4(6):946–54. https://doi.org/10.1161/01.str.4.6.946 [published Online First: 1973/11/01].

5. O'Donnell HC, Rosand J, Knudsen KA, et al. Apolipoprotein E genotype and the risk of recurrent lobar intracerebral hemorrhage. N Engl J Med. 2000;342(4):240–5. https://doi.org/10.1056/NEJM200001273420403 [published Online First: 2000/01/29].

6. Ariesen MJ, Claus SP, Rinkel GJ, et al. Risk factors for intracerebral hemorrhage in the general population: a systematic review. Stroke. 2003;34(8):2060–5. https://doi.org/10.1161/01.STR.0000080678.09344.8D [published Online First: 2003/07/05].

7. Sturgeon JD, Folsom AR, Longstreth WT, Jr., et al. Risk factors for intracerebral hemorrhage in a pooled prospective study. Stroke. 2007;38(10):2718–25. https://doi.org/10.1161/STROKEAHA.107.487090 [published Online First: 2007/09/01].

8. Suh I, Jee SH, Kim HC, et al. Low serum cholesterol and haemorrhagic stroke in men: Korea Medical Insurance Corporation Study. Lancet. 2001;357(9260):922–5. https://doi.org/10.1016/S0140-6736(00)04213-6 [published Online First: 2001/04/06].

9. Juvela S, Hillbom M, Palomaki H. Risk factors for spontaneous intracerebral hemorrhage. Stroke. 1995;26(9):1558–64. https://doi.org/10.1161/01.str.26.9.1558 [published Online First: 1995/09/01].

10. Thrift AG, Donnan GA, McNeil JJ. Heavy drinking, but not moderate or intermediate drinking, increases the risk of intracerebral hemorrhage. Epidemiology. 1999;10(3):307–12. [published Online First: 1999/05/07].

11. Yano K, Reed DM, MacLean CJ. Serum cholesterol and hemorrhagic stroke in the Honolulu Heart Program. Stroke. 1989;20(11):1460–5. https://doi.org/10.1161/01.str.20.11.1460 [published Online First: 1989/11/01].

12. Iso H, Jacobs DR, Jr., Wentworth D, et al. Serum cholesterol levels and six-year mortality from stroke in 350,977 men screened for the multiple risk factor intervention trial. N Engl J Med. 1989;320(14):904–10. https://doi.org/10.1056/NEJM198904063201405 [published Online First: 1989/04/06].

13. Goldstein LB, Amarenco P, Szarck M, et al. Hemorrhagic stroke in the Stroke Prevention by Aggressive Reduction in Cholesterol Levels study. Neurology. 2008;70(24 Pt 2):2364–70. https://doi.org/10.1212/01.wnl.0000296277.63350.77 [published Online First: 2007/12/14].

14. Amarenco P, Bogousslavsky J, Callahan A, 3rd, et al. High-dose atorvastatin after stroke or transient ischemic attack. N Engl J Med. 2006;355(6):549–59. https://doi.org/10.1056/NEJMoa061894 [published Online First: 2006/08/11].

15. Qureshi AI, Suri MA, Safdar K, et al. Intracerebral hemorrhage in blacks. Risk factors, subtypes, and outcome. Stroke. 1997;28(5):961–4. https://doi.org/10.1161/01.str.28.5.961 [published Online First: 1997/05/01].

16. Gunel M, Awad IA, Finberg K, et al. A founder mutation as a cause of cerebral cavernous malformation in Hispanic Americans. N Engl J Med. 1996;334(15):946–51. https://doi.org/10.1056/NEJM199604113341503 [published Online First: 1996/04/11].

17. Kuriyama S, Kusaka Y, Fujimura M, et al. Prevalence and clinicoepidemiological features of moyamoya disease in Japan: findings from a nationwide epidemiological survey. Stroke. 2008;39(1):42–7. https://doi.org/10.1161/STROKEAHA.107.490714 [published Online First: 2007/12/01].

18. Labovitz DL, Halim A, Boden-Albala B, et al. The incidence of deep and lobar intracerebral hemorrhage in whites, blacks, and Hispanics. Neurology. 2005;65(4):518–22. https://doi.org/10.1212/01.wnl.0000172915.71933.00 [published Online First: 2005/08/24].

19. Qureshi AI, Suri MF, Nasar A, et al. Changes in cost and outcome among US patients with stroke hospitalized in 1990 to 1991 and those hospitalized in 2000 to 2001. Stroke. 2007;38(7):2180–4. https://doi.org/10.1161/STROKEAHA.106.467506 [published Online First: 2007/05/26].

20. Taylor TN, Davis PH, Torner JC, et al. Lifetime cost of stroke in the United States. Stroke. 1996;27(9):1459–66. https://doi.org/10.1161/01.str.27.9.1459 [published Online First: 1996/09/01].

21. Fisher CM. Pathological observations in hypertensive cerebral hemorrhage. J Neuropathol Exp Neurol. 1971;30(3):536–50. https://doi.org/10.1097/00005072-197107000-00015 [published Online First: 1971/07/01].

22. Gebel JM, Jr., Jauch EC, Brott TG, et al. Relative edema volume is a predictor of outcome in patients with hyperacute spontaneous intracerebral hemorrhage. Stroke. 2002;33(11):2636–41. https://doi.org/10.1161/01.str.0000035283.34109.ea [published Online First: 2002/11/02].

23. Gingrich MB, Junge CE, Lyuboslavsky P, et al. Potentiation of NMDA receptor function by the serine protease thrombin. J Neurosci. 2000;20(12):4582–95. [published Online First: 2000/06/14].

24. Butcher KS, Baird T, MacGregor L, et al. Perihematomal edema in primary intracerebral hemorrhage is plasma derived. Stroke. 2004;35(8):1879–85. https://doi.org/10.1161/01.STR.0000131807.54742.1a [published Online First: 2004/06/05].

25. Tejima E, Zhao BQ, Tsuji K, et al. Astrocytic induction of matrix metalloproteinase-9 and edema in brain hemorrhage. J Cereb Blood Flow Metab. 2007;27(3):460–8. https://doi.org/10.1038/sj.jcbfm.9600354 [published Online First: 2006/06/22].

26. Aronowski J, Hall CE. New horizons for primary intracerebral hemorrhage treatment: experience from

preclinical studies. Neurol Res. 2005;27(3):268–79. https://doi.org/10.1179/016164105X25225 [published Online First: 2005/04/23].

27. Wagner KR. Modeling intracerebral hemorrhage: glutamate, nuclear factor-kappa B signaling and cytokines. Stroke. 2007;38(2 Suppl):753–8. https://doi.org/10.1161/01.STR.0000255033.02904.db [published Online First: 2007/01/31].

28. Xi G, Keep RF, Hoff JT. Mechanisms of brain injury after intracerebral haemorrhage. Lancet Neurol. 2006;5(1):53–63. https://doi.org/10.1016/S1474-4422(05)70283-0 [published Online First: 2005/12/20].

29. Selim M, Foster LD, Moy CS, et al. Deferoxamine mesylate in patients with intracerebral haemorrhage (i-DEF): a multicentre, randomised, placebo-controlled, double-blind phase 2 trial. Lancet Neurol. 2019;18(5):428–38. https://doi.org/10.1016/S1474-4422(19)30069-9 [published Online First: 2019/03/23].

30. Kidwell CS, Saver JL, Mattiello J, et al. Diffusion-perfusion MR evaluation of perihematomal injury in hyperacute intracerebral hemorrhage. Neurology. 2001;57(9):1611–7. https://doi.org/10.1212/wnl.57.9.1611 [published Online First: 2001/11/14].

31. Mayer SA, Lignelli A, Fink ME, et al. Perilesional blood flow and edema formation in acute intracerebral hemorrhage: a SPECT study. Stroke. 1998;29(9):1791–8. https://doi.org/10.1161/01.str.29.9.1791 [published Online First: 1998/09/10].

32. Siddique MS, Fernandes HM, Arene NU, et al. Changes in cerebral blood flow as measured by HMPAO SPECT in patients following spontaneous intracerebral haemorrhage. Acta Neurochir Suppl. 2000;76:517–20. https://doi.org/10.1007/978-3-7091-6346-7_108 [published Online First: 2001/07/14].

33. Herweh C, Juttler E, Schellinger PD, et al. Evidence against a perihemorrhagic penumbra provided by perfusion computed tomography. Stroke. 2007;38(11):2941–7. https://doi.org/10.1161/STROKEAHA.107.486977 [published Online First: 2007/09/29].

34. Qureshi AI, Wilson DA, Hanley DF, et al. No evidence for an ischemic penumbra in massive experimental intracerebral hemorrhage. Neurology. 1999;52(2):266–72. https://doi.org/10.1212/wnl.52.2.266 [published Online First: 1999/02/05].

35. Zazulia AR, Diringer MN, Videen TO, et al. Hypoperfusion without ischemia surrounding acute intracerebral hemorrhage. J Cereb Blood Flow Metab. 2001;21(7):804–10. https://doi.org/10.1097/00004647-200107000-00005 [published Online First: 2001/07/04].

36. Brott T, Broderick J, Kothari R, et al. Early hemorrhage growth in patients with intracerebral hemorrhage. Stroke. 1997;28(1):1–5. https://doi.org/10.1161/01.str.28.1.1 [published Online First: 1997/01/01].

37. Fujii Y, Takeuchi S, Sasaki O, et al. Multivariate analysis of predictors of hematoma enlargement in spontaneous intracerebral hemorrhage. Stroke. 1998;29(6):1160–6. https://doi.org/10.1161/01.str.29.6.1160 [published Online First: 1998/06/17].

38. Fujitsu K, Muramoto M, Ikeda Y, et al. Indications for surgical treatment of putaminal hemorrhage. Comparative study based on serial CT and time-course analysis. J Neurosurg. 1990;73(4):518–25. https://doi.org/10.3171/jns.1990.73.4.0518 [published Online First: 1990/10/01].

39. Kazui S, Naritomi H, Yamamoto H, et al. Enlargement of spontaneous intracerebral hemorrhage. Incidence and time course. Stroke. 1996;27(10):1783–7. https://doi.org/10.1161/01.str.27.10.1783 [published Online First: 1996/10/01].

40. Ezzeddine MA, Suri MF, Hussein HM, et al. Blood pressure management in patients with acute stroke: pathophysiology and treatment strategies. Neurosurg Clin N Am. 2006;17(Suppl 1):41–56. https://doi.org/10.1016/s1042-3680(06)80006-9 [published Online First: 2007/11/29].

41. Tentschert S, Wimmer R, Greisenegger S, et al. Headache at stroke onset in 2196 patients with ischemic stroke or transient ischemic attack. Stroke. 2005;36(2):e1–3. https://doi.org/10.1161/01.STR.0000151360.03567.2b [published Online First: 2004/12/18].

42. Broderick JP, Brott TG, Duldner JE, et al. Volume of intracerebral hemorrhage. A powerful and easy-to-use predictor of 30-day mortality. Stroke. 1993;24(7):987–93. https://doi.org/10.1161/01.str.24.7.987 [published Online First: 1993/07/01].

43. Cheung RT, Zou LY. Use of the original, modified, or new intracerebral hemorrhage score to predict mortality and morbidity after intracerebral hemorrhage. Stroke. 2003;34(7):1717–22. https://doi.org/10.1161/01.STR.0000078657.22835.B9 [published Online First: 2003/06/14].

44. Hemphill JC, 3rd, Bonovich DC, Besmertis L, et al. The ICH score: a simple, reliable grading scale for intracerebral hemorrhage. Stroke. 2001;32(4):891–7. https://doi.org/10.1161/01.str.32.4.891 [published Online First: 2001/04/03].

45. Tuhrim S, Horowitz DR, Sacher M, et al. Validation and comparison of models predicting survival following intracerebral hemorrhage. Crit Care Med. 1995;23(5):950–4. https://doi.org/10.1097/00003246-199505000-00026 [published Online First: 1995/05/01].

46. Tuhrim S, Horowitz DR, Sacher M, et al. Volume of ventricular blood is an important determinant of outcome in supratentorial intracerebral hemorrhage. Crit Care Med. 1999;27(3):617–21. https://doi.org/10.1097/00003246-199903000-00045 [published Online First: 1999/04/13].

47. Rost NS, Smith EE, Chang Y, et al. Prediction of functional outcome in patients with primary intracerebral hemorrhage: the FUNC score. Stroke.

2008;39(8):2304–9. https://doi.org/10.1161/STROKEAHA.107.512202 [published Online First: 2008/06/17].

48. Hwang DY, Dell CA, Sparks MJ, et al. Clinician judgment vs formal scales for predicting intracerebral hemorrhage outcomes. Neurology. 2016;86(2):126–33. https://doi.org/10.1212/WNL.0000000000002266 [published Online First: 2015/12/18].

49. Kidwell CS, Chalela JA, Saver JL, et al. Comparison of MRI and CT for detection of acute intracerebral hemorrhage. JAMA. 2004;292(15):1823–30. https://doi.org/10.1001/jama.292.15.1823 [published Online First: 2004/10/21].

50. Zhu XL, Chan MS, Poon WS. Spontaneous intracranial hemorrhage: which patients need diagnostic cerebral angiography? A prospective study of 206 cases and review of the literature. Stroke. 1997;28(7):1406–9. https://doi.org/10.1161/01.str.28.7.1406 [published Online First: 1997/07/01].

51. Flint AC, Roebken A, Singh V. Primary intraventricular hemorrhage: yield of diagnostic angiography and clinical outcome. Neurocrit Care. 2008;8(3):330–6. https://doi.org/10.1007/s12028-008-9070-2 [published Online First: 2008/03/06].

52. Hoh BL, Cheung AC, Rabinov JD, et al. Results of a prospective protocol of computed tomographic angiography in place of catheter angiography as the only diagnostic and pretreatment planning study for cerebral aneurysms by a combined neurovascular team. Neurosurgery. 2004;54(6):1329–40; discussion 40–2. https://doi.org/10.1227/01.neu.0000125325.22576.83 [published Online First: 2004/05/26].

53. Becker KJ, Baxter AB, Bybee HM, et al. Extravasation of radiographic contrast is an independent predictor of death in primary intracerebral hemorrhage. Stroke. 1999;30(10):2025–32. https://doi.org/10.1161/01.str.30.10.2025 [published Online First: 1999/10/08].

54. Goldstein JN, Fazen LE, Snider R, et al. Contrast extravasation on CT angiography predicts hematoma expansion in intracerebral hemorrhage. Neurology. 2007;68(12):889–94. https://doi.org/10.1212/01.wnl.0000257087.22852.21 [published Online First: 2007/03/21].

55. Kim J, Smith A, Hemphill JC, 3rd, et al. Contrast extravasation on CT predicts mortality in primary intracerebral hemorrhage. AJNR Am J Neuroradiol. 2008;29(3):520–5. https://doi.org/10.3174/ajnr.A0859 [published Online First: 2007/12/11].

56. Wada R, Aviv RI, Fox AJ, et al. CT angiography "spot sign" predicts hematoma expansion in acute intracerebral hemorrhage. Stroke. 2007;38(4):1257–62. https://doi.org/10.1161/01.STR.0000259633.59404.f3 [published Online First: 2007/02/27].

57. Morotti A, Brouwers HB, Romero JM, et al. Intensive blood pressure reduction and spot sign in intracerebral hemorrhage: a secondary analysis of a randomized clinical trial. JAMA Neurol.

2017;74(8):950–60. https://doi.org/10.1001/jamaneurol.2017.1014 [published Online First: 2017/06/20].

58. Jauch EC, Lindsell CJ, Adeoye O, et al. Lack of evidence for an association between hemodynamic variables and hematoma growth in spontaneous intracerebral hemorrhage. Stroke. 2006;37(8):2061–5. https://doi.org/10.1161/01.STR.0000229878.93759.a2 [published Online First: 2006/06/24].

59. Kazui S, Minematsu K, Yamamoto H, et al. Predisposing factors to enlargement of spontaneous intracerebral hematoma. Stroke. 1997;28(12):2370–5. https://doi.org/10.1161/01.str.28.12.2370 [published Online First: 1997/12/31].

60. Ohwaki K, Yano E, Nagashima H, et al. Blood pressure management in acute intracerebral hemorrhage: relationship between elevated blood pressure and hematoma enlargement. Stroke. 2004;35(6):1364–7. https://doi.org/10.1161/01.STR.0000128795.38283.4b [published Online First: 2004/05/01].

61. Powers WJ, Zazulia AR, Videen TO, et al. Autoregulation of cerebral blood flow surrounding acute (6 to 22 hours) intracerebral hemorrhage. Neurology. 2001;57(1):18–24. https://doi.org/10.1212/wnl.57.1.18 [published Online First: 2001/07/11].

62. Anderson CS, Heeley E, Huang Y, et al. Rapid blood-pressure lowering in patients with acute intracerebral hemorrhage. N Engl J Med. 2013;368(25):2355–65. https://doi.org/10.1056/NEJMoa1214609 [published Online First: 2013/05/30].

63. Hemphill JC 3rd, Greenberg SM, Anderson CS, et al. Guidelines for the Management of Spontaneous Intracerebral Hemorrhage: a guideline for healthcare professionals from the American Heart Association/American Stroke Association. Stroke. 2015;46(7):2032–60. https://doi.org/10.1161/STR.0000000000000069.

64. Qureshi AI, Palesch YY, Barsan WG, et al. Intensive blood-pressure lowering in patients with acute cerebral hemorrhage. N Engl J Med. 2016;375(11):1033–43. https://doi.org/10.1056/NEJMoa1603460 [published Online First: 2016/06/09].

65. Arima H, Heeley E, Delcourt C, et al. Optimal achieved blood pressure in acute intracerebral hemorrhage: INTERACT2. Neurology. 2015;84(5):464–71. https://doi.org/10.1212/WNL.0000000000001205 [published Online First: 2015/01/02].

66. Chung PW, Kim JT, Sanossian N, et al. Association between Hyperacute stage blood pressure variability and outcome in patients with spontaneous intracerebral hemorrhage. Stroke. 2018;49(2):348–54. https://doi.org/10.1161/STROKEAHA.117.017701 [published Online First: 2018/01/06].

67. Manning L, Hirakawa Y, Arima H, et al. Blood pressure variability and outcome after acute intracerebral haemorrhage: a post-hoc analysis of INTERACT2, a randomised controlled trial. Lancet

Neurol. 2014;13(4):364–73. https://doi.org/10.1016/S1474-4422(14)70018-3 [published Online First: 2014/02/18].

68. Qureshi AI, Huang W, Lobanova I, et al. Outcomes of intensive systolic blood pressure reduction in patients with intracerebral hemorrhage and excessively high initial systolic blood pressure: post hoc analysis of a randomized clinical trial. JAMA Neurol. 2020. https://doi.org/10.1001/jamaneurol.2020.3075 [published Online First: 2020/09/09].

69. Whelton PK, Carey RM, Aronow WS, et al. 2017 ACC/AHA/AAPA/ABC/ACPM/AGS/APhA/ASH/ASPC/NMA/PCNA guideline for the prevention, detection, evaluation, and management of high blood pressure in adults: a report of the American College of Cardiology/American Heart Association Task Force on Clinical Practice Guidelines. J Am Coll Cardiol. 2018;71(19):e127–e248. https://doi.org/10.1016/j.jacc.2017.11.006 [published online first: 2017/11/18].

70. Broderick J, Connolly S, Feldmann E, et al. Guidelines for the management of spontaneous intracerebral hemorrhage in adults: 2007 update: a guideline from the American Heart Association/American Stroke Association Stroke Council, High Blood Pressure Research Council, and the Quality of Care and Outcomes in Research Interdisciplinary Working Group. Stroke. 2007;38(6):2001–23. https://doi.org/10.1161/STROKEAHA.107.183689 [published Online First: 2007/05/05].

71. Balami JS, Buchan AM. Complications of intracerebral haemorrhage. Lancet Neurol. 2012;11(1):101–18. https://doi.org/10.1016/S1474-4422(11)70264-2 [published Online First: 2011/12/17].

72. Sarode R, Matevosyan K, Bhagat R, et al. Rapid warfarin reversal: a 3-factor prothrombin complex concentrate and recombinant factor VIIa cocktail for intracerebral hemorrhage. J Neurosurg. 2012;116(3):491–7. https://doi.org/10.3171/2011.11.JNS11836 [published Online First: 2011/12/20].

73. Fang MC, Chang Y, Hylek EM, et al. Advanced age, anticoagulation intensity, and risk for intracranial hemorrhage among patients taking warfarin for atrial fibrillation. Ann Intern Med. 2004;141(10):745–52. https://doi.org/10.7326/0003-4819-141-10-200411160-00005 [published Online First: 2004/11/17].

74. A randomized trial of anticoagulants versus aspirin after cerebral ischemia of presumed arterial origin. The Stroke Prevention in Reversible Ischemia Trial (SPIRIT) Study Group. Ann Neurol. 1997;42(6):857–65. https://doi.org/10.1002/ana.410420606 [published Online First: 1997/12/24].

75. Flibotte JJ, Hagan N, O'Donnell J, et al. Warfarin, hematoma expansion, and outcome of intracerebral hemorrhage. Neurology. 2004;63(6):1059–64. https://doi.org/10.1212/01.wnl.0000138428.40673.83 [published Online First: 2004/09/29].

76. Goldstein JN, Thomas SH, Frontiero V, et al. Timing of fresh frozen plasma administration and rapid correction of coagulopathy in warfarin-related intracerebral hemorrhage. Stroke. 2006;37(1):151–5. https://doi.org/10.1161/01.STR.0000195047.21562.23 [published Online First: 2005/11/25].

77. Ansell J, Hirsh J, Poller L, et al. The pharmacology and management of the vitamin K antagonists: the Seventh ACCP Conference on Antithrombotic and Thrombolytic Therapy. Chest. 2004;126(3 Suppl):204S–33S. https://doi.org/10.1378/chest.126.3_suppl.204S [published Online First: 2004/09/24].

78. Guidelines on oral anticoagulation: third edition. Br J Haematol. 1998;101(2):374–87. https://doi.org/10.1046/j.1365-2141.1998.00715.x [published Online First: 1998/06/03].

79. Lankiewicz MW, Hays J, Friedman KD, et al. Urgent reversal of warfarin with prothrombin complex concentrate. J Thromb Haemost. 2006;4(5):967–70. https://doi.org/10.1111/j.1538-7836.2006.01815.x [published Online First: 2006/05/13].

80. Makris M, Greaves M, Phillips WS, et al. Emergency oral anticoagulant reversal: the relative efficacy of infusions of fresh frozen plasma and clotting factor concentrate on correction of the coagulopathy. Thromb Haemost. 1997;77(3):477–80. [published Online First: 1997/03/01].

81. Yasaka M, Sakata T, Minematsu K, et al. Correction of INR by prothrombin complex concentrate and vitamin K in patients with warfarin related hemorrhagic complication. Thromb Res. 2002;108(1):25–30. https://doi.org/10.1016/s0049-3848(02)00402-4 [published Online First: 2003/02/15].

82. Dornbos D, 3rd, Nimjee SM. Reversal of systemic anticoagulants and antiplatelet therapeutics. Neurosurg Clin N Am. 2018;29(4):537–45. https://doi.org/10.1016/j.nec.2018.06.005 [published Online First: 2018/09/19].

83. Huttner HB, Schellinger PD, Hartmann M, et al. Hematoma growth and outcome in treated neurocritical care patients with intracerebral hemorrhage related to oral anticoagulant therapy: comparison of acute treatment strategies using vitamin K, fresh frozen plasma, and prothrombin complex concentrates. Stroke. 2006;37(6):1465–70. https://doi.org/10.1161/01.STR.0000221786.81354.d6 [published Online First: 2006/05/06].

84. Baker RI, Coughlin PB, Gallus AS, et al. Warfarin reversal: consensus guidelines, on behalf of the Australasian Society of Thrombosis and Haemostasis. Med J Aust. 2004;181(9):492–7. [published Online First: 2004/11/02].

85. Hanley JP. Warfarin reversal. J Clin Pathol. 2004;57(11):1132–9. https://doi.org/10.1136/jcp.2003.008904 [published Online First: 2004/10/29].

86. Perzborn E, Roehrig S, Straub A, et al. Rivaroxaban: a new oral factor Xa inhibitor. Arterioscler Thromb Vasc Biol. 2010;30(3):376–81. https://doi.

org/10.1161/ATVBAHA.110.202978 [published Online First: 2010/02/09].

87. Potpara TS, Polovina MM, Licina MM, et al. Novel oral anticoagulants for stroke prevention in atrial fibrillation: focus on apixaban. Adv Ther. 2012;29(6):491–507. https://doi.org/10.1007/s12325-012-0026-8 [published Online First: 2012/06/12].

88. Granger CB, Alexander JH, McMurray JJ, et al. Apixaban versus warfarin in patients with atrial fibrillation. N Engl J Med. 2011;365(11):981–92. https://doi.org/10.1056/NEJMoa1107039 [published Online First: 2011/08/30].

89. Poulakos M, Walker JN, Baig U, et al. Edoxaban: A direct oral anticoagulant. Am J Health Syst Pharm. 2017;74(3):117–29. https://doi.org/10.2146/ajhp150821 [published Online First: 2017/01/27].

90. Morris TA. New synthetic antithrombotic agents for venous thromboembolism: pentasaccharides, direct thrombin inhibitors, direct Xa inhibitors. Clin Chest Med. 2010;31(4):707–18. https://doi.org/10.1016/j.ccm.2010.06.006 [published Online First: 2010/11/05].

91. Eerenberg ES, Kamphuisen PW, Sijpkens MK, et al. Reversal of rivaroxaban and dabigatran by prothrombin complex concentrate: a randomized, placebo-controlled, crossover study in healthy subjects. Circulation. 2011;124(14):1573–9. https://doi.org/10.1161/CIRCULATIONAHA.111.029017 [published Online First: 2011/09/09].

92. Crowther M, Crowther MA. Antidotes for novel oral anticoagulants: current status and future potential. Arterioscler Thromb Vasc Biol. 2015;35(8):1736–45. https://doi.org/10.1161/ATVBAHA.114.303402 [published Online First: 2015/06/20].

93. Connolly SJ, Milling TJ, Jr., Eikelboom JW, et al. Andexanet Alfa for acute major bleeding associated with factor Xa inhibitors. N Engl J Med. 2016;375(12):1131–41. https://doi.org/10.1056/NEJMoa1607887 [published Online First: 2016/08/31].

94. Siegal DM, Curnutte JT, Connolly SJ, et al. Andexanet Alfa for the reversal of factor Xa inhibitor activity. N Engl J Med. 2015;373(25):2413–24. https://doi.org/10.1056/NEJMoa1510991 [published Online First: 2015/11/13].

95. Frontera JA, Bhatt P, Lalchan R, et al. Cost comparison of andexanet versus prothrombin complex concentrates for direct factor Xa inhibitor reversal after hemorrhage. J Thromb Thrombolysis. 2020;49(1):121–31. https://doi.org/10.1007/s11239-019-01973-z [published Online First: 2019/10/31].

96. Van der Wall SJ, Lopes RD, Aisenberg J, et al. Idarucizumab for dabigatran reversal in the management of patients with gastrointestinal bleeding. Circulation. 2019;139(6):748–56. https://doi.org/10.1161/CIRCULATIONAHA.118.036710 [published Online First: 2018/12/28].

97. Schiele F, van Ryn J, Canada K, et al. A specific antidote for dabigatran: functional and structural char-acterization. Blood. 2013;121(18):3554–62. https://doi.org/10.1182/blood-2012-11-468207 [published Online First: 2013/03/12].

98. Pollack CV, Jr., Reilly PA, Eikelboom J, et al. Idarucizumab for dabigatran reversal. N Engl J Med. 2015;373(6):511–20. https://doi.org/10.1056/NEJMoa1502000 [published Online First: 2015/06/23].

99. Naidech AM, Bendok BR, Garg RK, et al. Reduced platelet activity is associated with more intraventricular hemorrhage. Neurosurgery. 2009;65(4):684–8; discussion 88. https://doi.org/10.1227/01.NEU.0000351769.39990.16 [published Online First: 2009/10/17].

100. Naidech AM, Bernstein RA, Levasseur K, et al. Platelet activity and outcome after intracerebral hemorrhage. Ann Neurol. 2009;65(3):352–6. https://doi.org/10.1002/ana.21618 [published Online First: 2009/04/01].

101. Naidech AM, Jovanovic B, Liebling S, et al. Reduced platelet activity is associated with early clot growth and worse 3-month outcome after intracerebral hemorrhage. Stroke. 2009;40(7):2398–401. https://doi.org/10.1161/STROKEAHA.109.550939 [published Online First: 2009/05/16].

102. Naidech AM, Rosenberg NF, Bernstein RA, et al. Aspirin use or reduced platelet activity predicts craniotomy after intracerebral hemorrhage. Neurocrit Care. 2011;15(3):442–6. https://doi.org/10.1007/s12028-011-9557-0 [published Online First: 2011/05/14].

103. Baharoglu MI, Cordonnier C, Al-Shahi Salman R, et al. Platelet transfusion versus standard care after acute stroke due to spontaneous cerebral haemorrhage associated with antiplatelet therapy (PATCH): a randomised, open-label, phase 3 trial. Lancet. 2016;387(10038):2605–13. https://doi.org/10.1016/S0140-6736(16)30392-0 [published Online First: 2016/05/15].

104. Martin M, Conlon LW. Does platelet transfusion improve outcomes in patients with spontaneous or traumatic intracerebral hemorrhage? Ann Emerg Med. 2013;61(1):58–61. https://doi.org/10.1016/j.annemergmed.2012.03.025 [published Online First: 2012/07/31].

105. Ducruet AF, Hickman ZL, Zacharia BE, et al. Impact of platelet transfusion on hematoma expansion in patients receiving antiplatelet agents before intracerebral hemorrhage. Neurol Res. 2010;32(7):706–10. https://doi.org/10.1179/174313209X459129 [published Online First: 2010/09/08].

106. Nishijima DK, Zehtabchi S, Berrong J, et al. Utility of platelet transfusion in adult patients with traumatic intracranial hemorrhage and preinjury antiplatelet use: a systematic review. J Trauma Acute Care Surg. 2012;72(6):1658–63. https://doi.org/10.1097/TA.0b013e318256dfc5 [published Online First: 2012/06/15].

107. Beshay JE, Morgan H, Madden C, et al. Emergency reversal of anticoagulation and anti-

platelet therapies in neurosurgical patients. J Neurosurg. 2010;112(2):307–18. https://doi.org/10.3171/2009.7.JNS0982 [published Online First: 2009/08/12].

108. McMillian WD, Rogers FB. Management of pre-hospital antiplatelet and anticoagulant therapy in traumatic head injury: a review. J Trauma. 2009;66(3):942–50. https://doi.org/10.1097/TA.0b013e3181978e7b [published Online First: 2009/03/12].

109. Naidech AM, Liebling SM, Rosenberg NF, et al. Early platelet transfusion improves platelet activity and may improve outcomes after intracerebral hemorrhage. Neurocrit Care. 2012;16(1):82–7. https://doi.org/10.1007/s12028-011-9619-3 [published Online First: 2011/08/13].

110. Flordal PA, Sahlin S. Use of desmopressin to prevent bleeding complications in patients treated with aspirin. Br J Surg. 1993;80(6):723–4. https://doi.org/10.1002/bjs.1800800616 [published Online First: 1993/06/01].

111. Schwarz S, Hafner K, Aschoff A, et al. Incidence and prognostic significance of fever following intracerebral hemorrhage. Neurology. 2000;54(2):354–61. https://doi.org/10.1212/wnl.54.2.354 [published Online First: 2000/02/11].

112. Fogelholm R, Murros K, Rissanen A, et al. Admission blood glucose and short term survival in primary intracerebral haemorrhage: a population based study. J Neurol Neurosurg Psychiatry. 2005;76(3):349–53. https://doi.org/10.1136/jnnp.2003.034819 [published Online First: 2005/02/18].

113. Kimura K, Iguchi Y, Inoue T, et al. Hyperglycemia independently increases the risk of early death in acute spontaneous intracerebral hemorrhage. J Neurol Sci. 2007;255(1–2):90–4. https://doi.org/10.1016/j.jns.2007.02.005 [published Online First: 2007/03/14].

114. van den Berghe G, Wouters P, Weekers F, et al. Intensive insulin therapy in critically ill patients. N Engl J Med. 2001;345(19):1359–67. https://doi.org/10.1056/NEJMoa011300 [published Online First: 2002/01/17].

115. Vespa P, Boonyaputthikul R, McArthur DL, et al. Intensive insulin therapy reduces microdialysis glucose values without altering glucose utilization or improving the lactate/pyruvate ratio after traumatic brain injury. Crit Care Med. 2006;34(3):850–6. https://doi.org/10.1097/01.CCM.0000201875.12245.6F [published Online First: 2006/03/01].

116. Gregory PC, Kuhlemeier KV. Prevalence of venous thromboembolism in acute hemorrhagic and thromboembolic stroke. Am J Phys Med Rehabil. 2003;82(5):364–9. https://doi.org/10.1097/01.PHM.0000064725.62897.A5 [published Online First: 2003/04/22].

117. Lacut K, Bressollette L, Le Gal G, et al. Prevention of venous thrombosis in patients with acute intracerebral hemorrhage. Neurology. 2005;65(6):865–9. https://doi.org/10.1212/01.wnl.0000176073.80532.a2 [published Online First: 2005/09/28].

118. Boeer A, Voth E, Henze T, et al. Early heparin therapy in patients with spontaneous intracerebral haemorrhage. J Neurol Neurosurg Psychiatry. 1991;54(5):466–7. https://doi.org/10.1136/jnnp.54.5.466 [published Online First: 1991/05/01].

119. Gregson BA, Mendelow AD, Investigators S. International variations in surgical practice for spontaneous intracerebral hemorrhage. Stroke. 2003;34(11):2593–7. https://doi.org/10.1161/01.STR.0000097491.82104.F3 [published Online First: 2003/10/18].

120. Mendelow AD, Gregson BA, Fernandes HM, et al. Early surgery versus initial conservative treatment in patients with spontaneous supratentorial intracerebral haematomas in the International Surgical Trial in Intracerebral Haemorrhage (STICH): a randomised trial. Lancet. 2005;365(9457):387–97. https://doi.org/10.1016/S0140-6736(05)17826-X.

121. Mendelow AD, Gregson BA, Rowan EN, et al. Early surgery versus initial conservative treatment in patients with spontaneous supratentorial lobar intracerebral haematomas (STICH II): a randomised trial. Lancet. 2013;382(9890):397–408. https://doi.org/10.1016/S0140-6736(13)60986-1.

122. Mendelow AD, Teasdale GM, Barer D, et al. Outcome assignment in the International Surgical Trial of Intracerebral Haemorrhage. Acta Neurochir (Wien). 2003;145(8):679–81; discussion 81. https://doi.org/10.1007/s00701-003-0063 9 [published Online First: 2003/10/02].

123. Prasad KS, Gregson BA, Bhattathiri PS, et al. The significance of crossovers after randomization in the STICH trial. Acta Neurochir Suppl. 2006;96:61–4. https://doi.org/10.1007/3-211-30714-1_15 [published Online First: 2006/05/05].

124. Vespa P, Hanley D, Betz J, et al. ICES (intraoperative stereotactic computed tomography-guided endoscopic surgery) for brain hemorrhage: a multicenter randomized controlled trial. Stroke. 2016;47(11):2749–55. https://doi.org/10.1161/STROKEAHA.116.013837.

125. Hanley DF, Thompson RE, Muschelli J, et al. Safety and efficacy of minimally invasive surgery plus alteplase in intracerebral haemorrhage evacuation (MISTIE): a randomised, controlled, open-label, phase 2 trial. Lancet Neurol. 2016;15(12):1228–37. https://doi.org/10.1016/S1474-4422(16)30234-4 [published Online First: 2016/10/19].

126. Fiorella D, Arthur A, Bain M, et al. Minimally invasive surgery for intracerebral and intraventricular hemorrhage: rationale, review of existing data and emerging technologies. Stroke. 2016;47(5):1399–406. https://doi.org/10.1161/STROKEAHA.115.011415 [published Online First: 2016/04/07].

127. Bauer AM, Rasmussen PA, Bain MD. Initial single-center technical experience with the BrainPath system for acute intracerebral hemorrhage evacuation.

Oper Neurosurg (Hagerstown). 2017;13(1):69–76. https://doi.org/10.1227/NEU.0000000000001258.

128. Zhou X, Chen J, Li Q, et al. Minimally invasive surgery for spontaneous supratentorial intracerebral hemorrhage: a meta-analysis of randomized controlled trials. Stroke. 2012;43(11):2923–30. https://doi.org/10.1161/STROKEAHA.112.667535.

129. Xia Z, Wu X, Li J, et al. Minimally invasive surgery is superior to conventional craniotomy in patients with spontaneous Supratentorial intracerebral hemorrhage: a systematic review and meta-analysis. World Neurosurg. 2018;115:266–73. https://doi.org/10.1016/j.wneu.2018.04.181.

130. Scaggiante J, Zhang X, Mocco J, et al. Minimally invasive surgery for intracerebral hemorrhage. Stroke. 2018;49(11):2612–20. https://doi.org/10.1161/STROKEAHA.118.020688.

131. Mould WA, Carhuapoma JR, Muschelli J, et al. Minimally invasive surgery plus recombinant tissue-type plasminogen activator for intracerebral hemorrhage evacuation decreases perihematomal edema. Stroke. 2013;44(3):627–34. https://doi.org/10.1161/STROKEAHA.111.000411 [published Online First: 2013/02/09].

132. Hanley DF, Thompson RE, Rosenblum M, et al. Efficacy and safety of minimally invasive surgery with thrombolysis in intracerebral haemorrhage evacuation (MISTIE III): a randomised, controlled, open-label, blinded endpoint phase 3 trial. Lancet. 2019;393(10175):1021–32. https://doi.org/10.1016/S0140-6736(19)30195-3.

133. Awad IA, Polster SP, Carrion-Penagos J, et al. Surgical performance determines functional outcome benefit in the Minimally Invasive Surgery Plus Recombinant Tissue Plasminogen Activator for Intracerebral Hemorrhage Evacuation (MISTIE) procedure. Neurosurgery. 2019;84(6):1157–68. https://doi.org/10.1093/neuros/nyz077 [published Online First: 2019/03/21].

134. Kellner CP, Song R, Pan J, et al. Long-term functional outcome following minimally invasive endoscopic intracerebral hemorrhage evacuation. J Neurointerv Surg. 2020;12(5):489–94. https://doi.org/10.1136/neurintsurg-2019-015528.

135. Vitt JR, Sun CH, Le Roux PD, et al. Minimally invasive surgery for intracerebral hemorrhage. Curr Opin Crit Care. 2020;26(2):129–36. https://doi.org/10.1097/MCC.0000000000000695.

136. Labib MA, Shah M, Kassam AB, et al. The safety and feasibility of image-guided BrainPath-mediated Transsulcul hematoma evacuation: a multicenter study. Neurosurgery. 2017;80(4):515–24. https://doi.org/10.1227/NEU.0000000000001316.

Seizures and Status Epilepticus

10

Joseph I. Sirven, Luca Farrugia, and Christian Rosenow

Introduction

Seizures are one of the most dramatic events that occur in all of medicine and are immediately perceived by the lay public as an emergency. However, not all seizures are true emergencies. Seizures become emergencies when an individual is either in danger of harming himself or herself, or alternatively if the seizure continues for a long period of time for which immediate medical attention is necessary.

Seizures account for an estimated 1–2% of emergency department visits with higher numbers of emergency department visits among infants and toddlers, males, and African Americans [1]. Although seizures are very common, with 11% of the population having a seizure at some point in their lifetime, epilepsy occurs in only 3% of the population [2]. Thus, most people who have a seizure do not have epilepsy, but rather symptomatic seizures, defined as those caused by well-defined acute insults, such as brain tumor, head injury, and intracranial bleeding. A provoked seizure is caused by an identifi-

able transient disturbance, such as an electrolyte abnormality (e.g., hypocalcemia).

Emergency department physicians encounter a number of clinical scenarios involving seizures: new-onset seizures, breakthrough seizures in patients with known epilepsy, and conditions that can mimic seizures. Because no sign, symptom, or test clearly differentiates a seizure from a nonseizure event (e.g., syncope, pseudoseizure), the clinical history remains the most important tool in distinguishing seizures from their mimickers.

Seizures

When evaluating a patient who has just experienced a seizure, the physician should first verify that the patient has normal vital signs and adequate oxygenation and that there is no further seizure activity. There is no standardized algorithm for the evaluation of every patient with a first seizure. However, the American Academy of Neurology in collaboration with the American Epilepsy Society has provided evidence-based guidelines as to what the first-time seizure evaluation should include [3]. The history should initially focus on determining whether a seizure actually occurred and evaluating the circumstances and characteristics of the event. It should be determined whether there was an aura or a postictal period. Every attempt should be made to interview observers and EMS to obtain a clear description of the seizure to avoid misdiagnosing nonseizure events. It is also essential to

J. I. Sirven (✉)
Department of Neurology, Division of Epilepsy, Mayo Clinic, Jacksonville, FL, USA
e-mail: Sirven.Joseph@mayo.edu

L. Farrugia · C. Rosenow
Department of Neurology, Division of Epilepsy, Mayo Clinic, Phoenix, AZ, USA
e-mail: Farrugia.Luca@mayo.edu;
Rosenow.Christian@mayo.edu

© The Author(s), under exclusive license to Springer Nature Switzerland AG 2021
K. L. Roos (ed.), *Emergency Neurology*, https://doi.org/10.1007/978-3-030-75778-6_10

conduct a thorough medical review of potential etiologies of seizures, including sleep deprivation, alcohol consumption, illicit drug use, medical conditions, and prescription medications and any over-the-counter agents, including stimulants and herbals/botanicals. The physical examination should include a thorough neurologic and mental status evaluation. The differential diagnosis of seizures is listed in Table 10.1.

Diagnostic Testing

Diagnostic testing can be helpful in corroborating the diagnosis and establishing an etiology (Table 10.2). Laboratory testing is essential and

Table 10.1 Differential diagnosis of seizures

Syncope
Migraine with aura
Hypoglycemia
Psychogenic nonepileptic attacks
Panic attacks
Paroxysmal movement disorders
Acute dystonic reactions
Hemifacial spasms
Nonepileptic myoclonus
Sleep disorders
Parasomnias
Cataplexy
Hypnic jerks
Transient ischemic attack
Transient global amnesia

for the first seizure should include toxicology screening looking for potential agents that may cause seizures, such as cocaine and other stimulants. A complete blood cell count, urinalysis, and chest X-ray are important to assess for infection. Electrolytes also need to be evaluated and should include glucose, sodium, potassium, calcium, and magnesium. Lumbar puncture is indicated in the setting of a seizure and fever to rule out a CNS infection. Neuroimaging studies are a standard of care for epilepsy. Either computed tomography (CT) with contrast or an MRI needs to be performed; however, non-contrast CT is not considered a thorough-enough imaging study for patients with seizures. If a patient has a known history of epilepsy and is on anti-seizure medications (AEDs), checking serum levels of those medications is helpful to assess compliance as breakthrough seizures often occur in the setting of low concentrations of AEDs. Last but not least, an electroencephalogram is essential to the first seizure workup. The purpose of the EEG is to assess for potential recurrence of seizures if the seizure has stopped and to rule out status epilepticus if the patient has not returned to baseline.

Therapy

If a patient has had a single seizure, therapy with an AED is often not necessary unless there is an

Table 10.2 Diagnostic testing for seizures

Diagnostic test	Assessing for	Comments
Toxicology screen	Positive agents known to cause seizures	Look for stimulant agents such as cocaine, alcohol, and illicit agents
Electrolyte panel	Metabolic derangements	Hypoglycemia, hyponatremia, hypernatremia, hypocalcemia, and hypomagnesemia may all cause seizures
Arterial blood gas	Hypoxia	Hypoxia is a common cause of seizures
Urinalysis	Urinary tract infection	
Chest X-ray	Pulmonary infection	
MRI or CT with contrast	Any structural lesion	The preferred study is MRI of the brain. If a CT, then the study needs to be with contrast
Electroencephalogram	Epileptiform discharges	Must be performed for a first seizure
Serum antiepileptic drug levels	Subtherapeutic levels	Should be assessed only in patients with a history of seizures and currently on AED therapy
Lumbar puncture	Central nervous system infection	Spinal fluid should be analyzed in patients with seizures and fever and in those who are immunocompromised

obvious structural lesion or overt epileptogenic abnormalities on the EEG, such as a focal or generalized interictal sharp/spike wave. If the patient has more than one seizure or has a high probability of recurrence due to an underlying condition [4], then therapy should be initiated. In the emergency department or hospital setting, a benzodiazepine, such as lorazepam or diazepam, is often appropriate for short-term control. If one is looking to initiate an AED with the idea of having the patient remain on the AED for some time, then an intravenous AED may be more appropriate, such as fosphenytoin, phenobarbital, valproic acid, levetiracetam, or lacosamide. Further discussion on the emergency treatment of seizure is discussed in the therapy section of this chapter.

Status Epilepticus (SE)

The term "status epilepticus" was first used in 1868 to describe grand mal seizures occurring in rapid succession without complete recovery between convulsions [5]. Research in status epilepticus since then has advanced our understanding from the old concept of "just a cluster of severe seizures" to a self-sustaining unique pathophysiological condition with a potentially poor prognosis.

Definitions

The definition of status epilepticus has evolved over the years. The Epilepsy Foundation of America's Working Group on Status Epilepticus defines status epilepticus as "continuous seizure activity (partial or generalized, convulsive or nonconvulsive) lasting 30 min or more or intermittent seizure activity lasting 30 min or more during which consciousness is not regained" [6]. Furthermore, SE has recently been defined as failure of seizure termination mechanisms or aberrant activation of seizure initiation mechanisms for prolonged periods of time [7]. The cutoff time limit at 30 min comes from multiple scientific sources of evidence:

(a) Experiments in animals have shown status epilepticus becoming self-sustaining within 15–30 min.
(b) Status epilepticus-induced damages become distinct after 30 min of seizure activity.
(c) There is a time-dependent development of pharmacoresistance as seizures progress.

As the prognosis of status epilepticus changes with a delay in starting treatment, a narrower time window should be used for defining SE for treatment purposes. Thus, to stress the urgency of starting treatment in all patients in SE, continuous or intermittent convulsive seizures lasting more than 5 min, or nonconvulsive seizures lasting more than 10 minutes without full recovery of consciousness between seizures, is the new definition of SE [8]. The rationale for 5 min has been adopted in other operational (treatment oriented) definitions and is based on the pathophysiology [9].

Subtle status epilepticus is a term suggested by Treiman to represent the maintained electroencephalographic expression of seizures with or without the presence of convulsive signs, yet the prognostic and therapeutic implications of that stage are still those of convulsive status epilepticus [10]. Sometimes subtle status epilepticus may appear de novo after a severe insult to the brain. The greater the degree of encephalopathy present, the more subtle is the convulsive activity.

Lowenstein et al. [11] proposed that continuous, generalized convulsive seizures be defined as status epilepticus when they last more than 5 min and when two or more seizures occur during which the patient does not return to baseline consciousness. Generalized convulsive status epilepticus (GCSE) has been conceptualized into three distinct phases to capture the transition from isolated seizures to status epilepticus and in the development of time-dependent pharmacoresistance. Figure 10.1 illustrates this theoretical construct of status.

Status epilepticus has been classified in many ways based on either the symptomatology of the seizures, epilepsy syndromes, or a treatment-oriented scheme. The World Health Organization

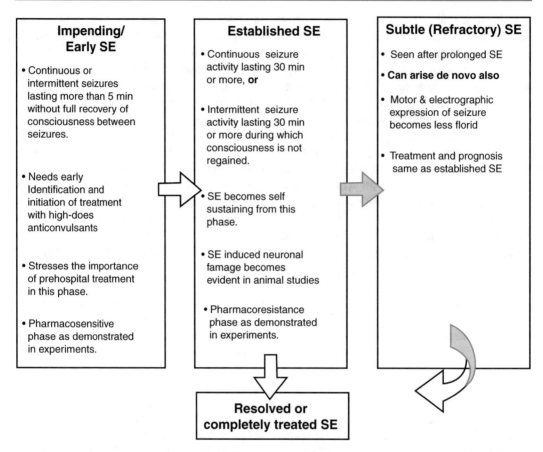

Fig. 10.1 Status epilepticus (SE) can best be understood as a spectrum of three phases each with distinct pathophysiology and unique therapeutic strategies. The *arrows* demonstrate the typical order in which these phases manifest. SE typically begins in an early phase characterized by discrete seizures without intervening recovery. It then progresses to established SE which implies at least 30 min of seizures without recovery. After established SE, the condition can either resolve after treatment or it can lead to subtle or refractory SE. Refractory SE can either resolve with treatment or continue unabated until death

and the International League Against Epilepsy (ILAE) have classified status epilepticus on the basis of clinical semiology and electroencephalographic classification (Table 10.3). Overt GCSE is easily recognized as recurrent generalized convulsions without full recovery of neurologic function between seizures.

The term *partially treated status epilepticus* refers to the cessation of clinical seizures or only subtle symptoms, but the continuance of electrographic seizures. Epidemiological studies suggest 10% of patients treated for status epilepticus remain in this group. Experimental studies suggest uncontrolled firing alone can kill neurons.

Table 10.3 Classification of status epilepticus (as per WHO and ILAE) [1]

Generalized SE	Partial or focal SE
Convulsive	Simple partial attacks
	Partial elementary
Tonic–clonic	Motor
Tonic	Sensory
Clonic	Somatomotor
Myoclonic	Dysphasic
Nonconvulsive	Continuous partial epilepsy
Absence status	(Epilepsia partialis continua)
	Complex partial attacks
Unilateral SE: hemiclonic SE	
Nonclassifiable SE	
Erratic SE	

Refractory status epilepticus is defined as seizures lasting longer than 2 h or seizures recurring at a rate of two or more episodes per hour without recovery to baseline between seizures, despite treatment with conventional antiepileptic drugs (AEDs) [12]. However, in clinical practice, status epilepticus is often considered to be refractory in any patient who has not responded to first-line AEDs. The likelihood of response to another add-on AED decreases with the failure of the first AED.

Epidemiology

Status epilepticus epidemiological studies are difficult to assess as status epilepticus occurs not only in people with epilepsy but also in individuals with acute systemic and neurologic illness. Nevertheless a handful of retrospective and prospective epidemiological studies conducted in different communities have contributed to our understanding of status epilepticus. The annual estimates of status epilepticus in the UK, the USA, and worldwide are approximately 14,000, 150,000, and 3 million cases, respectively.

In the Richmond study, partial status epilepticus with secondary generalization was the most common seizure type in both children and adults, while generalized tonic–clonic status epilepticus was the major form of status epilepticus as the final seizure type. Approximately 69% of adults with status epilepticus and 64% of children with status epilepticus presented with partial status epilepticus as the initial seizure type. When seizures did not secondarily generalize, simple partial status epilepticus was more common than partial complex status epilepticus in both children and adults [13].

Approximately one-fifth to one-half of all status epilepticus cases are reported to be refractory status epilepticus, which means around 50,000–60,000 per year alone in the USA [14]. Refractory status epilepticus is associated with an increased length of hospital stay and functional disability. Nonconvulsive status epilepticus (NCSE) and focal motor seizures at onset are risk factors for refractory status epilepticus.

The age-specific incidence curve of status epilepticus is U-shaped as is the incidence of recurrence of status epilepticus. The highest incidence occurs in young children (less than 1 year old, approx. 160/100,000 population) and the elderly (greater than 85 years, approx. 111/100,000 population). Some studies have demonstrated a higher incidence of status epilepticus among males compared to females with a ratio of 1.5–2:1 [15]. The higher incidence of status epilepticus among the elderly is worrisome because concurrent medical conditions are more frequent and management is often complicated and thus the prognosis worse. The estimated cost of status epilepticus in the USA is $4 billion per year and more than $90 billion worldwide.

The risk of recurrent status epilepticus is highest among individuals who have already experienced one episode of status epilepticus when compared with those with seizures who have never experienced status epilepticus. In one series, recurrence was much more common during the first year of life. Recurrence rates in the pediatric, adult, and elderly population were 35%, 7%, and 10%. Of note, recurrence rates are highest in female patients and those with SE refractory to the first anti-seizure medication [16]. Overall 13% of patients experienced repeat episodes of status epilepticus [17]. Status epilepticus recurrence is highest (about 80%) in those with progressive symptomatic status epilepticus [18, 19].

Etiology

The profile of etiologic risk factors is different in children and adults. In adults the most common causes of status epilepticus are lower antiepileptic drug levels in individuals with epilepsy (34%), remote symptomatic causes (24%), and acute or remote cerebrovascular disease (22%). In children the most common causes of status epilepticus are infection with fever (52%), remote symptomatic causes (SE occurring more than 1 week following brain insult; 39%), and lower antiepileptic drug levels in individuals with epi-

Table 10.4 Etiology of status epilepticus in different age groups

Etiology in adults	Etiology in pediatric age group
Lower antiepileptic drug level (34%)	Systemic infection with fever (52%)
Remote symptomatic causes (24%)	Remote symptomatic causes (39%)
Cerebrovascular disease (22%)	Lower antiepileptic drug levels (21%)
Metabolic	Cerebrovascular accident
Hypoxia	Metabolic
Alcohol-related	Idiopathic
Tumor	Hypoxia
Systemic infection with fever	Anoxia
Anoxia	CNS infection
Trauma	Drug overdose
Drug overdose	Trauma
CNS infection	Tumor
Idiopathic	Hemorrhage
Hemorrhage	

lepsy (21%). Etiologies in different age groups are further detailed in Table 10.4 [15].

One notable point with regard to etiology is that a significant number of patients with no history of epilepsy can present with status epilepticus. A study based on a twin registry at the Virginia Commonwealth University suggested a role for genetics in status epilepticus [20].

Pathophysiology

Status epilepticus occurs when there is a failure of the mechanism that terminates a single seizure, thereby leading to prolonged or multiple self-sustaining seizures. There are no studies that have shown proof that seizures become self-sustaining in human beings, but studies in experimental animals have theorized some possibilities. Understanding the mechanisms involved in the transformation from isolated seizures to self-sustaining status epilepticus might help us to prevent intractable status epilepticus and the consequences of status epilepticus, which are brain damage and epileptogenesis. Three impor-

tant basic mechanisms are associated with status epilepticus:

1. *From isolated seizure to status epilepticus*: Experimental hypotheses that explain the transition from isolated seizure to status epilepticus include marked changes in ionic channels (shift of sodium, chloride, and calcium), adenosine formation/release, electrical synchronization, and failure of GABA-mediated inhibition [21]. Neurologic insults either lower the seizure threshold or result in excessive excitation or failure in inhibitory mechanisms. Some of the mechanisms which are responsible for termination of seizures are blockade of N-methyl-D-aspartate (NMDA) channels by magnesium, activation of K+ conductances and thus repolarization of neurons and neuropeptide Y [22], and change in GABA-A receptors. Failure in either of these terminating mechanisms can lead to status epilepticus. In addition, the activation of the NMDA receptor by the excitatory neurotransmitter glutamate may be required for the propagation of seizure activity [23]. This NMDA receptor-initiated propagation has been hypothesized to be due to activation of AMPA receptors, leading to GluA1 subunit expression at glutamatergic synapses, indicating AMPA-R may be a potential therapeutic target [24].

Once self-sustaining status epilepticus is established, it is maintained by underlying changes that do not depend on continuous seizure activity, and it is easily stopped by only a few drugs, all of which directly or indirectly inhibit glutamatergic neurotransmission [25]. Maladaptive changes in the form of increased expression of proconvulsive neuropeptides (substance P, neurokinin B) and depletion of inhibitory neuropeptides (neuropeptide Y, galanin, somatostatin) that contribute to a state of raised excitability have been described.

2. *Time-dependent pharmacoresistance*: Another important finding in comparative studies is the progressive time-dependent

development of pharmacoresistance. This has been attributed to an alteration in the functional properties of GABA receptors present in the hippocampal dentate granule cells. Kapur and MacDonald showed that the anticonvulsant potency of benzodiazepines can decrease by 20 times within 30 min of self-sustaining status epilepticus [26]. Mazarati and Wasterlain showed a mechanistic shift from inadequate GABAergic inhibitory receptor-mediated transmission to excessive NMDA excitatory receptor-mediated transmission in an animal model [27]. Anticonvulsants like phenytoin also lose potency, but more slowly. Translocation of calmodulin from the membrane to the cytosol has been associated with phenytoin resistance [28]. There is no evidence of development of pharmacoresistance in human beings, although epidemiological studies suggest early treatment is much more effective than late treatment.

3. *Seizure-induced neuronal injury and death*: Continuous seizures, even in the absence of convulsive activity, cause neuronal loss resulting from excessive neuronal firing through excitotoxic mechanisms [29]. Additionally, apoptosis is likely to play a role in cell death during status epilepticus [30]. It is important to note that in experiments where systemic factors are controlled, there is still damage to the brain. Decreased neuronal density in the hippocampi of patients who died from status epilepticus has been reported [31]. In animal studies, neuronal damage has been demonstrated in the substantia nigra pars reticularis after 30 min of seizure activity and in the third and fourth layer of the cerebral cortex and CA-1, CA-4 sublayers of the hippocampus after 45–60 min of seizure [32]. Neuron-specific enolase, a marker of neuronal death, is increased in the serum of patients after status epilepticus [33]. Given the probability of cerebral injury, it is imperative for the clinician to recognize and treat status epilepticus expeditiously.

Systemic Changes with Status Epilepticus and Complications

The systemic effects of status epilepticus are a consequence of the massive catecholamine release that occurs together with excessive muscular activity. Lothman divided these progressive changes into two phases: the first phase lasts up to 30 min after seizure initiation; the second phase continues after the initial 30 min (Fig. 10.2) [34]. As a result of sympathetic overdrive, the body responds to GCSE with both systemic and cerebral complications. Systemic complications are more limited with NCSE. It is important to anticipate the possible complications of status epilepticus as they are the fundamental reason for the high morbidity and mortality associated with status epilepticus. There are numerous complications secondary to status epilepticus as detailed in Table 10.5 [35].

Clinical Presentation

For practical purposes status epilepticus can be subclassified into convulsive status (focal or generalized) and nonconvulsive status (complex partial attacks or absence seizures) based on the clinical manifestations of the seizure activity. Moreover, a newly described subtype of status epilepticus has been described named new-onset refractory status epilepticus (NORSE).

Convulsive Status Epilepticus
GCSE is the most common and serious form of status epilepticus. The evolution of this form of status epilepticus from overt to subtle GCSE has been well described in experimental and clinical studies. Clinical features of subtle GCSE are profound coma with convulsive activity limited to nystagmoid movement of the eyes or intermittent brief clonic twitches of the extremities or trunk and bilateral ictal discharges on the EEG [36]. *Generalized myoclonic status epilepticus* is predominantly seen in children. Convulsive *simple*

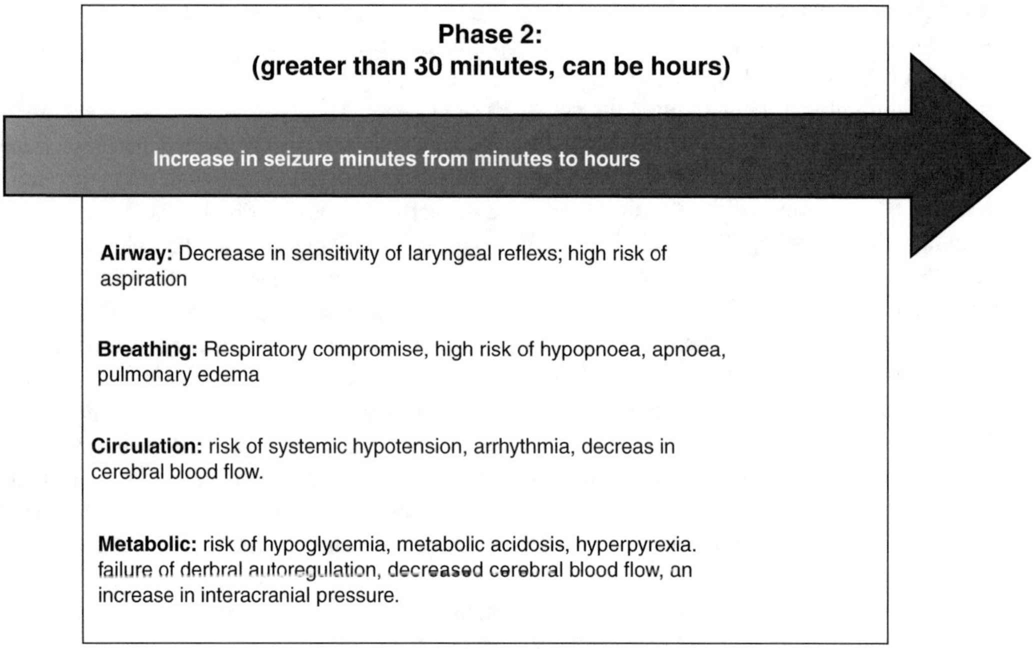

Phase 2:
(greater than 30 minutes, can be hours)

Increase in seizure minutes from minutes to hours

Airway: Decrease in sensitivity of laryngeal reflexs; high risk of aspiration

Breathing: Respiratory compromise, high risk of hypopnoea, apnoea, pulmonary edema

Circulation: risk of systemic hypotension, arrhythmia, decreas in cerebral blood flow.

Metabolic: risk of hypoglycemia, metabolic acidosis, hyperpyrexia. failure of derbral autoregulation, decreased cerebral blood flow, an increase in interacranial pressure.

Fig. 10.2 The systemic consequences of persistent seizures are outlined below. The ABCs of critical care must be managed during SE

partial status epilepticus (i.e., *epilepsia partialis continua*) is characterized by repeated partial motor seizures, preserved consciousness, and preserved neurovegetative regulations. Repeated clonic jerks with localization depending on the localization of the epileptogenic lesion in the primary motor cortex are the cardinal clinical feature [37].

Nonconvulsive Status Epilepticus

The definition and clinical features of NCSE are more heterogeneous and controversial. The semiological spectrum of NCSE ranges from negative symptoms (coma, catatonia, aphasia, amnesia, confusion) to positive symptoms (agitation, automatisms, delirium, delusion, psychosis) [38]. Apart from absence status epilepticus and complex partial status epilepticus (CPSE), the term NCSE has often been applied to patients who are severely obtunded or comatose with minimal or no motor movements. Thus definitions of NCSE should include (1) unequivocal electrographic

seizure activity, (2) periodic epileptiform discharges or rhythmic discharges with clinical seizure activity, and (3) rhythmic discharges with either clinical or electrographic response to treatment [39].

In a series of 570 critically ill patients monitored to detect subclinical seizures or for unexplained depressed level of consciousness, 18% were having nonconvulsive seizures and 10% were in NCSE [40]. *Typical absence status epilepticus* involves prolonged absence attacks with continuous or discontinuous 3-Hz spike and wave occurring in patients with generalized epilepsy. Isolated impairment of consciousness, at times with subtle jerks of the eyelids, is the essential symptom. The term *complex partial status epilepticus* implies a prolonged epileptic episode in which focal fluctuating or frequently recurring electrographic epileptic discharges, arising in temporal or extra temporal regions, result in a confusional state with variable clinical symptoms. Clinical features include clouding of conscious-

Table 10.5 Systemic and CNS complications of status epilepticus

System	Complications
Cardiovascular	Arrhythmias
	Arrest
	Tachycardia, bradycardia
	Congestive heart failure
	Hypertension, hypotension
Respiratory	Apnea
	Pulmonary edema
	Adult respiratory distress syndrome
	Nosocomial infection
	Aspiration
	Laryngeal spasm
	Respiratory acidosis
	Pulmonary embolus
Central nervous system	Cerebral edema
	Carbon dioxide narcosis
	Cerebral hypoxia
	Cerebral hemorrhage
Metabolic	Metabolic acidosis
	Hyperkalemia
	Hyponatremia
	Hypo/hyperglycemia
	Dehydration
Renal	Renal tubular acidosis
	Acute nephritic syndrome
	Oliguria/anuria
	Uremia
	Rhabdomyolysis
	Myoglobinuria
Endocrine	Hypopituitarism
	Elevated prolactin
	Elevated vasopressin
	Elevated plasma cortisol
	Weight loss
Miscellaneous	Disseminated intravascular clotting
	Loss of intestinal mobility
	Pandysautonomia
	Multiple organ dysfunction syndrome
	Fractures

ness, various automatisms (oroalimentary, gestural), and language disturbances. *Electrical status epilepticus during sleep* is characterized by spike-and-wave discharges in 85–100% of nonrapid eye movement (REM) sleep. This is associated with certain epilepsy syndromes such as Landau–Kleffner and Lennox–Gastaut syndromes [41].

New-Onset Refractory Status Epilepticus (NORSE)

New-onset refractory status epilepticus (NORSE) is defined as refractory status epilepticus without an obvious cause after initial investigations; "initial" typically refers to 1–2 days, which is adequate time to rule out strokes, brain masses, drug overdoses, and herpes encephalitis [42]. Refractory status epilepticus (SE) is a condition in which patients suddenly experience continuous seizures or a flurry of very frequent seizures (the definition of "SE") that do not respond to standard anticonvulsant medications (the definition of "refractory"). Seizures are thought to be due to an excess of pro-inflammatory molecules in the brain, perhaps triggered by a simple viral infection, although no clear cause has ever been demonstrated. Affected individuals are most often treated for weeks in an intensive care unit because they require prolonged anesthesia with coma-inducing drugs to control their seizures. NORSE carries a high rate of complications and mortality, but a significant proportion of patients do eventually recover. Epilepsy and cognitive issues are common among survivors although a small minority of them eventually return to a normal.

NORSE has been described mostly in young adults, but it can occur at any age during adulthood. Similar conditions, called febrile illness-related epilepsy syndrome (FIRES) and idiopathic hemiconvulsion–hemiplegia and epilepsy syndrome (IHHES), have been described in school-aged children and infants, respectively. Some authors now believe that these different syndromes might be the expression of a common disease.

As NORSE is not always clearly reported in series of patients with SE, but often as either "unknown cause" or "possible brain infection," it is difficult to provide an accurate estimate of its incidence. However, it is likely that it is responsible for at least 10–20% of cases of SE that do not respond to standard anticonvulsant medications [42]. This proportion can reach 50–70% when considering only cases of SE that do not respond to a first trial of coma-inducing anesthetic agents (known as "super-refractory" or "malignant" SE) and/or last more than 1 week ("prolonged" SE) [42].

Investigations in Patients with Status Epilepticus

The diagnosis of status epilepticus is often clinical. Investigations are done to find the etiology of the status epilepticus, to define the type of status epilepticus syndrome, and to differentiate from other acute neurologic conditions that can simulate complex partial status epilepticus (intoxications, encephalitis, metabolic disorders, pseudostatus). These diagnostic assessments are important but should not delay treatment. A summary of the diagnostic tests obtained from different guidelines and systematic review is presented in Table 10.6.

Management

Management of status epilepticus is divided into three categories: prehospital management, management in the acute setting (emergency department and intensive care unit), and management of prolonged status epilepticus, which is predominantly performed in the intensive care unit.

Prehospital Management [43]

The result of early treatment of status epilepticus in the ambulance, home, or at a care facility is that seizures are more likely to respond and that overall treatment costs and outcome may be improved. The intravenous administration of lorazepam (4 mg IV) or diazepam (5 mg), if lorazepam is not available, by paramedics is reasonably safe and is the best documented treatment in the prehospital setting in adults. A class I trial showed that intramuscular midazolam dosed at 10 mg is as effective as 4 mg intravenous lorazepam or 10 mg intravenous diazepam in the pre-

hospital management of status epilepticus especially when intravenous drug administration routes are not available or feasible [44]. In children, intravenous lorazepam or intramuscular midazolam is considered the first-line treatment [45]. If intravenous access is not obtained, nasal midazolam is effective in terminating seizures and is preferred to rectal diazepam [46, 47]. The intramuscular administration of lorazepam seems to be safe and fast acting in adults, and the oral administration of midazolam is effective in adults with disabilities (level C evidence) and in children (level C evidence). Rectal diazepam is safe and effective in adults in the prehospital care of patients with frequent seizures [48].

Management in the Emergency Department and Intensive Care Unit

Airway, arterial blood gas monitoring, and ECG and blood pressure monitoring are vital during the course of treatment. The presence of hypoxia and respiratory acidosis is an indication for intubation in most cases. In one-third of adults in status epilepticus, arterial pH falls below 7, primarily due to lactic acidosis from skeletal muscle convulsive activity. Respiratory acidosis responds well to oxygen and control of convulsive activity. Maintain cerebral perfusion pressure (CPP) above 60 mmHg. The systolic pressure should be maintained above 120 mm Hg if possible and should not be allowed to fall below 90 mm Hg, even if this requires the use of vasopressors. Prevent cerebral edema as much as possible with attention to brain tissue oxygenation and electrolyte balance. Cerebral edema can be treated with a 10–20% mannitol infusion (0.5–1.5 g/kg/dose, in 15–30 minutes, after ruling out the presence of cerebral hemorrhage). Should this fail, assisted respiration can be considered with hyperventilation and IV pentobarbital. Corticosteroids do not seem to be effective for treating cerebral edema due to status epilepticus. Hyperglycemia, which is secondary to catecholamine release, does not need correction in most cases and is not as harmful to the brain during status epilepticus as in ischemia, as circulation can carry lactate out of

Table 10.6   Diagnostic tests in patient with status epilepticus

Tests	Indication	Comments
Electrolytes (e.g., sodium, calcium, phosphorus, magnesium, glucose)	Performed according to suspected etiology and patient history	Abnormalities averaged 6% in children
Serum AED level	In children and probably also in adults who are treated chronically with AEDs (level B)	Low levels of AEDs are found in up to 32% of epileptics with SE
Toxicology study	Performed whenever there is no evident etiology at the first examination (level C)	Frequency of ingestion as a diagnosis in children was at least 3.6%. Both blood and urine should be sent. Routine test as "triage" discouraged
Blood culture	Insufficient data to support or refute whether blood cultures should be done on a routine basis (level U evidence). Perform if there is a strong suspicion of systemic infection or in cases of febrile SE in infants	The yield of blood culture was 2.5% in children with SE
Lumbar puncture	Insufficient data to support or refute whether LP should be done on a routine basis (level U evidence). However it is always necessary in neonatal SE	The yield was 12% in children with febrile SE and bacterial meningitis. Twenty percent of the patients may have nonspecific reactive pleocytosis in the CSF after SE
Cranial CT scan	Considered when there are clinical indications or if the etiology is unknown (level C). It is essential in cases of SE involving partial attacks and in patients with evidence of focality in the first neurologic assessment. Better than MRI in emergency as it detects almost all structural pathologies which require emergency neurosurgical interventions	Insufficient evidence to support or refute recommending routine neuroimaging (level U). Complex partial SE, simple partial SE, and generalized convulsive SE require scan. Contrast-enhanced CT is necessary when non-contrast-enhanced CT suggests vascular anomaly or isodense subdural hematoma
Cerebral MRI	Insufficient evidence to support or refute recommending routine neuroimaging (level U). It should be performed to supplement the information provided by the cranial CT scan and in all cases of cryptogenic diagnosis with normal cranial CT results	Better than CT in nonemergency for cerebral structural evaluation. Diagnostic yield is high
Electroencephalography	Indicated to define the electroclinical type of SE, to guide maintenance antiepileptic treatment, and in defining a possible evolving epileptic syndrome. It is indicated when nonconvulsive or subtle SE is suspected and in patients who have received a long-acting paralytic agent or who are in drug-induced coma (level C)	Generally an urgent test, especially when there are doubts concerning the origin of the paroxysmal episode (nonepileptic paroxysmal disorders or pseudo status)
Genetic and congenital metabolic error studies	Insufficient evidence to support or refute whether such studies should be done routinely (level U). In children, metabolic studies recommended when the initial evaluation reveals no etiology and there is a preceding history suggestive of a metabolic disorder	Nonconvulsive SE has been associated with ring chromosome 20 syndrome

Classification of recommendations (as from American Academy of Neurology) [1]
Level A rating requires at least two consistent Class I studies
Level B rating requires at least one Class I study or at least two consistent Class II studies
Level C rating requires at least one Class II study or two consistent Class III studies
Level U means data inadequate or conflicting; given current knowledge, test is unproven
Summarized from American Academy of Neurology practice parameter guideline and review article by Perias et al. [1]

the brain. Some studies suggest mild acidosis is an anticonvulsant and neuroprotective [49]. Hypoglycemia in adults is treated by an initial bolus of 50 mL of 50% glucose after the IV administration of 100 mg of thiamine (to prevent the possible development of Wernicke encephalopathy). In children, an initial bolus of 2 mL/kg of 25% glucose is recommended.

Pharmacotherapy of Status Epilepticus

Intravenous benzodiazepines, which work through enhancing gamma-aminobutyric acid (GABA) inhibition of repetitive neuronal firing, are the first-choice antiepileptic drug, with an efficacy of at least 79% in stopping the seizure. Phenytoin, valproate, and levetiracetam are considered as second-line, whereas barbiturates, lacosamide, and lidocaine are some of the third-line drugs. In order to prevent seizure recurrence, administration of second-line drugs is recommended even if convulsions have stopped [50]. Detailed descriptions of these drugs are provided in Table 10.7 [51, 52, 77]. A large randomized trial comparing 20 mg/kg of fosphenytoin, 40 mg/kg of valproate, and 60 mg/kg of levetiracetam in benzodiazepine-resistant status epilepticus failed to show any differences between these three drug regimens and doses. There are many protocols/drug regimens for the manage-

Table 10.7 Summary of some of the common drugs used in the treatment of status epilepticus

Generic name/ common route of administration	Loading dose	Maintenance dose	Half-life/time to peak concentration	Comments
First-line drugs Diazepam/IV Lorazepam/IV Midazolam/IV Midazolam IM Clonazepam/IV	0.15 mg/kg at 5 mg/min 0.1 mg/kg at 2 mg/min 10 mg 0.2 mg/kg by slow IV push 0.015 mg/kg	Not typically used as maintenance therapy Repeat to max of 2 mg/min 0.75–10 mg/kg/ min for 12–24 h	28–54 h/peaks in 2–30 min 8–25 h/peaks in 30–120 min 3 h/peaks in 30 min 18–39 h/peaks in 10–30 min	Diazepam gel peaks in 45–90 min, but therapeutic level is maintained for 8 h compared to 2 h for IV diazepam Longer-acting anticonvulsant effect than diazepam. 26% hypotension and less than 20% respiratory depression in VA cooperative study [54] Low peak concentration due to poor bioavailability, use in acute seizure not recommended. Respiratory depression noted. Can be given IM Main disadvantages are bronchorrhea/ bronchoplegia. Limited clinical experience
Second-line drugs Phenytoin/IV Fosphenytoin/IV Valproate/IV Levetiracetam/ IV Lacosamide/IV	20 mg/kg at 50 mg/kg (max of 30 mg/kg) 40 mg/kg at 50 mg/kg (max of 30 mg/kg) phenytoin equivalents 20–40 mg/kg 1500–3000 mg over 25 min 200 mg over 30–60 min	<50 mg/min (reduce to 0.3 mg/ kg/min in elderly, critically ill, and liver disease patients) <50 mg/min phenytoin equivalents 4–8 mg/kg tid 1500 mg PO bid 200 mg PO bid	24 h (wide variation)/peaks after 15 min 24 h (wide variation)/peaks in 20 min 15 h/peaks in 20 min 12 h 12 h	Heart rate, blood pressure, and the ECG should always be monitored because of the risk of cardiac arrhythmia and hypotension. It precipitates when mixed with most parenteral solutions except physiologic saline solution and often causes phlebitis at the infusion site Can be given orally High price when compared with PHT, does not produce respiratory depression or alter consciousness Not to be used in children with acute liver disease or patients with inherited metabolic disorders Not FDA approved for status Not FDA approved for status. PR prolongation on EKG is possible

Table 10.7 (continued)

Generic name/common route of administration	Loading dose	Maintenance dose	Half-life/time to peak concentration	Comments
Third-line drugs Phenobarbital/IV Paraldehyde/IV, rectal, nasogastric tube Lidocaine/IV Propofol/IV Pentobarbital/IV *Thiopental/IV*	20 mg/kg at 30–50 mg/min (max of 30 mg/kg) 100–200 mg/kg diluted to 5% solution 1.5–2 mg/kg 1–2 mg/kg by slow IV push 10–15 mg/kg 100–200 mg	2–4 mg/kg qd 20 mg/kg/h (0.4 mL/kg/h of a 5% solution) 0.6–9.0 mg/kg/h (max 300 mg/h) 2–15 mg/kg/h 0.5–1 mg/kg/h 3–5 mg/kg/h	96 h/peaks in 3–60 min 6 h/peaks immediately with IV, with other route taking 30–120 min 2 h/peaks within 4–8 min 2 h/peaks in 5 min 10–20 h 12–36 h	Longest half-life which is influenced by age; neonates have the highest. In VA study, reported side effects were hypotension (34.1%), hypoventilation (13.2%), and cardiac rhythm disturbances (3.3%) [54] Bioavailability of rectal route is 80%. The IV solution must be 5% or less because of reduced solubility (7.8%) at body temperature. Pulmonary edema, pulmonary hemorrhage, and right heart failure are some of the side effects Dose-dependent CNS depression. Can cause bradycardia and hypotension Monitoring with continuous EEG and blood pressure in ICU setting recommended. Bradycardia and hypotension are frequent side effects Effects monitored by regular EEGs, measuring the frequency of paroxysm-suppression intervals, and BP monitoring. Hypotension and respiratory depression common Induces coma requiring artificial respiration in an ICU. Use is associated with a high morbidity and mortality rate and should therefore only be used for 24–48 h

ment of status epilepticus. The American Academy of Neurology in collaboration with the Epilepsy Foundation recommends use of an algorithm for management of status epilepticus as noted in Fig. 10.3 [53]. More than the use of specific drug or drug order, the most important factor in status epilepticus termination is the rapid use of effective drugs in adequate doses, based on estimated weights and mg/kg requirements.

Some of the less commonly used antiepileptic drugs which have been tried in status epilepticus, especially refractory status epilepticus, are:

(a) *Magnesium* [55]: It is useful in seizures due to eclampsia and hypomagnesemia. In eclampsia, target level of serum magnesium is 3.5–6.0 mEq/L. This level is achieved by infusion of 5 g of magnesium sulfate over 5–30 minutes, followed by 1 g/h of continuous infusion.

(b) *Nonnarcotic anesthetics*: Isoflurane, etomidate, and ketamine have been used in treating refractory SE. Clinical trials with these are limited. Etomidate has a high risk of adrenal insufficiency due to acute hemorrhage of the adrenal glands [56], whereas there is considerable risk of respiratory depression, apnea, and laryngospasm with ketamine [57].

(c) *Pyridoxine*: This drug has been used in refractory status epilepticus in children under 3 years of age with a history of chronic epilepsy or in established neonatal status epilepticus or refractory status epilepticus in infants [58].

(d) *Newer antiepileptics*: Topiramate [59], levetiracetam [60], perampanel [61], brivaracetam [62], and clobazam [63] have all been used for the treatment of refractory status epilepticus.

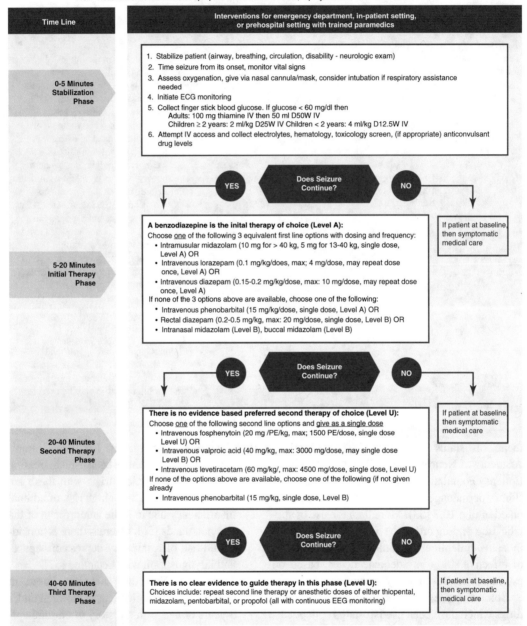

Proposed Algorithm for Convulsive Status Epilepticus

From "Treatment of Covulsive Status Epileptius un children and Adults," *Epiley Currents* 16.1 - Jan/Feb 2016

Time Line	Interventions for emergency department, in-patient setting, or prehospital setting with trained paramedics

0-5 Minutes Stabilization Phase	1. Stabilize patient (airway, breathing, circulation, disability - neurologic exam)
	 2. Time seizure from its onset, monitor vital signs
	 3. Assess oxygenation, give via nasal cannula/mask, consider intubation if respiratory assistance needed
	 4. Initiate ECG monitoring
	 5. Collect finger stick blood glucose. If glucose < 60 mg/dl then
	     Adults: 100 mg thiamine IV then 50 ml D50W IV
	     Children ≥ 2 years: 2 ml/kg D25W IV Children < 2 years: 4 ml/kg D12.5W IV
	 6. Attempt IV access and collect electrolytes, hematology, toxicology screen, (if appropriate) anticonvulsant drug levels

Does Seizure Continue? YES → / NO →

If patient at baseline, then symptomatic medical care

| **5-20 Minutes Initial Therapy Phase** | **A benzodiazepine is the inital therapy of choice (Level A):**
 Choose <u>one</u> of the following 3 equivalent first line options with dosing and frequency:
 • Intramusular midazolam (10 mg for > 40 kg, 5 mg for 13-40 kg, single dose, Level A) OR
 • Intravenous lorazepam (0.1 mg/kg/does, max; 4 mg/dose, may repeat dose once, Level A) OR
 • Intravenous diazepam (0.15-0.2 mg/kg/dose, max: 10 mg/dose, may repeat dose once, Level A)
 If none of the 3 options above are available, choose one of the following:
 • Intravenous phenobarbital (15 mg/kg/dose, single dose, Level A) OR
 • Rectal diazepam (0.2-0.5 mg/kg, max: 20 mg/dose, single dose, Level B) OR
 • Intranasal midazolam (Level B), buccal midazolam (Level B) |

Does Seizure Continue? YES → / NO →

If patient at baseline, then symptomatic medical care

| **20-40 Minutes Second Therapy Phase** | **There is no evidence based preferred second therapy of choice (Level U):**
 Choose <u>one</u> of the following second line options and <u>give as a single dose</u>
 • Intravenous fosphenytoin (20 mg /PE/kg, max; 1500 PE/dose, single dose Level U) OR
 • Intravenous valproic acid (40 mg/kg, max: 3000 mg/dose, may single dose Level B) OR
 • Intravenous levetiracetam (60 mg/kg/, max: 4500 mg/dose, single dose Level U)
 If none of the options above are available, choose one of the following (if not given already
 • Intravenous phenobarbital (15 mg/kg, single dose, Level B) |

Does Seizure Continue? YES → / NO →

If patient at baseline, then symptomatic medical care

| **40-60 Minutes Third Therapy Phase** | **There is no clear evidence to guide therapy in this phase (Level U):**
 Choices include: repeat second line therapy or anesthetic doses of either thiopental, midazolam, pentobarbital, or propofol (all with continuous EEG monitoring) |

If patient at baseline, then symptomatic medical care

Disclaimer: This clinical algorithm/guideline is designed to assist clinicians by providing an analytic framework for evaluatin and treating patients with status epilepticus. It is not intended to establish a community standard of care, replace a clinician's medical judgment, or establish a protocol for all patients. The clinical conditions contemplated by this algorithm/guideline will not fit or work with all patients. Approcaches not covered in this algortihm/guideline may be appropriate.

2016 © Epilepsy curents

Fig. 10.3 The American Epilepsy Society in collaboration with the Epilepsy Foundation proposed algorithm for management of status epilepticus in adults and children

Some of the antiepileptic drugs used in specific types of status epilepticus are summarized below:

(a) *Generalized convulsive status epilepticus*: intravenous lorazepam or phenobarbital or diazepam–phenytoin combinations are acceptable initial treatments. In 20–35% of patients, initial therapy will fail. Fosphenytoin or phenytoin is an attractive second choice and general anesthesia is a third choice.

(b) *Typical absence status epilepticus (NCSE)*: intravenous or oral benzodiazepines as initial treatment.

(c) *Complex partial status epilepticus (NCSE)*: oral, rectal, or intravenous benzodiazepines as initial treatment (protocol similar to GCSE).

(d) *NCSE in coma*: intravenous benzodiazepines and phenytoin (fosphenytoin) or phenobarbital together with anesthetic agents.

(e) *Atypical absence status epilepticus (NCSE)*: oral or intravenous valproic acid.

(f) *Electrical status epilepticus during sleep*: oral clobazam.

(g) *Myoclonic status (following hypoxia, in non-progressive encephalopathies)*: clonazepam, piracetam.

(h) *Status epilepticus in neonates*: phenobarbital is the most frequently used in neonatal seizures [64].

Management of Refractory Status Epilepticus

Refractory status epilepticus requires aggressive treatment; however, optimal treatment has not been defined. Refractory status epilepticus is best managed with a multidisciplinary team in the intensive care unit with continuous monitoring of hemodynamic parameters and EEG [50]. Without EEG the response to AED treatment is difficult to verify, as subclinical, electrographic seizure activity can be detected in up to 48% of patients after the cessation of clinical symptoms of GCSE. However, it should be noted that a delay in obtaining an EEG should not withhold treatment. Complications should be aggressively managed. Continuous intravenous anesthetics (midazolam, propofol, thiopental, pentobarbital) are commonly used in refractory GCSE. In a meta-analysis of continuous intravenous anesthetics, the overall rates were similar in mid-

azolam- and propofol-treated patients, and ultimate treatment failure was less common with pentobarbital (3%) than with midazolam (21%) or propofol (20%) [65].

Ketamine is an N-methyl-D-aspartase (NMDA) antagonist that has promise as a treatment for refractory status epilepticus. Glutamate antagonists might be particularly helpful in the later phases of status epilepticus, when gamma-aminobutyric (GABA) agonists or promoters (e.g., benzodiazepines and barbiturates) have lost some effectiveness and excessive glutamatergic activity may perpetuate seizures. A typical loading dose of ketamine is 2 mg/kg, followed by an infusion of 1.5 to 5 mg/kg/hr, but higher doses may have significant side effects, and optimal treatment has not yet been defined [66, 67, 68].

Different surgical options for refractory status epilepticus have been reported in the literature including focal resections, corpus callosotomy, hemispherectomy, and subpial transection. Vagus nerve stimulation has also been reported to be useful in a few cases. Low-frequency stimulation through subdural electrodes has been used to suppress seizures in refractory status epilepticus.

For conditions like NORSE or autoimmune conditions like NMDA encephalitis, immunomodulatory therapy is appropriate as early institution of immunomodulatory therapies (e.g., glucocorticoids, intravenous *immunoglobulin*) may improve outcomes [42]. The proportion of cases of GCSE that are ultimately identified as having an autoimmune or paraneoplastic etiology ranges from 2% to 6%, with the higher estimate drawn from cases of refractory status epilepticus [68, 69, 70]. The diagnosis and treatment of paraneoplastic and autoimmune encephalitis are discussed in detail elsewhere.

Prognosis

The mortality of status epilepticus varies from 11% to 34% with rates higher in adults (15–49%) than in children (3–9%) [71, 72]. The case fatality in the first month after status epilepticus was 21% and is primarily in those with acute symptomatic status epilepticus associated with illnesses that have a high mortality [73]. In the adult population, status epilepticus is often secondary to anoxia, hypoxia, stroke, metabolic abnormalities, brain tumor, or head injury, which has the highest mortality. In children, higher mortality is associated with severe acute encephalopathies and progressive encephalopathies. The lowest mortality rate is found in febrile and idiopathic status epilepticus.

Etiology, time from onset of status epilepticus to the administration of medical treatment, duration of seizures, age, and response to early treatment are some of the variables that predict the outcome of status epilepticus. Recurrence of status epilepticus is also associated with increased morbidity with some cases leading to the development of subsequent epilepsy and progression to intractable epilepsy. Other serious comorbidities include cognitive deficits, such as a decline in short-term memory and intelligence quotient (IQ) scores [73, 74]. The risk of unprovoked seizures is 3.3 times higher after acute symptomatic status epilepticus (41%) than after single seizures (13%), and the risk of developing a febrile seizure is seven times higher in status epilepticus than after simple febrile convulsions [75, 76].

Summary

Status epilepticus is a major medical and neurological emergency. Incidence shows variations with ethnicity (highest among blacks), gender (male higher), and age (highest among children and elderly population). Etiology is different in adults and children. A notable point with regard to etiology is that an individual with no history of epilepsy can present with status epilepticus. Continuous, generalized convulsive seizures are considered to be status epilepticus when they last more than 5 minutes or there are two or more seizures during which the patient does not return to baseline consciousness. The evolution of status epilepticus in different phases has been well described. Early treatment of status epilepticus is required as time-dependent pharmacoresistance has been described in animal studies. Even with current best practice, 50% of patients with refractory GCSE will die. Therefore there is an urgent need for new treatment options that can stop seizures more effectively and safely than current drugs.

References

1. Pallin DJ, Espinola JA, Leung DY, Hopper DC, Camargo CA Jr. Seizure visits in US emergency departments: epidemiology and potential disparities in care. Int J Emerg Med. 2008;1(2):97–105.
2. Hauser WA, Annegers JF, Rocca WA. Descriptive epidemiology of epilepsy: contributions of population-based studies from Rochester. Minnesota Mayo Clin Proc. 1996;71:576–86.
3. Krumholtz A, Wiebe S, Gronseth G, Gloss D, Sanchez A, Kabir A, Liferidge A, Martello J, Kanner A, Shinnar S, Hopp J, French J. Evidence – based guideline: first seizure in adults. Neurology. 2015;84(16):1705–13.
4. Fields MC, Labovitz DL, French JA. Hospital-onset seizures: an inpatient study. JAMA Neurol. 2013;70(3):360–4.
5. Trousseau A. Lectures on Clinical medicine Delivered at the Hotel Dieu, Paris, 1868. Vol 1 (P V Bazire, trans) London: New Sydenham Society; 1868.
6. Dodson WE, DeLorenzo RJ, Pedley TA, Shinnar S, Treiman DM, Wannamaker BB. The treatment of convulsive status epilepticus: recommendations of the Epilepsy Foundation of America's Working Group on Status Epilepticus. J Am Med Assoc. 1993;270:854–9.
7. Trinka E, Cock H, Rossetti AO, Sheffer IE, Shinnar S, Shorvon S, Lowenstein DH. A definition and classification of status epilepticus—report of the ILAE task force on classification of status epilepticus. Epilepsia. 2015;56(10):1515–23.
8. Trinka E, Hofler J, Leitinger M, Brigo F. Pharmacotherapy for status epilepticus. Drugs. 2015;75:1499–521.
9. Chen JWY, Wasterlain CG. Status epilepticus: pathophysiology and management in adults. Lancet Neurol. 2006;5:246–56.
10. Treiman DM, Meyers PD, Walton NY, Collins JF. A comparison of four treatments for generalized convulsive status epilepticus. N Engl J Med. 1998;339:792–8.
11. Lowenstein D, Bleck T, Macdonald R. It's time to revise the definition of status epilepticus. Epilepsia. 1999;40:120–2.
12. Bleck TP. Refractory status epilepticus. Curr Opin Crit Care. 2005;11:117–20.
13. DeLorenzo RJ, Hauser WA, Towne AR, et al. A prospective population-based epidemiologic study of status epilepticus in Richmond, Virginia. Neurology. 1996;46:1029–35.
14. Rossetti AO, Lowenstein DH. Management of refractory status epilepticus in adults. Lancet Neurol. 2011;10(10):922–30.

15. Logroscino G, Hesdorffer DC, Cascino G, Annegers JF, Hauser WA. Time trends in incidence, mortality, and case fatality after first episode of status epilepticus. Epilepsia. 2001;42:1031–5.
16. Sculier C, Gainza-Lein M, Fernandez IS, Loddenkemper T. Long-term outcomes of status epilepticus: a critical assessment. Epilepsia. 2018;59(Suppl 2):155–269.
17. DeLorenzo RJ, Pellock JM, Towne AR, Boggs JG. Epidemiology of status epilepticus. J Clin Neurophysiol. 1995;12:316–25.
18. Hesdorffer DC, Logroscino G, Hauser WA, Cascino G. Risk of and predictors for recurrence in status epilepticus. Epilepsia. 1995;36(Suppl 4):149.
19. Shinnar S, Maytal J, Krasnoff L, Moshe SL. Recurrent status epilepticus in children. Ann Neurol. 1992;31:598–604.
20. Corey LA, Pellock JM, Boggs JG, Miller LL, DeLorenzo RJ. Evidence for a genetic predisposition for status epilepticus. Neurology. 1998;50(2):558–60.
21. Kapur J, Lothman EW. NMDA receptor activation mediates the loss of GABAergic inhibition induced by recurrent seizures. Epilepsy Res. 1990;5:103–11.
22. Vezzani A, Ravizza T, Moneta D, et al. Brain-derived neurotrophic factor immunoreactivity in the limbic system of rats after acute seizures and during spontaneous convulsions: temporal evolution of changes as compared to neuropeptide Y. Neuroscience. 1999;90:1445–61.
23. Kamphius W, de Rijk TC, Talamini LM, Lopes da Silva FH. Rat hippocampal kindling induces changes in the glutamate receptor mRNA expression patterns in dentate granule neurons. Eur J Neurosci. 1994;6:1119–27.
24. Joshi S, Kapur J. Mechanism of status epilepticus: AMPA receptor hypothesis. Epilepsia. 2018;59(Suppl2):78–81.
25. Gerfin-Moser A, Grogg F, Rietschin L, Thompson SM, Streit P. Alterations in glutamate but not GABAA receptor subunit expression as a consequence of epileptiform activity in vitro. Neuroscience. 1995;67:849–65.
26. Kapur J, Macdonald RL. Rapid seizure-induced reduction of benzodiazepine and Zn2+ sensitivity of hippocampal dentate granule cell GABAA receptors. J Neurosci. 1997;17:7532–40.
27. Mazarati AM, Wasterlain CG. N-methyl-D-aspartate receptor antagonists abolish the maintenance phase of self-sustaining status epilepticus in rate. Neurosci Lett. 1999;265:187–90.
28. Mazarati AM, Baldwin RA, Sankar R, Wasterlain CG. Time-dependent decrease in the effectiveness of antiepileptic drugs during the course of self-sustaining status epilepticus. Brain Res. 1998;814:179–85.
29. Sloviter RS. Decreased hippocampal inhibition and a selective loss of interneurons in experimental epilepsy. Science. 1987;235:73–6.
30. Pollard H, Charriaut-Marlangue C, Cantagrel S, et al. Kainate-induced apoptotic cell death in hippocampal neurons. Neuroscience. 1994;63:7–18.
31. Corsellis JA, Bruton CJ. Neuropathology of status epilepticus in humans. Adv Neurol. 1983;34:129–39.
32. Nevander G, Ingvar M, Auer R, Siesjö BK. Status epilepticus in well-oxygenated rats causes neuronal necrosis. Ann Neurol. 1985;18(3):281–90.
33. DeGiorgio CM, Correale JD, Gott PS, et al. Serum neuron-specific enolase in human status epilepticus. Neurology. 1995;45:1134–7.
34. Lothman E. The biochemical basis and pathophysiology of status epilepticus. Neurology. 1990;40(Suppl1):13–23.
35. Simon RP. Physiologic consequences of status epilepticus. Epilepsia. 1985;26(Suppl 1):S58–66.
36. Treiman DM, DeGiorgio CM, Salisbury S, Wickboldt C. Subtle generalized convulsive status epilepticus. Epilepsia. 1984;25:653.
37. Treiman DM. Status epilepticus. Ballieres Clin Neurol. 1996;5:821–39.
38. Jirsch J, Hirsch LJ. Nonconvulsive seizures: developing a rational approach to the diagnosis and management in the critically ill population. Clin Neurophysiol. 2007;118:1660.
39. Walker MC. Diagnosis and treatment of nonconvulsive status epilepticus. CNS Drugs. 2001;15(12):931–9.
40. Pandian JD, Cascino GD, So EL, Manno E, Fulgham JR. Digital video electroencephalographic monitoring in the neurological-neurosurgical intensive care unit: clinical features and outcome. Arch Neurol. 2004;61:1090–4.
41. Yan Liu X, Wong V. Spectrum of epileptic syndromes with electrical status epilepticus during sleep in children. Pediatr Neurol. 2000;22(5):371–9.
42. Gaspard N, Foreman BP, Alvarez V, et al. New-onset refractory status epilepticus: etiology, clinical features, and outcome. Neurology. 2015;85:1604.
43. Alldredge BK, Gelb AM, Isaacs SM, et al. A comparison of lorazepam, diazepam, and placebo for the treatment of out-of-hospital status epilepticus. N Engl J Med. 2001;345:631–7.
44. Silbergleit R, Durkaslski V, Lowenstein D, Conwit R, Pancioli A, colleagues. Intramuscular versus intravenous therapy for prehospital status epilepticus. NEJM. 2012;366:591–600.
45. McTague A, Martland T, Appleton R. Drug management for acute tonic-clonic convulsions including convulsive status epilepticus in children. Cochrane Database Syst Rev. 2018;1:CD001905.
46. Harbord MG, Kyrkou NE, Kyrkou MR, et al. Use of intranasal midazolam to treat acute seizures in paediatric community settings. J Paediatr Child Health. 2004;40:556–8.
47. McIntyre J, Robertson S, Norris E, et al. Safety and efficacy of buccal midazolam versus rectal diazepam for emergency treatment of seizures in children: a randomised controlled trial. Lancet. 2005;366:205.
48. Fakhoury T, Chumley A, Bensalem-Owen M. Effectiveness of diazepam rectal gel in adults with acute repetitive seizures and prolonged seizures: a single-center experience. Epilepsy Bchav. 2007;11:357.

49. Giffard RG, Monyer H, Christine CW, Choi DW. Acidosis reduces NMDA receptor activation, glutamate neurotoxicity, and oxygen glucose deprivation neuronal injury in cortical cultures. Brain Res. 1990;506:339–42.

50. Brophy GM, Bell R, Claassen J, et al. Guidelines for the evaluation and management of status epilepticus. Neurocrit Care. 2012;17:3.

51. Chapman MG, Smith M, Hirsch NP. Status epilepticus. Anesthesia. 2001;56:648–59.

52. Lowenstein DH. The Management of Refractory Status Epilepticus: an update. Epilepsia. 2007;47(Suppl 1):35–40.

53. Glauser T, Shinnar S, Gloss D, Alldredge B, et al. Proposed algorithm for treatment of convulsive status epilepticus in children and adults. Epilepsy Curr. 2016;16(1):48–61. https://doi.org/10.5698/1535-7597-16.1.48.

54. Treiman DM, Meyers PD, Walton NY, et al. A comparison of four treatments for generalized convulsive status epilepticus Veterans affairs status epilepticus cooperative study group. N Engl J Med. 1998;339:792–8.

55. (The Collaborative Eclampsia Trialists): Which anticonvulsants for women with eclampsia? Evidence from the Collaborative Eclampsia trial. Lancet. 1995;345:1455–63.

56. Brown JK, Hussain IH. Status epilepticus. II Treatment. Dev Med Child Neurol. 1991;33:97–109.

57. Mewasingh LD, Sekhara T, Aeby A, et al. Oral ketamine in paediatric non-convulsive status epilepticus. Seizure. 2003;12:483–9.

58. Appleton R, Choonara I, Martland T, et al. The treatment of convulsive status epilepticus in children. The status epilepticus working party, members of the status epilepticus working party. Arch Dis Child. 2000;83:415–9.

59. Kahriman M, Minecan D, Kutluay E, et al. Efficacy of topiramate in children with refractory status epilepticus. Epilepsia. 2003;44:1353–6.

60. Rossetti AO, Bromfield EB. Determinants of success in the use of oral levetiracetam in status epilepticus. Epilepsy Behav. 2006;8:651–4.

61. Ho C, Lin C, Lu Y, et al. Perampanel treatment for refractory status epilepticus in a neurological intensive care unit. Neurocrit Care. 2019;31(1):24–9.

62. Brigo F, Lattanzi S, Trinka E. Intravenous brivaracetam in the treatment of status epilepticus: A systematic review. CNS Drugs. 2019;33(8):771–81.

63. Sivakumar S, Ibrahim M, Parker D Jr, et al. Clobazam: an effective add-on therapy in refractory status epilepticus. Epilepsia. 2015;56:e83.

64. Bartha AI, Shen J, Katz KH, et al. Neonatal seizures: multicenter variability in current treatment practices. Pediatr Neurol. 2007;37:85.

65. Claassen J, Hirsch LJ, Emerson RG, Mayer SA. Treatment of refractory status epilepticus with pentobarbital, propofol, or midazolam: a systematic review. Epilepsia. 2002;43:146–53.

66. Walker MC. Treatment of nonconvulsive status epilepticus. Int Rev Neurobiol. 2007;81:287–97.

67. Basha MM, Alqallaf A, Shah AK. Drug-induced EEG pattern predicts effectiveness of ketamine in treating refractory status epilepticus. Epilepsia. 2015;56:e44.

68. Fujikawa DG. Starting ketamine for neuroprotection earlier than its current use as an anesthetic/antiepileptic drug late in refractory status epilepticus. Epilepsia. 2019;60:373.

69. Khawaja AM, DeWolfe JL, Miller DW, Szaflarski JP. New-onset refractory status epilepticus (NORSE)–the potential role for immunotherapy. Epilepsy Behav. 2015;47:17.

70. Spatola M, Novy J, Du Pasquier R, et al. Status epilepticus of inflammatory etiology: a cohort study. Neurology. 2015;85:464.

71. Chin RF, Neville BG, Peckham C, et al. Incidence, cause, and short-term outcome of convulsive status epilepticus in childhood: prospective population-based study. Lancet. 2006;368:222.

72. Kravljanac R, Jovic N, Djuric M, et al. Outcome of status epilepticus in children treated in the intensive care unit: a study of 302 cases. Epilepsia. 2011;52:358.

73. DeLorenzo RJ, Towne AR, Pellock JM, Ko D. Status epilepticus in children, adults and the elderly. Epilepsia. 1992;33(Suppl 4):S15–25.

74. Dodrill CB, Wilensky AJ. Intellectual impairment as an outcome of status epilepticus. Neurology. 1990;40(5 Suppl 2):23–7.

75. Hesdorffer DC, Logroscino G, Cascino G, Annegers JF, Hauser WA. Risk of unprovoked seizure after acute symptomatic seizure: effect of status epilepticus. Ann Neurol. 1998;44:908–12.

76. Annegers JF, Hauser WA, Elveback LR, Kurland LT. The risk of epilepsy following febrile convulsions. Neurology. 1979;29:297–303.

77. Kapur J, Elm J, Chamberlain J, et al. Randomized trial of three anticonvulsant medications for status epilepticus. NEJM. 2019;381:22.

Central Nervous System Infections

11

Karen L. Roos

Meningitis

Meningitis is the most worrisome illness in the patient who presents to the emergency department with fever and headache. The classic triad of meningitis is fever, headache, and meningismus, which is resistance to passive flexion of the neck due to pain. A stiff neck is the pathognomonic sign of meningeal irritation from any process.

Viral Meningitis

The clinical presentation of viral meningitis is fever, headache, nausea, photophobia, and meningismus. Individuals with viral meningitis appear acutely ill and complain of a severe headache but are typically awake and alert. They may be lethargic, but are not stuporous or comatose. They do not present with seizures or focal neurological deficits.

The most common viruses to cause meningitis are the enteroviruses. The enteroviruses are the coxsackieviruses, the echoviruses, and the viruses identified by number (enteroviruses 68–71). Herpes simplex virus type 2 (HSV-2), the human immunodeficiency virus (HIV-1), and the

K. L. Roos (✉)
The John and Nancy Nelson Professor of Neurology, Indiana University School of Medicine, Indianapolis, IN, USA
e-mail: kroos@iupui.edu

arthropod-borne viruses are also fairly common etiologic agents of meningitis.

Bacterial Meningitis

Patients with bacterial meningitis have either a subacute illness that has progressed over 24–72 h or a fulminant illness that developed over several hours. The initial symptoms of bacterial meningitis include any of the following: fever, headache, lethargy, stupor, confusion, nausea, vomiting, and photophobia. It is the altered level of consciousness that is the single symptom that distinguishes the patient with bacterial meningitis from the patient with viral meningitis. Seizures occur in 40% of patients with bacterial meningitis and typically occur in the first week of illness. In children, symptoms of bacterial meningitis are often preceded by an upper respiratory tract infection or an otitis media [1]. Nuchal rigidity may be absent early in the course of the illness; therefore, the absence of a stiff neck should not exclude the diagnosis of bacterial meningitis [2]. In both children and adults, vomiting is a frequent, but often overlooked, symptom of bacterial meningitis.

Predisposing and associated conditions for bacterial meningitis are as follows: (1) pneumonia; (2) otitis, mastoiditis, or sinusitis; (3) diabetes; (4) alcoholism; (5) head trauma with basilar skull fracture; (6) asplenia; (7) congenital or acquired deficiency in the terminal common complement pathway (C3 and C5 to C9) or hypo- or agammaglobulinemia; and (8) endocarditis. It is important to note that the predisposing and associated conditions are often not known at the time of presentation.

The most common causative organisms of bacterial meningitis are *Streptococcus pneumoniae* and *Neisseria meningitidis*. The incidence of meningitis due to *N. meningitidis* has decreased with the vaccination of children and adolescents with the tetravalent (serogroups A, C, W-135, and Y) meningococcal glycoconjugate vaccine. The vaccine does not contain serogroup B, which is responsible for one third of cases of meningococcal disease [3]. There are two serogroup B meningococcal vaccines. The Advisory Committee on Immunization Practices (ACIP) recommends vaccination of adolescents and young adults 16–23 years of age with a serogroup B meningococcal vaccine.

Meningitis due to otitis, mastoiditis, or sinusitis may be due to *Streptococci* spp. (including *S. pneumoniae*), gram-negative anaerobes, *S. aureus*, *Haemophilus* sp., or Enterobacteriaceae. Patients with congenital or acquired deficiency in the terminal common complement pathway (C3 and C5 to C9), immunoglobulin deficiency, or asplenia are at risk for meningitis due to *N. meningitidis* or *S. pneumoniae*. Patients with defects of cell-mediated immunity are at risk for meningitis due to *Listeria monocytogenes*. Meningitis complicating endocarditis may be due to viridans streptococci, *S. aureus*, *S. bovis*, the HACEK group (*Haemophilus* sp., *Actinobacillus actinomycetemcomitans*, *Cardiobacterium hominis*, *Eikenella corrodens*, *and Kingella kingae*), or enterococci. Meningitis in the postneurosurgical patient and/or the patient with a ventriculostomy may be due to staphylococci, gram-negative bacilli, or anaerobes.

The presence of a diffuse erythematous maculopapular and/or petechial rash on the trunk and lower extremities, in the mucous membranes and conjunctiva, and occasionally on the palms and soles is typical of meningococcemia. It is the location of the rash on the trunk and lower extremities that should raise a concern for menin-

gococcemia. A viral exanthem typically appears as a maculopapular rash on the head and neck.

Aseptic Meningitis

Aseptic meningitis is an old term that is of little use today. The criteria for aseptic meningitis were described by Wallgren in 1925 and are as follows: (1) acute onset; (2) fever, headache, and meningismus; (3) CSF abnormalities typical of meningitis with a predominance of either lymphocytes and mononuclear cells or polymorphonuclear leukocytes; (4) absence of bacteria by smear and by culture of cerebrospinal fluid; (5) no parameningeal focus of infection; and (6) self-limited benign course [4–6]. The term aseptic meningitis can really only be applied to viral meningitis, meningitis following posterior fossa surgery, meningitis associated with inflammatory diseases (systemic lupus erythematosus, sarcoidosis, Sjögren's syndrome, etc.), and medication-induced meningitis and, as such, should be labeled by these terms rather than as an "aseptic meningitis." In medication-induced meningitis, meningitis following posterior fossa surgery, and sarcoidosis, the CSF glucose concentration may be low.

Lyme Disease

Lyme disease is due to the spirochete *Borrelia burgdorferi*. Patients with meningitis due to *B. burgdorferi* complain of headache and fatigue, and some have myalgias and arthralgias. A unilateral or bilateral facial nerve palsy (less often cranial nerves III, IV, VI, and VIII) may be present or a painful radiculopathy. Inquire about and examine the patient for the classic erythema migrans lesion.

Tuberculous Meningitis

Suspect tuberculous meningitis in the patient with either several weeks of headache, fever, and night sweats or a fulminant presentation with fever, altered mental status, and focal neurological deficits.

Differential Diagnosis

The differential diagnosis of the triad of fever, headache, and stiff neck is bacterial or viral meningitis, fungal meningitis, tuberculous meningitis, syphilitic meningitis, drug-induced aseptic meningitis, carcinomatous or lymphomatous meningitis, and aseptic meningitis. If the presentation is that of headache and stiff neck, subarachnoid hemorrhage is in the differential diagnosis [7]. When impaired consciousness, focal neurological deficits, or new-onset seizures are added to the classic triad, the differential diagnosis includes viral encephalitis, intracranial venous thrombosis, tick-borne bacterial infections, and infectious intracranial mass lesions. The differential diagnosis in HIV-infected patients who present with meningeal signs includes, in addition to meningitis caused by HIV, meningitis caused by *Cryptococcus neoformans*, *Mycobacterium tuberculosis*, and *Treponema pallidum*.

Initial Management

The patient with fever and headache should be managed as if they have bacterial meningitis until bacterial meningitis is ruled out. Recommendations for initial management include adjunctive and antimicrobial therapy and the diagnostic studies that have the highest yield for distinguishing between bacterial and viral meningitis. Those diagnostic studies include Gram's stain and bacterial blood cultures, serum procalcitonin and C-reactive protein, and spinal fluid analysis. Serum procalcitonin (>2 ng/mL) and C-reactive protein (>40 mg/L) are significantly higher in patients with bacterial meningitis than in those with viral meningitis and can help in diagnosis when the results of spinal fluid analysis are available.

Empiric antimicrobial therapy for bacterial meningitis includes antibiotic therapy, as well as acyclovir for herpes simplex virus encephalitis as that is in the differential diagnosis and doxycycline for a tick-borne bacterial infection during the season when ticks are biting.

The most common causative organisms of community-acquired bacterial meningitis in children and adults are *S. pneumoniae* and *N. meningitidis*. Empiric therapy of bacterial meningitis is based on predisposing and associated conditions (Table 11.1) and based on the possibility that a penicillin- and cephalosporin-resistant strain of *S. pneumoniae* is the causative organism. In infants older than 1 month of age, children, and adults up to the age of 55, empiric therapy includes a third- or fourth-generation cephalosporin, either ceftriaxone (pediatric dose, 80–100 mg/kg/day in a 12-h dosing interval; adult dose, 2 g every 12 h) or cefotaxime (pediatric dose, 225–300 mg/kg/day in a 6- or 8-h dosing interval; adult dose, 8–12 g/day in a 4- to 6-h dosing interval) plus vancomycin (pediatric dose, 40–60 mg/kg/day in a 6- or 12-h dosing interval; adult dose, 45–60 mg/kg/day in an 8-h dosing interval).

Metronidazole (1500–2000 mg/day in an 8-h dosing interval) is added to the empiric regimen to cover anaerobic bacteria in patients with the predisposing conditions of otitis, mastoiditis, sinusitis, neurosurgical procedures, and head trauma. Ampicillin should be added to the empiric regimen for coverage of *L. monocytogenes* in individuals over the age of 55 years and in individuals with impaired cell-mediated immunity due to a chronic illness, organ transplantation, pregnancy, malignancy, immunosuppressive therapy, or AIDS, if they have not been on trimethoprim–sulfamethoxazole prophylactic therapy. Gentamicin is added to ampicillin in critically ill patients with *L. monocytogenes* meningitis. The dose of ampicillin is 2 g every 4 h, and the dose of gentamicin is 7.5 mg/kg/day in an 8-h dosing interval.

Meropenem is a carbapenem antibiotic, and the combination of meropenem plus vancomycin can be recommended as empiric therapy for bacterial meningitis in children and adults when *Streptococcus pneumoniae*, *Haemophilus influenzae*, *Listeria monocytogenes*, or aerobic gram-negative bacilli (including *Pseudomonas aeruginosa* and *Escherichia coli*) are possible meningeal pathogens based on predisposing and

Table 11.1 Empiric antibiotic therapy based on predisposing and associated conditions

Predisposing condition	Bacterial pathogen	Antibiotic
Neonate	Group B streptococcus, *Escherichia coli*, *Listeria monocytogenes*	Ampicillin plus cefotaxime or an aminoglycoside
Children and adults—community acquired	*Streptococcus pneumoniae* and *Neisseria meningitidis*	Third- or fourth-generation cephalosporin plus vancomycin
Otitis, mastoiditis, sinusitis	Streptococci spp., gram-negative anaerobes (*Bacteroides* sp., *Fusobacterium* sp.), *S. aureus*, *Haemophilus* sp., Enterobacteriaceae	Third- or fourth-generation cephalosporin plus vancomycin plus metronidazole
Adults over the age of 55 and those with chronic illness	*S. pneumoniae*, gram-negative bacilli, *N. meningitidis*, *L. monocytogenes*, *Haemophilus influenzae*	Third- or fourth-generation cephalosporin plus vancomycin plus ampicillin
Endocarditis	Viridans streptococci, *S. aureus*, *Streptococcus bovis*, HACEK group, enterococci	Third- or fourth-generation cephalosporin plus vancomycin
Immunosuppressed	*S. pneumoniae*, *L. monocytogenes*, *H. influenzae*	Third- or fourth-generation cephalosporin plus vancomycin plus ampicillin
Postneurosurgical	Staphylococci, gram-negative bacilli	Vancomycin plus meropenem or vancomycin plus ceftazidime
Intraventricular device	Staphylococci, gram-negative bacilli, anaerobes	Vancomycin plus meropenem plus metronidazole or vancomycin plus ceftazidime plus metronidazole

associated conditions. Meropenem should not be used as monotherapy.

Prior to or with the first dose of antibiotic, dexamethasone (infants and children 2 months of age and older, 0.15 mg/kg of body weight intravenously every 6 h for 2–4 days; adults, 10 mg intravenously every 6 h for 4 days) should be administered in patients with possible pneumococcal meningitis. Dexamethasone is administered either 15–20 min before the first dose of an antimicrobial agent or with the first dose of an antimicrobial agent.

In patients in whom herpes simplex virus encephalitis is suspected, acyclovir 10 mg/kg every 8 h is added to the empiric regimen. Doxycycline 100 mg every 12 h can be added to the empiric regimen during tick season if tick-borne bacterial infections are suspected. Doxycycline is relatively contraindicated in pregnant and lactating women and in children younger than 8 years of age.

Neuroimaging

A head CT scan prior to lumbar puncture is recommended in patients with any of the following criteria: an abnormal level of consciousness, a new-onset seizure, a focal neurological deficit, an immunocompromised state, papilledema, or poorly visualized fundi. A CT scan prior to LP should also be obtained in patients from an endemic area for cysticercosis who are at risk for an intraventricular cyst with associated edema.

The primary argument against imaging prior to lumbar puncture is that imaging delays the lumbar puncture by 2–3 h and subsequently delays the initiation of antimicrobial therapy. Obtain blood cultures, initiate adjunctive and antimicrobial therapy, obtain a cranial CT if any of the above criteria are met, and then perform spinal fluid analysis.

Spinal Fluid Analysis

The CSF abnormalities characteristic of bacterial meningitis are:

- An opening pressure >180 mm H_2O.
- A polymorphonuclear pleocytosis. The CSF should be examined promptly after it is

obtained because white blood cells in the CSF begin to lyse after about 90 min.

- A low glucose concentration. A glucose concentration of <40 mg/dL occurs in approximately 58% of patients with bacterial meningitis. A normal CSF-to-serum glucose ratio is 0.6. A CSF-to-serum glucose ratio of less than 0.31 is seen in approximately 70% of patients with bacterial meningitis.
- An elevated protein concentration.
- Gram's stain is positive in identifying the organism in 60–90% of cases of bacterial meningitis [8]. However, the probability of detecting bacteria on a Gram's stain specimen depends on the number of organisms present. Most smears will be positive when the CSF bacterial concentration is >10⁵ CFU/mL. Only 25% of smears are positive when the bacterial concentration is 10^3 CFU/mL or less [1].
- Latex agglutination tests, which detect the antigens of common meningeal pathogens, are no longer routinely available or recommended for the rapid determination of the bacterial etiology of meningitis
- Cerebrospinal fluid PCR assays have been developed to detect bacterial nucleic acid in CSF. The CSF multiplex PCR pathogen assays detect the nucleic acid of *S. pneumoniae*, *N. meningitidis*, *Escherichia coli*, *Streptococcus agalactiae*, *Haemophilus influenzae*, and *L. monocytogenes*, in addition to seven viruses and *Cryptococcus neoformans* [9].
- The sensitivity and specificity of bacterial PCRs have not been defined, and therefore there is a risk of false-negative and false-positive results. PCR will not replace culture as culture is critical for antimicrobial sensitivity testing.

The CSF abnormalities typical of viral meningitis are:

- A normal opening pressure
- A lymphocytic pleocytosis
- A normal or mildly decreased glucose concentration

- A normal or mildly elevated protein concentration

Table 11.2 provides a list of cerebrospinal fluid diagnostic studies for the patient with suspected meningitis. The basic studies that should be performed on CSF in every patient with fever, headache, and meningismus are the following: (1) cell count with differential, (2) glucose and protein concentration, (3) Gram's stain and bacterial culture, (4) viral culture for enteroviruses, (5) a multiplex PCR pathogen assay if available, and if not, the reverse transcriptase PCR for enteroviruses, and PCR for herpes simplex virus-1 (HSV-1) and herpes simplex virus-2 (HSV-2). The remaining diagnostic tests listed in Table 11.2 should be obtained depending on the time of the year (i.e., if mosquitoes are biting), place of residence and travel history (i.e., fungal antigens and antibodies, *B. burgdorferi* antibodies), and risk factors (i.e., HIV, herpes simplex

Table 11.2 Cerebrospinal fluid studies for meningitis

Cell count with differential
Glucose and protein concentration
Stain and culture
   Gram's stain and bacterial culture
   India ink and fungal culture
   Viral culture
   Acid-fast smear and *M. tuberculosis* culture
Antigens
   Cryptococcal polysaccharide antigen
   Histoplasma polysaccharide antigen
Polymerase chain reaction:
CSF multiplex PCR assay
Specific meningeal pathogen PCRs:
   Reverse transcriptase PCR for enteroviruses
   PCR for herpes simplex virus types 1 and 2
   PCR for West Nile virus
   PCR for Epstein–Barr virus
   PCR for varicella zoster virus
   PCR for *M. tuberculosis*
   PCR for HIV RNA
Antibodies
   Herpes simplex virus (serum/CSF antibody ratio of <20:1)
   Varicella zoster virus IgM and IgG antibody index
   Arthropod-borne viruses (West Nile virus IgM)
   Borrelia burgdorferi antibody index
   C. immitis complement fixation antibody
   VDRL, FTA-ABS

virus-2, VDRL). Meningitis due to *M. tuberculosis* is a consideration in the patient with a fulminant presentation and in the patient with a subacute course of illness.

A Gram's stain on CSF can be completed within minutes. When positive, the physician is paged with the results. Table 11.3 lists the appearance of the organism on Gram's stain. Never send tube #1 for Gram's stain as the CSF in tube #1 is at risk for being contaminated by *Staphylococcus epidermidis* that is normally found on the skin. This will result in a false-positive result of gram-positive cocci in CSF.

There may initially be a predominance of polymorphonuclear leukocytes in enteroviral meningitis early in the disease course with a transition to a lymphocytic pleocytosis within 24 h. Enteroviruses can either be isolated in CSF culture or detected in CSF by the reverse transcriptase polymerase chain reaction (RT-PCR) technique or both. Serology should be sent to detect a fourfold increase in IgG between acute and convalescent sera obtained 4 weeks later. Herpes simplex virus type 2 DNA can be detected in CSF by PCR. CSF culture is positive for HSV-2 in the majority of cases of meningitis associated with primary genital herpes, but is rarely positive in cases of

meningitis associated with recurrent episodes of genital herpes. Similarly, PCR for HSV-2 is rarely positive in cases of recurrent episodes of HSV-2 meningitis. HIV-1 RNA levels can be measured in CSF, and the virus can be cultured from CSF.

In meningitis due to an arthropod-borne virus, there may be a polymorphonuclear leukocytosis early in infection with a shift to a lymphocytic or mononuclear pleocytosis during the first week of illness. Patients with West Nile virus meningitis may have a persistent CSF neutrophilic pleocytosis. There is a CSF PCR test available for West Nile virus, but the sensitivity and specificity have not been defined. The best diagnostic test for West Nile virus meningitis is the detection of West Nile virus IgM in CSF, but this may not be positive until 7 days after the onset of symptoms. The identification of an arthropod-borne virus as the causative agent of meningitis is often dependent on serology. According to the Centers for Disease Control and Prevention, a confirmed case of arboviral meningitis is defined as a febrile illness with mild neurological symptoms during a period when arboviral transmission is likely to occur plus at least one of the following criteria: (1) fourfold or greater increase in serum antibody titer between acute and convalescent sera; (2) viral isolation from tissue, blood, or CSF; or (3) specific immunoglobulin M (IgM) antibody to an arbovirus in the CSF.

It is important to emphasize that IgM immunoglobulins do not cross the blood-brain barrier. The presence of pathogen-specific IgM in CSF is evidence of intrathecal antibody production unless the lumbar puncture introduced blood into the CSF. IgG immunoglobulins do cross the blood-brain barrier from serum, and thus the interpretation of pathogen-specific IgG in CSF requires the use of the antibody index. The CSF antibody index is the ratio of:

Table 11.3 Appearance of the organism on Gram's stain

Organism	Gram's stain
Neisseria meningitidis	Biscuit- or kidney-shaped gram-negative diplococci
Streptococcus pneumoniae	Gram-positive lancet-shaped diplococci which tend to associate in pairs rather than in short chains
Escherichia coli	Gram-negative bacilli
Pseudomonas aeruginosa	Gram-negative bacilli
Listeria monocytogenes	Gram-positive rod[a]
Staphylococcus aureus	Gram-positive cocci
Staphylococcus epidermidis	Gram-positive cocci

[a]*Listeria monocytogenes* may appear coccoid on Gram's stains of clinical specimens, particularly CSF, and are often mistaken for pneumococci. *Listeria monocytogenes* resembles diphtheroids and may thus be dismissed as a contaminant

$$ \text{pathogen - specific IgG in CSF / pathogen - specific IgG in serum} \, (\text{numerator}) $$

$$ \text{total IgG in CSF / total IgG in serum} \, (\text{denominator}) $$

The antibody index is generally considered positive when the ratio is greater than 1.0.

The diagnosis of Lyme disease meningitis typically begins with a serum ELISA (enzyme-linked immunosorbent assay) to measure antibody to *B. burgdorferi*. A positive result is confirmed with a Western blot. Examination of the CSF demonstrates a lymphocytic pleocytosis with a normal glucose concentration and a mild to moderately elevated protein concentration. Intrathecal anti-*Borrelia burgdorferi* antibodies can be detected. The demonstration of anti-*Borrelia burgdorferi* antibodies in CSF should not be regarded as definitive evidence of neurologic Lyme disease based on the assumption that the presence of antibodies in CSF is evidence of intrathecal antibody production. The determination of the intrathecal production of antibodies to an organism requires more than the detection of antibodies in CSF, as IgG antibodies can be passively transferred from serum to CSF, and Lyme antibodies may persist in the CSF for years. An antibody index is recommended to detect the intrathecal production of antibodies. The antibody index is the ratio of (anti-Borrelia IgG in CSF/anti-Borrelia IgG in serum) to (total IgG in CSF/total IgG in serum) [10]. The antibody index is, in general, considered positive when the result is >1.3–1.5.

The CSF abnormalities characteristic of asymptomatic and symptomatic syphilitic meningitis are a mononuclear pleocytosis, a slightly elevated protein concentration, and a positive VDRL. A positive CSF FTA-ABS is not diagnostic of neurosyphilis, but a negative FTA-ABS is evidence against the diagnosis.

In tuberculous meningitis, the CSF glucose concentration is typically only mildly decreased (35–40 mg/dL).

Therapy of Bacterial Meningitis

Once the meningeal pathogen has been identified, antibiotic therapy is modified. Table 11.4 lists the recommended antibiotics based on bacterial pathogen, and therapy should be further modified when the results of antimicrobial sensitivity testing are available. Table 11.5 is a list of the recommended dose.

The Infectious Diseases Society of America (IDSA) practice guidelines for the management of bacterial meningitis [11] and the European Federation of Neurological Societies (EFNS) guideline on the management of community-acquired bacterial meningitis [12] recommend the use of dexamethasone (0.15 mg/kg every 6 h for 2–4 days) in adults with suspected or proven pneumococcal meningitis. The first dose should be administered

Table 11.4 Recommendations for specific antibiotic therapy in bacterial meningitis

Microorganism	Antibiotic
Streptococcus pneumoniae	
Penicillin-susceptible MIC <0.1 mg/L	Penicillin G or ceftriaxone or cefotaxime
Penicillin-tolerant (MIC 0.1–1.0 mg/L)	Ceftriaxone or cefotaxime
Penicillin-resistant (MIC >1 mg/L) or cefotaxime or ceftriaxone MIC ≥1 mg/L	Ceftriaxone or cefotaxime or meropenem plus vancomycin
Neisseria meningitidis	Penicillin G or ampicillin Ceftriaxone or cefotaxime for penicillin-resistant strains
Listeria monocytogenes	Ampicillin Ampicillin plus gentamicin (see text)
Streptococcus agalactiae (group B streptococci)	Ampicillin or penicillin G or cefotaxime
Escherichia coli and other Enterobacteriaceae	Ceftriaxone or cefotaxime or meropenem
Pseudomonas aeruginosa	Meropenem or ceftazidime
Staphylococcus aureus	
Methicillin susceptible	Nafcillin or oxacillin
Methicillin resistant	Vancomycin
Staphylococcus epidermidis	Vancomycin or linezolid
Haemophilus influenzae	Ceftriaxone or cefotaxime
Gram-positive anaerobic bacteria—*Actinomyces*, *Propionibacterium* species Gram-negative anaerobic bacteria—*Fusobacterium*, *Bacteroides* species	Metronidazole

Table 11.5 Recommended dose of antibiotic therapy

Antibiotic agent	Total daily dosage (dosing interval in hours)
Ampicillin	Neonate: 150 mg/kg/day (q8 h) Infants and children: 300 mg/kg/day (q6 h) Adult: 12 g/day (q4–6 h)
Cefepime	Infants and children: 150 mg/kg/day (q8 h) Adult: 6 g/day (q8 h)
Cefotaxime	Neonate: 100–150 mg/kg/day (q8–12 h) Infants and children: 225–300 mg/kg/day (q6–8 h) Adult: 8–12 g/day (q4–6 h)
Ceftriaxone	Infants and children: 80–100 mg/kg/day (q12 h) Adult: 4 g/day (q12 h)
Gentamicin	Neonate: 5 mg/kg/day (q12 h) Infants and children: 7.5 mg/kg/day (q8 h) Adult: 7.5 mg/kg/day (q8 h)
Meropenem	Infants and children: 120 mg/kg/day (q8 h) Adult: 6 g/day (q8 h)
Metronidazole	Infants and children: 30 mg/kg/day (q6 h) Adult dose: 1500–2000 mg/day (q6 h)
Nafcillin	Neonates: 75 mg/kg/day (q8–12 h) Infants and children: 200 mg/kg/day (q6 h) Adult: 12 g/day (q4 h)
Penicillin G	Neonates: 0.15–0.2 mU/kg/day (q8–12 h) Infants and children: 0.3 mU/kg/day (q4–6 h) Adult: 24 million units/day (q4–6 h)
Rifampin	Infants and children: 10–20 mg/kg/day (q12–24 h) Adults: 600–1200 mg/day (q12 h)
Vancomycin[a]	Neonates: 20–30 mg/kg/day (q8–12 h) Infants and children: 60 mg/kg/day (q6 h) Adults: 45–60 mg/kg/day (q6–12 h)
Chemoprophylaxis *Neisseria meningitidis*	Rifampin 600 mg twice daily for 2 days or ceftriaxone 250 mg intramuscular

[a]Intraventricular vancomycin administration: children, 10 mg/day; adults, 20 mg/day

10–20 min before, or at least concomitant with, the first dose of antimicrobial agent. The EFNS Task Force recommends, in addition to the above, that dexamethasone be administered to children with suspected pneumococcal or *H. influenzae* type b meningitis. The IDSA practice guidelines recommend adjunctive therapy with dexamethasone in infants and children with *H. influenzae* type b meningitis, but recognize that there is controversy concerning the use of adjunctive dexamethasone therapy in infants and children with pneumococcal meningitis. The recommendation is that the potential benefits be weighed against the potential risks. The IDSA practice guidelines also acknowledge that "some authorities would initiate dexamethasone in all adults with suspected bacterial meningitis because the etiology of meningitis is not always ascertained at initial evaluation" [11].

Therapy of Viral Meningitis

Viral meningitis is treated with nonsteroidal anti-inflammatory agents and amitriptyline. The initial lumbar puncture is often therapeutic in relieving the headache for several hours, but the headache returns and, in the case of enteroviral meningitis, may be quite troublesome for weeks to come.

Therapy of Lyme Disease Meningitis

Lyme disease meningitis in adults and children ≥8 years of age is treated with doxycycline 200–400 mg/day in two divided doses for 10–14 days.

Therapy of Syphilitic Meningitis

Syphilitic meningitis is treated with intravenous aqueous crystalline penicillin G 3–4 mU every 4 h for 10–14 days.

Encephalitis

Encephalitis should be suspected in every patient with fever and headache and one or more of the following: an altered level of consciousness, behavioral abnormalities or confusion, new-onset seizure activity, and focal neurological deficits. Fever is expected, but fever is never a constant clinical feature.

Encephalitis may be due to reactivation of a latent herpesvirus infection that was acquired in childhood (herpes simplex virus-1 and varicella zoster virus), primary infection with a herpesvirus, an arthropod-borne virus, a tick-borne bacterial infection, or rabies.

Epidemiologic clues that are helpful in establishing the etiologic agent of the encephalitis include the season of the year, occupational exposures and recreational activities, travel history, the immune status of the patient, recent or chronic illness and its treatment (i.e., the risk of PML with hematologic malignancies and with immunomodulating agents), vaccination history, and prevalence of disease in the local community [13].

Herpes Simplex Virus-1

Herpes simplex virus-1 encephalitis presents with a subacute progression of fever, hemicranial headache, behavioral abnormalities, focal seizure activity, and focal neurologic deficits, most often dysphasia or hemiparesis. In addition to fever and headache, confusion and word finding difficulties are the most common signs.

Mosquito-Borne Viruses

Mosquito-borne viral infections may cause a mild febrile illness with headache, an aseptic meningitis, or an encephalitis. The onset of symptoms of encephalitis may be preceded by an influenza-like prodrome of fever, malaise, myalgias, and nausea and vomiting. These symptoms may be followed by confusion and seizures. Patients with West Nile virus encephalitis may have tremor or a maculopapular or roseolar rash. Patients with West Nile virus encephalitis or St. Louis virus encephalitis may have an acute asymmetric flaccid weakness due to anterior horn cell disease (a poliomyelitis-like syndrome, acute flaccid paralysis) or parkinsonian features.

Varicella Zoster Virus

Varicella zoster virus encephalitis occurs when previously acquired latent virus reactivates. Varicella zoster virus encephalitis due to the reactivation of latent varicella zoster virus can follow the cutaneous eruption of zoster, or occur in association with a diffuse varicella-like rash or occur without a varicella rash or a recent history of shingles. Approximately 40% of patients with varicella zoster virus encephalitis have no history of zoster or a varicella rash.

The characteristic clinical presentation of varicella zoster virus encephalitis is headache, malaise, confusion, and focal neurologic symptoms and signs. Varicella zoster virus encephalitis is due to ischemic and hemorrhagic infarctions of the cortical and subcortical gray matter and white matter. Multinucleated giant cells, inclusion bodies, herpesvirus particles, varicella zoster virus DNA, and antigen can be found in affected cerebral arteries. Vasculopathy may be recurrent and present with TIAs months after acute zoster [14]. Zoster reactivation may also cause demyelinating lesions or a ventriculitis and periventriculitis with hydrocephalus, altered mental status, and trouble with gait.

Tick-Borne Bacterial Infections

The most common tick-borne infection to cause encephalitis is *Rickettsia rickettsii* (Rocky Mountain spotted fever). Rocky Mountain spotted fever presents with fever, headache, altered mental status (stupor, confusion, delirium, and coma), seizures, and focal neurologic deficits. A petechial rash is characteristic of Rocky Mountain spotted fever. The rash of Rocky Mountain spotted fever consists initially of 1–5-mm pink macules that are often noted first on the wrists and ankles then spread centrally to the chest, face, and abdomen. The rash of Rocky Mountain spotted fever usually does not involve the mucous membranes. Petechial lesions in the axilla and around the ankles accompanied by lesions on the palms and soles of the feet are characteristic of Rocky Mountain spotted fever. The macules will initially blanch with pressure, but after a few days, they become fixed and turn dark red or purple. Diagnosis can be made by biopsy of the lesions.

Ehrlichia typically cause a mild illness, but two human ehrlichioses may cause fever, headache, and an altered mental status. The headache is often intense [15]. Ehrlichia are bacteria that infect mononuclear cells and polymorphonuclear leukocytes. Human monocytic ehrlichiosis is caused by *Ehrlichia chaffeensis*, and human granulocytic anaplasmosis is caused by *Anaplasma phagocytophilum*.

Epstein–Barr Virus

Encephalitis can complicate acute Epstein–Barr virus infection, occur as a parainfectious immune-mediated demyelinating disorder, or present as an encephalomyeloradiculitis.

Rabies

Rabies due to the bite of a bat presents with focal neurological deficits (hemiparesis or hemisensory deficits), choreiform movements, myoclonus, seizures, and hallucinations. Phobic spasms are not a cardinal feature of bat rabies.

Differential Diagnosis

An encephalopathy is in the differential diagnosis of every patient with an altered level of consciousness or acute confusional state. An encephalopathy may be infectious, autoimmune, metabolic, toxic, ischemic, or anoxic. Although the specific diagnostic tests for encephalitis are serology, magnetic resonance imaging, specifi-

Table 11.6 Routine tests for encephalopathy

Metabolic	Infectious	Toxic
Electrolytes	CBC with differential	Serum and urine tox screens
Glucose	Blood cultures	
Creatinine	Chest X-ray	
Liver function tests	Urinalysis	
Ammonia	Urine culture	

Table 11.7 Serological tests for encephalitis

IgM and IgG antibodies for
St. Louis encephalitis virus
West Nile encephalitis virus[a]
Eastern equine encephalitis virus
Western equine encephalitis virus
Japanese encephalitis virus
Dengue virus
Epstein–Barr virus (VCA IgM and IgG and EBNA)
Varicella zoster virus
Herpes simplex virus-1
Rabies virus
HIV
Tick-borne bacterial infection
IgG and IgM by indirect immunofluorescence for Rocky Mountain spotted fever[b]
Ehrlichia chaffeensis, *Anaplasma phagocytophilum*

[a]West Nile virus IgM and IgG antibody titers that are positive by ELISA should be confirmed by the more specific plaque-reduction neutralization assay and cell culture
[b]In addition to the indirect fluorescent antibody test for rickettsial infections, there are enzyme-linked immunosorbent assays and flow immunoassays available, as well as PCR

cally fluid attenuated inversion recovery (FLAIR) and diffusion-weighted imaging (DWI), and spinal fluid analysis, routine tests for encephalopathy should be sent as outlined in Table 11.6.

Initial Management
Initial management should be Gram's stain of blood, blood cultures, and complete blood count (CBC) with differential. This is followed by empiric therapy for bacterial and viral encephalitis and a tick-borne infection and includes dexamethasone, a third- or fourth-generation cephalosporin, vancomycin, ampicillin (for patients meeting the criteria described above), acyclovir, and doxycycline.

Diagnosis

Serology

Table 11.7 is a list of serological tests for encephalitis. The determination of which tests to send should be individualized for each patient based on the season of the year, the area where the patient lives or has traveled to, the patient's occupation and recreational activities, and the patient's risk factors. It is important to obtain acute serology (IgM and IgG) in the Emergency Room for a broad range of pathogens, so that 4 weeks later, convalescent serology can be obtained to detect a fourfold or greater increase in virus-specific IgG antibodies.

During mosquito season, serological testing should be done to detect IgM and IgG antibodies to St. Louis encephalitis virus, West Nile encephalitis virus, and any other mosquito-borne viruses that are endemic in the area in which the patient has lived or traveled to. West Nile virus IgM and IgG antibody titers that are positive by enzyme-linked immunosorbent assay should be confirmed by the more specific plaque-reduction neutralization assay and cell culture. Serology should also be sent for rabies virus IgM and IgG if there is any possibility of exposure to a bat.

During the season when ticks are biting, serological testing to detect IgG and IgM by indirect fluorescent antibodies (IFA) and PCR assays for Rocky Mountain spotted fever should be obtained. Serial samples over a number of days are recommended to detect a rise in the antibody titer. The serological tests for rickettsial infections have a low sensitivity early in the disease [16]. Not all patients will have a serological response. Skin lesions should be biopsied. The diagnosis of infection with either *E. chaffeensis* or *A. phagocytophilum* is made by serology and by the examination of blood smears for morulae, which are Ehrlichia inclusion bodies, in mononuclear cells (*E. chaffeensis*) or polymorphonuclear leukocytes (*A. phagocytophilum*).

Use serology to diagnose acute Epstein–Barr virus infection. Acute Epstein–Barr virus infection is confirmed by the detection of antiviral capsid antigen (VCA) IgM antibodies and the absence of antibodies to virus-associated nuclear antigen (anti-EBNA IgG). Virus capsid antigen IgG antibodies develop after IgM antibodies. In subsequent serum samples (collected 36 days after the onset of illness), there should be a decrease in the VCA IgG antibody titer and an increase in anti-EBNA IgG. The detection of IgG antibodies against viral capsid antigen but no EBNA antibodies is also evidence of recent infection.

Neuroimaging

Herpes Simplex Virus-1

MR fluid attenuated inversion recovery (FLAIR), T2-weighted images, and diffusion-weighted sequences demonstrate an abnormal lesion of increased signal intensity in the temporal lobe in 90% of adult patients with herpes simplex virus encephalitis at 48 h from symptom onset (Fig. 11.1a, b).

Mosquito-Borne Virus

In encephalitis due to the flaviviruses (Japanese encephalitis virus, West Nile virus, St. Louis encephalitis virus, and Powassan virus), hyperintense lesions on T2-weighted and FLAIR images may be seen in the thalami, substantia nigra, and basal ganglia.

Varicella Zoster Virus

On neuroimaging in varicella zoster virus encephalitis, there may be evidence of ischemic and hemorrhagic infarctions of the cortical and subcortical gray matter and white matter, demyelinating lesions, or periventricular enhancement.

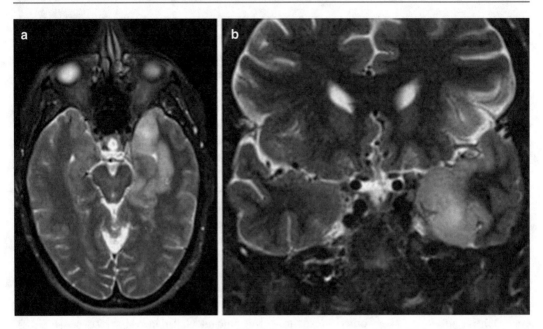

Fig. 11.1 (**a**) Axial and (**b**) coronal T2-weighted MRI demonstrating a lesion of increased signal intensity in the left anteromedial temporal lobe in HSV-1 encephalitis. (Courtesy of Darren O'Neill M.D.)

JC Virus

In progressive multifocal leukoencephalopathy, there are one or more nonenhancing subcortical white matter hyperintensities on T2 and FLAIR sequences.

Spinal Fluid Analysis

The characteristic findings on lumbar puncture in viral encephalitis are an increased opening pressure, a lymphocytic pleocytosis, a mild to moderate increase in the protein concentration, and a normal (or rarely mildly decreased) glucose concentration. Virus-specific IgM antibodies and PCR are both recommended. There are both CSF multiplex PCR assays and specific viral pathogen PCRs. The CSF multiplex PCR assays typically test for herpes simplex virus-1, herpes simplex virus-2, enteroviruses, human herpesvirus-6, cytomegalovirus, and varicella zoster virus. Approximately 10 ccs of CSF should be saved for future testing. This may be necessary if the CSF multiplex assay fails to detect the nucleic acid of the suspected virus based on clinical presentation and neuroimaging, and further testing

for a specific viral PCR would be useful, and/or CSF is needed for metagenomic next-generation sequencing to aid with diagnosis.

Herpes Simplex Virus-1

The CSF HSV-1 polymerase chain reaction (PCR) may be falsely negative in the first 72 h of symptoms of HSV encephalitis, and detection rates decrease 10 days after the onset of symptoms. Antibodies to HSV-1 can be detected in CSF beginning at about day 8 after the onset of symptoms and for approximately 3 months. A serum/CSF antibody ratio of less than 20:1 is diagnostic of recent HSV-1 encephalitis.

Mosquito-Borne Viruses

Patients with West Nile virus encephalitis may have a CSF lymphocytic or neutrophilic pleocytosis. The best test for West Nile virus encephalitis or myelitis is the CSF IgM antibody test. This may take a week or longer to be positive. Serum West Nile virus IgM and IgG are evidence of exposure to the virus but cannot be used to make a diagnosis of West Nile virus encephalitis. The CSF PCR for West Nile virus nucleic acid has a poor sensitivity but a 100% specificity.

The diagnosis of the other mosquito-borne viral infections is made by demonstrating a four-fold or greater increase in IgG between acute and convalescent sera obtained 4 weeks later.

Tick-Borne Bacterial Infections

In Rocky Mountain spotted fever, human monocytic ehrlichiosis, and human granulocytic anaplasmosis, there is a CSF lymphocytic pleocytosis, but it is often low grade.

Varicella Zoster Virus

The best test for varicella zoster virus encephalitis is the detection of varicella zoster virus IgM antibodies in CSF. The CSF VZV PCR has a 25–67% sensitivity in reported series. ·

Pitfalls

Epstein–Barr virus DNA can be found in peripheral blood latently infected mononuclear cells and may be positive in CSF in any CNS inflammatory disorder.

The detection of HHV-6 nucleic acid in CSF is not definitive evidence that HHV-6 is the etiological organism of the encephalitis. Send CSF for HHV-6 IgM.

Pearl

A rhombencephalitis (brainstem encephalitis), presenting with cranial nerve deficits and ataxia, may be due to HSV-1, enterovirus A-71, *L. monocytogenes*, flavivirus (West Nile virus, St. Louis encephalitis virus, Powassan virus, Japanese encephalitis virus), or rabies.

Table 11.8 Cerebrospinal fluid diagnostic studies for encephalitis

Cell count with differential
Glucose and protein concentration
Stain and culture
    Gram's stain and bacterial culture
    India ink and fungal culture
    Viral culture
    Acid-fast smear and *M. tuberculosis* culture
Antigens
    Cryptococcal polysaccharide antigen
    Histoplasma polysaccharide antigen
Polymerase chain reaction
    CSF multiplex PCR assays
    Specific meningeal pathogen PCRs:
        Reverse transcriptase PCR for enteroviruses
        PCR for herpes simplex virus types 1 and 2
        PCR for West Nile virus
        PCR for Epstein–Barr virus
        PCR for varicella zoster virus
        PCR for JC virus
        PCR for *M. tuberculosis*
        PCR for CMV
        PCR for HIV RNA
        RT-PCR for rabies virus
Metagenomic next-generation sequencing (mNGS)[a]
Antibodies
    Herpes simplex virus (serum/CSF antibody ratio of <20:1)
    Varicella zoster virus
    Arthropod-borne viruses
    C. immitis complement fixation antibody
    Rabies virus

[a]Metagenomic next-generation sequencing (mNGS) allows for the detection of the nucleic acid of a number of infectious agents in CSF. Given the sensitivity of this technology, there is a risk of false-positive results requiring confirmation of the results by independent pathogen-specific techniques

Table 11.8 is a list of the cerebrospinal fluid diagnostic studies for encephalitis.

Therapy

Herpes simplex virus-1 encephalitis is treated with acyclovir 10 mg/kg every 8 h for 21 days.

Varicella zoster virus encephalitis is treated with acyclovir 10–15 mg/kg every 8 h for a minimum of 14 days.

The tick-borne bacterial infections are treated with doxycycline 100 mg every 12 h for a minimum of 7 days and for at least 48 h after defervescence.

A number of agents have been investigated for the treatment of mosquito-borne viral encephalitis, many of which have been specifically investigated for West Nile virus encephalitis. These agents include ribavirin, interferon, and intravenous immunoglobulin containing high titers of anti-West Nile virus antibodies. None of these agents has been shown to be efficacious to date.

Parainfectious or Postinfectious Encephalitis

Parainfectious or postinfectious immune-mediated encephalitis occurs within days to weeks of a viral infection, such as H1N1, or a vaccination [17]. This is an acute monophasic, inflammatory disorder of the central nervous system. It is primarily a disease of white matter, but gray matter may also be affected. There is typically an abrupt onset of multifocal neurological deficits and an altered level of consciousness days to weeks after a viral illness or vaccination. On T2-weighted and FLAIR magnetic resonance imaging, there are bilateral, asymmetric areas of increased signal abnormality in the subcortical white matter, cerebellum, periventricular white matter, and brainstem. On T1 imaging, the lesions enhance in a nodular, spotty, ring, or heterogeneous pattern after the administration of gadolinium. Spinal fluid analysis demonstrates a lymphocytic or mononuclear pleocytosis, a normal glucose concentration, and an elevated protein concentration. Myelin basic protein and oligoclonal bands may be detected. Therapy is with intravenous high-dose corticosteroids. Plasma exchange is recommended for patients who do not respond to treatment with corticosteroids.

Infectious Mass Lesions

A brain abscess or a subdural empyema may present with fever, headache, focal neurological deficits, and an altered level of consciousness. The causative organism of an infectious mass lesion can be predicted from the suspected source of infection (i.e., sinusitis, otitis media, dental infections, trauma, and neurosurgical procedures), but in general, empiric antimicrobial therapy is initiated with a combination of a third- or fourth-generation cephalosporin, vancomycin, and metronidazole (see Table 11.5). Neuroimaging demonstrates the lesion. A subdural empyema requires emergent neurosurgical evacuation as the evolution of an empyema tends to be remarkably rapid once infection is established in the subdural space. As the empyema enlarges, there is a significant risk of increased intracranial pressure from the expanding mass lesion and brain herniation. Identification of the causative organism or organisms of a brain abscess is made by stereotactic aspiration, Gram's stain, and culture of the purulent contents of the lesion, and of a subdural empyema, by Gram's stain and culture of the pus at the time of surgical evacuation of the empyema. Once the organism has been identified and the results of antimicrobial sensitivity testing are known, antimicrobial therapy is modified accordingly (see Table 11.5).

Neurocysticercosis is a cause of an infectious mass lesion or lesions. The most common clinical presentation is a new-onset seizure. On occasion, the presentation may be headache. A lesion of neurocysticercosis progresses through four stages, but only a lesion in the vesicular or colloidal stage requires antiparasitic therapy. A lesion in the vesicular stage appears as a cyst with a nodule in the center. The nodule/s is the scolex of the parasite/s (Fig. 11.2). As the lesion progresses to the colloidal stage, there will be enhancement post the administration of contrast, and the lesion is surrounded by edema (Fig. 11.3). As the parasite dies and the lesion progresses to the granulo-nodular stage, post the administration of contrast, the lesion will often have a homogeneous ring-enhancing appearance with no surrounding edema. Finally the lesion calcifies and the parasite is no longer viable. Lesions in the vesicular or colloidal stage are treated with albendazole 15 mg/kg/day in two divided doses for 14 days. Prednisone or dexamethasone is begun before anticysticidal therapy to reduce the host inflammatory response. When more than two lesions are pres-

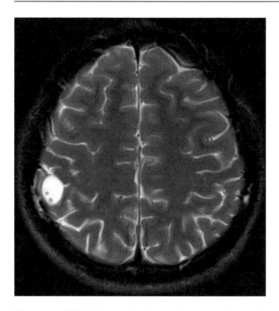

Fig. 11.2   T2 MR image of a lesion of neurocysticercosis in the vesicular stage

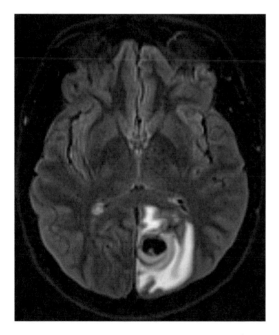

Fig. 11.3   FLAIR MR image of a lesion of neurocysticercosis in the colloidal stage

ent, praziquantel 50 mg/kg/day is added to prednisone and albendazole for a 14-day course of therapy. Antiepileptic therapy is continued indefinitely.

Spinal Epidural Abscess

A spinal epidural abscess is a purulent infection in the space outside the dura but within the spinal canal. An epidural abscess may develop from hematogenous spread of infection from a remote site of infection, by direct extension from a contiguous infection such as a skin or soft tissue infection, or by inoculation of microorganisms into the epidural space during an invasive spinal procedure. Risk factors for spinal epidural abscess include diabetes mellitus, intravenous drug abuse, trauma, an immunocompromised state, and invasive procedures (injections in the epidural space, spinal catheters, and spinal operations) [18]. An epidural abscess is more common in the posterior epidural space of the spinal canal, but those associated with osteomyelitis/discitis have been reported to be more common in the anterior epidural space [19].

The clinical presentation of a spinal epidural abscess was described by Heusner in 1948 [20]. The initial symptom is back pain at the spinal level of the epidural abscess. About 50% of patients have fever. Back pain is followed by radicular pain due to nerve root compression. This is followed by the development of a neurological deficit with paresis of appendicular musculature, loss of sensation below the level of the lesion, and loss of bowel and bladder control. Finally, there is paraplegia and loss of all sensory modalities below the level of the lesion.

The most common causative organisms of a spinal epidural abscess are *S. aureus*, coagulase-negative staphylococci, and gram-negative bacilli [21]. Spinal cord injury is due to either direct mechanical compression from the abscess or a result of ischemia from septic thrombophlebitis or a combination of these. A spinal epidural abscess may develop in the dorsal or ventral epidural space (Fig. 11.4) [21].

Magnetic resonance imaging with gadolinium is the procedure of choice to demonstrate a spinal epidural abscess. The erythrocyte sedimentation rate and C-reactive protein are almost always elevated, and there is often evidence of a peripheral leukocytosis.

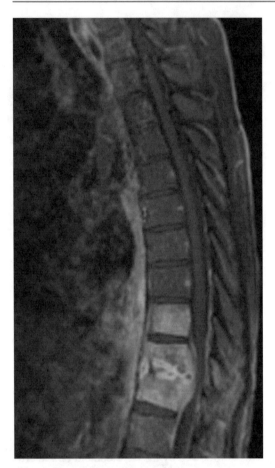

Fig. 11.4 Sagittal T1 postcontrast MRI demonstrating extensive abnormal enhancement within the bone marrow intervertebral disk space and ventral epidural space at the T10–11 level, compatible with discitis/osteomyelitis and associated ventral epidural abscess. Marked resultant mass effect and compression of the distal thoracic spinal cord. Abnormal enhancement also present within the T9 vertebral body. (Courtesy of Darren O'Neill M.D.)

Empiric antibiotic therapy is initiated with vancomycin and a third- or fourth-generation cephalosporin. Emergency laminectomy with evacuation of the purulent material allows for decompression of the spinal cord and identification of the organism. Antimicrobial therapy is modified when the organism has been identified and the results of antimicrobial sensitivity testing are known. The preoperative neurological examination is the most important predictor of outcome. In patients who have been paralyzed for greater than 24–36 h, emergency decom-pressive surgery is less likely to change their prognosis as the paralysis is more likely to be irreversible [22].

References

1. Klein JO, Feigin RD, McCracken GH. Report of the task force on diagnosis and management of meningitis. Pediatrics. 1986;78S:959–82.
2. Valmari P, Peltola H, Ruuskanen O, et al. Childhood bacterial meningitis: initial symptoms and signs related to age, and reasons for consulting a physician. Eur J Pediatr. 1987;146:515–8.
3. Gardner P. Prevention of meningococcal disease. N Engl J Med. 2006;355:1466–73.
4. Connolly KJ, Hammer SM. The acute aseptic meningitis syndrome. Infect Dis Clin N Am. 1990;4:599–622.
5. Adair CV, Gauld RL, Smadel JE. Aseptic meningitis, a disease of diverse etiology: clinical and etiologic studies on 854 cases. Ann Intern Med. 1953;39:675–704.
6. Wallgren A. Une nouvelle maladie infectieuse du systeme nerveux central: (meningite aseptique aique). Acta Pediatr. 1925;4:158–82.
7. Schut ES, de Gans J, van de Beek D. Community-acquired bacterial meningitis in adults. Pract Neurol. 2008;8:8–23.
8. Marton KL, Gean AD. The spinal tap: a new look at an old test. Ann Intern Med. 1986;104:840–8.
9. Radmard S, Reid S, Ciryam P, Boubour A, et al. Clinical utilization of the FilmArray Meningitis/Encephalitis (ME) multiplex polymerase chain reaction (PCR) Assay. Front Neurol. 2019;10:281.
10. Blanc F, Jaulhac B, Fleury M, de Seze J. Relevance of the antibody index to diagnose Lyme neuroborreliosis among seropositive patients. Neurology. 2007;69:953–8.
11. Tunkel AR, Hartman BJ, Kaplan SL, Kaufman BA, et al. Practice guidelines for the management of bacterial meningitis. Clin Infect Dis. 2004;39:1267–84.
12. Chaudhuri A, Martin PM, Kennedy PGE, Andrew Seaton R, et al. EFNS guideline on the management of community-acquired bacterial meningitis: report of an EFNS task force on acute bacterial meningitis in older children and adults. Eur J Neurol. 2008;15:649–59.
13. Tunkel AR, Glaser CA, Bloch KC, Sejvar JJ, Marra CM, Roos KL, Hartman BJ, Kaplan SL, Scheld WM, Whitley RJ. The management of encephalitis: clinical practice guidelines by the Infectious Diseases Society of America. Clin Infect Dis. 2008;47:303–27.
14. Gilden DH, Cohrs RJ, Mahalingam R. VZV vasculopathy and postherpetic neuralgia: progress and perspective on antiviral therapy. Neurology. 2005;64:21–5.
15. Sexton DJ, Dasch GA. Rickettsial and ehrlichial infections. In: Roos KL, editor. Principles of neurologic infectious diseases. New York: McGraw-Hill; 2005. p. 327–42.

16. Kirkland KB, Wilkerson WE, Sexton DJ. Therapeutic delay and mortality in cases of Rocky Mountain spotted fever. Clin Infect Dis. 1995;20:1118–21.

17. Akins PT, Belko J, Uyeki TM, Axelrod Y, et al. H1N1 encephalitis with malignant edema and review of neurologic complications from influenza. Neurocrit Care. 2010;13:396–406.

18. Reihsaus E, Waldbaur H, Seeling W. Spinal epidural abscess: a meta-analysis of 915 patients. Neurosurg Rev. 2000;232:175–204.

19. Lury K, Smith JK, Castillo M. Imaging of spinal infections. Semin Roentgenol. 2006;41(4):363–79.

20. Heusner AP. Nontuberculous spinal epidural infections. N Engl J Med. 1948;239:845.

21. Darouiche RO. Spinal epidural abscess. N Engl J Med. 2006;355:2012–20.

22. Darouiche RO. Spinal epidural abscess and subdural empyema. In: Roos KL, Tunkel AR, editors. Bacterial infections of the central nervous system, handbook of clinical neurology. Edinburgh: Elsevier; 2010. p. 91–100.

Guillain-Barré Syndrome

12

Kelsey Satkowiak and A. Gordon Smith

History and Epidemiology

Octave Landry first described ten cases of ascending paralysis in 1859 with varying degrees of sensory involvement. Pathologic studies of nerves were not done with these initial cases, but subsequently Louis Dumenil provided a description of the peripheral nerve pathology seen in similar cases of ascending paralysis [1]. It was not until 1916, when Guillain, Barré, and Strohl noted two soldiers who had acute flaccid paralysis and areflexia with spontaneous recovery, that this condition was termed "Guillain-Barré syndrome" [2]. These soldiers were also noted to have an elevated protein concentration in the cerebrospinal fluid, and this formed the classic description of Guillain-Barré syndrome: acute ascending, symmetric weakness with decreased reflexes and albuminocytologic dissociation.

Guillain-Barré syndrome (GBS) is the most common cause of acute flaccid paralysis since the development of a vaccine against poliomyelitis has eradicated that disease in industrialized nations. The actual incidence of GBS is somewhat unclear as data is lacking from developing regions of the world, but is approximately 1.1 per 100,000 people per year based on a systemic review including European and North American data [3]. It is more common with increasing age. The average incidence is estimated to be 0.6 per 100,000 people per year in children and up to 2.6 per 100,000 per year in those over 80 years old, with a male to female predominance of 1.5:1 [3, 4]. Seasonal variation in incidence is reported in some countries, with winter months being a more likely time to develop GBS than summer [5]. This is felt to be related to increased frequency of viral prodromes based on season.

Geographic Variability

There are regional differences in the clinical presentation of Guillain-Barré syndrome. In North America and European countries, the most common presentation is that of an acute inflammatory demyelinating polyradiculoneuropathy (AIDP) [4]. AIDP accounts for 90% or more of US cases, with axonal and cranial nerve variants accounting for most of the remainder. This is different from China, Japan, and Central/South America where axonal variants account for 30–50% of cases [4]. This variability may be secondary to differences in immunogenic exposure, endemic infection, or genetic predispositions. One example of geographic variability led to the recognition of the acute motor axonal variant (AMAN). An increased incidence of Guillain-Barré syndrome was observed in children and young adults in the summer months in Northern China in the early

K. Satkowiak · A. G. Smith (✉)
Department of Neurology, Division of
Neuromuscular Medicine, Virginia Commonwealth
University, Richmond, VA, USA
e-mail: Kelsey.Satkowiak@vcuhealth.org;
gordon.smith@vcuhealth.org

1990s. The majority of patients had a primary axonal process and serologic evidence of a recent *Campylobacter jejuni* infection [6, 7]. The recognition of AMAN provided evidence supporting the concept of molecular mimicry which will be discussed later and associated a specific infection with development of GBS.

Infections

An antecedent infection is commonly associated with Guillain-Barré syndrome. Patients often report having a viral prodrome in the 4 weeks leading up to onset of their neurologic symptoms. Respiratory complaints of cough and fever are the most common (38–50%) followed by gastrointestinal symptoms (17–27%) [8, 9]. *Campylobacter jejuni* has consistently been the most commonly identified antecedent infectious agent, followed by cytomegalovirus [10]. Other infections reported vary by geographic location as one would expect and include Influenza A and B, Epstein-Barr virus, herpes simplex virus, Hepatitis A and E, dengue virus, rubella virus, *Mycoplasma pneumoniae*, and *Haemophilus influenzae* [10, 11]. Zika virus is a mosquito-borne RNA flavivirus that has more recently been associated with Guillain-Barré syndrome. In late 2013 until 2014, French Polynesia experienced a large outbreak of Zika virus infections, and a case-control study demonstrated increased incidence of GBS. Out of the 41 patients diagnosed with GBS during the study period, 98% had anti-Zika virus IgM or IgG [12]. Similarly, South America experienced an outbreak of Zika virus in 2015 and 2016 and reported an increased incidence of GBS during that time frame [13]. Electrophysiologically, these patients most often had the acute motor axonal neuropathy variant (AMAN) of GBS [12, 13].

In late 2019, SARs-CoV-2 was identified as causing the clinical syndrome of COVID-19. By March 2020 the World Health Organization declared the illness a pandemic, and clinicians have since reported a number of neurologic complications associated with infection by the virus,

including Guillain-Barré syndrome. In one case series, a father and daughter presented similarly with acute sensory changes and ascending weakness in the setting of respiratory illness that had spread throughout their family and were later diagnosed with COVID-19 by PCR [14]. A number of other case reports have been published with similar presentations. COVD-19 has been associated with numerous GBS variants including AIDP, AMAN, acute motor and sensory axonal neuropathy (AMSAN), and the Miller Fisher syndrome variant (MFS) [14–18]. Patients included in these case reports often experienced prodromal anosmia and ageusia, well-known manifestations of COVID-19 infection. Some cases of GBS from COVID-19 appear to be para-infectious, with patients still experiencing acute illness from COVID-19 when weakness begins, whereas others have a clear antecedent infection that resolves by the time neurologic symptoms begin.

Vaccines

There is controversy regarding whether vaccinations have a causal relationship to Guillain-Barré syndrome. An older preparation of the rabies vaccination derived from the suckling mouse brain or mature sheep brain has been reported to induce Guillain-Barré syndrome [19–21]. One study compared sera from patients who developed GBS after receiving the rabies vaccine to that from patients with sporadic GBS. Antibodies to myelin basic protein as well as Schwann cells were found only in those patients who had received the rabies vaccine [21]. This formulation of rabies vaccine is no longer used, and there is no data to suggest newer versions, derived from chick embryo cells, increase GBS risk [22]. The best studied association is in the setting of the H1N1 influenza vaccination program in 1976. Over 40 million people were vaccinated for H1N1 during a severe outbreak of disease in a 10-week time frame. Among these individuals there was an apparent increase of GBS. An initial retrospective study calculated a rate of 8.8 cases per million in people who had been vaccinated in the preceding 6 weeks [23]. The attributable risk of vaccine-related GBS in that study was estimated to be just less than one case per 100,000 vaccines, primarily within 5 weeks of getting the vaccination [23]. This study has been reanalyzed, and it is still felt that there was an increased risk of developing GBS in the weeks following this H1N1 vaccination [24]. Fortunately, modern H1N1 vaccines have not been associated with an increased risk of GBS [25]. In fact, the risk of developing GBS after influenza infection is higher than that from any ongoing association with the vaccination [26]. A case-control study from the United Kingdom showed that the relative risk of GBS within 90 days of influenza vaccine was 0.76 (95% confidence interval 0.41–1.40) compared to a relative risk of 7.35 (95% confidence interval 4.36–12.38) in the 90 days following influenza infection [27]. Annual influenza vaccines should not be avoided over concern for developing GBS.

In terms of safety data for vaccines in general, a Cochrane review suggested immunizations should not be given in the acute phase of Guillain-Barré syndrome and possibly up to a year after that diagnosis [28]. There are sporadic reports of increased incidence of Guillain-Barré syndrome from other authors secondary to vaccines for hepatitis and tetanus [25, 29, 30]. Other studies have not found such associations [22, 28, 31]. A recent case-control study published in China, evaluating patients over a 4-year span, found no increased cases of Guillain-Barré syndrome in patients vaccinated for hepatitis A or B, influenza, varicella, rabies, diphtheria, pertussis, tetanus, or MMR [32]. At this point, the 1976 influenza vaccination has been the only vaccination with a correlation strong enough to support a causative exposure.

Whether patients with a history of GBS should have an otherwise indicated influenza vaccine should be decided on an individual basis. The package insert from influenza vaccines in the United States recommends that if GBS has occurred within 6 weeks of a prior influenza vaccine the risks and benefits of administration of the vaccine again should be carefully considered. There are data suggesting the risk of recurrent

GBS is likely low. Among 550 patients with GBS identified over an 11-year period in northern California, 958 vaccines were administered to 279 individuals (including 405 influenza vaccines given to 107 patients). During the follow-up period, six patients (1.1%) developed recurrent GBS, none following a vaccine. Of the 550 patients, 18 had GBS within 6 weeks of an influenza vaccine, 2 of whom had a future influenza vaccine without GBS recurrence [33].

Other Triggers

A number of other triggers for GBS have been recognized. Surgery has been associated with an increased risk of Guillain-Barré syndrome in a recent nationwide French study [34]. This study evaluated patients who underwent surgery and were hospitalized with GBS from 2009 to 2014. While all surgeries had some association, orthopedic procedures or those procedures involving digestive organs were more closely linked with developing neurologic symptoms [34]. This supports the earlier literature from Massachusetts General Hospital, which reported cases of post-surgical polyneuritis after surgical trauma [35]. In addition to surgery, there are case reports of GBS occurring after trauma and pregnancy, although it is not clear if incidence in these situations is greater than that of the general population [36, 37].

Pathogenesis

Guillain-Barré syndrome is an autoimmune disorder and is characterized by activation of an immune response in the absence of any direct invasion of affected tissues by a microbial entity or tumor. There is clearly a combination of environmental exposures and genetic predisposition that leads to a dysregulated immune response. Self-tolerance, which is the ability of the human adaptive immune system to avoid attacking self-antigens, breaks down by some series of events. Regulatory T cells (Tregs) are the cells that classically help maintain self-tolerance. During acute illness with GBS, these cells are decreased in serum as identified by flow cytometry [38]. In clinically stable patients who have received IVIG, these Treg levels recover [38, 39].

Molecular Mimicry

Molecular mimicry is an important disease mechanism in some GBS subtypes. It occurs due to structural similarities between epitopes on infectious organisms or exogenous agents and human proteins expressed in peripheral nerves. Because of these structural similarities, antibodies and T cells that become activated in response to exogenous materials may attack self-protein. This phenomenon is a well-established mechanism in the pathogenesis of AMAN and MFS. Many cases of GBS are associated with an identified antecedent infection, with *C. jejuni* being the most common. Animal studies show that the specific bacterial strain of *C. jejuni* associated with AMAN has sialic acid in its wall that mimics human GM1 ganglioside [40, 41]. Similarly, the bacterial strains of *C. jejuni* associated with the Miller Fisher variant of GBS can carry GQ1b, GT1a, or GD3-like epitopes [41, 42] (the specific role of anti-ganglioside antibodies is discussed below).

There is less evidence supporting molecular mimicry in AIDP, which is not generally associated with ganglioside antibodies. However, there are cases in which antibodies against galactocerebroside (anti-Gal- C) occur in patients with AIDP after infection with *M. pneumoniae* [43–46]. Galactocerebroside is expressed in human myelin. Anti-Gal-C antibodies in animal models bind to several glycolipids on *M. pneumoniae*, suggesting a similar structure is present in the bacteria and supporting molecular mimicry as a possible cause in these cases of AIDP [47]. As not all cases of Guillain-Barré syndrome are associated with antecedent infections, there are certainly other pathogenetic mechanisms that have yet to be identified. The extent to which end-organ damage related to the novel COVID-19 infection may be related to molecular mimicry has yet to be determined.

Pathology

In all clinical variants of GBS, there is pathologic evidence of mononuclear inflammatory infiltration of the peripheral nervous system including the ventral and dorsal nerve roots, dorsal root ganglia, proximal and distal nerve trunks and distal nerve terminals, sympathetic chains and ganglia, and cranial nerves [48]. In AIDP, macrophages attack the plasma membrane of Schwann cells and the myelin sheath resulting in demyelination and, when severe enough, secondary axonal injury [49]. In AMAN, pathologic studies show macrophages infiltrating the periaxonal spaces [50, 51] (Fig. 12.1). There is nodal and axonal enlargement, and immunohistochemical staining has shown C3d complement deposition at the nodes

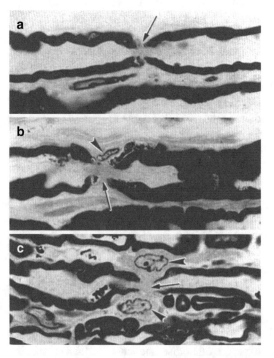

Fig. 12.1 GBS is characterized by macrophage invasion of the peripheral nerve. In a patient with AMAN, myelinated fibers from a dorsal root are normal (**a**, arrow points to a normal node of Ranvier). There is lengthening of the node of Ranvier in a longitudinal section from a ventral root (**b**) and further lengthening and infiltration by macrophages (arrowheads) in a more severely impacted fiber (Reproduced from Griffin et al. [51], with permission from Springer Nature)

of Ranvier, with a later finding of Wallerian degeneration [50]. Clinically speaking, there are reports of AMAN cases with quick onset of symptoms but also quick improvement such as the northern Chinese variant [6]. In these instances, it is likely that much of the weakness is due to functional and reversible axonal conduction failure in the nodal and perinodal regions rather than axonal loss [52, 53]. The concepts of conduction failure and conduction block will be discussed further in the electrophysiology section below. Similar to AMAN, AMSAN is characterized by macrophage infiltration of periaxonal spaces that result in severe axonal degeneration [54, 55]. Dorsal roots are also involved in AMSAN, but not AMAN.

Table 12.1 GBS variants and associated anti-ganglioside antibodies

Guillain-Barré syndrome variant	Antibody
AIDP	Gal-C
AMAN	GM1, GM1b, GD1a, Ga1Nac-GD1a
AMSAN	GM1, GM1b, GD1a
Miller Fisher	GQ1b, GT1a
Bickerstaff's encephalitis	GQ1b
Pharyngeal-cervical-brachial	GT1a
Overlap syndrome AIDP and Miller Fisher	GQ1b, GM1, GM1b, GD1a, GA1Nac-GD1a

Numerous anti-ganglioside antibodies are associated with variants of Guillain-Barré syndrome. Anatomical variation in gangliosides throughout the nervous system may be the reason for these patterns. Data adapted from Hughes and Ang [4, 46]

Anti-ganglioside Antibodies

Gangliosides are glycosphingolipids that contain at least one sialic acid linked to a carbohydrate moiety. They are found in cells and fluids throughout the body and are in a high abundance in the nervous system [56]. The nomenclature for gangliosides is based on the number of sialic acid molecules present. For example, the "M" in GM1 denotes "mono" indicating one sialic acid molecule, and in GD1 the "D" is for "duo" for two sialic acid molecules (T is for three and Q for 4). Gangliosides have diverse functions, but those localized to cell surfaces play a role in cell-cell recognition, adhesion, and signal transduction [57]. Antibodies against gangliosides have repeatedly been found in the axonal variants of GBS, but only antibodies to galactocerebroside have been found in AIDP [46] (Table 12.1). The idea that exogenous gangliosides are immunogenic has been deduced from a series of patients developing flaccid weakness after ganglioside injections as a nonspecific pain treatment. In one study, patients who developed GBS after these injections had elevated titers of antibodies against GM1 in their blood, a finding absent in patients who did not develop GBS [58]. The mechanism of injury is complicated, given that direct injection of anti-ganglioside antibodies does not directly cause neurologic disease [59]. Part of the

pathology may involve prevention of normal nerve recovery, as it was found that in animal models with peripheral nerve injury, passive transfer of anti-ganglioside antibodies severely inhibited the normal regeneration of injured axons [60].

Specific anti-ganglioside antibodies can be seen with more than one GBS variant and in other peripheral neuropathies. For example, both AMAN and multifocal motor neuropathy with partial motor conduction block are associated with anti-GM1 antibodies. The strongest association between a specific ganglioside antibody and a clinical subtype is for MFS with over 85% of patients having anti-GQ1b antibodies [61]. GQ1b is highly concentrated in the neuromuscular junction of the oculomotor, trochlear, and abducens cranial nerves which may account for the ophthalmoplegia seen in this condition [62]. The majority of AMAN patients who have significant motor symptoms have anti-GM1 antibodies. Antibodies can also occur against complexes of gangliosides rather than just one ganglioside. Antibody complexes to GQ1b/GM1 have been identified in Miller Fisher syndrome, for example, in cases where patients are seronegative to GQ1b alone [63]. It is felt that these complexes are involved in complement activation and axonal injury similar to single ganglioside antibodies, and it appears that patients with antibodies against complexes may have more severe disease, perhaps related to greater activation of the complement cascade [47].

Clinical Features

The classic and well-known presentation of GBS is that of progressive, proximal, and distal flaccid weakness and areflexia in a patient with a preceding infection. While most patients have this pattern of involvement, the spectrum of clinical symptoms and exam findings is broader, including paresthesia, pain, dysautonomia, and respiratory insufficiency (physiologic and anatomic variants will be discussed below). The most commonly used diagnostic criteria for GBS were developed in the late 1970s by the National Institute of Neurological Disorders and Stroke (NINDS) and apply primarily to the motor/paralytic forms. The clinical features required and supportive of GBS were reviewed and reaffirmed by Asbury and Cornblath in 1990 [64] (Table 12.2). By definition, the time to maximal weakness in GBS is 4 weeks or less. Approximately 50% of patients will reach their clinical nadir in 2 weeks, 80% by 3 weeks, and 90% by 4 weeks [64, 65]. This differentiates it from chronic inflammatory demyelinating polyradiculoneuropathy (CIDP), where symptoms progress over 8 weeks or more. There is controversy regarding classification of those patients who experience a nadir between 4 and 8 weeks. Some suggest this represents a distinct entity, subacute inflammatory demyelinating polyradiculopathy (SIDP) which has been identified in both the adult and pediatric population [66, 67]. Others have suggested this pattern exists on the spectrum of GBS or acute CIDP. Guillain-Barré syndrome has a variable recovery over the course of weeks to months. While weakness is the primary complaint and finding in GBS, patients typically report sensory symptoms or paresthesias that occur early in the course of their disease, prior to any weakness. Once weakness develops it is classically symmetric and is the symptom that prompts medical evaluation due to functional decline. Given that GBS affects proximal roots as well as more distal nerve segments, weakness does not always ascend from the feet upward and can manifest first in more proximal muscles. Bilateral facial weakness may be the first motor

Table 12.2 NINDS clinical criteria helpful in diagnosing Guillain-Barré syndrome

Required in diagnosis	Strongly supportive of diagnosis	Casting doubt on diagnosis	Rules out diagnosis, if present
Progressive motor weakness of more than one limb Areflexia or hyporeflexia	Symptoms that cease to progress by 4 weeks Recovery starting 2–4 weeks after progression stops Relative symmetry Mild objective sensory involvement Cranial nerve/facial involvement Autonomic dysfunction Absence of fever EMG/NCS with some evidence of slowing or conduction block during illness CSF with elevated protein and <10 mononuclear lymphocyte cells/mm^3	Marked asymmetry of weakness Significant sphincter, bowel, or bladder dysfunction at onset A sharp sensory level on exam CSF with the presence of polymorphonuclear leukocytes or with >50 mononuclear lymphocyte cells/mm^3	Recent history of hexacarbon abuse such as huffing paint or sniffing glue Abnormalities in porphyrin metabolism Recent diphtheritic infection Features of lead neuropathy/lead intoxication Purely sensory presentation A diagnosis of poliomyelitis, botulism, toxic neuropathy, or functional weakness

Contents of this table are adapted from Asbury and Cornblath who updated the original NIND criteria in 1990 [64]
EMG electromyography, *NCS* nerve conduction study, *CSF* cerebrospinal fluid

manifestation and be more symptomatic than lower extremity weakness. Bulbar weakness or respiratory insufficiency from diaphragmatic weakness can also occur and is one of the most dangerous presentations if patients are not promptly evaluated. One prospective study showed that the factors which most strongly predict respiratory insufficiency and mechanical ventilation within 1 week of onset of symptoms included low Medical Research Council (MRC) sum score at admission, fewer days between onset of weakness and admission, and facial and/or bulbar weakness at admission [68]. Considering epidemiological studies and therapeutic trial data, about 25–50% of patients who develop GBS will be weak enough to require mechanical ventilation [69, 70].

Areflexia is a core feature of GBS. The symptomatic and weak limbs are most likely to be areflexic, and as such proximal reflexes in the arms may be normal if symptoms are only present in the lower extremities. Normal reflexes in a clinically weak limb are unusual but occasionally observed. One retrospective study found that the presence of reflexes significantly delayed the time to diagnosis of GBS and thus negatively impacted patient outcomes [71].

Neuropathic pain is common and often unrecognized and undertreated. Retrospective data suggest 66–75% of GBS have neuropathic pain which can be severe or debilitating [72, 73]. Acutely, aching back and leg pain is common, possibly related to the radicular inflammation that occurs. Pain can persist outside of the acute phase, and patients can experience chronic symptoms in the extremities or back that may be related to axon loss and regeneration [30]. In this chronic phase, pain is more prominent in patients who had more severe weakness, functional disability, and fatigue during the acute phase of symptoms. Both AIDP and axonal variants can result in significant pain [74].

Dysautonomia is a common clinical feature, particularly in severe forms of GBS. Features of sympathetic or parasympathetic dysfunction can be present due to underlying small fiber injury. Patients with dysautonomia have been found to have a decreased intraepidermal nerve fiber den-

sity, and these changes may predict increased likelihood of long-term disability [73, 75]. A recent retrospective review of 187 patients with GBS found that ileus (42%), hypertension (39%), hypotension (37%), fever (29%), heart rate variability (27%), and urinary retention (24%) were the most common features of autonomic dysfunction [76]. Similar to previous data, patients who had a higher GBS disability score at admission were more likely to develop autonomic complications [76, 77].

Clinical Variants

Acute Inflammatory Demyelinating Polyradiculoneuropathy (AIDP)

In Europe and North America, AIDP is the most common form of GBS. It presents as described above with sensory symptoms or pain (back and radicular), progressive symmetric weakness, areflexia, and frequent facial weakness. The presence of dysautonomia is also not uncommon. Without electrodiagnostic testing, it is not possible to tell the difference between demyelinating and axonal forms of GBS. Generally speaking, AIDP tends to have a quicker recovery as remyelination is faster than axonal regeneration.

Acute Motor Axonal Neuropathy (AMAN) and Acute Motor and Sensory Axonal Neuropathy (AMSAN)

These variants were first described in the 1980s when several cases of GBS were noted to have nerve biopsies consistent with axonal damage and lacking inflammation [54]. Since that time, the axonal variants have been classified as AMAN if patients have only motor nerve involvement or AMSAN if they have both motor and sensory nerve involvement. Nerve conduction studies demonstrate low compound muscle action potential (CMAP) and sensory nerve action potential (SNAP) amplitudes (CMAP only in AMAN, both in AMSAN) without significantly slowed conduction velocities, conduction block, temporal dispersion, or prolonged distal or F-wave latencies. Electromyography may show early denervation, which is less likely to be seen in AIDP. Geographically, these variants are less common in Europe and North America, but more frequently occur in Asia and Central and South America. As previously mentioned, AMAN gained recognition in the 1990s when a large outbreak occurred in China in children associated with *C. jejuni* infections [7, 78]. These patients had significantly decreased CMAP amplitudes with preserved SNAPs [7]. Patients not only had a very quick onset of ascending weakness but also a rapid recovery with almost complete resolution of symptoms. It has since been suggested that these children may have had distal conduction block rather than widespread axonal degeneration, which made recovery swifter. Cases of AMSAN tend to have severe involvement of sensory and motor fibers, a more prolonged course, and significant residual symptoms [78].

Miller Fisher Syndrome and Related Disorders

Miller Fisher syndrome (MFS) is the most well-known cranial nerve GBS variant and was first described in the 1950s. The classic presentation includes ataxia, ophthalmoplegia, and areflexia, but other less common clinical features include facial nerve palsy, pupillary abnormalities, or ptosis [79, 80]. In clinical practice patients may present with double vision as their first complaint. The majority of patients with MFS have a full recovery from symptoms, and for this reason immunotherapy is controversial [80]. Electrodiagnostic testing often shows reduced SNAP amplitudes and facial motor CMAP amplitudes. CMAP amplitudes in the limbs may be reduced and minimal F-wave latencies prolonged. Compared to GBS, patients tend to have more axonal rather than demyelinating features, but both can be seen [81]. Antibodies to GQ1b are present in approximately 85% of cases [61].

Some patients who do not have the classic triad of symptoms are considered to have Miller Fisher syndrome-related disorders; this can be thought of as a spectrum of disease and includes those with central nervous system involvement, such as Bickerstaff's encephalitis. This condition was first described by Bickerstaff and Cloake in 1951 in three patients with drowsiness, ophthalmoplegia, and ataxia. They noted as more cases came to light that some of these patients also had extensor plantar responses in an otherwise flaccid paresis, suggesting central nervous system involvement [82]. In a more recent study of 62 cases of patients with clinical presentations consistent with Bickerstaff's encephalitis, 66% had positive anti-GQ1B antibodies [42]. Patients with this condition generally have a monophasic illness that improves significantly over time, similar to the majority of GBS cases. Autopsy studies have shown lymphocytic infiltrates in the CNS and axonal degeneration in the peripheral nerves [83].

Pharyngeal-Cervical-Brachial Variant

The pharyngeal-cervical-brachial GBS is much less common and can have significant early bulbar dysfunction as implied by its name [84, 85]. This variant can also be associated with neck and shoulder weakness, facial/extraocular weakness, or ataxia, showing significant overlap with Miller Fisher syndrome. Retrospective chart reviews have revealed that approximately 30% of patients have a preceding *C. jejuni* infection [42]. About one third of the time, this variant is associated with anti-ganglioside antibodies, including GT1a, GQ1b, GM1, GM1b, GD1a, or GalNAc-GD1a [42]. More recently, anti-GM3 has also been associated with this variant [86].

Guillain-Barré Syndrome in Children

Guillain-Barré syndrome is less common in the pediatric population than in adults, with an incidence of up to 0.75–0.8 per 100,000 per year in those under 18 years of age [3, 87]. Infants and young children can have clinical presentations that include hypotonia, poor feeding, irritability due to neuropathic pain, and an overall decrease in level of activity that may appear to look like altered mental status. In the acute phase of disease, and at the nadir of symptoms, 75% of children can no longer walk unaided, 30% are quadriplegic, up to 50% can have cranial nerve involvement, and 15–20% have respiratory compromise or autonomic dysfunction [88, 89]. Electrophysiologic findings are similar to those observed in adults. Children tend to recover quicker with less long-term residual deficits than adults and overall lower mortality rate of 1–2% [90–92].

Prognosis

Guillain-Barré syndrome is monophasic in the majority of patients, with only 5% of patients reporting a recurrence [93]. The recovery process is slow and typically begins 2 to 4 weeks after onset of symptoms, but can be delayed up to 6 months. Speed of recovery also depends on the degree of underlying axonal injury, as axonal regeneration is a more time-consuming process. About 80% of patients recover with only mild residual symptoms or signs such as hyporeflexia, but 5–10% can have severe residual weakness. Despite treatment updates over the years and supportive care in developed countries, the mortality ranges from 3% to 8% [69, 94]. Prognosis is generally good for those with a classic course, but can be less so for those who experience worsening of symptoms after initial treatment or who go on to have an eventual diagnosis of CIDP. Table 12.3 shows features associated with poor prognosis in GBS (Table 12.3). Notable features include older age, axonal variants, prominent dysautonomia, and pre-existing cardiac or pulmonary conditions that could complicate respiratory status [95–97]. The Modified Erasmus GBS Outcome Score (mEGOS) is a functional outcome model based on severity of MRC sum score, presence or absence of preceding diarrhea, and age [95]. This model was created to be applied at the time of admission or up to 7 days after admission and helps predict the probability of walking up to 6 months after discharge. Common causes of death in GBS include respiratory complications such as ventilator-associated pneumonia and cardiovascular complications such as myocardial infarction, arrhythmia, or pulmonary embolism, or autonomic dysfunction [8, 94]. Fatigue can persist in those who otherwise have complete motor recovery.

Table 12.3 Clinical features associated with a worse prognosis in Guillain-Barré syndrome

Increased age, >40–50
Pre-existing cardiac or pulmonary disease
Rapid progression of symptoms; short duration from symptom onset to non-ambulatory
Preceding infections, diarrheal>respiratory
Axonal variants
Autonomic instability
Ventilation requirement
CMAPs <20% of normal
High-grade deficits on the GBS disability scale

Data adapted and summarized from Vandenberg, Winer, Walgaard, Visser, Cornblath, and colleagues [8, 68, 94, 96, 97]

CMAP compound motor action potential

Localization and Differential Diagnosis

A large number of central and peripheral nervous system disorders can present with progressive weakness. It is paramount to perform a thorough neurologic physical exam in order to localize the likely neuroanatomic site of injury. Central nervous system conditions such as encephalomyelitis and rhomboencephalitis need to be considered when encountering Miller Fisher syndrome-Bickerstaff's brainstem encephalitis spectrum disorders, and transverse myelitis or structural myelopathy may need to be considered in the evaluation of paralytic variants. Infections of the anterior horn may cause a flaccid paralysis and include West Nile virus, poliomyelitis in areas that are still endemic, and nonpolio enteroviruses [98]. The distribution of weakness is an important diagnostic clue. Distal predominant weakness suggests the possibility of an acute polyneuropathy that may be toxic or acquired, whereas proximal predominant weakness may suggest a myopathy or defect in neuromuscular junction transmission. Asymmetric weakness is unusual in GBS but is typical in infectious etiologies, neuropathies secondary to vasculitis, or diabetic lumbosacral radiculoplexus neuropathy

(DLRPN or "diabetic amyotrophy"). Tone and reflexes aid in determining if weakness is from a central or peripheral cause. Once weakness has been localized to the peripheral nervous system, a sensory exam can often distinguish a muscle or neuromuscular junction problem from a peripheral nerve, plexus, or root problem.

Neuromuscular junction disease can certainly cause rapidly progressive proximal weakness. In children and infants, botulism can cause such a presentation and is associated with autonomic manifestations, such as constipation and pupillary dilation. In adults, myasthenia gravis can present with acute weakness, although should not have any sensory features, which differentiates it from GBS. If the presentation is acute but purely sensory in nature, GBS is unlikely to be the underlying etiology. Objective physical exam evidence of sensory loss in the proximal limbs and trunk would be more consistent with a sensory neuronopathy for which there are a limited number of etiologies including paraneoplastic syndromes (e.g., anti-Hu), Sjogren's syndrome, or pyridoxine toxicity [99]. Nerve conduction studies demonstrate non-length-dependent loss of SNAP amplitudes or absent responses with normal CMAPs. Rarely, GBS presents as a sensory syndrome, but in this case, the NCS would demonstrate sensory and motor involvement with demyelination. Finally, acute severe myopathies such as the immune-mediated necrotizing myopathies, acute myositis, or rhabdomyolysis may present with acute weakness. These conditions should be easily differentiated from GBS by lack of sensory findings and relatively normal nerve conduction studies.

Diagnostic Evaluation

The diagnosis of GBS is largely clinical, based on the presence of proximal and distal weakness with hypo- or areflexia with a nadir in less than 4 weeks. However, one does have to keep in mind an awareness of the broad spectrum of presentations. Ancillary testing such as blood work, cerebrospinal fluid analysis, and nerve conduction studies with needle electromyography can help confirm the diagnosis and in some cases aid in prognostication. Often early in the course of the disease, these ancillary tests are normal, and so treatment should not be withheld if clinical judgment supports the diagnosis.

If a preceding infection occurred, appropriate studies may be performed to identify infectious etiologies. For example, antecedent diarrheal illness may prompt serology and stool culture for *C. jejuni*. Other studies may include acute or convalescent serology for Epstein-Barr virus (EBV), cytomegalovirus (CMV), or *M. pneumoniae*. Testing for serum anti-ganglioside antibodies can be obtained in specific clinical situations (e.g., anti GQ1b in a patient with MFS) as discussed in the pathogenesis section. Appropriate PCR of the serum, CSF, or stool can identify any ongoing infections that may be contributing to the presentation. In patients presenting with an asymmetric polyradiculopathy pattern, HIV, CMV, Lyme disease, and diphtheria should be considered [100] (Table 12.4). Tick paralysis is a cause of acute flaccid paralysis that may mimic GBS. It can progress for days until the tick is removed [101]. A careful skin exam should be done in patients with flaccid paralysis who have had ample outdoor exposure and in all children when GBS is less likely to be causing their acute weakness. If there is concern for workplace/environmental exposures or toxic ingestions, clinicians may consider obtaining a serum drug screen or heavy metal screen (arsenic, mercury, thallium, lead). Patients with systemic signs of organ dysfunction or autoimmune disease may benefit from checking serum inflammatory markers such as a Westergren sedimentation rate, C reactive protein, anti-nuclear antibody, anti-Sjogren's syndrome A and B antibodies (SSA, SSB), anti-neutrophil cytoplasmic antibodies (ANCA), and cryoglobulins [102]. In a patient presenting with a GBS-like syndrome with associated photosensitivity and GI complaints, porphobilinogen and delta-aminolevulinic acid concentrations may be measured to evaluate for possible acute porphyria.

Table 12.4 Infections mimicking GBS and their associated diagnostic findings

Syndrome	Pattern	Lab workup	EMG/NCS	Other features
Botulism	In children Symmetric, descending, motor but no sensory, pupillary dilation	Normal CSF Positive stool culture for botulism	Low-amplitude CMAP from presynaptic defect	Possible exposure to canned food or honey
Poliomyelitis	Asymmetric, motor but no sensory, muscle tenderness, bulbar and respiratory dysfunction	CSF ↑ cell count, ↑ protein Positive stool cultures for polio	Normal SNAPs, low-amplitude CMAP	Several days after acute viral illness
West Nile	Asymmetric, motor but no sensory unless occurring as a myelitis Parkinsonian rigidity may be present	CSF ↑ cell count, ↑ protein MRI with T2 hyperintensity of anterior horn cells	Normal SNAPs, low-amplitude CMAP	Mosquito borne May have febrile illness during onset
HIV sero-conversion	Asymmetric, motor and sensory, often with encephalitis	CSF ↑ cell count, ↑ protein Increased HIV viral load	Axonal or demyelinating damage to sensory and motor NCS	
Lyme disease	Motor>sensory symptoms, cranial neuropathies, meningitis, asymmetric weakness	CSF ↑ cell count, ↑ protein, positive CSF or serum Lyme IgG	Axonal damage on NCS	Months after tick bite/ infection
Diphtheria	Bulbar symptoms, prolonged and often biphasic course, autonomic features	CSF may have ↑ cell count and protein	Demyelinating damage with prolonged latency and reduced CV on NCS	Follows a severe pharyngeal infection Multiorgan failure
Tick paralysis	Ascending weakness, sensory and motor, autonomic	CSF normal	Demyelinating with conduction block, reduced amplitudes Normal RNS	

Above are the common clinical presentations, serum/CSF studies, and electrodiagnostic findings associated with infections that mimic GBS. Data is adapted from Soloman, Grattan-Smith, Logina, and colleagues [98, 100, 101]
CSF cerebrospinal fluid, *CMAP* compound muscle action potential, *SNAP* sensory nerve action potential, *NCS* nerve conduction study, *RNS* repetitive nerve stimulation, *NMJ* neuromuscular junction, *CV* conduction velocity

Cerebrospinal Fluid

The classic finding on analysis of CSF in patients with GBS is an elevated CSF protein concentration or CSF-to-serum albumin ratio in the absence of a pleocytosis (so-called albuminocytologic dissociation). This increase in the protein concentration is a manifestation of the disruption of the blood-brain barrier, and early in the course of the disease, it may not be elevated. A large cohort study of approximately 450 GBS patients showed that an increased CSF concentration was significantly affected by timing of the lumbar puncture. Overall, 64% of patients had abnormally elevated protein concentrations [103]. Only 49% of patients had an elevation on day 1 of admission,

53% had an elevation by day 3, and up to 88% by the end of 3 weeks [103]. Results also showed that 85% of patients had a normal cell count (<5 cells/mm³), while 15% had a mild pleocytosis (always <50 cells/mm³) [103]. Obtaining CSF in GBS patients may have the most utility in excluding other infections or inflammatory etiologies, and an elevation of the CSF cell count >50 cells/mm³ would support an alternative diagnosis. HIV-associated GBS is often associated with a pleocytosis; thus, GBS patients with elevated CSF white blood cell counts should be evaluated for HIV. Patients with viral polyradiculopathies due to Lyme disease (Bannwarth's lymphocytic meningoradiculitis), neurolymphomatosis, or leptomeningeal malignancy may all have a significant pleocytosis. While some patients with autopsy confirmed GBS had a polymorphonuclear pleocytosis, this is exceedingly rare and should prompt the clinician to consider other etiologies [104].

Electrophysiology

Electrophysiology can help determine if patients have axonal or demyelinating forms of GBS and aid in determining prognosis. Similar to cerebrospinal fluid studies, nerve conduction studies may be normal if performed early in the disease course, and repeating the study in 1–2 weeks from onset of symptoms may be useful in defining the primary pathophysiology. Early NCS findings in AIDP are prolonged F-wave latencies or absent F-waves with intact distal responses suggesting more proximal injury near the nerve root and a "sural sparing" pattern of reduced SNAP amplitudes [105]. This pattern is also termed "normal sural abnormal median" because distal upper extremity SNAP amplitudes are reduced or the responses absent while the sural sensory responses in the leg are relatively preserved. This pattern is seen in both AIDP and chronic inflammatory demyelinating polyradiculoneuropathy (CIDP) but not in other forms of peripheral neuropathy (e.g., diabetic neuropathy) [106, 107]. Other features indicating a primary demyelinating pathophysiology include prolonged distal motor latencies, slowed motor conduction velocities and partial motor conduction block, and/or abnormal temporal dispersion [108].

The axonal injury seen in AMAN manifests as low CMAP amplitudes. In AMSAN both CMAP and SNAP amplitudes are reduced, or the responses are absent. Most patients with AIDP develop some degree of secondary axonal injury, and when severe this may prevent recognition of the primary underlying pathophysiology. Once axonal damage is present, needle electromyography demonstrates fibrillation potentials and positive sharp waves (although these findings are not seen until 2–3 weeks following axon injury). In MFS nerve conduction studies may be normal or SNAP amplitudes may be reduced [109]. Miller Fisher syndrome can be associated with demyelinating or axonal findings on NCS, although axonal injury tends to be more common overall [81, 109, 110].

The electrodiagnostic criteria for GBS vary depending on the clinical subtype and are largely used as a tool for research. For chronic inflammatory demyelinating polyradiculoneuropathy (CIDP), the European Federation of Neurological Societies and Peripheral Nerve Society developed a task force to review and publish evidence-based guidelines to aid in electrodiagnosis in 2005 [111]. As is the case with CIDP, there are many sets of electrodiagnostic criteria for GBS. One main difference between older and newer criteria is the concept of reversible conduction failure (RCF) that can change the appearance of nerve conduction studies over time. Reversible conduction failure occurs in AMAN and AMSAN patients when abnormal CMAP amplitude reduction and conduction block or slowing quickly recover on repeat studies [52, 112]. Reversible conduction failure is thought to be related to functional conduction failure related to the activity of antibodies or other mediators in the nodal and perinodal regions (e.g., anti-GM1 antibodies in some patients with AMAN). In the recent set of criteria proposed by Uncini and colleagues, RCF is felt to occur when two or more nerves display >150% increase in distal CMAP amplitude without an increase in CMAP duration on repeat testing [113]. In addition, isolated F-wave absence that recovers without increased minimal latency and proximal to distal CMAP amplitude ratios of <0.7 which improve more than 0.2 on repeat NCS without temporal dispersion would be consistent with RCF [113]. Table 12.5 summarizes two sets of formal electrodiagnostic criteria, an older set by Hadden and colleagues and the newer set from Uncini and colleagues which takes into consideration repeating diagnostic studies [113, 114] (Table 12.5).

Table 12.5 Examples of electrodiagnostic criteria for Guillain-Barré syndrome

	Hadden and colleagues	Uncini and colleagues
AIDP	*At least one finding present in two different nerves, or two findings present in one nerve if the others are inexcitable; dCMAP must be >10% LLN:* F-wave latency >120% ULN pCMAP/dCMAP ratio < 0.5 and dCMAP ≥20% LLN DML >110% ULN (120% if dCMAP <100% LLN) Motor CV <90% LLN (85% if dCMAP <50% LLN)	*Initial or repeat study must have the following in ≥2 nerves*: F-response latency >120% ULN pCMAP/dCMAP duration ratio > 130% dCMAP duration >120% ULN DML >130% ULN Motor CV <70% LLN *OR one of the above in one nerve plus*: Abnormal ulnar SNAP amplitude with normal sural SNAP amplitude Absent F-waves in two nerves with dCMAP >20% LLN
AMAN	No features of demyelination in any nerve with dCMAP ≥10% LLN, and only one demyelinating feature present if dCMAP <10% LLN dMAP <80% LLN in at least two nerves	*Initial or repeat study should have no features of AIDP in any nerve and the initial study should have at least one of the following in ≥2 nerves*: Isolated F-wave absence (or <20% persistence) pCMAP/dCMAP amplitude ratio <0.7 dCMAP<80% LLN *At repeat study at least one of the following is present in two nerves*: Persistent or further reduction in dCMAP amplitude pCMAP/dCMAP amplitude ratio <0.7 at initial test that recovers due to decrease of dCMAP without increased temporal dispersion (dCMAP duration ≤120% ULN and pCMAP/dCMAP duration ratio ≤130%)

Table 12.5 (continued)

	Hadden and colleagues	Uncini and colleagues
AMSAN		*Same criteria as AMAN plus at initial study*: SNAP amplitudes <50% LLN in at least 2 nerves *At repeat study*: Evidence for axonal degeneration and reversible conduction failure in motor nerves Evidence of axonal degeneration and RCF in sensory nerves

Uncini's criteria consider both an initial and repeat electrodiagnostic study, and for this reason, the criteria also include evidence of reversible conduction failure as a parameter to identify. In both sets of criteria, inexcitable nerves are those with absent dCMAP, or dCMAP present in only one nerve with amplitude <10% of normal. Data adapted from Uncini and Hadden [113, 114]

dCMAP compound muscle action potential amplitude after distal stimulation, *pCMAP* compound muscle action potential after proximal stimulation, *LLN* lower limit of normal, *ULN* upper limit of normal, *SNAP* sensory nerve action potential, *CV* conduction velocity, *RCF* reversible conduction failure

Imaging

MRI of the lumbar spine may demonstrate post-contrast enhancement of the nerve roots (Fig. 12.2) [115]. While this supports an inflammatory process and breakdown of the blood-brain barrier, it is nonspecific and can be seen in other infectious, inflammatory, or autoimmune conditions. Peripheral nerve ultrasound is a newer imaging approach being studied in different acquired polyneuropathies and may be useful in AIDP diagnosis. Ultrasound-identified nerve enlargement can be present early in the course of GBS and may aid in diagnosis when nerve conduction studies still appear normal in the acute setting [116–118].

Fig. 12.2 Magnetic resonance imaging with and without gadolinium contrast may demonstrate nerve root enhancement in AIDP. In this 5-year-old patient with AIDP, a T1-weighted image without contrast appears normal (**a**). Sagittal (**b**) and axial (**c**) T1-weighted images following contrast administration demonstrate nerve root enhancement (arrows). (Reproduced from Iwata F, et al. MR imaging in Guillain-Barre syndrome. Pediatr Radiol. 1969 with permission from Springer Nature)

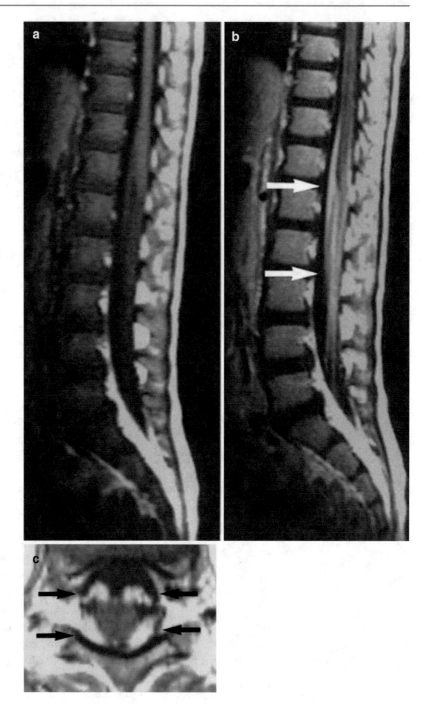

Treatment

The treatment approach in patients with Guillain-Barré syndrome is twofold: One priority is to quickly provide immunologic therapy to address the underlying disease process, improve neuro-

logic outcome, and hasten recovery. The other aspect of treatment relates to supportive care for the cardiac, respiratory, autonomic, and infectious complications that can occur. In the randomized controlled trials that have been done to establish evidence-based immunologic therapies

Table 12.6 The Guillain-Barré syndrome disability scale

Score	Disability
0	Healthy
1	Minor symptoms or signs of neuropathy but capable of manual work and running
2	Able to walk 10 meters or more without support of a cane but incapable of working or running
3	Able to walk 10 meters with a stick (cane), appliance, or support
4	Confined to bed or chair bound
5	Requiring assisted ventilation for at least part of a day
6	Death

This scale is used as a marker of response in many treatment trials for GBS. It is adapted from Hughes [4]

for Guillain-Barré syndrome, most patients received immunomodulating treatment within 2 weeks of moderate to severe symptom development (defined as loss of ambulation). The GBS disability scale was used for enrollment and as a primary outcome measure in these trials (Table 12.6). The French Cooperative study looked at patients only mildly affected (those who remained ambulatory), but who received treatments, and found that there was faster motor recovery with immunologic therapy [119]. However, if only mild symptoms are present in a patient, treatment may not be necessary, and clinicians should weigh the pros and cons. Below are the specific therapies that have been studied. Of note, there have not been randomized controlled trials assessing the most beneficial timing of treatment in Miller Fisher syndrome. In general, for all variants, early treatment is preferred.

Plasma Exchange

Plasma exchange (PLEX) was first proposed as a potential GBS therapy in several case reports published in the 1970s [120]. Plasma exchange is presumed to work by removing circulating serum antibodies, immune complexes, components of complement, and cytokines. Early trials primarily enrolled patients with severe enough disease that they were non-ambulatory or required assistance to walk. In most cases, patients were treated within 2 weeks of symptom onset with 200 ml/kg–250 ml/kg and 3–5 exchanges over 5–10 days [119, 121–124]. While not always statistically significant in clinical trials, plasma exchange consistently showed benefit in improving patient symptoms compared to controls. Participants receiving exchanges had improvement of the GBS severity score at 1 month compared to controls by at least 1 point [123, 125]. In addition, the percentage of patients who were able to eventually ambulate independently was consistently found to be higher in the plasma exchange groups [119, 121, 122, 125]. In one study, there was a trend toward shortened hospital stays and reduced time requiring ventilatory support with a respirator in those that received plasma exchange [121].

While most experts recommend five plasma exchange treatments, with some recommending fewer exchanges for those with milder disease, the number needed to achieve optimal efficacy for an individual patient is unclear. The French Cooperative Group study endeavored to address this clinical question. They randomized 556 GBS patients based on severity to 0 versus 2 exchanges for those with mild disease (ambulatory), 2 versus 4 for those with moderate disease (unable to stand without assistance), and 4 versus 6 for those with severe GBS (mechanically ventilated). In those with mild GBS, two exchanges improved the time to recovery from a median of 8 to 4 days. Patients with moderate GBS receiving four exchanges experienced a reduced time to walk with assistance from a median of 24 to 20 days compared to those receiving two and also had a higher rate of recovering full strength at 1 year (64% vs. 46%). However, ventilated patients did no better with six exchanges compared to four. The authors concluded that ambulatory patients with GBS can be treated with two exchanges but those with moderate or severe disease should be treated with four [125]. Most experts continue to use five exchanges for those patients with moderate to severe weakness based on the original GBS trials, although patients with mild disease can be treated with two.

There are several adverse effects associated with plasma exchange including bloodstream or skin infections and line complications. Other side effects include labile blood pressure due to fluid shifts, cardiac arrhythmias, or venous thrombus and pulmonary embolism [119, 124].

Intravenous Immunoglobulin (IVIG)

There are no placebo-controlled trials of intravenous immunoglobulin (IVIG) in adults with GBS given PLEX was widely being used by the time of the first IVIG trials. Several studies have compared IVIG to PLEX for GBS in adults and showed that either treatment approach is acceptable. In these studies, a dose of 0.4 g/kg of intravenous immunoglobulin daily for 5 days showed similar outcomes as plasma exchange in terms of improvement of strength, time to recovery, time to unaided walking, or discontinuation of mechanical ventilation [126–128]. In addition to monotherapy with IVIG or plasma exchange, combined therapy has also been studied (IVIG given after plasma exchange) and generally yields no additional benefit [128]. Data also support efficacy of IVIG in pediatric GBS patients [129, 130].

Intravenous immunoglobulin is better tolerated and causes less adverse reactions than plasma exchange and is now often selected as first choice of treatment for acute Guillain-Barré syndrome given the comparable efficacy. Many experts administer the full 2 g/kg dose over 2–3 days depending on the patient's cardiac function and fluid status. Side effects of IVIG include nausea/vomiting, aseptic meningitis, exacerbation of chronic renal failure, erythema at the infusion site, and myocardial infarction [128]. In addition, general malaise or flu-like symptoms can occur.

Nonresponders

While PLEX and IVIG are effective treatments for GBS, many patients do not have an observable clinical response to either treatment. One question that often arises is whether a second round of immunotherapy should be given for ongoing symptoms. This question was addressed in the International Second IVIG dose (ISID) study. The nonrandomized ISID study compared outcomes among patients who received a second course of IVIG versus those only treated with one course among patients participating in the International GBS Outcome Study (IGOS), a large international observational study. Outcomes were no different between the two groups [131]. A prospective randomized trial, the Second IVIG course in GBS (the SID-GBS trial), is taking place in the Netherlands to further examine whether a second course of IVIG can improve outcome in patients with severe disease [132]. In clinical practice some experts (but not others) will repeat a course of IVIG or plasma exchange 1–2 weeks after the initial treatment if patients continue to progress or have very severe weakness.

Treatment-Related Fluctuations

Treatment-related fluctuations (TRFs) are defined as a clinical deterioration that occurs after a patient has had stabilization of his or her disease or has at least had initial improvement. Treatment-related fluctuations are felt to be due to circulating factors or antibodies which remain active once the initial immune therapy has worn off. After administration of IVIG, for example, IgG concentration in the serum rises quickly but also falls quickly in the first 7 days after treatment before clearance slows down [133]. If antibodies are still present at that time, symptoms may worsen (Fig. 12.3). Treatment-related fluctuations occur in approximately 10% of GBS patients within 60 days of initial presentation [134–136]. Sometimes it can be difficult to determine if a patient has a TRF, recurrence of GBS, or the acute onset of CIDP. The number of exacerbations, time to symptom nadir, and GBS disability score can help differentiate between these entities. Acute CIDP should be suspected with deterioration occurring after 8 weeks of symptom onset or when there are three or more episodes of deterioration [137]. Table 12.7 helps identify characteristics consistent with TRF vs. recurrent GBS (Table 12.7).

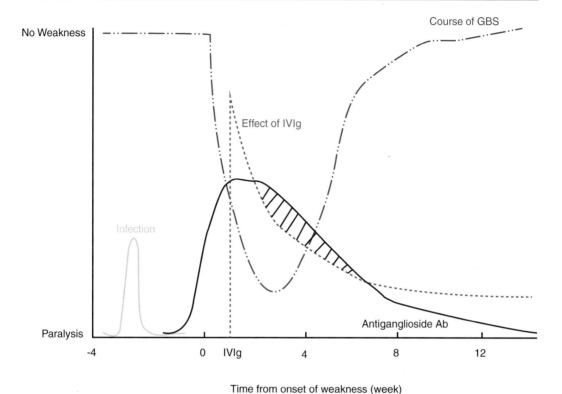

Fig. 12.3 Treatment-related fluctuations may be related to the duration of effect of GBS therapies relative to the duration of the autoimmune process. This figure displays changes of antibody titers in GBS with the superimposed effect of IVIG. If antibody titers are still elevated after treatment (shown by the shaded area), further clinical deterioration may occur. This would be considered a treatment-related fluctuation. Additional immunosuppressive therapy may help reduce remaining antibodies and improve symptoms in this case. The original data on treatment-related fluctuations was adapted from Van Doorn [30], and the data regarding IVIG pharmacokinetics was adapted from Bonilla [133]

Table 12.7 Characteristics used to differentiate recurrent GBS, treatment-related fluctuations, and acute onset CIDP

	GBS-TRF	GBS recurrence	CIDP
Average time from onset of disease to exacerbation of symptoms	<2 months	>2 months (after complete resolution of symptoms; rare)	>2 months
Time to symptom nadir (days)	8		26
Number of exacerbations within 2 years from onset	≤2		≥3
GBS disability score at nadir	≥3, more severe		Broad range, though less severe than GBS-TRF

This data is extracted from a study by Rut et al., representing analysis of the difference in timing, number of exacerbations, and severity in symptoms to help differentiate disease entities. This study looked at those diagnosed with AIDP or CIDP and recorded characteristics and course of disease in the subset who had AIDP with TRF or acute onset CIDP [137].
TRF Treatment-related fluctuations, *CIDP* chronic inflammatory demyelinating polyradiculoneuropathy

Emerging Therapies

Up to 50% of GBS patients do not respond to either PLEX or IVIG, and thus there is an urgent need for new therapies [128]. Given evidence that complement may play an important role in disease pathogenesis, there has been interest in exploring the potential role for complement inhibitors. Eculizumab is a monoclonal antibody that inhibits the activity of C5 convertase, which prevents the formation of terminal complement (C5b-9). In mouse models with respiratory failure and neuropathy induced by injection of anti-GQ1b antibodies, this drug prevented manifestations of neurologic disease compared to controls [138]. A phase 2 double-blinded placebo-controlled trial of IVIG with eculizumab versus placebo in Japan found that 61% of those in the active treatment arm were able to walk independently at 4 weeks compared to 45% in the placebo group. While this primary endpoint did not meet statistical significance, 6 months following treatment, 74% of treated patients were able to run versus 18% of those treated with placebo. Eculizumab was found to be well tolerated [139]. Eculizumab is in phase 3 trials now for Guillain-Barré syndrome as well as for CIDP. Another monoclonal antibody against complement, anti-C1q, was found in mouse models of GBS to attenuate the complement cascade, reduce immune cell recruitment and axonal injury, and improve respiratory function [140]. This drug (ANX005) has been studied in phase 1 trials in the United States as an add-on treatment to IVIG, similar to eculizumab. The reassuring safety profile has prompted phase 2 trials that are currently recruiting [141, 142].

Rituximab is a chimeric monoclonal antibody that targets CD20. It has been studied in refractory CIDP cases with antinodal antibodies and has improved functional outcomes. No clinical trials have formally assessed efficacy of rituximab in refractory GBS. One case report noted significant improvement in muscle strength in a patient with myelodysplastic syndrome and GBS treated with rituximab [143]. There are also case reports to suggest that rituximab itself could induce Guillain-Barre syndrome [144, 145]. The anti-CD52 monoclonal antibody alemtuzumab has also been reported to improve strength in a patient with chronic lymphocytic leukemia and GBS refractory to both IVIG and PLEX [146]. In this case report, the patient was also noted to have positive GQ1b antibodies, which disappeared after treatment with alemtuzumab [146].

Fc receptors are proteins found on the surface of cells that aid in immune system function, such as lymphocytes, natural killer cells, macrophages, and neutrophils. FcRn, one of the neonatal Fc receptors in humans, has been found to promote stability of IgG and prevent breakdown. Blockage of this receptor decreases both appropriate antibody and autoantibody IgG levels in animal models [147]. In GBS mouse models with pathogenic IgG autoantibodies, blocking FcRn can reduce nerve injury [148]. For this reason, a number of anti-FcRn antibodies are being studied in clinical trials of autoimmune conditions. Multiple FcRn inhibitors are being evaluated in early phase trials for CIDP, and this is a promising therapeutic strategy for GBS [149–151].

Another agent that is being studied with interest is hypersialylated IgG. During animal in vivo characterization, hypersialylated IgG displayed more consistent and stronger anti-inflammatory effects than standard intravenous immunoglobulin [152]. Hypersialylated IgG may also upregulate gene expression of IL-33, which serves to protect nerves from antibody-mediated injury in animal models [153]. A phase 1 study is underway using hypersialylated IgG in TTP, but there are no current trials in GBS.

Supportive Care and Symptomatic Treatment

Symptomatic treatment and supportive care are essential components of GBS therapy. Patients with GBS also require very attentive medical and neurological monitoring with special attention to strength, respiratory, and cardiovascular function.

Respiratory

Monitoring respiratory strength and providing early support are of the utmost importance. One quarter of GBS patients presenting with impaired ambulation eventually require ventilatory support [4]. It is paramount to recognize early signs of respiratory distress and use objective parameters to help measure respiratory function [154] (Table 12.8). Bedside spirometry should be followed closely, with special attention to forced vital capacity and maximum inspiratory/expiratory pressures. These values should be periodically repeated and the values trended in individuals with rapidly progressing weakness or significant bulbar complaints. The decision to intubate a patient should be based on the trajectory of change as well as the absolute values. The Erasmus GBS Respiratory Insufficiency score (EGRIS score) can help predict when a patient should be moved to an intensive care unit due to impending need for ventilatory support [155].

Table 12.8 Clinical warning signs and objective measures of respiratory distress

Warning signs
  Bulbar weakness with dysphagia
  Dysphonia
  Rapid shallow breathing
  Tachycardia
  Weak cough
  Staccato speech
  Accessory muscle use
  Paradoxical breathing
  Orthopnea
  Weakness of trapezius and neck muscles
  Single breath count less than 20
  Cough after swallowing
Objective measures
  Force vital capacity (FVC) <15 mL/kg, or <1 L, or a 50% drop from previous
  Maximum inspiratory pressure >−30 cm H_2O
  Maximum expiratory pressure <40 cm H_2O
  Desaturation or nocturnal desaturation

Familiarity of the signs and symptoms of respiratory dysfunction can help providers anticipate the need for intubation and mechanical ventilation. Above are warning signs as well as objective measures of impending respiratory failure. This table uses data adapted from Mehta's paper on neuromuscular respiratory failure [154].

FVC Forced vital capacity

When respiratory parameters fall below the values listed in Table 12.8, consideration should be given to elective intubation. Preemptive intubation can be less traumatic for both patients and families. Arterial blood gases can be obtained; however, hypoxemia or hypercarbia may be late findings in neuromuscular respiratory failure, and values may be normal even in patients who are imminently decompensating. Once patients have been intubated, continued monitoring of pulmonary function tests should take place to predict when they may be able to be weaned from ventilation and extubated. A negative inspiratory force of less than 50 cm H_2O and vital capacity improvement of greater than 4 ml/kg from the values prior to intubation suggest a successful extubation [156]. If intubation is prolonged due to inability to wean from the ventilator, tracheostomy should be considered.

Autonomic Dysfunction

Dysautonomia, which occurs in approximately one third of patients with GBS, can cause significant morbidity and mortality by manifesting in multiple organ systems [76]. Continuous cardiac monitoring should be considered in all patients, and a baseline ECG should be obtained early in the admission. Heart rate variability can be seen, and atropine or transcutaneous pacing may be needed for patients that develop tachycardia or heart block, respectively. If hemodynamic instability develops, care should be taken to use short-acting agents for management, given blood pressure can change very rapidly and patients may be more sensitive to certain medications. Table 12.9 lists drugs commonly associated with increased autonomic instability in GBS (Table 12.9). Hypotension can be addressed with fluids, placing the patient in the Trendelenburg position, or using short-acting vasopressive agents. If hypertension occurs, it should be treated with intravenous agents that are short-acting and those which can be titrated quickly such as esmolol or nicardipine [157]. Diarrhea, constipation, and urinary retention or urgency

Table 12.9 Drugs associated with increased autonomic instability in Guillain-Barre syndrome

Exaggerated hypotensive response	Exaggerated hypertensive response	Tendency to provoke arrhythmia
Phentolamine	Phenylephrine	Succinylcholine
Nitroglycerin	Ephedrine	
Edrophonium	Dopamine	
Thiopental	Isoproterenol	
Morphine sulfate		
Furosemide		

The drugs listed in this table should be avoided or used with caution. Data adapted from Dalos et al. [157]

may occur, and medication regimens or catheters may be required to address the abnormal bowel or bladder function.

Pain

As mentioned previously, pain can be seen early as a presenting symptom of GBS, but for many patients, it is present in the chronic recovery phase. This is a symptom that is often overlooked, particularly in critically ill patients who are intubated, when communication is difficult. Treatment of pain involves using standard neuropathic pain agents, and less commonly opioids. In one small randomized controlled study, 18 patients admitted and intubated with GBS were either given gabapentin or placebo for pain. Patient-reported pain scores were reduced, as was the use of opioid medications for pain in the group that received gabapentin at 15 mg/kg/day [158]. In another prospective trial, 12 adults received either carbamazepine or placebo via a PEG tube at a dose of 100 mg every 8 hours. In this small study, patients also had significantly lower self-reported pain ratings and required less opioids on the days they received carbamazepine [159]. Given the severity of the discomfort patients with GBS experience, opioids are sometimes necessary for treatment. In this case, special attention should be paid to gastrointestinal dysmotility or autonomic dysfunction from opioid use.

It is worth mentioning that corticosteroid therapy has been studied as a modality of treatment for GBS. Several randomized controlled trials have showed no statistically significant difference in speed of recovery or prognosis in GBS patients receiving IV steroids compared to controls [160–163]. Despite this, corticosteroids can be used for treating acute pain early in the course of the disease and have been reported as effective in both adult and pediatric populations [164, 165].

Mobility and Physical Therapy

As with most conditions causing acute weakness, physical therapy is extremely important both acutely and in recovery. In the hospital setting and early in the course of disease, therapy helps prevent complications such as decubitus ulcers, contractures, and deep venous thrombosis. After discharge and in the chronic recovery phase, continued exercise is felt to be important, although there is limited data showing this benefit. One study examined 16 GBS patients with severe fatigue and 4 patients with CIDP and found improved fatigue, physical fitness, functional outcomes, and quality of life in those that completed a 12-week bike training program [166]. Another case report showed improved fatigue and functional outcome in a patient who completed a 16-week cardiovascular training regimen 3 years after his acute weakness from Guillain-Barré syndrome [167]. There is currently an ongoing prospective, observer blinded trial evaluating the efficacy and cost-effectiveness of a 12-week tailored home exercise program versus advice and usual care in those with immune-mediated neuropathies [168].

Conclusion

Guillain-Barré syndrome classically presents with symmetric proximal and distal weakness, areflexia, and CSF albuminocytologic disassociation. Guillain-Barré syndrome is the most common neuromuscular cause of acute weakness. AIDP is the most common form in the United States. Variant syndromes include axonal variants (AMSAN and AMAN), MFS-related disorders, and pharyngeal cervical brachial variant. Strong clinical trial evidence supports the efficacy of IVIG and PLEX, but supportive treatment, attentive monitoring, and general medical care and pain management are also essential. Ongoing research to better understand the pathophysiology of Guillain-Barré syndrome is leading to numerous targeted treatment trials and immunomodulatory therapies with several promising agents in the therapeutic pipeline.

References

1. Dumenil L. Paralysie peripherique du movement et du sentiment portant sur les cuatre members. Atrophie des rameaux nerveux des parties paralysies. Gaz Hebd Med. 1864;1:203–6.
2. Guillain G, Barré JA, Strohl A. Sur un syndrome de radiculo-névrite avec hyperalbuminose du liquide céphalo-rachidien sans réaction cellulaire. Remarques sur les caractères cliniques et graphiques des réflexes tendineux. Ann Med Interne (Paris). 1999;150(1):1462–70.
3. Sejvar JJ, Baughman AL, Wise M, Morgan OW. Population incidence of Guillain-Barré syndrome: a systematic review and meta-analysis. Neuroepidemiology. 2011;36:123–33.
4. Hughes RAC, Cornblath DR. Guillain-Barré syndrome. Lancet. 2005;366(9497):1653–66.
5. Webb AJS, Brain SAE, Wood R, Rinaldi S, Turner MR. Seasonal variation in Guillain-Barré syndrome: a systematic review, meta-analysis and Oxfordshire cohort study. J Neurol Neurosurg Psychiatry. 2015;86(11):1196–201.
6. Ho TW, Mishu B, Li CY, Gao CY, Cornblath DR, Griffin JW, et al. Guillain-barré syndrome in Northern China relationship to Campylobacter jejuni infection and anti-glycolipid antibodies. Brain. 1995;118(3):597–605.
7. McKhann GM, Cornblath DR, Ho T, Griffin JW, Li CY, Bai AY, et al. Clinical and electrophysiological aspects of acute paralytic disease of children and young adults in northern China. Lancet. 1991;338(8767):593–7.
8. Winer JB, Hughes RAC, Anderson MJ, Jones DM, Kangro H, Watkinsh RPF. A prospective study of acute idiopathic neuropathy. II. Antecedent events. J Neurol Neurosurg Psychiatry. 1988;51(5):613–8.
9. Koga M, Yuki N, Hirata K. Antecedent symptoms in Guillain-Barré syndrome: an important indicator for clinical and serological subgroups. Acta Neurol Scand. 2001;103(5):278–87.
10. Hadden RDM, Karch H, Hartung HP, Zielasek J, Weissbrich B, Schubert J, et al. Preceding infections, immune factors, and outcome in Guillain-Barré syndrome. Neurology. 2001;56(6):758–65.
11. Hao Y, Wang W, Jacobs BC, Qiao B, Chen M, Liu D, et al. Antecedent infections in Guillain-Barré syndrome: a single-center, prospective study. Ann Clin Transl Neurol. 2019;6(12):2510–7.
12. Cao-Lormeau VM, Blake A, Mons S, Lastère S, Roche C, Vanhomwegen J, et al. Guillain-Barré Syndrome outbreak associated with Zika virus infection in French Polynesia: a case-control study. Lancet. 2016;387(10027):1531–9.
13. Parra B, Lizarazo J, Jiménez-Arango JA, Zea-Vera AF, González-Manrique G, Vargas J, et al. Guillain-Barré syndrome associated with Zika virus infection in Colombia. N Engl J Med. 2016;375(16):1513–23.
14. Paybast S, Gorji R, Mavandadi S. Guillain-Barré syndrome as a neurological complication of novel COVID-19 infection: a case report and review of the literature. Neurologist. 2020;25(4):101–3.
15. Sedaghat Z, Karimi N. Guillain Barre syndrome associated with COVID-19 infection: a case report. J Clin Neurosci. 2020;76:233–5.
16. Rodríguez Y, Novelli L, Rojas M, De Santis M, Acosta-Ampudia Y, Monsalve DM, et al. Autoinflammatory and autoimmune conditions at the crossroad of COVID-19. J Autoimmun. 2020;114:102506.
17. Farzi MA, Ayromlou H, Jahanbakhsh N, Bavil PH, Janzadeh A, Shayan FK. Guillain-Barré syndrome in a patient infected with SARS-CoV-2, a case report. J Neuroimmunol. 2020;346:577294.
18. Gutiérrez-Ortiz C, Méndez A, Rodrigo-Rey S, San Pedro-Murillo E, Bermejo-Guerrero L, Gordo-Mañas R, et al. Miller Fisher syndrome and polyneuritis cranialis in COVID-19. Neurology. 2020;95(5):601–5.
19. Toro G, Vergara I, Romén G. Neuroparalytic accidents of Antirabies vaccination with suckling mouse brain vaccine: clinical and pathologic study of 21 cases. Arch Neurol. 1977;34(11):694–700.
20. Appelbaum E, Nelson J. Neurological complications following antirabies vaccination. J Am Med Assoc. 1953;151(3):188–91.
21. Hemachudha T, Griffin DE, Chen WW, Johnson RT. Immunologic studies of rabies vaccination-induced Guillain-Barré syndrome. Neurology. 1988;38(3):375–8.
22. Haber P, Sejvar J, Mikaeloff Y, DeStefano F. Vaccines and Guillain-Barré syndrome. Drug Safety. 2009;32:309–23.
23. Schonberger LB, Bregman DJ, Sullivan-bolyai JZ, Keenlyside RA, Ziegler DW, Retailliau HF, et al. Guillain-Barre syndrome following vaccination in the national influenza immunization program, United States, 1976–1977. Am J Epidemiol. 1979;110(2):105–23.
24. Safranek TJ, Lawrence DN, Kuriand LT, Culver DH, Wiederholt WC, Hayner NS, et al. Reassessment of the association between Guillain-Barré syndrome

and receipt of swine influenza vaccine in 1976–1977: Results of a two-state study. Am J Epidemiol. 1991;133(9):940–51.

25. Lasky T, Terracciano GJ, Magder L, Koski CL, Ballesteros M, Nash D, et al. The Guillain-Barré syndrome and the 1992–1993 and 1993–1994 influenza vaccines. N Engl J Med. 1998;339(25):1797–802.

26. Lehmann HC, Hartung HP, Kieseier BC, Hughes RAC. Guillain-Barré syndrome after exposure to influenza virus. Lancet Infect Dis. 2010;10:643–51.

27. Stowe J, Andrews N, Wise L, Miller E. Investigation of the temporal association of Guillain-Barré syndrome with influenza vaccine and influenza-like illness using the United Kingdom general practice research database. Am J Epidemiol. 2009;169(3):382–8.

28. Hughes R, Rees J, Smeeton N, Winer J. Vaccines and Guillain-Barre syndrome. BMJ. 1996;312:1475.

29. Souayah N, Nasar A, Suri MFK, Qureshi AI. Guillain-Barre syndrome after vaccination in United States. A report from the CDC/FDA Vaccine Adverse Event Reporting System. Vaccine. 2007;25(29):5253–5.

30. van Doorn PA, Ruts L, Jacobs BC. Clinical features, pathogenesis, and treatment of Guillain-Barré syndrome. Lancet Neurol. 2008;7:939–50.

31. Pritchard J, Mukherjee R, Hughes RAC. Risk of relapse of Guillain-Barré syndrome or chronic inflammatory demyelinating polyradiculoneuropathy following immunisation [7]. J Neurol Neurosurg Psychiatry. 2002;73:348–9.

32. Chen Y, Zhang J, Chu X, Xu Y, Ma F. Vaccines and the risk of Guillain-Barré syndrome. Eur J Epidemiol. 2020;35(4):363–70.

33. Baxter R, Lewis N, Bakshi N, Vellozzi C, Klein NP. Recurrent Guillain-Barré syndrome following vaccination. Clin Infect Dis. 2012;54(6):800–4.

34. Rudant J, Dupont A, Mikaeloff Y, Bolgert F, Coste J, Weill A. Surgery and risk of Guillain-Barré syndrome. Neurology. 2018;91(13):e1220–7.

35. Arnason BG, Asbury AK. Idiopathic polyneuritis after surgery. Arch Neurol. 1968;18(5):500–7.

36. Myers TR, McCarthy NL, Panagiotakopoulos L, Omer SB. Estimation of the incidence of Guillain-Barré syndrome during pregnancy in the United States. Open Forum Infect Dis. 2019;6(3):1–3.

37. Jia H, Tian Y, Wu Y-M, Li B. Two cases of Guillain-Barré syndrome after cerebral hemorrhage or head trauma. Neuroimmunol Neuroinflammation. 2017;4(4):61–4.

38. Chi L-J, Wang H-B, Zhang Y, Wang W-Z. Abnormality of circulating CD4+CD25+ regulatory T cell in patients with Guillain-Barré syndrome. J Neuroimmunol. 2007;192(1–2):206–14.

39. Maddur MS, Rabin M, Hegde P, Bolgert F, Guy M, Vallat JM, et al. Intravenous immunoglobulin exerts reciprocal regulation of Th1/Th17 cells and regula-

tory T cells in Guillain–Barré syndrome patients. Immunol Res. 2014;60(2–3):320–9.

40. Yuki N, Yamada M, Koga M, Odaka M, Susuki K, Tagawa Y, et al. Animal model of axonal Guillain-Barré syndrome induced by sensitization with GM1 ganglioside. Ann Neurol. 2001;49(6):712–20.

41. Yuki N, Susuki K, Koga M, Nishimoto Y, Odaka M, Hirata K, et al. Carbohydrate mimicry between human ganglioside GM1 and Campylobacter jejuni lipooligosaccharide causes Guillain-Barré syndrome. Proc Natl Acad Sci U S A. 2004;101(31):11404–9.

42. Odaka M, Yuki N, Hirata K. Anti-GQ1b IgG antibody syndrome: clinical and immunological range. J Neurol Neurosurg Psychiatry. 2001;70(1):50–5.

43. Mori M, Kuwabara S, Miyake M, Dezawa M, Adachi-Usami E, Kuroki H, et al. Haemophilus influenzae has a GM1 ganglioside-like structure and elicits Guillain-Barre syndrome. Neurology. 1999;52(6):1282–4.

44. Koga M, Yuki N, Tai T, Hirata K. Miller Fisher syndrome and Haemophilus influenzae infection. Neurology. 2001;57(4):686–91.

45. Susuki K, Odaka M, Mori M, Hirata K, Yuki N. Acute motor axonal neuropathy after Mycoplasma infection: evidence of molecular mimicry. Neurology. 2004;62(6):949–56.

46. Ang CW, Tio-Gillen AP, Groen J, Herbrink P, Jacobs BC, Van Koningsveld R, et al. Cross-reactive anti-galactocerebroside antibodies and Mycoplasma pneumoniae infections in Guillain-Barré syndrome. J Neuroimmunol. 2002;130(1–2):179–83.

47. Kusunoki S, Kaida KI. Antibodies against ganglioside complexes in Guillain-Barré syndrome and related disorders. J Neurochem. 2011;116:828–32.

48. Asbury AK, Arnason BG, Adams RD. The inflammatory lesion in idiopathic polyneuritis: Its role in pathogenesis. Medicine (United States). 1969;48(3):173–215.

49. Prineas JW. Pathology of the Guillain-Barré syndrome. Ann Neurol. 1981;9(1 S):6–19.

50. Hafer-Macko C, Hsieh ST, Yan Li C, Ho TW, Sheikh K, Cornblath DR, et al. Acute motor axonal neuropathy: an antibody-mediated attack on axolemma. Ann Neurol. 1996;40(4):635–44.

51. Griffin JW, Li CY, Macko C, Ho TW, Hsieh ST, Xue P, et al. Early nodal changes in the acute motor axonal neuropathy pattern of the Guillain-Barré syndrome. J Neurocytol. 1996;25(1):33–51.

52. Kuwabara S, Bostock H, Ogawara K, Sung JY, Kanai K, Mori M, et al. The refractory period of transmission is impaired in axonal Guillain-Barré syndrome. Muscle Nerve. 2003;28(6):683–89.

53. Hiraga A, Mori M, Ogawara K, Hattori T, Kuwabara S. Differences in patterns of progression in demyelinating and axonal Guillain-Barré syndromes. Neurology. 2003;61(4):471–4.

54. Feasby TE, Gilbert JJ, Brown WF, Bolton CF, Hahn AF, Koopman WF, et al. An acute axonal form of Guillain-Barrée polyneuropathy. Brain. 1986;109(6):1115–26.

55. Griffin JW, Li CY, Ho TW, Tian M, Gao CY, Xue P, et al. Pathology of the motor-sensory axonal Guillain-Barré syndrome. Ann Neurol. 1996;39(1):17–26.

56. Yu RK, Tsai YT, Ariga T, Yanagisawa M. Structures, biosynthesis, and functions of gangliosides-an overview. J Oleo Sci. 2011;60:537–44.

57. Anderson RGW. The caveolae membrane system. Ann Rev Biochem. 1998;67:199–225.

58. Illa I, Ortiz N, Gallard E, Juarez C, Grau JM, Dalakas MC. Acute axonal Guillain-Barré syndrome with IgG antibodies against motor axons following parenteral gangliosides. Ann Neurol. 1995;38(2):218–24.

59. Dasgupta S, Li D, Yu RK. Lack of apparent neurological abnormalities in rabbits sensitized by gangliosides. Neurochem Res. 2004;29(11 SPEC. ISS.):2147–52.

60. Lehmann HC, Lopez PHH, Zhang G, Ngyuen T, Zhang J, Kieseier BC, et al. Passive immunization with anti-ganglioside antibodies directly inhibits axon regeneration in an animal model. J Neurosci. 2007;27(1):27–34.

61. Nishimoto Y, Odaka M, Hirata K, Yuki N. Usefulness of anti-GQ1b IgG antibody testing in Fisher syndrome compared with cerebrospinal fluid examination. J Neuroimmunol. 2004;148(1–2):200–5.

62. Chiba A, Kusunoki S, Obata H, Machinami R, Kanazawa I. Ganglioside composition of the human cranial nerves, with special reference to pathophysiology of Miller Fisher syndrome. Brain Res. 1997;745(1–2):32–36.

63. Ito H, Hatanaka Y, Fukami Y, Harada Y, Kobayashi R, Okada H, et al. Anti-ganglioside complex antibody profiles in a recurrent complicated case of GQ1b-seronegative miller fisher syndrome and Bickerstaff brainstem encephalitis: A case report. BMC Neurol. 2018;18(1):1–4.

64. Asbury AK, Cornblath DR. Assessment of current diagnostic criteria for Guillain-Barré syndrome. Ann Neurol. 1990;27(1 S):21–4.

65. Löffel NB, Rossi LN, Mumenthaler M, Lütschg J, Ludin HP. The Landry-Guillain-Barré syndrome. Complications, prognosis and natural history in 123 cases. J Neurol Sci. 1977;33(1–2):71–9.

66. Oh SJ, Kurokawa K, De Almeida DF, Ryan HF, Claussen GC. Subacute inflammatory demyelinating polyneuropathy. Neurology. 2003;61(11):1507–12.

67. Rodriguez-Casero MV, Shield LK, Kornberg AJ. Subacute inflammatory demyelinating polyneuropathy in children. Neurology. 2005;64(10):1786–8.

68. Walgaard C, Lingsma HF, Ruts L, Drenthen J, Van Koningsveld R, Garssen MJP, et al. Prediction of respiratory insufficiency in Guillain-Barré syndrome. Ann Neurol. 2010;67(6):781–7.

69. Rees JH, Thompson RD, Smeeton NC, Hughes RAC. Epidemiological study of Guillain-Barré syndrome in south east England. J Neurol Neurosurg Psychiatry. 1998;64(1):74–7.

70. Hughes RAC, Hadden RDM, Rees JII, Swan A V., Beghi E, Bogliun G, et al. The Italian Guillain-Barre study group. The prognosis and main prognostic indicators of Guillain-Barre syndrome: A multicentre prospective study of 297 patients (multiple letters) [1]. Brain. 1998;121:2053–61.

71. Dubey D, Kapotic M, Freeman M, Sawhney A, Rojas JC, Warnack W, et al. Factors contributing to delay in diagnosis of Guillain-Barré syndrome and impact on clinical outcome. Muscle Nerve. 2016;53(3):384–7.

72. Pentland B, Donald SM. Pain in the Guillain-Barré syndrome: a clinical review. Pain. 1994;59(2):159–64.

73. Ruts L, Van Doorn PA, Lombardi R, Haasdijk ED, Penza P, Tulen JHM, et al. Unmyelinated and myelinated skin nerve damage in Guillain-Barré syndrome: Correlation with pain and recovery. Pain. 2012;153(2):399–409.

74. Ruts L, Drenthen J, Jongen JLM, Hop WCJ, Visser GH, Jacobs BC, et al. Pain in Guillain-Barré syndrome: a long-term follow-up study. Neurology. 2010;75(16):1439–47.

75. Pan CL, Tseng TJ, Lin YH, Chiang MC, Lin WM, Hsieh ST. Cutaneous innervation in Guillain-Barré syndrome: pathology and clinical correlations. Brain. 2003;126(2):386–97.

76. Chakraborty T, Kramer CL, Wijdicks EFM, Rabinstein AA. Dysautonomia in Guillain-Barré Syndrome: s. Neurocrit Care. 2020;32(1):113–20.

77. Zochodne DW. Autonomic involvement in Guillain–Barre syndrome: a review. Muscle Nerve. 1994;17(10):289–99.

78. Feasby TE, Hahn AF, Brown WF, Bolton CF, Gilbert JJ, Koopman WJ. Severe axonal degeneration in acute Guillain-Barré syndrome: evidence of two different mechanisms? J Neurol Sci. 1993;116(2):185–92.

79. Fisher M. An unusual variant of acute idiopathic polyneuritis (syndrome of ophthalmoplegia, ataxia and areflexia). N Engl J Med. 1956;255(2):57–65.

80. Mori M, Kuwabara S, Fukutake T, Yuki N, Hattori T. Clinical features and prognosis of Miller Fisher syndrome. Neurology. 2001;56(8):1104–6.

81. Fross RD, Daube JR. Neuropathy in the miller fisher syndrome: clinical and electrophysiologic findings. Neurology. 1987;37(9):1493–8.

82. Bickerstaff ER. Brain stem encephalitis (Bickerstaff's encephalitis). 1978. 605–9 p.

83. Al-din AN, Anderson M, Bickerstaff ER, Harvey I. Brainstem encephalitis and the syndrome of miller fisher a clinical study. Brain. 1982;105(3):481–95.

84. Ropper AH. Unusual clinical variants and signs in Guillain-Barré Syndrome. Arch Neurol. 1986;43(11):1150–2.

85. Nagashima T, Koga M, Odaka M, Hirata K, Yuki N. Continuous spectrum of pharyngeal-cervical-brachial variant of Guillain-Barré syndrome. Arch Neurol. 2007;64(10):1519–23.

86. Quintas S, López Ruiz R, Ramos C, Vivancos J, Zapata-Wainberg G. Pharyngeal-cervical-brachial variant of Guillain-Barré syndrome with predominant bulbar palsy and anti-GM3 IgG antibodies. Neurol Sci. 2018;39:1291–2.

87. Morris AMS, Elliott EJ, D'Souza RM, Antony J, Kennett M, Longbottom H. Acute flaccid paralysis in Australian children. J Paediatr Child Health. 2003;39(1):22–6.

88. Korinthenberg R, Trollmann R, Felderhoff-Müser U, Bernert G, Hackenberg A, Hufnagel M, et al. Diagnosis and treatment of Guillain-Barré Syndrome in childhood and adolescence: an evidence- and consensus-based guideline. Europ J Paediatr Neurol. 2020;25:5–16.

89. Bradshaw DY, Jones HR. Guillain-Barré syndrome in children: clinical course, electrodiagnosis, and prognosis. Muscle Nerve. 1992;15(4):500–6.

90. Ryan MM. Guillain-Barré syndrome in childhood. J Paediatri Child Health. 2005;41:237–41.

91. Delanoe C, Sebire G, Landrieu P, Huault G, Metral S. Acute inflammatory demyelinating polyradiculopathy in children: clinical and electrodiagnostic studies. Ann Neurol. 1998;44(3):350–6.

92. Jones HR. Childhood Guillain-Barre syndrome: clinical presentation, diagnosis, and therapy. J Child Neurol. 1996;11:4–12.

93. Kuitwaard K, Bos-Eyssen ME, Blomkwist-Markens PH, Van Doorn PA. Recurrences, vaccinations and long-term symptoms in GBS and CIDP. J Peripher Nerv Syst. 2009;14(4):310–5.

94. Van Den Berg B, Bunschoten C, Van Doorn PA, Jacobs BC. Mortality in Guillain-Barré syndrome. Neurology. 2013;80(18):1650–4.

95. Walgaard C, Lingsma HF, Ruts L, Van Doorn PA, Steyerberg EW, Jacobs BC. Early recognition of poor prognosis in Guillain-Barré syndrome. Neurology. 2011;76(11):968–75.

96. Visser LH, Schmitz PIM, Meulstee J, Van Doorn PA, Van Der Meché FGA. Prognostic factors of Guillain-Barre syndrome after intravenous immunoglobulin or plasma exchange. Neurology. 1999;53(3):598–604.

97. Cornblath DR, Mellits ED, Griffin JW, McKhann GM, Albers JW, Miller RG, et al. Motor conduction studies in Guillain-Barré syndrome: Description and prognostic value. Ann Neurol. 1988;23(4):354–9.

98. Solomon T, Willison H. Infectious causes of acute flaccid paralysis. Curr Opin Infect Dis. 2003;16:375–81.

99. Gwathmey KG. Sensory neuronopathies. Muscle Nerve. 2016;53:8–19.

100. Logina I, Donaghy M. Diphtheritic polyneuropathy: a clinical study and comparison with Guillain-Barré syndrome. J Neurol Neurosurg Psychiatry. 1999;67:433–8.

101. Grattan-Smith PJ, Morris JG, Johnston HM, Yiannikas C, Malik R, Russell R, et al. Clinical and neurophysiological features of tick paralysis. Brain. 1997;120(11):1975–87.

102. Crone C, Krarup C. Diagnosis of acute neuropathies. J Neurol. 2007;254:1151–69.

103. Fokke C, Van Den Berg B, Drenthen J, Walgaard C, Van Doorn PA, Jacobs BC. Diagnosis of Guillain-Barré syndrome and validation of Brighton criteria. Brain. 2014;137(1):33–43.

104. Rauschka H, Jellinger K, Lassmann H, Braier F, Schmidbauer M. Guillain-Barré syndrome with marked pleocytosis or a significant proportion of polymorphonuclear granulocytes in the cerebrospinal fluid: neuropathological investigation of five cases and review of differential diagnoses. Europ J Neurol. 2003;10:479–86.

105. Albers JW, Kelly JJ. Acquired inflammatory demyelinating polyneuropathies: clinical and electrodiagnostic features. Muscle Nerve. 1989;12:435–51.

106. Bromberg MB, Albers JW. Patterns of sensory nerve conduction abnormalities in demyelinating and axonal peripheral nerve disorders. Muscle Nerve. 1993;16(3):262–6.

107. Derksen A, Ritter C, Athar P, Kieseier BC, Mancias P, Hartung HP, et al. Sural sparing pattern discriminates Guillain-Barré syndrome from its mimics. Muscle Nerve. 2014;50(5):780–4.

108. Brown WF, Feasby TE. Conduction block and denervation in Guillain-Barré polyneuropathy. Brain. 1984;107(1):219–39.

109. Jamal GA, Ballantyne JP. The localization of the lesion in patients with acute ophthalmoplegia, ataxia and areflexia (miller fisher syndrome): A serial multimodal neurophysiological study. Brain. 1988;111(1):95–114.

110. Scelsa SN, Herskovitz S. Miller Fisher syndrome: axonal, demyelinating or both? Electromyogr Clin Neurophysiol. 2000;40(8):497–502.

111. Hughes RAC, Bouche P, Cornblath DR, Evers E, Hadden RD, Hahn AF, et al. European Federation of Neurological Societies/Peripheral Nerve Society Guideline* on management of chronic inflammatory demyelinating polyradiculoneuropathy. Report of a joint task force of the European Federation of Neurological Societies and the Peripheral Nerve Society. J Peripheral Nerv Syst. 2005;10:326–32.

112. Uncini A, Manzoli C, Notturno F, Capasso M. Pitfalls in electrodiagnosis of Guillain-Barré syndrome subtypes. J Neurol Neurosurg Psychiatry. 2010;81(10):1157–63.

113. Uncini A, Ippoliti L, Shahrizaila N, Sekiguchi Y, Kuwabara S. Optimizing the electrodiagnostic accuracy in Guillain-Barré syndrome subtypes: criteria sets and sparse linear discriminant analysis. Clin Neurophysiol. 2017;128(7):1176–83.

114. Hadden RDM, Cornblath DR, Hughes RAC, Zielasek J, Hartung HP, Toyka KV, et al. Electrophysiological classification of Guillain-Barre syndrome: clinical associations and outcome. Ann Neurol. 1998;44(5):780–8.

115. Iwata F, Utsumi Y. MR imaging in Guillain-Barre syndrome. Pediatr Radiol. 1997;27(1):36–8.

116. Telleman JA, Grimm A, Goedee S, Visser LH, Zaidman CM. Nerve ultrasound in polyneuropathies. Muscle Nerve. 2018;57(5):716–28.

117. Grimm A, Décard BF, Axer H. Ultrasonography of the peripheral nervous system in the early stage of Guillain-Barré syndrome. J Peripher Nerv Syst. 2014;19(3):234–41.

118. Razali SNO, Arumugam T, Yuki N, Rozalli FI, Goh KJ, Shahrizaila N. Serial peripheral nerve ultrasound in Guillain-Barré syndrome. Clin Neurophysiol. 2016;127(2):1652–6.

119. French Cooperative Group. Efficiency of plasma exchange in Guillain-Barré syndrome: role of replacement fluids. French Cooperative Group on Plasma Exchange in Guillain-Barré syndrome. Ann Neurol. 1987;22(6):753–61.

120. Brettle RP, Gross M, Legg NJ, Lockwood M, Pallis C. Treatment of acute polyneuropathy by plasma exchange. Lancet. 1978;312:1100.

121. Färkkilä M, Kinnunen E, Haapanen E, Iivanainen M. Guillain-Barré syndrome: quantitative measurement of plasma exchange therapy. Neurology. 1987;37(5):837–40.

122. Greenwood RJ, Hughes RAC, Bowden AN, Gordon NS, Millac P, Davis JN, et al. Controlled trial of plasma exchange in acute inflammatory polyradiculoneuropathy. J Clin Apher. 1985;2(4):877–9.

123. Osterman PO, Lundemo G, Pirskanen R, Fagius J, Pihlstedt P, Sidén Å, et al. Beneficial effects of plasma exchange in acute inflammatory polyradiculoneuropathy. Lancet. 1984;324(8415):1296–9.

124. Plasmapheresis and acute Guillain-Barré syndrome. Neurology. 1985;35(8):1096–104.

125. Raphaël JC, Chevret S, Chastang C, Jars-Guincestre MC. Appropriate number of plasma exchanges in Guillain-Barre syndrome. Ann Neurol. 1997;41(3):298–306.

126. Van Der Meché FGA. The Guillain-Barre syndrome: Plasma exchange or immunoglobulins intravenously. J Neurol Neurosurg Psychiatry. 1994;57(SUPPL):293–5.

127. Bril V, Ilse WK, Pearce R, Dhanani A, Sutton D, Kong K. Pilot trial of immunoglobulin versus plasma exchange in patients with Guillain-Barré syndrome. Neurology. 1996;46(1):100–3.

128. Hughes RAC. Randomised trial of plasma exchange, intravenous immunoglobulin, and combined treatments in Guillain-Barre syndrome. Lancet. 1997;349(9047):225–30.

129. Gürses N, Uysal S, Çetinkaya F, Işek I, Kalayci AG. Intravenous immunoglobulin treatment in children with guillain-barre syndrome. Scand J Infect Dis. 1995;27(3):241–3.

130. Korinthenberg R, Schessl J, Kirschner J, Mönting JS. Intravenously administered immunoglobulin in the treatment of childhood Guillain-Barré syndrome: a randomized trial. Pediatrics. 2005;116(1):2004–1324.

131. Verboon C, Van Den Berg B, Cornblath DR, Venema E, Gorson KC, Lunn MP, et al. Original research: second IVIg course in Guillain-Barré syndrome with poor prognosis: the non-randomised ISID study. J Neurol Neurosurg Psychiatry. 2020;91(2):113–21.

132. Walgaard C, Jacobs BC, Lingsma HF, Steyerberg EW, Cornblath DR, van Doorn PA, et al. Second IVIg course in Guillain-Barré syndrome patients with poor prognosis (SID-GBS trial): protocol for a double-blind randomized, placebo-controlled clinical trial. J Peripher Nerv Syst. 2018;23(4):210–5.

133. Bonilla FA. Pharmacokinetics of immunoglobulin administered via intravenous or subcutaneous routes. Immunol Allergy Clin North America. 2008;28:803–19.

134. Kleyweg RP, Van Der Meche FGA. Treatment related fluctuations in Guillain-Barre syndrome after high-dose immunoglobulins or plasma-exchange. J Neurol Neurosurg Psychiatry. 1991;54(11):957–60.

135. Ropper AH, Albers JW, Addison R. Limited relapse in Guillain-Barré syndrome after plasma exchange. Arch Neurol. 1988;45(3):314–5.

136. Visser LH, Van Der Meché FGA, Meulstee J, Van Doorn PA. Risk factors for treatment related clinical fluctuations in Guillain-Barré syndrome. J Neurol Neurosurg Psychiatry. 1998;64(2):242–4.

137. Ruts L, Van Koningsveld R, Van Doorn PA. Distinguishing acute-onset CIDP from Guillain-Barré syndrome with treatment related fluctuations. Neurology. 2005;65(1):1680–6.

138. Halstead SK, Zitman FMP, Humphreys PD, Greenshields K, Verschuuren JJ, Jacobs BC, et al. Eculizumab prevents anti-ganglioside antibody-mediated neuropathy in a murine model. Brain. 2008;131(5):1197–208.

139. Misawa S, Kuwabara S, Sato Y, Yamaguchi N, Nagashima K, Katayama K, et al. Safety and efficacy of eculizumab in Guillain-Barré syndrome: a multicentre, double-blind, randomised phase 2 trial. Lancet Neurol. 2018;17(6):519–29.

140. McGonigal R, Cunningham ME, Yao D, Barrie JA, Sankaranarayanan S, Fewou SN, et al. C1q-targeted inhibition of the classical complement pathway prevents injury in a novel mouse model of acute motor axonal neuropathy. Acta Neuropathol Commun. 2016;4:1–16.

141. Lansita JA, Mease KM, Qiu H, Yednock T, Sankaranarayanan S, Kramer S. Nonclinical development of ANX005: a humanized Anti-C1q Antibody for treatment of autoimmune and neurodegenerative diseases. Int J Toxicol. 2017;36(6):449–62.

142. A Clinical Study of ANX005 and IVIG in Subjects With Guillain Barré Syndrome (GBS) – Full Text View – ClinicalTrials.gov [Internet]. [cited 2020 Oct 14]. Available from: https://clinicaltrials.gov/ct2/show/NCT04035135?cond=guillain+barre+syndrome&draw=2.

143. Ostronoff F, Perales MA, Stubblefield MD, Hsu KC. Rituximab-responsive Guillain-Barré syndrome following allogeneic hematopoietic SCT. Bone Marrow Transplant. 2008;42(1):71–2.

144. Marino D, Farina P, Jirillo A, De Franchis G, Simonetto M, Aversa SML. Neurological syndrome after R-CHOP chemotherapy for a non-Hodgkin

lymphoma: What is the diagnosis? Int J Hematol. 2011;94(5):461–2.

145. Carmona A, Alonso JD, de las Heras M, Navarrete A. Guillain-Barre syndrome in a patient with diffuse large B-cell lymphoma, and rituximab maintenance therapy. An association beyond anecdotal evidence? Clin Transl Oncol. 2006;8(10):764–6.

146. Tzachanis D, Hamdan A, Uhlmann EJ, Joyce RM. Successful treatment of refractory guillain-barré syndrome with alemtuzumab in a patient with chronic lymphocytic leukemia. Acta Haematol. 2014;132(2):240–3.

147. Vaccaro C, Zhou J, Ober RJ, Ward ES. Engineering the Fc region of immunoglobulin G to modulate in vivo antibody levels. Nat Biotechnol. 2005;23(10):1283–8.

148. Zhang G, Bogdanova N, Gao T, Sheikh KA. Elimination of activating Fcγ receptors in spontaneous autoimmune peripheral polyneuropathy model protects from neuropathic disease. PLoS One. 2019;14(8):1–13.

149. Smith B, Kiessling A, Lledo-Garcia R, Dixon KL, Christodoulou L, Catley MC, et al. Generation and characterization of a high affinity anti-human FcRn antibody, rozanolixizumab, and the effects of different molecular formats on the reduction of plasma IgG concentration. MAbs. 2018;10(7):1111–30.

150. Kiessling P, Lledo-Garcia R, Watanabe S, Langdon G, Tran D, Bari M, et al. The FcRn inhibitor rozanolixizumab reduces human serum IgG concentration: a randomized phase 1 study. Sci Transl Med. 2017;9(414):1–12.

151. A Study to Assess Long-term Safety, Tolerability and Efficacy of Rozanolixizumab in Subjects With Chronic Inflammatory Demyelinating Polyradiculoneuropathy – Full Text View – ClinicalTrials.gov [Internet]. [cited 2020 Oct 14]. Available from: https://clinicaltrials.gov/ct2/show/NCT04051944?type=Intr&cond=cidp&draw=2&rank=3.

152. Washburn N, Schwabb I, Ortiz D, Bhatnagar N, Lansing JC, Medeiros A, et al. Controlled tetra-Fc sialylation of IVIg results in a drug candidate with consistent enhanced anti-inflammatory activity. Proc Natl Acad Sci U S A. 2015;112(11):297–306.

153. Zhang G, Massaad CA, Gao T, Pillai L, Bogdanova N, Ghauri S, et al. Sialylated intravenous immunoglobulin suppress anti-ganglioside antibody mediated nerve injury. Exp Neurol. 2016;282:49–55.

154. Mehta S. Neuromuscular disease causing acute respiratory failure. Respiratory Care. 2006;51(9):1016–21.

155. Chung HK. Comparison between EGRIS and outcome of Guillain-Barre syndrome: retrospective study in one center (P06.144). Neurology. 2012;78(Meeting Abstracts 1):144.

156. Nguyen TN, Badjatia N, Malhotra A, Gibbons FK, Qureshi MM, Greenberg SA. Factors predicting extubation success in patients with Guillain- Barré syndrome. Neurocritical Care. 2006;5:230–4.

157. Dalos NP, Borel C, Hanley DF. Cardiovascular autonomic dysfunction in Guillain-Barré syndrome: therapeutic implications of Swan-Ganz monitoring. Arch Neurol. 1988;45(1):115–7.

158. Pandey CK, Bose N, Garg G, Singh N, Baronia A, Agarwal A, et al. Gabapentin for the treatment of pain in Guillain-Barré syndrome: a double-blinded, placebo-controlled, crossover study. Anesth Analg. 2002;95(6):1719–23.

159. Pandey CK, Raza M, Tripathi M, Navkar D V., Kumar A, Singh UK. The comparative evaluation of gabapentin and carbamazepine for pain management in Guillain-Barré syndrome patients in the intensive care unit. Anesth Analg. 2005;101(1):220–5.

160. Singh NK, Gupta A. Do corticosteroids influence the disease course or mortality in Guillain – Barre' Syndrome? J Assoc Physicians India. 1996;44(1):22–4.

161. Bansal BC, Sood AK, Gupta AK, Yadav P. Role of steroids in the treatment of Guillain Barre syndrome – a controlled trial. Neurol India. 1986;34(5):329–35.

162. Guillain-Barré Syndrome Steroid Trial Group. Double-blind trial of intravenous methylprednisolone in Guillain-Barré syndrome. Lancet. 1993;341(8845):586–90.

163. Hughes RAC, Newsom-Davis JM, Perkin GD, Pierce JM. Controlled trial of prednisolone in acute polyneuropathy. Lancet. 1978;312(8093):750–3.

164. Kabore R, Magy L, Boukhris S, Mabrouk T, Lacoste M, Vallat JM. Contribution of corticosteroid to the treatment of pain in the acute phase of Guillain-Barré syndrome. Revue Neurologique. 2004;160:821–3.

165. Kajimoto M, Koga M, Narumi H, Inoue H, Matsushige T, Ohga S. Successful control of radicular pain in a pediatric patient with Guillain-Barré syndrome. Brain Dev. 2015;37(9):897–900.

166. Garssen MPJ, Bussmann JBJ, Schmitz PIM, Zandbergen A, Welter TG, Merkies ISJ, et al. Physical training and fatigue, fitness, and quality of life in Guillain-Barré syndrome and CIDP. Neurology. 2004;63(12):2393–5.

167. Pitetti KH, Barrett PJ, Abbas D. Endurance exercise training in Guillain-Barre Syndrome. Arch Phys Med Rehabil. 1993;74(7):761–5.

168. White CM, Hadden RD, Robert-Lewis SF, McCrone PR, Petty JL. Observer blind randomised controlled trial of a tailored home exercise programme versus usual care in people with stable inflammatory immune mediated neuropathy. BMC Neurol. 2015;15(1):1–9.

Spinal Cord Compression and Myelopathies

13

William F. Schmalstieg and Brian G. Weinshenker

Acute myelopathies are potentially devastating conditions that may result in irreversible loss of mobility and control of bodily functions. Many etiologies of acute myelopathy are treatable, and rapid diagnosis and institution of appropriate treatment can prevent or reduce the extent of permanent damage to the spinal cord. Delays in the diagnosis and treatment of acute cord syndromes are frequent and may contribute to loss of neurologic function [1]. Furthermore, some inflammatory conditions that cause myelopathy may relapse and may benefit from maintenance prophylactic therapies. Therefore, assessment of the risk of relapse is important even when spontaneous or treatment-induced remission occurs.

This chapter considers the clinical presentation, evaluation, and management of acute and subacute spinal cord disorders and includes a diagnostic algorithm to distinguish compressive and noncompressive myelopathies and also to distinguish among the various noncompressive etiologies (Fig. 13.1). The key elements are high index of suspicion and confirmation, primarily with neuroimaging, but occasionally supported by other laboratory studies. The chapter concludes with treatment recommendations.

Pathophysiology

A review of spinal anatomy informs a discussion of the pathophysiology and clinical presentation of acute disorders of the cord. The spinal cord extends between the medulla and the conus medullaris, which is opposite the L1 vertebral body. Much of the substance of the cord is composed of large myelinated tracts, the most clinically relevant of which include:

1. Lateral corticospinal tracts carrying ipsilateral motor fibers
2. Spinothalamic tracts carrying contralateral pain and temperature sensation
3. Dorsal columns carrying ipsilateral joint position and vibratory sensation

The arterial vascular supply of the spinal cord consists of a single anterior spinal artery and two posterior spinal arteries, which originate from the vertebral arteries. The anterior spinal artery is also supplied by multiple segmental arteries arising from the thoracic and abdominal aorta. The anterior spinal artery supplies the lateral corticospinal and spinothalamic tracts, whereas the dorsal columns are supplied by the posterior spinal arteries. The venous drainage of the cord is through the epidural venous plexus.

W. F. Schmalstieg (✉)
Department of Neurology, University of Minnesota, Minneapolis, MN, USA
e-mail: wschmals@umn.edu

B. G. Weinshenker
Department of Neurology, Mayo Clinic, Rochester, MN, USA
e-mail: weinb@mayo.edu

© The Author(s), under exclusive license to Springer Nature Switzerland AG 2021
K. L. Roos (ed.), *Emergency Neurology*, https://doi.org/10.1007/978-3-030-75778-6_13

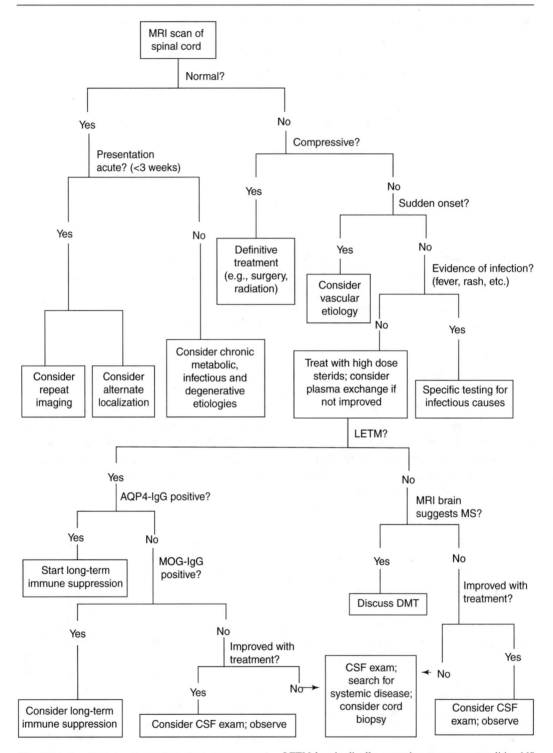

Fig. 13.1 Approach to diagnosis and management of acute and subacute myelopathies. *AQP4* aquaporin-4, *CSF* cerebrospinal fluid, *DMT* disease-modifying therapy, *LETM* longitudinally extensive transverse myelitis, *MS* multiple sclerosis, *MOG* myelin oligodendrocyte glycoprotein, *NMO* neuromyelitis optica

The cord is surrounded by the meninges (pia, arachnoid, and dura mater), which are in turn encircled by the vertebrae. The vertebral bodies are anterior to the cord, the pedicles lateral, and the laminae and spinous processes posterior.

Compressive lesions, such as epidural abscess or metastases, obstruct the epidural venous plexus, which impairs venous drainage leading to vasogenic edema and in turn an inflammatory cascade mediated, in part, by prostaglandins and other inflammatory cytokines. Simultaneously, the combination of external mechanical compression and internal swelling of the cord disrupts axonal conduction. Subsequent inflammation then leads to localized demyelination and frank ischemia of the cord [2].

Vascular occlusions or other vascular anomalies can cause acute cord injury. The portion of the cord supplied by the anterior spinal artery is particularly vulnerable. Restricted flow of the feeding vessels to this artery may produce watershed ischemia, particularly at the caudal regions of the anterior spinal cord supplied by the dominant radicular artery of Adamkiewicz. Ischemia of the spinal cord may occur during surgical cross-clamping of the aorta. Other potential causes of anterior spinal artery occlusion include aortic dissection, atherosclerosis, cardiac embolism, hypercoagulable states, and fibrocartilaginous embolism from intervertebral disk fragments. Another uncommon but important vascular anomaly associated with myelopathy is dural arteriovenous fistula, an abnormal connection of a dural artery to a vein that results in venous hypertension, resulting in damage to the cord. Dural fistulas result in distension of veins on the surface of the spinal cord, which is an important radiologic sign of this entity that is often evident on MRI of the lumbar spine.

As elaborated in the section on differential diagnosis, a wide variety of demyelinating, inflammatory, and infectious conditions can produce intrinsic damage to the substance of the spinal cord. A detailed description of the underlying pathophysiology of each of these conditions is beyond the scope of this text, and in many of these conditions, the pathogenesis is poorly understood.

Antibodies targeting the aquaporin-4 (AQP4) water channel (AQP4-IgG) are now known to account for an important portion of cases formerly diagnosed with "idiopathic transverse myelitis." Neuromyelitis optica spectrum disorders (NMOSD) are inflammatory diseases characterized by recurrent, severe attacks of optic neuritis and longitudinally extensive transverse myelitis (associated with an acute T2 lesion longer than three vertebral segments on MRI sagittal images) [3]. Some individuals with NMOSD have spatially limited presentations, for example, recurrent attacks of transverse myelitis without optic neuritis. In 15% of patients with AQP4-IgG-associated myelopathy, a lesion shorter than three vertebral segments occurs at the initial presentation of NMOSD, but the majority of patients have a longitudinally extensive lesion [4]. AQP4 channels are highly expressed at the astrocytic end feet of the blood-brain barrier. AQP4 antibodies are pathogenic and not merely markers of autoimmunity or disease severity. Brain MRI lesions in patients with NMO occur in regions known to express high levels of AQP4 [5]. Additionally, transfer of pooled IgG antibodies from NMO-IgG-positive patients to rats reproduces lesions similar to those seen in human NMO [6, 7]. Antibody- and complement-mediated cytotoxicity to astrocytes occurs in vitro in the presence of AQP4 autoantibodies and active complement and may account for the tissue damage seen in pathologic samples from patients with NMO [8]. Additional mechanisms that may contribute to injury caused by AQP4-specific autoantibodies include disruption of potassium and glutamate homeostasis due to the physical association of AQP4 with an inward rectifying potassium channel and the excitatory amino acid transporter EAAT2 [8].

A subset of patients with longitudinally extensive myelitis have serum antibodies against myelin oligodendrocyte glycoprotein (MOG), a minor myelin protein [9]. Myelitis associated with MOG-IgG is usually longitudinally extensive, as it is with AQP4-IgG, but often is associated with less edema and enhancement and may occasionally be associated with multiple simultaneous lesions. Relapses that occur in this antibody-defined patient subgroup usually consist of recurrent optic neuritis, and recurrent myelitis is rare [10]. A potential pathogenic role of this antibody, possibly via complement-mediated oligodendrocytopathy, has been suggested but is not clearly established [11].

Differential Diagnosis

The differential diagnosis of acute myelopathy is extensive, including structural, vascular, demyelinating, infectious, inflammatory, neoplastic, and paraneoplastic conditions (Table 13.1).

Table 13.1 Etiologies of acute and subacute myelopathies

External compression
  Metastatic spinal cord compression
  Epidural abscess
  Spinal stenosis
  Disk herniation
  Spinal fracture
  Extramedullary hematopoiesis
  Epidural lipomatosis
  Atlantoaxial instability
Syrinx
Vascular
  Spinal cord infarct
  Intraspinal hematoma
  Dural arteriovenous fistula
Demyelinating
  Multiple sclerosis
  Neuromyelitis optica spectrum disorders (AQP4-IgG positive and "seronegative")
  Myelin oligodendrocyte glycoprotein antibody (MOG-IgG)-associated disorder
  Idiopathic transverse myelitis
  Acute disseminated encephalomyelitis
Infectious viruses
  Herpesviruses
  Arboviruses (including West Nile virus)
  Acute flaccid myelitis (Enteroviruses D68, A71, Echoviruses and Coxsackieviruses)
  Enteroviruses 70 and 71
  Adenovirus
  HIV
  HTLV-1
  Poliomyelitis
  Rabies

Table 13.1 (continued)

Infectious-bacterial
  Syphilis
  Tuberculosis
  Lyme disease (rare)
Infectious-parasitic
  Schistosomiasis
  Strongylosis
Parainfectious
  Mycoplasma
  Chlamydia
  SARS-CoV-2
Inflammatory
  Sjögren syndrome
  Systemic lupus erythematosus
  Wegener granulomatosis
  Behçet disease
Sarcoidosis
Toxic/metabolic
  Nitrous oxide toxicity
  Copper deficiency
  Vitamin B12 deficiency (rare)
Iatrogenic
  Radiation myelitis
  Postvaccination myelitis
  Intrathecal chemotherapy
Neoplasia
  Intradural, extramedullary tumors (meningioma, neurofibroma)
  Intramedullary tumors (astrocytoma, ependymoma)
  Lymphomatoid granulomatosis
  Intravascular lymphoma
Paraneoplastic myelitis

Structural

External compression of the spinal cord is an important and treatable cause of acute myelopathy. Recognition of these conditions with MR imaging is usually considered straightforward. A typical example of cord compression in the setting of vertebral metastasis from a primary lung carcinoma is displayed in Fig. 13.2. It is essential to have a high index of suspicion for these disorders as few symptoms aside from pain may be present initially and neurologic deterioration can occur rapidly.

Spinal cord compression in the setting of congenital spinal canal stenosis and/or degenerative

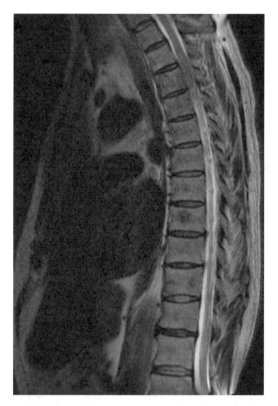

Fig. 13.2 Thoracic spinal cord compression caused by metastatic lung carcinoma, sagittal T2 MRI

disk disease usually presents with subacute or chronic symptoms, although acute presentations can occur in the setting of trauma or acute disk herniation. Magnetic resonance imaging readily detects these abnormalities.

Occasionally, patients with myelopathy resulting from spinal canal stenosis, often due to a combination of congenital and acquired pathologies, may have longitudinally extensive cord signal abnormalities on MRI. These intrinsic cord abnormalities may distract the clinician from considering the significance of spinal stenosis that may be compressing the cord and producing a subacute ischemic myelopathy. Cord compression may be erroneously attributed to cord edema from an intramedullary lesion rather than to primary compression due to spinal stenosis. Often, the syndrome is diagnosed as neuromyelitis optica, transverse myelitis, sarcoidosis, or spinal

cord tumor. However, myelopathy secondary to stenosis usually evolves over several months, whereas transverse myelitis (either idiopathic or related to NMO) does so over days to weeks. In addition, gadolinium enhancement associated with stenosis tends to be quite focal and localized to the area of maximal compression, whereas enhancement in longitudinally extensive myelitis or tumor often extends over several vertebral segments (Fig. 13.3) [12, 13].

Uncommon causes of extradural compression include extramedullary hematopoiesis, epidural lipomatosis, and atlantoaxial instability. Extramedullary hematopoiesis associated with beta thalassemia, myelodysplastic syndromes, and polycythemia vera may rarely result in epidural cord compression. Symptoms typically evolve over one to several months [14]. Epidural lipomatosis is a condition in which excess fat deposits form in the epidural space and may compress the spinal cord, especially in patients with preexisting spinal stenosis. Risk factors include endogenous or exogenous corticosteroid excess, obesity, and diabetes mellitus [15]. This condition often causes slowly progressive neurologic symptoms, but there are several reports of acute myelopathy related to epidural fat deposition [16]. Atlantoaxial instability is usually associated with an underlying condition and most commonly occurs in patients with rheumatoid arthritis or trisomy 21 [17, 18]. Patients with atlantoaxial dislocation may present with progressive myelopathy or acute spinal cord injury.

Symptomatic spinal cord syrinx is usually a hydromyelia that complicates Chiari type 1 malformation; it presents with a slowly progressive central cord syndrome, characterized by early deep, poorly localized pain followed by loss of pain and temperature sensation at the level of the lesion and by progressive segmental lower motor neuron symptoms at the level of the lesion and upper motor neuron symptoms below the lesion [19]. When a syrinx is present in the cervical cord, weakness appears initially in the upper limbs as the motor pathways to the arms are medial to those supplying the trunk and legs.

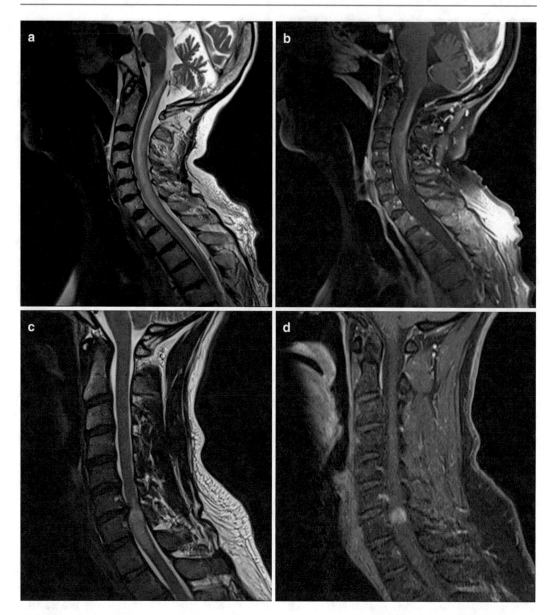

Fig. 13.3 Comparison of MR imaging in transverse myelitis and compressive stenosis with longitudinally extensive intramedullary lesion; compressive stenosis is associated with a focal ring pattern of gadolinium enhancement at the point of maximal cord compression.

(a) Transverse myelitis associated with NMOSD, sagittal T2 MRI. (b) Transverse myelitis associated with NMOSD, sagittal T1 MRI with gadolinium. (c). Compressive stenosis, sagittal T2 MRI. (d) Compressive stenosis, sagittal T1 MRI with gadolinium

Patients with this condition may present for acute evaluation when motor symptoms become bothersome or when painless injuries, especially burns, occur. Rarely, acute myelopathy due to syrinx presents after neck trauma [20] or Valsalva maneuver [21].

Vascular

In the absence of a compressive lesion, the sudden onset of severe impairment of motor and spinothalamic sensory functions with relative preservation of dorsal column sensory modalities suggests a stroke in the distribution of the anterior spinal artery. This is a feared complication of surgical manipulation of the thoracic or abdominal aorta and in that context is readily identified. However, cord infarction may occur spontaneously and occasionally without clearly identifiable risk factors that aid in the diagnosis.

MRI findings suggestive of anterior spinal cord infarction include central T2 hyperintensity affecting the ventral gray matter of the cord, often as paired lesions ("owl eyes"). The posterior cord is usually spared. Gadolinium enhancement is variable, and absence of enhancement in the setting of a sudden-onset myelopathy is more suggestive of infarct than an inflammatory process [22]. Figures 13.4 and 13.5 display the evolution of a typical cord infarct. A high index of suspicion is required, because specific confirmation with vascular imaging is not usually successful.

Intraspinal hematomas are uncommon. The commonest cause of spontaneous hematoma is an underlying vascular malformation, especially cavernous angioma [23]. These conditions can occur as a rare but serious consequence of lumbar puncture, especially in patients treated with anticoagulant drugs. A study of 342 patients who were anticoagulated with heparin after lumbar puncture demonstrated a 2% risk of spinal hematoma, whereas there were no hematomas in a matched cohort of patients who were not anticoagulated [24]. Patients with a recent history of spinal surgery, epidural anesthesia, or coagulopathy are also at risk. Hemorrhage into the subarachnoid, subdural, or epidural spaces can occur, with epidural hematoma being the most common [24]. Patients present with new, severe spinal pain and rapidly progressive neurologic deficits. These conditions can be readily identified with MR imaging.

A high index of suspicion for spinal arteriovenous fistula (AVF) is necessary as this is a treatable cause of progressive myelopathy. In the majority of cases, this condition produces a myelopathy that evolves over months. Some patients present with a stepwise course with repeated episodic deterioration related to upright posture or to minor exertion. Although this disorder is most common in men in the seventh decade of life, this potentially reversible process should be considered in all patients with an otherwise unexplained progressive or subacute myelopathy [25]. Abnormal high T2 signal in the cord extending into the conus and gadolinium enhancement are typical but nonspecific MRI findings of spinal dural AVF. Presence of a focal nonenhancing area within a long segment of intense holocord enhancement ("missing piece sign") occurs in slightly less than half of cases and may provide a valuable clue to diagnosis [26]. The absence of any abnormal T2 signal is distinctly unusual in patients with dural AVF and suggests an alternate diagnosis. Detection of flow voids representing dilated veins on the surface of the spinal cord is a specific finding (Fig. 13.6), but may be seen in less than 50% of patients on standard MR imaging. Prone-supine myelography is highly sensitive for detection of dilated veins, but the invasive nature of the procedure and substantial false-positive rate limit the usefulness of myelography as a screening tool [25]. In patients with a stepwise or progressive myelopathy and radiologic findings suggestive of dural AV fistula, comprehensive spinal angiography may be warranted. Fistulae producing a progressive myelopathy may be found as high as the brainstem, and

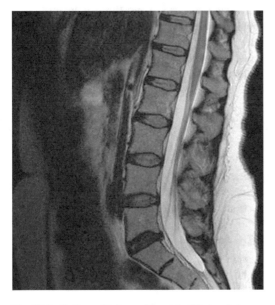

Fig. 13.4 Early cord infarct with patchy T2 signal change and swelling of the distal spinal cord, sagittal T2 MRI

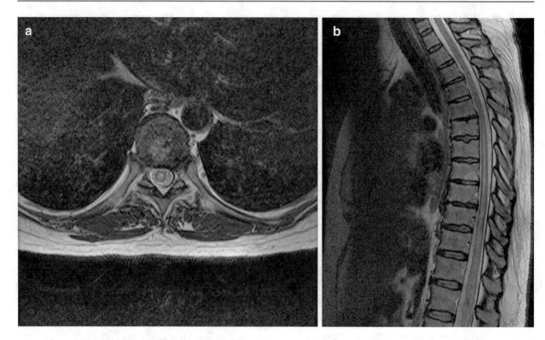

Fig. 13.5 Established cord infarct with central T2 hyperintensity. (**a**) Axial T2 MRI. (**b**) Sagittal T2 MRI

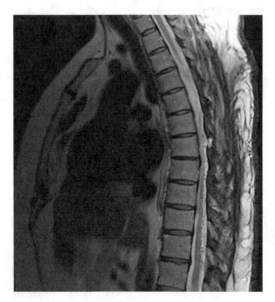

Fig. 13.6 Characteristic flow voids due to dilation of veins on the surface of the spinal cord in the setting of dural AVF, sagittal T2 MRI

accordingly one needs to be determined to detect the abnormality in cases where the clinical and screening radiologic features strongly suggest that a fistula is present.

Demyelinating Disease

Demyelinating diseases account for a substantial percentage of acute myelopathies. Distinguishing patients who have or are at risk to develop multiple sclerosis (MS) from those with less common demyelinating disorders is important for the prognosis of the patient and for selection of appropriate therapy to prevent recurrence.

In a patient presenting with a new, incomplete myelopathy, the following features on spinal MRI suggest that it is likely MS-related (Fig. 13.7):

1. Clearly circumscribed, focal T2 hyperintensity.
2. Affects only part of the cord in axial cross section, usually but not exclusively in the periphery of the spinal cord.
3. Extends over less than two vertebral segments.
4. Minimal or no cord swelling is present [27].

A careful history may elicit previous episodic neurologic symptoms suggestive of past MS

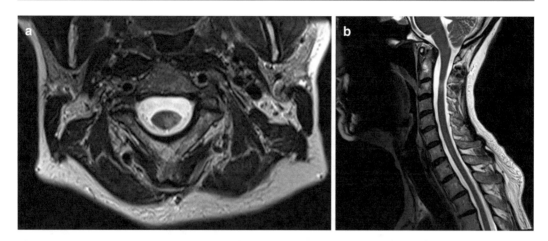

Fig. 13.7 Typical cord lesion caused by multiple sclerosis. (**a**) Axial T2 MRI. (**b**) Sagittal T2 MRI

exacerbations and support the diagnosis. MRI scan of the brain may detect typical brain lesions of multiple sclerosis (focal, T2 hyperintense lesions that are periventricular, juxtacortical, or located in the brainstem). However, nonspecific brain lesions are common due to definable (e.g., migraine, cigarette smoking) and nondefinable causes, and therefore such lesions should not be assumed to be pathognomonic of MS. Additionally, brain lesions are common in NMOSD and do not exclude that diagnosis [28].

CSF analysis to detect oligoclonal bands, preferably by isoelectric focusing, confirms a diagnosis of MS or predicts its eventual diagnosis independent of MRI findings [29]. Cerebrospinal fluid (CSF) examination is often performed, although it may be unnecessary to do so in patients with a high pretest probability of having MS based on clinical and radiographic evidence. Nevertheless, as oligoclonal bands are not present in all patients with MS and occur in other inflammatory, infectious, and neoplastic conditions, presence of oligoclonal bands should not be regarded as "diagnostic" of MS, and the result of this study should not be used to guide treatment decisions in isolation.

Certain "red flags" should prompt consideration of demyelinating processes distinct from MS. These include CSF nucleated cell count greater than 50/μL and neutrophilic predominance among CSF white blood cells, as well as cord lesions that do not meet the criteria described

above for MS. In particular, longitudinally extensive cord signal change extending over three or more vertebral segments is unusual in MS. Disorders that should be considered in this circumstance include NMOSD, myelin oligodendrocyte glycoprotein antibody-associated disease (MOGAD), acute disseminated encephalomyelitis (ADEM), idiopathic transverse myelitis, infectious myelopathies, sarcoidosis, and many other diseases mentioned in Table 13.1.

All patients with longitudinally extensive transverse myelitis (LETM) should be screened for AQP4-IgG and for MOG-IgG when AQP4-IgG is negative. The sensitivity of AQP4-IgG for NMOSD is approximately 75%, and specificity of this varies depending on the assay used, from 95% for ELISA to 99% for cell-based assays, although this will vary based on the clinical likelihood of the diagnosis [30].

Brain MRI is helpful in the evaluation of suspected NMOSD as brain MRI lesions are common in this condition. In one series of 60 NMOSD patients, 60% had an abnormal brain MRI [28]. MRI lesions have been reported in NMOSD in regions of the brain known to express high levels of aquaporin-4, including the hypothalamus and periventricular regions [5]. However, brain lesions in NMOSD patients usually differ from lesions that are characteristic of MS.

CSF findings of NMOSD differ from those of MS; oligoclonal bands are infrequent in NMOSD, and pleocytosis exceeding 50 WBC/

µL and neutrophilic pleocytosis occur in approximately 25% of cases in the context of an acute attack [31]. Occasional patients have CSF AQP4-IgG antibodies despite having negative results in serum [32].

Recent international consensus criteria for diagnosis of NMOSD have been liberalized and no longer require optic neuritis and myelitis for diagnosis. Any compatible acute syndrome including optic neuritis, myelitis, area postrema syndrome (episode of otherwise unexplained hiccups or nausea and vomiting), brainstem syndrome, or diencephalic or cerebral syndromes in a patient with demonstrated AQP4-IgG qualifies for diagnosis of NMOSD, as long as other mimics are considered and excluded [33]. Detection of AQP4-IgG in the setting of a single episode of LETM strongly predicts subsequent relapse; one series demonstrated a 55% risk of further episodes of myelitis and/or optic neuritis within 1 year in patients with a LETM who were seropositive for AQP4-IgG [34].

Patients who are seronegative for AQP4-IgG may still qualify for a diagnosis of NMOSD, but the criteria are more rigorous. They must have at least two sites of CNS involvement, one of which is spinal cord, optic nerve, or area postrema, and certain MRI criteria must be satisfied; in the case of myelitis, a contiguous spinal cord lesion extending over ≥3 vertebral segments (Fig. 13.8) is required.

Acute myelopathy may occur in the setting of ADEM, a multifocal demyelinating disorder of the CNS that typically occurs after an infectious syndrome or recent vaccination; it is more common in children than in adults. In the classic presentation, MRI demonstrates multifocal gadolinium-enhancing CNS lesions. The most specific criterion that distinguishes ADEM from MS, and is required for the diagnosis, is encephalopathy [35].

Recently it has become apparent that a subset of patients with clinical syndromes resembling attacks of NMO [9] or ADEM [36] have serum and/or CSF antibodies against native, conformationally intact myelin oligodendrocyte glycoprotein (MOG-IgG). Most authors regard MOG-antibody-associated disease as a separate

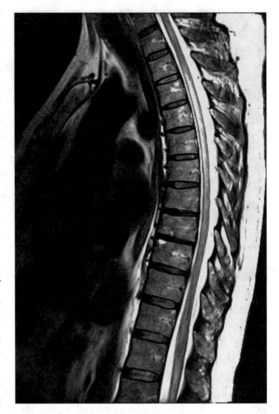

Fig. 13.8 Longitudinally extensive cord signal change associated with NMOSD, sagittal T2 MRI

clinical entity that is distinct from both MS and AQP4 antibody-positive NMOSD [37]. MOGAD is highly responsive to corticosteroids and may be less likely to relapse than MS or AQP4 antibody-positive NMOSD [38]. However, some patients with MOGAD have a severe, relapsing course associated with incapacitating neurologic disability [39]. MOG-IgG and AQP4-IgG should be investigated in those presenting with a first episode of LETM; as detection of both in the same patient is extremely rare, testing MOG-IgG only if AQP4-IgG is not detected is a reasonable practice.

Patients with a symmetric, severe acute myelopathy ("complete transverse myelitis") and/or isolated LETM with negative AQP4 and MOG-IgG antibodies may have an isolated inflammatory demyelinating transverse myelitis (i.e., idiopathic transverse myelitis) or another infectious, inflammatory, or neoplastic condition. As discussed below, serum and CSF testing may reveal evidence of a parainfectious cause in these patients; when such testing is unrevealing, clinical and radiographic follow-up is important. In patients in this group who display ongoing clinical deterioration beyond 3 weeks or have worsening findings on MRI, investigations to rule out other causes such as tumor or neurosarcoidosis may be appropriate, including spinal cord biopsy. However, spinal cord biopsy carries significant risk of neurologic injury and may be noninformative because of the small samples that can be obtained, so it should be regarded as a last approach and only when the clinical situation is dire and all other modalities have been exhausted, including search for related pathology (e.g. primary tumor, systemic sarcoidosis) and empiric therapy has failed.

Infectious

In addition to compression by an extrinsic infectious lesion such as an epidural abscess, some pathogens can produce acute or subacute myelopathies by direct infection of the cord or by inducing a parainfectious, presumably autoimmune process.

Clinical features that should prompt an increased level of suspicion for an infectious process include current or recent presence of fever, meningismus, rash, symptoms of systemic illness, recent travel, or immunosuppression. Although nonspecific, CSF pleocytosis (particularly if greater than 50 WBCs/μL) suggests this possibility. However, patients with parainfectious myelopathy often do not recall or have symptoms of a recent illness. In a review of 23 patients with parainfectious myelopathy confirmed by serological or CSF studies, only 9 (39%) recalled symptoms consistent with an infectious process in the previous month [40].

Viral infection can result in spinal cord pathology via at least two mechanisms. These include direct viral infection of neural tissue and parainfectious, presumably immune-mediated inflammation.

The nervous system is not the site of initial infection in most viruses that cause symptoms when they invade the CNS, with many of these being transmitted hematogenously via arthropod vectors (e.g., West Nile virus,) or acquired through the gastrointestinal (e.g., poliomyelitis, coxsackieviruses) or respiratory tracts (e.g., enterovirus 68) [41]. CNS invasion occurs in a small minority of infections with these viruses. In most cases, the mechanisms by which viruses enter the CNS from the periphery and the factors predisposing to this complication are poorly understood. Several of these viruses characteristically produce an acute flaccid myelitis with sparing of sensory function. Poliomyelitis is the classic example of such a condition. Poliomyelitis is now extraordinarily rare in developed countries, although it may be imported from endemic regions [42], and limited person-to-person spread in an undervaccinated community has been reported in recent years [43]. Similar clinical presentations have been associated with epidemics of enterovirus 70 (acute hemorrhagic conjunctivitis) and enterovirus 71 (hand, foot, and mouth disease) [44], as well as West Nile virus [45]. Since 2014, an increasing number of cases of acute flaccid myelitis have been observed in children, and a relationship to enterovirus D68 is strongly suspected [46]. Unfortunately, the prognosis for motor recovery in these cases is frequently poor.

Rabies is unique among human viral CNS infections in that neurons are the typical site of initial infection, usually in the peripheral nervous system after a bite from an infected animal, with retrograde transport of virus to the CNS. More rarely, transmission has been reported through the olfactory epithelium [47] and after transplant of the cornea or solid organs from an infected donor [48, 49]. Locally acquired infections in the United States are usually due to exposure to bats, and occasionally a history of a bite is not evident [50]. In the developing world, dogs remain the primary vector [51]. A minority of cases of rabies present as an ascending flaccid paralysis with spinal cord signal change [50]. The prognosis of human rabies is dismal, but early recognition of infection should be sought as rare cases of survival have been reported in recent years [52].

Certain herpes viruses, particularly varicella zoster, typically persist in the dorsal root ganglia after initial infection and may invade the CNS directly after viral reactivation. In other cases, herpes virus infections may cause spinal cord inflammation indirectly by an immune-mediated, parainfectious mechanism. A clear distinction between a parainfectious etiology and direct infection of the CNS may not be possible in some cases, and thus CSF PCR testing for herpes viruses (herpes simplex virus 1 and 2, Epstein-Barr virus, varicella zoster virus, cytomegalovirus, human herpesvirus-6) is appropriate in an unexplained myelopathy as these viruses may be treatable with specific antiviral therapies [40]. Many other viruses have been implicated as causes of parainfectious myelitis, including adenoviruses, measles [40], hepatitis C [53], SARS-CoV-2 (COVID-19) [54], and dengue [55].

Parainfectious myelitis may occur in association with recent bacterial infections, often with *Chlamydia* and *Mycoplasma* species [40]. Myelitis can occur in *Mycobacterium tuberculosis* infection either due to direct involvement of the cord or on a compressive basis in the setting of vertebral involvement (Pott disease). Bacterial myelitis can also occur, albeit rarely, with *Treponema pallidum* (syphilis) [56] or *Borrelia burgdorferi* (Lyme disease) infections [57].

Fungal and parasitic infections are rare causes of acute myelitis, but should be considered in patients at risk due to immunosuppression and/or travel exposures. Infections associated with acute myelopathies include schistosomiasis [58], strongylosis, candidiasis [40], and blastomycosis [59].

Inflammatory

In addition to inflammatory demyelinating diseases, other systemic inflammatory disorders can produce acute or subacute myelopathies. Myelopathy can occur as a complication of Sjögren syndrome or systemic lupus erythematosus. However, antibodies associated with these syndromes (e.g., ANA, SS-A) are encountered in patients with NMOSD and may occur in other inflammatory demyelinating diseases. A serological survey of 153 patients with NMOSD found ANA and SS-A antibodies in 44% and 16%,

respectively [60]. Accordingly, diagnoses of lupus or Sjögren syndrome-induced myelitis should not be made unless specific diagnostic criteria for these diseases are met and a serological test for AQP4-IgG is negative.

Behçet disease is a chronic, relapsing inflammatory disorder characterized by recurrent oral aphthous ulcers and other systemic manifestations including recurrent genital ulcerations and eye and skin lesions [61]. Spinal cord and other nervous system involvement occurs in a minority of patients with this condition, either due to direct formation of lesions in the CNS or secondary to infarct from involvement of major vascular structures [62]. Presence of a positive pathergy test (development of a nodule ≥ 2 mm in diameter 24–48 h after subcutaneous insertion of a sterile needle) is accepted as a supportive criterion for diagnosis of this disease, but this test is insensitive and does not establish a diagnosis in isolation [61]. Spinal MRI often shows a distinctive central cord lesion with T2 hypointense core and T2 hyperintense rim ("bagel sign") [63], but confident diagnosis requires presence of other characteristic systemic features.

Sarcoidosis is a non-necrotizing granulomatous inflammatory process that can involve multiple organ systems. Neurological involvement occurs in approximately 5% of cases [64]. Spinal cord involvement is one of the commonest sites of CNS involvement in neurosarcoidosis, and one recent single-center series showed that in approximately 80% of patients with spinal cord involvement, this was the initial clinical manifestation of sarcoidosis [65]. Usually, the onset is over months, but it may present more acutely in some patients. In the absence of systemic symptoms, the diagnosis of neurosarcoidosis is often difficult. Spinal imaging findings may include several patterns, but the commonest is a longitudinally extensive myelitis that can be best distinguished from other causes of myelitis with long lesions by virtue of dorsal subpial gadolinium enhancement as well as enhancement of the central canal; on axial images it gives the appearance of a trident that is highly suggestive of neurosarcoidosis ("trident sign") [66]. Other patterns include "miliary" pattern with multiple nodular enhancing parenchymal lesions, meningeal enhancement, and nerve root enhancement [65]. Persistence of enhancement for greater than 2 months is more common in sarcoidosis than in demyelinating causes of inflammatory myelopathy [67]. CSF pleocytosis is common [65]. Oligoclonal bands in the CSF have been reported in 23–51% of cases; the presence of oligoclonal bands should not automatically lead to a diagnosis of MS [65, 68, 69]. Low CSF glucose and elevated CSF angiotensin-converting enzyme (ACE) levels are less common, but may suggest sarcoidosis when present as both findings are unusual in inflammatory demyelinating diseases [67]. Although neither sensitive nor specific, an elevated serum ACE level may suggest sarcoidosis as well. In patients with imaging findings suspicious for sarcoid and those with an otherwise unexplained myelopathy, it is helpful to search for evidence of systemic sarcoid in a lesion that could be biopsied (e.g., an enlarged lymph node). PET scanning is the most sensitive modality for detecting systemic sarcoidosis, although CT imaging of the chest may also demonstrate evidence of hilar lymphadenopathy. Blind conjunctival biopsy occasionally demonstrates characteristic noncaseating granulomatous inflammation. When systemic evidence for sarcoidosis cannot be demonstrated, but the diagnosis is highly suspected because of relatively specific MRI findings, empiric corticosteroid treatment for both therapeutic and diagnostic purposes is often the best approach; dramatic and sustained improvement may yield an incomplete but acceptable level of diagnostic certainty.

Toxic/Metabolic

Metabolic disorders affecting the cord usually produce a chronic myelopathy, although many patients will not complain of symptoms until a certain level of impairment develops. In most, careful history reveals that the symptoms of myelopathy are long-standing. Nevertheless, given that the diagnosis and treatment of these disorders is associated with minimal risk, obtaining limited metabolic studies such as serum vita-

min B12, methylmalonic acid, and copper levels is appropriate in the setting of unexplained subacute or chronic myelopathies.

Acute myelopathies have occurred secondary to toxic exposures from consumption of toxic dietary staples (e.g., cassava, *Lathyrus sativus*) or recreational substance abuse (e.g., tricresyl phosphate toxicity from consumption of adulterated "Jamaican ginger" extract); many of these conditions are of limited historical or geographic relevance [70]. An exception is myelopathy secondary to nitrous oxide exposure. Nitrous oxide can produce myelopathy via irreversible oxidation of cobalamin, resulting in secondary vitamin B12 deficiency [70]. Individuals with preexisting subclinical vitamin B12 deficiency are particularly vulnerable. This condition continues to occur secondary to recreational abuse [71] and rarely in patients receiving nitrous oxide anesthesia [72] or dental professionals working in poorly ventilated offices [71]. In recreational users, specific questioning about use of nitrous oxide is important as users may be reluctant to admit this habit and unaware of its toxic potential.

Iatrogenic

Patients who have undergone radiation treatment for cancer can develop radiation myelitis when the spinal cord is included in the radiation field. This condition can present acutely during radiation treatment or in a delayed fashion. In a patient with a history of cancer, it is essential to exclude direct metastatic involvement of the epidural space prior to attributing any myelopathy to radiation effect.

Autoimmune myelitis may occur after vaccinations. Classic descriptions of postvaccination encephalomyelitis occurred in individuals who received obsolete forms of rabies vaccination, but postvaccination myelitis has been reported after a host of other common vaccinations including influenza, pertussis, diphtheria-tetanus, MMR, and hepatitis B [73]. However, the onset of myelopathy after vaccination may be purely coincidental, and recent vaccination should not deter investigations to uncover other treatable causes.

Subacute myelopathy also may result from toxic effects of intrathecal chemotherapy with several agents including methotrexate, doxorubicin, vincristine, and cytarabine [70].

Neoplastic and Paraneoplastic

Intramedullary neoplasms such as astrocytomas and ependymomas and extramedullary, intradural tumors such as meningiomas and neurofibromas may become symptomatic with a subacute time course mimicking extradural tumors or transverse myelitis. These tumors are easily visualized on MRI, although they may sometimes be confused with inflammatory lesions. Biopsy is usually required to confirm the diagnosis.

Lymphoproliferative malignancies, such as lymphomatoid granulomatosis and intravascular lymphoma, can involve the spinal cord and evolve with a subacute time course. Confident diagnosis requires biopsy of the CNS or other involved sites, although in the case of lymphomatoid granulomatosis the presence of oligoclonal bands and positive CSF PCR for Epstein-Barr virus increases the index of suspicion.

Myelitis may occur as a paraneoplastic disease. The index of suspicion for a paraneoplastic process should be increased in patients with a known history of cancer and in smokers. A serum evaluation for paraneoplastic autoantibodies should be considered in these circumstances. Certain imaging patterns may also be suspicious for a paraneoplastic etiology; we have encountered a number of patients with hyperintense T2 lesions that appear confined within individual spinal tracts in this circumstance, often symmetrically on both sides of the cord (Fig. 13.9) [74]. Paraneoplastic syndromes may produce multifocal nervous system involvement mimicking other disorders such as NMO. In particular, collapsin response-mediator protein-5 (CRMP-5) IgG antibodies can cause autoimmune myelitis and optic neuritis [75, 76].

Alternate Localizations

When there is no spinal cord abnormality on neuroimaging in the context of an apparent acute myelopathy, the responsible lesion may be elsewhere in the nervous system. The primary item on the differential diagnosis in patients with bilateral motor and sensory symptoms is an acute

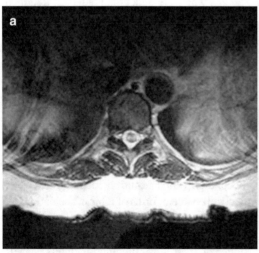
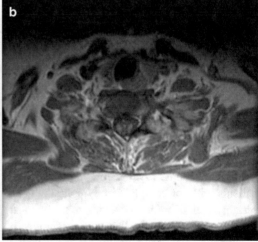

Fig. 13.9 Signal change in the central cord and lateral columns caused by paraneoplastic myelitis in the setting of renal cell carcinoma. (a) Axial T2 MRI. (b) Axial T1 MRI with gadolinium

neuropathy such as Guillain-Barré syndrome. In addition to ascending weakness, findings favoring this diagnosis include areflexia, absence of a defined sensory level, and elevated protein concentration in the CSF with a normal cell count. In patients with pure motor symptoms, myopathies and occasionally neuromuscular junction disorders can be mistaken for spinal cord disease. Parafalcine space-occupying lesions (e.g., meningioma) and bilateral anterior cerebral artery distribution infarcts occasionally present with bilateral lower limb weakness mimicking myelopathy as well.

However, the absence of an MRI abnormality should not automatically lead to the conclusion that the problem does not localize to the spinal cord. Subtle imaging abnormalities such as swelling of the cord in the absence of signal change, as occasionally seen in early cord infarct, or symptomatic epidural lipomatosis may be missed on initial review. The possibility of an "acute" presentation of a chronic metabolic, degenerative, or infectious disorder (e.g., AIDS myelopathy, tropical spastic paraparesis due to HTLV-I) should also be considered, although these conditions rarely evolve during short-term neurologic follow-up. Occasionally, patients with chronic myelopathies do not seek medical attention despite long-standing symptoms until they become associated with functional impairment and may describe new functional incapacity (e.g., inability to walk effectively) as an acute problem.

Epidemiology

Metastatic spinal cord compression is a common complication of advanced cancer, occurring in 2.5–6% of individuals with systemic malignancy ascertained in population-based studies [77, 78]. In approximately 20% of cases, cord compression is the presenting manifestation of cancer [79]. Metastases attributable to a specific cancer generally parallel the relative frequency of that cancer, with approximately half of cases attributable to carcinomas of the breast, prostate, and lung [77]. However, certain malignancies including renal cell carcinoma [77], multiple myeloma, and lymphoma [79] are disproportionately more likely to result in cord compression, whereas gastrointestinal cancers, including colorectal and pancreatic carcinoma, are disproportionately less likely to do so [78].

As MS is a relatively common disorder (prevalence estimated at 3.1 cases per 1000 in the US population [80]) and the majority of patients have imaging evidence of spinal cord involvement even at the time of diagnosis [81], MS is responsible for a substantial proportion of acute myelopathies. MS plaques in the cord often result in minimal symptoms and are asymptomatic in up to two-thirds of cases [82]. Milder myelopathic presentations with asymmetric motor and sensory involvement (i.e., "partial transverse myelitis") are the most common myelopathies that are manifestations of inaugural or established MS [83].

Other individual causes of nontraumatic, acute myelopathy are uncommon. A recent Australian series suggested an overall incidence of 24.6 cases of inflammatory myelitis per million per year, with approximately one quarter of these consistent with definite or possible "idiopathic transverse myelitis"; in most patients, inflammatory myelitis was the first symptom of MS, but not in those with long spinal cord lesions who did not have brain lesions [68]. By contrast, epidural abscess was diagnosed in 2 of 10,000 hospital admissions per year at an urban referral center [84]. Collectively, however, these less common entities constitute an important group of disorders that may need very specific treatment.

The etiology of new-onset, noncompressive myelopathy is often unclear at the time of presentation. A French series reported that the etiology of acute myelopathy could not be determined in 101 of 170 patients at onset [40]. However, careful investigation will usually reveal a cause of myelopathy. A recent series of 226 patients referred for evaluation of suspected inflammatory myelitis demonstrated that a defined etiology of myelopathy was present in 158 cases (69.9%). The most common etiologies included MS (75), vascular disorders (41), neurosarcoidosis (12), and NMOSD (12). Less than 20% of patients met criteria for "idiopathic transverse myelitis" [85]. Many patients with inflammatory disorders would likely benefit from maintenance therapies to prevent relapse. This result highlights the importance of diagnostic testing in cases of acute noncompressive myelopathy, as many patients with this type of presentation have treatable disorders with potential to result in serious future morbidity.

Demographics and Other Risk Factors

Age, gender, ethnicity, and race may suggest that a particular cause of acute myelopathy is more or less likely. Demographic features associated with selected causes of acute myelopathy are presented in Table 13.2 [25, 86–89]. Most causes of acute myelopathy are not restricted by demography, and age, gender, and ethnicity do not exclude any etiology from consideration in an individual patient.

Recognition of risk factors related to habits or other medical histories is equally important. Risk factors associated with particular causes of myelopathy are listed in Table 13.3.

Table 13.2 Demographic factors associated with specific causes of myelopathy

Metastatic spinal cord compression: prior history of malignancy, elderly patients and children; uncommon in young adults
Multiple sclerosis: median age of onset in third decade of life; more common in females
Neuromyelitis optica: relapsing form more common in women; non-Caucasians overrepresented in US patients relative to MS
Spinal cord infarct: increased risk with age; male sex
Dural arteriovenous fistula: most common in seventh decade of life; male predominance
Systemic lupus erythematosus/Sjögren syndrome: female predominance
Behçet disease: most common in patients of Middle Eastern and Far Eastern origin; more common in males of Middle Eastern origin and more severe in males
Sarcoidosis: more common in women; three–fourfold greater risk in African Americans compared to Caucasians

Table 13.3 Risk factors associated with specific causes of myelopathy

Cigarette smoking: metastatic spinal cord compression, paraneoplastic myelopathy, cord infarction
Injection drug use: epidural abscess
Nitrous oxide abuse: myelopathy due to induced vitamin B12 deficiency
Immunosuppression: epidural abscess, other infectious myelopathies
History of cancer: metastatic spinal cord compression, toxic myelopathy with history of intrathecal chemotherapy, radiation myelitis with history of radiotherapy
Obesity: epidural lipomatosis
Corticosteroid excess: epidural lipomatosis
GI malabsorption or surgery: myelopathy due to nutritional deficiency, including B12 and copper deficiency
Excess zinc ingestion: myelopathy due to copper deficiency

Clinical Features

Syndromes

Presentations of spinal cord disease are often described in terms of clinical syndromes. Spinal cord syndromes associated with specific etiologies are listed in Table 13.4. Although the type of clinical presentation seen may help to narrow the differential diagnosis, none of these syndromes are pathognomonic for any particular condition. Accordingly, recognition of other characteristic clinical features, imaging findings, and the results of other diagnostic studies are necessary for accurate diagnosis.

Brown-Séquard Syndrome

"Complete" Brown-Séquard syndrome refers to the clinical presentation seen with hemisection of the spinal cord. An affected patient has loss of motor function and dorsal column sensory modalities on the side of the lesion, with pain and temperature loss below the level of the lesion on the opposite side of the body due to disruption of the spinothalamic tract. The complete presentation is unusual; a "partial" Brown-Séquard syndrome with preservation of dorsal column sensory func-

Table 13.4 Etiologies of spinal cord syndromes

Brown-Séquard syndrome
Multiple sclerosis
Penetrating trauma
Metastatic cord compression
Epidural abscess
Parainfectious myelopathy
Anterior cord syndrome
Anterior spinal artery infarct
Disk herniation
Metastatic cord compression
Epidural abscess
Radiation myelitis
Trauma
Central cord syndrome
Syringomyelia
Intrinsic spinal cord tumor
Neuromyelitis optica
Transverse myelitis
Trauma
Posterior cord syndrome
Multiple sclerosis
Posterior spinal artery infarct
Tertiary syphilis
Subacute combined degeneration due to B12 or copper deficiency
Conus medullaris syndrome
Disk herniation
Metastatic cord compression
Intrinsic spinal cord tumor
Trauma
Dural arteriovenous fistula
Demyelinating disease
Complete cord syndrome
Idiopathic transverse myelitis
Neuromyelitis optica spectrum disorders
Trauma
Metastatic cord compression
Epidural abscess
Hemorrhage
Ischemia

tion is more common. This type of asymmetric presentation is often seen in demyelinating diseases, particularly MS, but can also occur early in the evolution of cord compression.

Anterior Cord Syndrome

In this presentation, the corticospinal and spinothalamic tracts are injured bilaterally with preservation of dorsal column sensory functions. This syndrome is seen with infarction of the anterior spinal artery but can also occur with compressive lesions.

Central Cord Syndrome

The characteristic evolution of a central cord syndrome in the setting of a syrinx was described earlier. Common features include deep, uncomfortable pain, loss of pain and temperature sensation at the level of the lesion due to disruption of the crossing fibers of the spinothalamic tracts, and impairment of motor function in the upper limbs prior to the lower limbs and trunk. In addition to syrinx and cord tumor, the features of central cord syndrome can occur with inflammatory demyelinating diseases, particularly neuromyelitis optica.

Posterior Cord Syndrome

Isolated involvement of the dorsal columns is most commonly seen in the setting of a chronic myelopathy; tabes dorsalis in the setting of tertiary syphilis is a classic example. This syndrome occasionally occurs due to infarction of a posterior spinal artery.

Conus Medullaris Syndrome

Myelopathy confined to the terminal portion of the spinal cord results in flaccid paralysis of the bladder and anal sphincters. The presentation may occur as a component of a more extensive cord lesion involving the conus or be quite isolated. There are multiple causes including compression, dural arteriovenous fistula, neoplasm, and demyelination. One needs to distinguish this presentation from a cauda equina syndrome. Compression or inflammation of the cauda equina produces lower motor neuron findings including weakness and reflex loss in the lower limbs corresponding to the involved nerve roots as well as sensory changes in the dermatomes innervated by involved sensory roots. Pain is usual in cauda equina syndrome; bowel and bladder involvement is variable depending on the levels involved.

Complete Cord Syndrome

The clinical picture of complete transection of the spinal cord at the level of the lesion (absence of all sensory modalities and motor function below the lesion) is described as the complete cord syndrome. This type of presentation occurs with severe idiopathic transverse myelitis and NMOSD and is also a common presentation of an extradural compressive lesion producing severe cord compression.

Symptoms

Although many symptoms of acute cord injury are nonspecific, certain symptoms are characteristic and suggestive of particular conditions.

Pain is not unique to cord compression, but is an important "red flag." In the majority of cases of metastatic SCC, pain precedes the onset of other neurologic symptoms. Pain in the thoracic region is particularly concerning, not only because the majority of metastatic cord compressions occur in this region [90] but also because "benign," musculoskeletal and radicular causes of pain in the thoracic spine are far less common than in the neck or low back. Pain that worsens at night or with recumbent position is also suggestive of cord compression.

A history of prior neurological symptoms is often informative in the diagnosis of inflammatory demyelinating diseases. A history of previous episodic visual, motor, urinary, or sensory disturbances lasting greater than 24 h may suggest previously unrecognized MS exacerbations. A history of clear worsening of neurologic symptoms in response to heat or a reproducible "shock-like" sensation traveling down the spine with forward flexion of the neck (Lhermitte sign) is quite suggestive of demyelination. Paroxysmal tonic spasms (brief, involuntary muscle contractions typically lasting from 15 to 60 s at a time) are a less common but highly specific indicator of an inflammatory demyelinating disease. A history of episodes of intractable vomiting or hiccups is now recognized as a common harbinger of NMO spectrum disorders [91, 92].

Time Course

Myelopathies can develop suddenly, acutely (<24 h to 3 weeks), subacutely (over weeks to months), or insidiously. Apoplectic onset of symptoms often suggests a vascular etiology such as an ischemic cord infarct or occasionally a hemorrhage. Compressive lesions can also present abruptly, as in the case of an acute disk herniation or a pathologic fracture in the setting of malignancy. Inflammatory disorders usually do not present instantaneously, but patients may awaken with new symptoms and thereby confound the determination of the mode of onset.

Many etiologies of myelopathy, such as demyelinating diseases, other inflammatory disorders, and cord compression, reach maximal severity over days to a few weeks. Other conditions that can present with a similar time course include parainfectious myelopathy, radiation myelitis, and paraneoplastic myelitis. Disorders that evolve over weeks or longer include spinal stenosis, dural arteriovenous fistula, chronic infections (e.g., HIV myelopathy, HTLV-I, tertiary syphilis), metabolic disorders, and intradural and intramedullary tumors.

Diagnosis

Neuroimaging and, to a lesser extent, other diagnostic studies are essential for accurate diagnosis of acute and subacute myelopathies given the lack of specificity of clinical and demographic features. A stepwise approach to diagnostic testing is discussed; specific features suggestive of particular disorders were presented earlier.

Spine MRI

MRI scan of the spine is the key diagnostic procedure in the assessment of acute cord lesions. MR imaging is superior to other modalities in visualizing soft tissue and is accordingly the procedure of choice in assessing inflammatory, vascular, infectious, and metabolic myelopathies. MRI has also supplanted CT myelography as the preferred procedure in cases of suspected cord compression. In metastatic SCC, MRI is equally sensitive and more specific than CT myelography [93, 94]. Additionally, myelography may result in neurologic deterioration in patients with severe compression who have complete block of the flow of myelographic dye.

Patients with cord compression may experience significant neurologic deterioration over a period of a few hours. When suspected, MR imaging should be obtained on an emergent basis and not delayed. If a compressive lesion is identified, definitive treatment with surgery or radiotherapy is indicated. Although additional testing to identify the underlying condition causing compression is important, treatment is urgently needed and should not be delayed to obtain additional testing; however, radiotherapy may not be provided until a definitive diagnosis of cancer is obtained at the time of surgery in patients without an established history of cancer. When abnormal signal is apparent within the substance of the cord, a review of the past history, clinical presentation, and imaging findings may suggest a particular diagnosis. However, in many cases further studies are necessary.

CSF Examination

A CSF examination is often the next step in the evaluation of a noncompressive myelopathy. CSF examination is usually not helpful in diagnosing the cause of spinal cord compression and may result in neurologic deterioration in patients with severe cord compression. Routine CSF studies should include cell count with differential, glucose and protein concentration, oligoclonal banding, and cytologic examination; it is often helpful to retain spinal fluid to allow for additional testing informed by the results of the initial screening tests.

Brain MRI

In cases of acute, noncompressive myelopathy, brain MR imaging is useful to detect features suggestive of demyelinating disease. In the setting of an asymmetric partial transverse myelitis, detection of brain lesions consistent with MS strongly suggests that the presentation is due to inflammatory demyelinating disease. In patients with a clinically isolated demyelinating syndrome, the finding of typical MS lesions on brain MRI predicts an approximately 90% chance of developing clinically definite MS in the future [95]. However, a normal brain MRI scan does not exclude the diagnosis of a demyelinating disease. It is also important to distinguish the typical periventricular, juxtacortical, and brainstem lesions of MS from nonspecific T2 signal abnormalities in the deep subcortical white matter, which do not have the same diagnostic implications when seen in isolation.

Blood/Serology

Serum AQP4-IgG and, if negative, MOG-IgG serologies should be obtained in patients with unexplained longitudinally extensive ($\geq$3 vertebral segments in length) signal abnormality regardless of whether or not a patient has a past history of optic neuritis. Cell-based assays using proteins expressed in native conformation and not denatured proteins are necessary to achieve both optimal specificity and sensitivity, especially for MOG-IgG [96]. Patients with a history of optic neuritis and partial transverse myelitis *without* longitudinally extensive cord signal change are *unlikely* to have NMOSD, although 15% of patients with AQP4-IgG have lesions shorter than three vertebral segments, and this may be even more common in patients who are on immunosuppression. MS is a more likely diagnosis for patients with short myelitis lesions, especially if these lesions are peripheral. MOG-IgG antibodies have somewhat lesser specificity than AQP4-IgG, and therefore, positive results in patients with a low pretest clinical probability of MOGAD should be viewed with suspicion [37].

In patients with isolated myelitis and otherwise normal CNS imaging, acute and convalescent viral serologies may yield evidence supporting a role of common pathogens associated with infectious and parainfectious myelopathy. CSF PCR and IgM studies may be a more reliable marker of recent infection. Detecting evidence of recent infection with herpes viruses is important as patients may respond to specific antiviral therapy with acyclovir and related antiviral agents. Even in cases where a positive result does not alter the treatment strategy, finding evidence of a recent infection may limit the need for additional diagnostic testing.

When an underlying systemic inflammatory disease is suspected, obtaining an antinuclear antibody (ANA), anti-double-stranded DNA antibodies, antibodies to extractable nuclear antigens (e.g., SS-A), and antineutrophil cytoplasmic antibodies (p-ANCA and c-ANCA) may be useful to screen for systemic inflammatory and vasculitic disorders. However, when clinical and radiographic findings strongly suggest an inflammatory demyelinating disease, a "positive" serologic result, such as a positive ANA, is unlikely to indicate an alternate diagnosis, especially considering the nonspecificity of this antibody. A "panel" of serologic markers of autoimmunity to screen for "mimics" of multiple sclerosis is not helpful and may be misleading given the high frequency of false-positive results when used as a screening test.

Blood/Others

Additional laboratory tests may be valuable in diagnosing the cause of a compressive myelopathy, although usually not essential to emergent management. In cases where cord compression is the initial manifestation of an occult cancer, prostate-specific antigen testing and monoclonal protein studies of the serum and urine (often pos-

itive in multiple myeloma and other plasma cell dyscrasias) may suggest an underlying malignancy. When epidural abscess is considered, blood cultures should be obtained from two separate sites, ideally prior to the institution of empiric antibiotic therapy. The yield of blood cultures in epidural abscess is approximately 60%, with the most common organism being *Staphylococcus aureus* [97].

Other Imaging Studies

In patients who are unable to undergo MRI because of implanted MRI-incompatible medical devices, presence of magnetic foreign bodies, or body habitus, CT myelography is an alternative imaging modality to exclude compression.

CT imaging of the chest, abdomen, and pelvis may reveal an underlying cancer in cases of occult malignancy presenting with cord compression. In noncompressive myelopathies that are atypical for demyelinating disease, CT imaging may also be useful to screen for lymphadenopathy suggestive of sarcoidosis or lymphoma. Positron emission tomography (PET) scan can detect metabolically active lymph nodes in cases of sarcoidosis as well as an otherwise occult malignancy in cases of cord compression or finding of a positive paraneoplastic autoantibody.

Treatment

Compressive

Despite availability of MR imaging, delays in the treatment of metastatic cord compression remain common. In one series of 301 patients, only 33% were ambulatory at the time of treatment, unchanged from the era prior to MR imaging. Most had experienced deterioration in motor function *after* initial presentation to a medical practitioner before definitive treatment was instituted [1]. Patients who are nonambulatory often remain so; nearly 40% of nonambulant patients remain unable to walk after treatment [98]. In contrast, 80–100% of spinal cord compression patients who are ambulatory at the time of treatment initiation remain ambulatory [77, 99–101]. Accordingly, rapid identification of cord compression and early definitive treatment are essential for optimal outcomes. Corticosteroids and surgical decompression were proven effective for treatment of metastatic spinal cord compression in controlled clinical trials, and the standard of care also includes radiotherapy.

A single placebo-controlled trial addressed the use of corticosteroids as an adjunct to radiation therapy in metastatic cord compression. The treatment group received 96 mg of intravenous (IV) dexamethasone at presentation and then 24 mg of oral dexamethasone four times daily for 3 days followed by taper. At the conclusion of treatment, 81% of the dexamethasone-treated group versus 59% of the placebo-treated group were ambulatory; at 6 months, 63% of patients in the treatment group versus 33% of the placebo-treated group were ambulatory [102]. Two small trials comparing high-dose dexamethasone (96–100 mg initial IV dose) to lower doses (10–16 mg) did not demonstrate a statistically significant difference in outcome between the two doses [103, 104].

Patchell and colleagues reported a randomized but nonblinded trial of direct decompressive surgery for metastatic cord compression followed by radiotherapy versus radiotherapy alone. Patients in the surgery group were more likely to remain ambulatory (84% versus 57%, p 0.001) and for a longer interval (median 122 days versus 13 days, p 0.003) compared to the radiotherapy only group. In patients unable to walk prior to treatment, a higher percentage of surgically treated patients regained that capacity (62% versus 19%, p 0.01). Patients with lymphoma were excluded as this tumor is considered highly radiosensitive, as were those who had been non-ambulatory for greater than 48 h. On the basis of this trial, surgery is recommended for symptomatic patients with spinal cord compression who would be able to tolerate it [98].

In patients who are poor surgical candidates due to baseline functional status or short life expectancy, radiotherapy alone is also beneficial in relieving pain and preserving ambulatory capacity [100]. No specific radiotherapy regimen has been proven superior. In the United States, patients often receive 30 Gy to the involved area in equal doses over 10 days. Some authors have advocated lower doses, with doses as low as 8 Gy in a single fraction appearing beneficial in a randomized trial [105].

The treatment of other causes of spinal cord compression is usually surgical. Although no controlled trials have addressed the issue of surgical versus medical management of epidural abscess, surgical decompression followed by antibiotic treatment is considered the standard of care for this condition [106]. Surgery is also indicated in patients with symptomatic compression on the basis of degenerative spine disease and/or a congenitally narrow spinal canal.

Vascular

No treatment of spinal cord infarction is proven effective, and management is supportive. In patients with evidence of spinal cord injury after aortic surgery, a protocol for hemodynamic augmentation of the blood pressure with vasopressors and use of lumbar drainage has been advocated. This strategy has not been validated in a clinical trial, but good outcomes have been reported with this protocol in patients presenting with delayed evidence of cord ischemia after surgery on the thoracic aorta [107]. Similar treatment might be considered in patients with early cord ischemia due to other causes, but efficacy has not been established. There are a limited number of reports of successful use of catheter-guided intra-arterial thrombolysis for cord infarction [108, 109]. The primary limitation of thrombolysis is the narrow window of opportunity for successful administration, especially considering the difficulties inherent in determining the etiology of an acute myelopathy and excluding contraindications to thrombolysis.

Dural arteriovenous fistulae and other spinal cord arteriovenous malformations should be treated with surgical or endovascular obliteration of the fistula. Improvement in functional status in these conditions can occur even when treatment has been delayed for up to several years [110].

Approach to Suspected Inflammatory and Other Myelopathies

Given the relative rarity of many causes of acute, noncompressive myelopathy and the difficult ethics of conducting controlled trials in patients with devastating acute neurologic conditions, there is a dearth of controlled clinical trial data for these disorders. We present a general approach to management in which empiric, early treatment is instituted, while additional diagnostic studies are conducted to refine the diagnosis.

After cord compression has been excluded by neuroimaging, clinicians must decide whether the history, clinical presentation, and imaging are sufficient to define a particular diagnosis. Often, the diagnosis is not immediately apparent. In most of these cases, initial treatment with high-dose steroids is appropriate. Traditionally, high-dose steroids were delivered intravenously (e.g., methylprednisolone 1 gram IV daily for 5 days), although recent studies have suggested that high-dose oral steroids at an equivalent dose (e.g., prednisone 1250 mg daily for 5 days) are equally effective [111]. Although corticosteroid treatment is of unproven benefit for many causes of acute myelopathy, the treatment is regarded to be highly effective for transverse myelitis of a variety of causes. Even if the diagnosis of a primary inflammatory process is incorrect, corticosteroids may be beneficial in reducing inflammation and edema and rarely would worsen the underlying disease process causing an acute myelopathy. Accordingly, most patients should be offered corticosteroid treatment empirically when an inflammatory myelopathy is being considered. In cases in which infectious etiologies are suspected, particularly bacterial and fungal infections, it is often best to defer steroid administration until the diagnosis of infection can be confirmed or refuted. Corticosteroid treatment causes clinical deterioration in patients with dural arteriovenous fistula, and therefore, when this diagnosis is seriously considered, corticosteroids should not be administered [112–114].

Patients who do not respond to initial steroid treatment and who do not have evidence of a non-inflammatory disorder, such as cord infarction, may benefit from plasma exchange. A randomized, sham-controlled trial of plasma exchange in patients with severe attacks of acute CNS demyelination unresponsive to high-dose steroids demonstrated a 42.1% rate of moderate or greater improvement with plasmapheresis as compared to 5.9% for sham treatment [115]. Factors reported to predict a beneficial response to plasma exchange include male sex, preservation of reflexes, and early onset of treatment [116]. When plasma exchange is employed, patients typically receive 5–7 exchanges, although no trials have established the optimum number of treatments.

In patients who stabilize or improve, assessment for an underlying demyelinating disease should be conducted as described previously. Patients with features suggestive of MS or a high risk of developing this condition should be considered for disease-modifying therapy. The institution of such therapies is not urgent and should be offered after careful consideration as to the nature of the underlying disorder, such as MS versus NMOSD. Multiple oral, injectable, and parenteral therapies are available, and there is no consensus as to whether early use of any particular group of treatments improves overall outcomes, although ongoing clinical trials addressing early use of "highly active" (i.e., parenteral) therapies versus an "escalation" approach may inform this decision in the near future. At present, we recommend selection of disease-modifying therapy based on patient risk factors, comorbidities, and patient preference [117].

Patients who meet diagnostic criteria for NMOSD or those seropositive for AQP4-IgG are at high risk for additional, clinically severe episodes of demyelination, and early institution of long-term immunosuppressant therapy for patients in these categories is indicated. Approved therapies for AQP4-IgG seropositive NMO include eculizumab [118] and inebilizumab [119]. Historically, other immune suppressants including azathioprine [120], mycophenolate mofetil [121], and rituximab have also been used [122]; there is insufficient evidence to establish whether one of these agents is superior as an initial treatment. There is no current consensus on whether to start long-term immune therapies in patients with MOG-IgG antibodies who have had a single clinical attack; those patients with a history of multiple relapses should be treated with immunosuppressive medications and not disease-modifying treatments for MS, except for anti-CD20 monoclonal antibodies, which may be appropriate.

Patients with subacute myelopathy who are not improving with treatment and have no diagnosis after a thorough search for infectious and systemic inflammatory disorders may be candidates for biopsy of the spinal cord; the primary goals are to exclude malignancy and identify certain inflammatory disorders with characteristic histology (e.g., neurosarcoidosis). When neuroimaging is highly suggestive, empiric long-term corticosteroid treatment for a presumptive diagnosis of neurosarcoidosis may be appropriate without biopsy, but such decisions are difficult and risk missing an alternate etiology that requires different treatment.

When a chronic inflammatory disorder such as sarcoidosis is identified, patients require initiation of treatment, usually with a prolonged course of moderate dose steroids (i.e., prednisone 1 mg/kg/day for one or more months, with gradual taper). Steroid-sparing immune-suppressive agents should also be considered in patients with an established chronic or relapsing course. Several immune therapies are anecdotally reported to be of benefit in sarcoidosis, with methotrexate, azathioprine, and mycophenolate mofetil among the most commonly employed [123, 124]. Tumor necrosis factor (TNF)-alpha inhibitors have shown promise for treatment of refractory disease [124]. Treatment with CD20 monoclonal antibodies (e.g., rituximab) has also been employed, with variable response [125, 126], and these should not be used as first-line agents for treatment of CNS sarcoidosis.

Conclusion

The initial priority in assessment of an acute or subacute myelopathy is to obtain neuroimaging to determine whether cord compression is present. Patients with symptomatic cord compression require urgent intervention, usually with surgical treatment. In patients with noncompressive cord signal abnormality, high-dose steroid therapy (e.g., methylprednisolone 1000 mg IV for 5 days) is appropriate in most cases of idiopathic, inflammatory, or demyelinating myelopathy. Subsequent investigations are guided by the history and clinical response. Patients who improve or stabilize within 3 weeks often have an inflammatory disease such as MS or NMOSD, a clinically isolated demyelinating syndrome, or idiopathic transverse myelitis. Brain MRI and CSF studies in these patients are helpful in determining the likelihood of future recurrence. In patients who continue to progress for greater than 3 weeks, one should consider neoplasm, chronic inflammatory disorders including sarcoidosis, and occult compression, such as may occur with spinal stenosis. If a diagnosis cannot be determined despite thoughtful investigations and the patient continues to worsen, biopsy may be required to determine the diagnosis and guide therapeutic intervention, but this should only be undertaken when there is a dire need to establish a diagnosis because of continuing deterioration and when all other informative diagnostic approaches have been exhausted.

References

1. Husband DJ. Malignant spinal cord compression: prospective study of delays in referral and treatment. Br Med J. 1998;317(7150):18–21.
2. Siegal T. Spinal cord compression: from laboratory to clinic. Eur J Cancer. 1995;31A(11):1748–53.
3. Lennon VA, Wingerchuk DM, Kryzer TJ, Pittock SJ, Lucchinetti CF, Fujihara K, et al. A serum autoantibody marker of neuromyelitis optica: distinction from multiple sclerosis. Lancet. 2004;364(9451):2106–12.
4. Flanagan EP, Weinshenker BG, Krecke KN, Lennon VA, Lucchinetti CF, McKeon A, et al. Short myclitis lesions in aquaporin-4-IgG-positive neuromy-

elitis optica spectrum disorders. JAMA Neurol. 2015;72(1):81–7.

5. Pittock SJ, Weinshenker BG, Lucchinetti CF, Wingerchuk DM, Corboy JR, Lennon VA. Neuromyelitis optica brain lesions localized at sites of high aquaporin 4 expression. Arch Neurol. 2006;63(7):964–8.

6. Bradl M, Misu T, Takahashi T, Watanabe M, Mader S, Reindl M, et al. Neuromyelitis optica: pathogenicity of patient immunoglobulin in vivo. Ann Neurol. 2009;66(5):630–43.

7. Kinoshita M, Nakatsuji Y, Kimura T, Moriya M, Takata K, Okuno T, et al. Neuromyelitis optica: passive transfer to rats by human immunoglobulin. Biochem Biophys Res Commun. 2009;386(4):623–7.

8. Hinson SR, Roemer SF, Lucchinetti CF, Fryer JP, Kryzer TJ, Chamberlain JL, et al. Aquaporin-4-binding autoantibodies in patients with neuromyelitis optica impair glutamate transport by down-regulating EAAT2. J Exp Med. 2008;205(11):2473–81.

9. Kitley J, Woodhall M, Waters P, Leite MI, Devenney E, Craig J, et al. Myelin-oligodendrocyte glycoprotein antibodies in adults with a neuromyelitis optica phenotype. Neurology. 2012;79(12):1273–7.

10. Dubey D, Pittock SJ, Krecke KN, Morris PP, Sechi E, Zalewski NL, et al. Clinical, radiologic, and prognostic features of myelitis associated with myelin oligodendrocyte glycoprotein autoantibody. JAMA Neurol. 2019;76(3):301–9.

11. Fang L, Kang X, Wang Z, Wang S, Wang J, Zhou Y, et al. Myelin oligodendrocyte glycoprotein-IgG contributes to oligodendrocytopathy in the presence of complement, distinct from astrocytopathy induced by AQP-4 IgG. Neurosci Bull. 2019;35(5):853–66.

12. Kelley BJ, Erickson BJ, Weinshenker BW. Compressive myelopathy mimicking transverse myelitis. Neurologist. 2010;16(2):120–2.

13. Flanagan EP, Krecke KN, Marsh RW, Giannini C, Keegan BM, Weinshenker BG. Specific pattern of gadolinium enhancement in spondylotic myelopathy. Ann Neurol. 2014;76(1):54–65.

14. Oustwani MB, Kurtides ES, Christ M, Ciric I. Spinal cord compression with paraplegia in myelofibrosis. Arch Neurol. 1980;37(6):389–90.

15. Al-Khawaja D, Seex K, Eslick GD. Spinal epidural lipomatosis—a brief review. J Clin Neurosci. 2008;15(12):1323–6.

16. Birmingham C, Tibbles C, Friedberg R. An unusual cause of spontaneous paralysis. J Emerg Med. 2009;36(3):290–5.

17. Kim DH, Hilibrand AS. Rheumatoid arthritis in the cervical spine. J Am Acad Orthop Surg. 2005;13(7):463–74.

18. Nader-Sepahi A, Casey AT, Hayward R, Crockard HA, Thompson D. Symptomatic atlantoaxial instability in Down syndrome. J Neurosurg. 2005;103(3 Suppl):231–7.

19. Patten J. Neurological differential diagnosis. 2nd ed. London: Springer; 1996.

20. Prattico F, Perfetti P, Gabrieli A, Longo D, Caroselli C, Ricci G. Chiari I malformation with syrinx: an unexpected diagnosis in the emergency department. Eur J Emerg Med. 2008;15(6):342–3.

21. Sullivan LP, Stears JC, Ringel SP. Resolution of syringomyelia and Chiari I malformation by ventriculoatrial shunting in a patient with pseudotumor cerebri and a lumboperitoneal shunt. Neurosurgery. 1988;22(4):744–7.

22. Zalewski NL, Rabinstein AA, Krecke KN, Brown RD Jr, Wijdicks EFM, Weinshenker BG, et al. Characteristics of spontaneous spinal cord infarction and proposed diagnostic criteria. JAMA Neurol. 2019;76(1):56–63.

23. Chao CH, Tsai TH, Huang TY, Lee KS, Hwang SL. Idiopathic spontaneous intraspinal intramedullary hemorrhage: a report of two cases and literature review. Clin Neurol Neurosurg. 2013;115(7):1134–6.

24. Ruff RL, Dougherty JH Jr. Complications of lumbar puncture followed by anticoagulation. Stroke. 1981;12(6):879 81.

25. Gilbertson JR, Miller GM, Goldman MS, Marsh WR. Spinal dural arteriovenous fistulas: MR and myelographic findings. Am J Neuroradiol. 1995;16(10):2049–57.

26. Zalewski NL, Rabinstein AA, Brinjikji W, Kaufmann TJ, Nasr D, Ruff MW, et al. Unique gadolinium enhancement pattern in spinal dural arteriovenous fistulas. JAMA Neurol. 2018;75(12):1542–5.

27. Polman CH, Reingold SC, Edan G, Filippi M, Hartung HP, Kappos L, et al. Diagnostic criteria for multiple sclerosis: 2005 revisions to the "McDonald Criteria". Ann Neurol. 2005;58(6):840–6.

28. Pittock SJ, Lennon VA, Krecke K, Wingerchuk DM, Lucchinetti CF, Weinshenker BG. Brain abnormalities in neuromyelitis optica. Arch Neurol. 2006;63(3):390–6.

29. Tintoré M, Rovira A, Río J, Tur C, Pelayo R, Nos C, et al. Do oligoclonal bands add information to MRI in first attacks of multiple sclerosis? Neurology. 2008;70(13 Pt 2):1079–83.

30. Melamed E, Levy M, Waters PJ, Sato DK, Bennett JL, John GR, et al. Update on biomarkers in neuromyelitis optica. Neurol Neuroimmunol Neuroinflamm. 2015;2(4):e134.

31. O'Riordan JI, Gallagher HL, Thompson AJ, Howard RS, Kingsley DP, Thompson EJ, et al. Clinical, CSF, and MRI findings in Devic's neuromyelitis optica. J Neurol Neurosurg Psychiatry. 1996;60(4):382–7.

32. Klawiter EC, Alvarez E, Xu J, Paciorkowski AR, Zhu L, Parks BJ, et al. NMO-IgG detected in CSF in seronegative neuromyelitis optica. Neurology. 2009;72(12):1101–3.

33. Wingerchuk DM, Banwell B, Bennett JL, Cabre P, Carroll W, Chitnis T, et al. International consensus diagnostic criteria for neuromyelitis optica spectrum disorders. Neurology. 2015;85(2):177–89.

34. Weinshenker BG, Wingerchuk DM, Vukusic S, Linbo L, Pittock SJ, Lucchinetti CF, et al.

Neuromyelitis optica IgG predicts relapse after longitudinally extensive transverse myelitis. Ann Neurol. 2006;59(3):566–9.

35. Wingerchuk DM. Postinfectious encephalomyelitis. Curr Neurol Neurosci Rep. 2003;3(3):256–64.

36. de Mol CL, Wong Y, van Pelt ED, Wokke B, Siepman T, Neuteboom RF, et al. The clinical spectrum and incidence of anti-MOG-associated acquired demyelinating syndromes in children and adults. Mult Scler. 2020;26(7):806–14.

37. Jarius S, Paul F, Aktas O, Asgari N, Dale RC, de Seze J, et al. MOG encephalomyelitis: international recommendations on diagnosis and antibody testing. J Neuroinflammation. 2018;15(1):134.

38. Cobo-Calvo A, Ruiz A, Maillart E, Audoin B, Zephir H, Bourre B, et al. Clinical spectrum and prognostic value of CNS MOG autoimmunity in adults: the MOGADOR study. Neurology. 2018;90(21):e1858–69.

39. Jurynczyk M, Messina S, Woodhall MR, Raza N, Everett R, Roca-Fernandez A, et al. Clinical presentation and prognosis in MOG-antibody disease: a UK study. Brain. 2017;140(12):3128–38.

40. Debette S, de Sèze J, Pruvo JP, Zephir H, Pasquier F, Leys D, et al. Long-term outcome of acute and subacute myelopathies. J Neurol. 2009;256(6):980–8.

41. Solomon T, Willison H. Infectious causes of acute flaccid paralysis. Curr Opin Infect Dis. 2003;16(5):375–81.

42. Stewardson AJ, Roberts JA, Beckett CL, Prime HT, Loh PS, Thorley BR, et al. Imported case of poliomyelitis, Melbourne, Australia, 2007. Emerg Infect Dis. 2009;15(1):63–5.

43. Alexander JP, Ehresmann K, Seward J, Wax G, Harriman K, Fuller S, et al. Transmission of imported vaccine-derived poliovirus in an under-vaccinated community in Minnesota. J Infect Dis. 2009;199(3):391–7.

44. Palacios G, Oberste MS. Enteroviruses as agents of emerging infectious diseases. J Neurovirol. 2005;11(5):424–33.

45. Li J, Loeb JA, Shy ME, Shah AK, Tselis AC, Kupski WJ, et al. Asymmetric flaccid paralysis: a neuromuscular presentation of West Nile virus infection. Ann Neurol. 2003;53(6):703–10.

46. Helfferich J, Knoester M, Van Leer-Buter CC, Neuteboom RF, Meiners LC, Niesters HG, et al. Acute flaccid myelitis and enterovirus D68: lessons from past and present. Eur J Pediatr. 2019;178(9):1305–15.

47. Mori I. Transolfactory neuroinvasion by viruses threatens the human brain. Acta Virol. 2015;59(4):338–49.

48. Houff SA, Burton RC, Wilson RW, Henson TE, London WT, Baer GM, et al. Human-to-human transmission of rabies virus by corneal transplant. N Engl J Med. 1979;300(11):603–4.

49. Lu XX, Zhu WY, Wu GZ. Rabies virus transmission via solid organs or tissue allotransplantation. Infect Dis Poverty. 2018;7(1):82.

50. Human rabies—Minnesota, 2007. MMWR Morb Mortal Wkly Rep. 2008;57(17):460–2.

51. Hampson K, Coudeville L, Lembo T, Sambo M, Kieffer A, Attlan M, et al. Estimating the global burden of endemic canine rabies. PLoS Negl Trop Dis. 2015;9(4):e0003709.

52. Willoughby RE Jr, Tieves KS, Hoffman GM, Ghanayem NS, Amlie-Lefond CM, Schwabe MJ, et al. Survival after treatment of rabies with induction of coma. N Engl J Med. 2005;352(24):2508–14.

53. Aktipi KM, Ravaglia S, Ceroni M, Nemni R, Debiaggi M, Bastianello S, et al. Severe recurrent myelitis in patients with hepatitis C viral infection. Neurology. 2007;68(6):468–9.

54. Sotoca J, Rodríguez-Álvarez Y. COVID-19-associated acute necrotizing myelitis. Neurol Neuroimmunol Neuroinflamm. 2020;7(5):e803.

55. Seet RC, Lim EC, Wilder-Smith EP. Acute transverse myelitis following dengue virus infection. J Clin Virol. 2006;35(3):310–2.

56. Chilver-Stainer L, Fischer U, Hauf M, Fux CA, Sturzenegger M. Syphilitic myelitis: rare, nonspecific, but treatable. Neurology. 2009;72(7):673–5.

57. Lesca G, Deschamps R, Lubetzki C, Levy R, Assous M. Acute myelitis in early Borrelia burgdorferi infection. J Neurol. 2002;249(10):1472–4.

58. Haribhai HC, Bhigjee AI, Bill PL, Pammenter MD, Modi G, Hoffmann M, et al. Spinal cord schistosomiasis. A clinical, laboratory and radiological study, with a note on therapeutic aspects. Brain. 1991;114(Pt 2):709–26.

59. Parr AM, Fewer D. Intramedullary blastomycosis in a child: case report. Can J Neurol Sci. 2004;31(2):282–5.

60. Pittock SJ, Lennon VA, de Seze J, Vermersch P, Homburger HA, Wingerchuk DM, et al. Neuromyelitis optica and non organ-specific autoimmunity. Arch Neurol. 2008;65(1):78–83.

61. International Study Group for Behcet's. Disease criteria for diagnosis of Behcet's disease. Lancet. 1990;335(8697):1078–80.

62. Serdaroglu P. Behcet's disease and the nervous system. J Neurol. 1998;245(4):197–205.

63. Uygunoglu U, Zeydan B, Ozguler Y, Ugurlu S, Seyahi E, Kocer N, et al. Myelopathy in Behçet's disease: the bagel sign. Ann Neurol. 2017;82(2):288–98.

64. Stern BJ, Krumholz A, Johns C, Scott P, Nissim J. Sarcoidosis and its neurological manifestations. Arch Neurol. 1985;42(9):909–17.

65. Murphy OC, Salazar-Camelo A, Jimenez JA, Barreras P, Reyes MI, Garcia MA, et al. Clinical and MRI phenotypes of sarcoidosis-associated myelopathy. Neurol Neuroimmunol Neuroinflamm. 2020;7(4):e722.

66. Zalewski NL, Krecke KN, Weinshenker BG, Aksamit AJ, Conway BL, McKeon A, et al. Central canal enhancement and the trident sign in spinal cord sarcoidosis. Neurology. 2016;87(7):743–4.

67. Flanagan EP, Kaufmann TJ, Krecke KN, Aksamit AJ, Pittock SJ, Keegan BM, et al. Discriminating

long myelitis of neuromyelitis optica from sarcoidosis. Ann Neurol. 2016;79(3):437–47.

68. McLean BN, Miller D, Thompson EJ. Oligoclonal banding of IgG in CSF, blood–brain barrier function, and MRI findings in patients with sarcoidosis, systemic lupus erythematosus, and Behcet's disease involving the nervous system. J Neurol Neurosurg Psychiatry. 1995;58(5):548–54.

69. Joseph FG, Scolding NJ. Neurosarcoidosis: a study of 30 new cases. J Neurol Neurosurg Psychiatry. 2009;80(3):297–304.

70. Kumar N. Metabolic myelopathies and myeloneuropathies. In: Noseworthy JH, editor. Neurologic therapeutics principles and practice. Milton Park: Informa Health Care; 2006. p. 1766–81.

71. Layzer RB. Myeloneuropathy after prolonged exposure to nitrous oxide. Lancet. 1978;2(8102):1227–30.

72. Schilling RF. Is nitrous oxide a dangerous anesthetic for vitamin B12-deficient subjects? J Am Med Assoc. 1986;255(12):1605–6.

73. Huynh W, Cordato DJ, Kehdi E, Masters LT, Dedousis C. Post-vaccination encephalomyelitis: literature review and illustrative case. J Clin Neurosci. 2008;15(12):1315–22.

74. Jacob A, Weinshenker BG. An approach to the diagnosis of acute transverse myelitis. Semin Neurol. 2008;28(1):105–20.

75. Cross SA, Salomao DR, Parisi JE, Kryzer TJ, Bradley EA, Mines JA, et al. Paraneoplastic autoimmune optic neuritis with retinitis defined by CRMP-5-IgG. Ann Neurol. 2003;54(1):38–50.

76. Keegan BM, Pittock SJ, Lennon VA. Autoimmune myelopathy associated with collapsin response-mediator protein-5 immunoglobulin G. Ann Neurol. 2008;63(4):531–4.

77. Bach F, Larsen BH, Rohde K, Børgesen SE, Gjerris F, Bøge-Rasmussen T, et al. Metastatic spinal cord compression. Occurrence, symptoms, clinical presentations and prognosis in 398 patients with spinal cord compression. Acta Neurochir. 1990;107(1–2):37–43.

78. Loblaw DA, Laperriere NJ, Mackillop WJ. A population-based study of malignant spinal cord compression in Ontario. Clin Oncol (R Coll Radiol). 2003;15(4):211–7.

79. Schiff D, O'Neill BP, Suman VJ. Spinal epidural metastasis as the initial manifestation of malignancy: clinical features and diagnostic approach. Neurology. 1997;49(2):452–6.

80. Wallin MT, Culpepper WJ, Campbell JD, Nelson LM, Langer-Gould A, Marrie RA, et al. The prevalence of MS in the United States: a population-based estimate using health claims data. Neurology. 2019;92(10):e1029–40.

81. Bot JC, Barkhof F, Polman CH, et al. Spinal cord abnormalities in recently diagnosed MS patients: added value of spinal MRI examination. Neurology. 2004;62(2):226–33.

82. Thorpe JW, Kidd D, Moseley IF, Kenndall BE, Thompson AJ, MacManus DG, et al. Serial gadolinium-enhanced MRI of the brain and spinal cord in early relapsing-remitting multiple sclerosis. Neurology. 1996;46(2):373–8.

83. Scott TF, Bhagavatula K, Snyder PJ, Chieffe C. Transverse myelitis. Comparison with spinal cord presentations of multiple sclerosis. Neurology. 1998;50(2):429–33.

84. Hlavin ML, Kaminski HJ, Ross JS, Ganz E. Spinal epidural abscess: a ten-year perspective. Neurosurgery. 1990;27(2):177–84.

85. Zalewski NL, Flanagan EP, Keegan BM. Evaluation of idiopathic transverse myelitis revealing specific myelopathy diagnosis. Neurology. 2018;90(2):e96–e102.

86. Jacob A, Matiello M, Wingerchuk DM, Lucchinetti CF, Pittock SJ, Weinshenker BG. Neuromyelitis optica: changing concepts. J Neuroimmunol. 2007;187(1–2):126–38.

87. Kural-Seyahi E, Fresko I, Seyahi N, Ozyazgan Y, Mat C, Hamuryudan V, et al. The long-term mortality and morbidity of Behcet syndrome: a 2-decade outcome survey of 387 patients followed at a dedicated center. Medicine (Baltimore). 2003;82(1):60–76.

88. Yurdakul S, Hamuryudan V, Yazici H. Behcet syndrome. Curr Opin Rheumatol. 2004;16(1):38–42.

89. Rybicki BA, Major M, Popovich J Jr, Maliarik MJ, Iannuzzi MC. Racial differences in sarcoidosis incidence: a 5-year study in a health maintenance organization. Am J Epidemiol. 1997;145(3):234–41.

90. Cole JS, Patchell RA. Metastatic epidural spinal cord compression. Lancet Neurol. 2008;7(5):459–66.

91. Takahashi T, Miyazawa I, Misu T, Takano R, Nakashima I, Fujihara K, et al. Intractable hiccup and nausea in neuromyelitis optica with anti-aquaporin-4 antibody: a herald of acute exacerbations. J Neurol Neurosurg Psychiatry. 2008;79(9):1075–8.

92. McKeon A, Lennon VA, Lotze T, Tenenbaum S, Ness JM, Rensel M, et al. CNS aquaporin-4 autoimmunity in children. Neurology. 2008;71(2):93–100.

93. Carmody RF, Yang PJ, Seeley GW, Seeger JF, Unger EC, Johnson JE. Spinal cord compression due to metastatic disease: diagnosis with MR imaging versus myelography. Radiology. 1989;173(1):225–9.

94. Williams MP, Cherryman GR, Husband JE. Magnetic resonance imaging in suspected metastatic spinal cord compression. Clin Radiol. 1989;40(3):286–90.

95. Brex PA, Ciccarelli O, O'Riordan JI, Sailer M, Thompson AJ, Miller DH. A longitudinal study of abnormalities on MRI and disability from multiple sclerosis. N Engl J Med. 2002;346(3):158–64.

96. Ramanathan S, Dale RC, Brilot F. Anti-MOG antibody. The history, clinical phenotype and pathogenicity of a serum biomarker for demyelination. Autoimmun Rev. 2016;15(4):307–24.

97. Curry WT Jr, Hoh BL, Amin-Hanjani S, Eskandar EN. Spinal epidural abscess: clinical presenta-

tion, management, and outcome. Surg Neurol. 2005;63(4):364–71. discussion 371

98. Patchell RA, Tibbs PA, Regine WF, Payne R, Saris S, Kryscio RJ, et al. Direct decompressive surgical resection in the treatment of spinal cord compression caused by metastatic cancer: a randomised trial. Lancet. 2005;366(9486):643–8.

99. Martenson JA Jr, Evans RG, Lie MR, Ilstrup DM, Dinapoli RP, Ebersold MJ, et al. Treatment outcome and complications in patients treated for malignant epidural spinal cord compression (SCC). J Neuro-Oncol. 1985;3(1):77–84.

100. Maranzano E, Latini P. Effectiveness of radiation therapy without surgery in metastatic spinal cord compression: final results from a prospective trial. Int J Radiat Oncol Biol Phys. 1995;32(4):959–67.

101. Maranzano E, Latini P, Beneventi S, Marafioti L, Piro F, Perrucci E, et al. Comparison of two different radiotherapy schedules for spinal cord compression in prostate cancer. Tumori. 1998;84(4):472–7.

102. Sorensen S, Helweg-Larsen S, Mouridsen H, Hansen HH. Effect of high-dose dexamethasone in carcinomatous metastatic spinal cord compression treated with radiotherapy: a randomised trial. Eur J Cancer. 1994;30A(1):22–7.

103. Vecht CJ, Haaxma-Reiche H, van Putten WL, de Visser M, Vries EP, Twijnstra A. Initial bolus of conventional versus high-dose dexamethasone in metastatic spinal cord compression. Neurology. 1989;39(9):1255–7.

104. Graham PH, Capp A, Delaney G, Goozee G, Hickey B, Turner S, et al. A pilot randomised comparison of dexamethasone 96 mg vs 16 mg per day for malignant spinal-cord compression treated by radiotherapy: TROG 01.05 Superdex study. Clin Oncol (R Coll Radiol). 2006;18(1):70–6.

105. Maranzano E, Trippa F, Casale M, Costantini S, Lupattelli M, Bellavita R, et al. 8 Gy single-dose radiotherapy is effective in metastatic spinal cord compression: results of a phase III randomized multicentre Italian trial. Radiother Oncol. 2009;93(2):174–9.

106. Darouiche RO. Spinal epidural abscess. N Engl J Med. 2006;355(19):2012–20.

107. Cheung AT, Weiss SJ, McGarvey ML, Stecker MM, Hogan MS, Escherich A, et al. Interventions for reversing delayed-onset postoperative paraplegia after thoracic aortic reconstruction. Ann Thorac Surg. 2002;74(2):413–9. discussion 420–411

108. Baba H, Tomita K, Kawagishi T, Imura S. Anterior spinal artery syndrome. Int Orthop. 1993;17(6):353–6.

109. Restrepo L, Guttin JF. Acute spinal cord ischemia during aortography treated with intravenous thrombolytic therapy. Tex Heart Inst J. 2006;33(1):74–7.

110. Kaut O, Urbach H, Klockgether T. Improvement of paraplegia caused by spinal dural arteriovenous fis-

tula by surgical obliteration more than 6 years after symptom onset. J Neurol Neurosurg Psychiatry. 2008;79(12):1408–9.

111. Lattanzi S, Cagnetti C, Danni M, Provinciali L, Silvestrini M. Oral and intravenous steroids for multiple sclerosis relapse: a systematic review and meta-analysis. J Neurol. 2017;264(8):1697–704.

112. Söderlund ME, Benisty S, Gaston A, Djindjian M, Cesaro P, Créange A. Can myelopathies secondary to arterio-venous dural fistulae be aggravated by intravenous corticosteroid therapy? Rev Neurol (Paris). 2007;163(2):23507.

113. McKeon A, Lindell EP, Atkinson JL, Weinshenker BG, Piepgras DG, Pittock SJ. Pearls and oysters: clues for spinal dural arteriovenous fistulae. Neurology. 2011;76(3):e10–2.

114. O'Keeffe DT, Mikhail MA, Lanzino G, Kallmes DF, Weinshenker BG. Corticosteroid-induced paraplegia—a diagnostic clue for spinal dural arterial venous fistula. JAMA Neurol. 2015;72(7):833–4.

115. Weinshenker BG, O'Brien PC, Petterson TM, Weis J, Stevens L, Peterson WK, et al. A randomized trial of plasma exchange in acute central nervous system inflammatory demyelinating disease. Ann Neurol. 1999;46(6):878–86.

116. Keegan M, Pineda AA, McClelland RL, Darby CH, Rodriguez M, Weinshenker BG. Plasma exchange for severe attacks of CNS demyelination: predictors of response. Neurology. 2002;58(1):143–6.

117. Rae-Grant A, Day GS, Marrie RA, Rabinstein A, Cree BAC, Gronseth GS, et al. Practice guideline recommendations summary: disease-modifying therapies for adults with multiple sclerosis: report of the Guideline Development, Dissemination, and Implementation Subcommittee of the American Academy of Neurology. Neurology. 2018;90(17):777–88.

118. Pittock SJ, Berthele A, Fujihara K, Kim HJ, Levy M, Palace J, et al. Eculizumab in aquaporin-4 positive neuromyelitis optica spectrum disorder. N Engl J Med. 2019;381(7):614–25.

119. Cree BAC, Bennett JL, Kim HJ, Weinshenker BG, Pittock SJ, Wingerchuk DM, et al. Inebilizumab for the treatment of neuromyelitis optica spectrum disorder (N-MOmentum): a double-blind, randomised placebo controlled phase 2/3 trial. Lancet. 2019;394(10206):1352–63.

120. Wingerchuk DM, Weinshenker BG. Neuromyelitis optica. Curr Treat Options Neurol. 2005;7(3):173–82.

121. Jacob A, Matiello M, Weinshenker BG, Wingerchuk DM, Lucchinetti C, Shuster E, et al. Treatment of neuromyelitis optica with mycophenolate mofetil: retrospective analysis of 24 patients. Arch Neurol. 2009;66(9):1128–33.

122. Jacob A, Weinshenker BG, Violich I, McLinskey N, Krupp L, Fox RJ, et al. Treatment of neuromyelitis

optica with rituximab: retrospective analysis of 25 patients. Arch Neurol. 2008;65(11):1443–8.

123. Fritz D, van de Beek D, Brouwer MC. Clinical features, treatment and outcome in neurosarcoidosis: systematic review and meta-analysis. BMC Neurol. 2016;16(1):220.

124. Gelfand JM, Bradshaw MJ, Stern BJ, Clifford DB, Wang Y, Cho TA, et al. Infliximab for the treatment of CNS sarcoidosis: a multi-institutional series. Neurology. 2017;89(20):2092–105.

125. Bomprezzi R, Pati S, Chansakul C, Vollmer T. A case of neurosarcoidosis successfully treated with rituximab. Neurology. 2010;75(6):568–70.

126. Lord J, Paz Soldan MM, Galli J, Salzman KL, Kresser J, Bacharach R, et al. Neurosarcoidosis: longitudinal experience in a single-center, academic healthcare system. J Neurol Neuroimmunol Neuroinflamm. 2020;7(4):e743.

Movement Disorder Emergencies

14

Robert L. Rodnitzky and Christopher L. Groth

Introduction

Movement disorders can be the source of significant occupational, social, and functional disability. In most circumstances the progression of these disabilities is gradual, but there are circumstances when onset is acute or progression of a known movement disorders is unexpectedly rapid. These sudden appearances or worsening of abnormal involuntary movements can be so severe as to be frightening to the patient and their family and disabling, or even fatal, if left untreated. This chapter reviews movement disorder syndromes that rise to this level of concern and that require an accurate diagnosis that will allow appropriate therapy that is sufficient to allay anxiety and prevent unnecessary morbidity.

Acute Parkinsonism

The sudden or subacute onset of significant parkinsonism, especially akinesia, is potentially very frightening to the affected patient and his/her family members. Of more concern is the potential for severe untreated akinesia to lead to

R. L. Rodnitzky (✉) · C. L. Groth
Neurology Department, Roy J. and Lucille A. Carver
College of Medicine, University of Iowa,
Iowa City, IA, USA
e-mail: robert-rodnitzky@uiowa.edu;
christopher-groth@uiowa.edu

serious complications, such as pulmonary embolism, aspiration, and pneumonia. Seven general etiologic categories of acute parkinsonism can be identified, and the likelihood of arriving at the correct clinical diagnosis can be greatly enhanced by systematically considering which one or combination of these etiologies may be at play in a given acutely parkinsonian patient. The seven etiologic categories of acute parkinsonism are as follows: (1) structural, (2) toxic, (3) impaired levodopa absorption, (4) iatrogenic, (5) infectious, (6) surgery, and (7) genetic.

Structural

The two most common structural causes of acute parkinsonism are stroke and hydrocephalus, although neither is extremely common in an absolute sense. Parkinsonism due to acute hydrocephalus is to be distinguished from the gradually evolving form of parkinsonism that can occur in patients with chronic hydrocephalus, especially normal pressure hydrocephalus. Acute parkinsonism can occur simultaneously with the development of acute hydrocephalus [1] but can also occur after shunt placement [2, 3] or shunt revision [4] in patients with long-standing hydrocephalus. The rapid onset of parkinsonism in acute hydrocephalus is probably due to direct compression or shearing force on the substantia nigra secondary to changing pressure dynamics of the rapidly enlarging ventricles [5]. Parkinsonism due to shunt revision or placement is due to rapidly shrinking ventricles with subsequent midbrain distortion [2]. The simultaneous occurrence of other signs of rostral midbrain dysfunction, along with parkinsonism, after shunting supports the notion that the postshunting findings are all due to mechanical distortion of the midbrain [6]. In patients whose akinesia appears to be related to acute hydrocephalus with acutely enlarging ventricles, shunting is indicated and could be lifesaving. Parkinsonism might be improved by this intervention or, as mentioned above, could be exacerbated. In parkinsonism related to acute hydrocephalus, persistent hydrocephalus, or shunt revision, levodopa therapy is usually effective both in the short term and over the long term [2, 4–6].

Acute cerebral infarction involving the striatum or the substantia nigra is another structural insult that can result in acute parkinsonism. The common term "vascular parkinsonism," as used today, refers to the gradual appearance of parkinsonian features, usually a parkinsonian gait, due to diffuse, bihemisphere small vessel ischemic disease. Large artery infarctions, on the other hand, produce unilateral or bilateral parkinsonism over a matter of days to months. When a striatal infarction is associated with significant hemiparesis, unilateral parkinsonism typically evolves once the hemiparesis begins to improve [7]. Striatal infarctions are relatively common, but only a small percentage result in parkinsonism [8]. Parkinsonism can also develop after infarction of the substantia nigra [9]. Infarction of the pedunculopontine nuclei in the brainstem can cause acute onset of gait freezing, similar to that seen in Parkinson's disease [10]. Therapy of infarction-related parkinsonism with levodopa is most effective in those cases where the pathology is in, or close to, the substantia nigra [11]. Somewhat paradoxically, stroke involving the tuberothalamic artery can improve parkinsonian tremor, presumably through damage to the ventrolateral thalamic nucleus, similar to the lesion of a therapeutic thalamotomy [12], or deep brain stimulation of this structure. Acute worsening of parkinsonism of any cause is sometimes mistak-

enly diagnosed as a stroke and in those instances has even been mistakenly treated with intravenous thrombolytic therapy [201].

Toxic

A variety of nonindustrial toxins can also cause acute parkinsonism. The more common toxic exposures that might present to a community emergency department are discussed here. Organophosphate insecticides, either through inadvertent ingestion on food or exposure in an agricultural setting, can cause acute, reversible parkinsonism. In these cases, treatment with levodopa [13] has been less effective than amantadine [14] and dopamine agonists [15]. Carbon monoxide (CO) poisoning results in subacute parkinsonism. In a large series of 242 CO poisoning cases, 10% of the individuals affected developed parkinsonism with a latency of 2–26 weeks (median 4 weeks) after the acute exposure [16]. Imaging of the brain in these patients reveals evidence of bilateral pallidal necrosis with symmetric hypodensity on CT scan and high signal intensity on FLAIR and T2-weighted MRI sequences [17]. There is, however, not a complete correlation between the appearance of pallidal necrosis on CT or MRI and parkinsonism in CO poisoning. Of 17 patients with CO-related parkinsonism in one series, only 47% had abnormal CT scans [16]. In this series, levodopa and anticholinergic drugs were not effective, but 81% of affected individuals recovered gradually over a 6-month period of time. Initial hyperbaric oxygen therapy of CO poisoning in the acute phase may reduce subsequent neurologic sequelae, but controlled studies of this therapeutic approach are still lacking [18]. Long-term exposure to ambient CO in the form of air pollution can also increase the risk of Parkinson's disease [202]. Purposeful or accidental ingestion of ethylene glycol or methanol can result in acute parkinsonian akinesia, often associated with hemorrhagic necrosis of the basal ganglia [19]. Levodopa therapy can improve the rigidity and bradykinesia associated with these two toxic exposures [19].

Impaired Levodopa Absorption

Gastric emptying is commonly slightly delayed in PD patients, but superimposed gastrointestinal disorders can further delay passage of levodopa through the pylorus resulting in a significant decrease in levodopa absorption in its main absorptive site in the jejunum. The consequence of such an acute or subacute decrease in levodopa absorption is an acute increase in parkinsonian symptoms, including akinesia due to delayed-on or no-on [203]. In these cases, identification and treatment of the comorbid gastrointestinal disorder is the first therapeutic measure that should be taken. In a review of 146 non-parkinsonian patients with acute gastroparesis, the 3 most common associated clinical features were abdominal pain, depression on antidepressant therapy, and gastroesophageal reflux [20]. Should recent onset or worsening of any of these comorbid conditions be present in the acutely akinetic PD patient, gastroparesis with resultant impaired levodopa absorption should be strongly suspected. Gastroparesis in PD patients has also been reported in the presence of acute duodenal ulcer and intestinal volvulus [21]. In addition to treating the primary medical cause of delayed gastric emptying, prokinetic agents can be useful to reduce gastric stasis. Domperidone, a peripheral dopamine receptor antagonist, is useful for this purpose but is not yet approved in the USA. Administering levodopa with a carbonated and/or caffeinated beverage may enhance passage of levodopa through the stomach and enhance absorption. Replacing an oral dopamine agonist with a transdermal agent, such as rotigotine [22], would be useful. For very severe absorptive dysfunction with significant akinesia such as after gastrointestinal surgery, subcutaneous apomorphine may prove useful [23], although in this circumstance, some patients become relatively refractory to all dopaminergic agents, including apomorphine [21]. In some PD patients, failure of the pyloric sphincter to relax is the cause of delayed gastric emptying and resultant delayed intestinal absorption of levodopa. A preliminary report of botulinum injection of this sphincter suggested that this therapy may result in several months of symptomatic improvement in reliable "on" responses to each levodopa dosage [204].

Iatrogenic

Extrapontine myelinolysis, typically due to very rapid correction of hyponatremia, can include striatal involvement and an attendant akinetic rigid state which may respond to levodopa therapy [205]. The inadvertent or ill-advised use of drugs that are dopamine receptor blocking agents (DRBA) can rapidly result in a severely exacerbated parkinsonian state in PD patients. Occasionally, non-PD patients or PD patients not yet known to have clinically apparent PD can be rendered acutely or subacutely akinetic by the administration of DRBAs, particularly if used at a high dosage. Among DRBAs, the typical antipsychotic agents, such as haloperidol, have the greatest potential to cause significant akinesia, but other classes of dopamine antagonists, including most of the atypical antipsychotic agents and the DRBA antiemetic drugs, such as prochlorperazine and metoclopramide, have this potential as well [24]. The most serious iatrogenic forms of acute akinesia are neuroleptic malignant syndrome (NMS) and the closely related condition known as parkinsonism-hyperpyrexia syndrome (PHS), as these conditions, left untreated, can result in major disability and are potentially fatal. Serotonin syndrome shares some clinical features with NMS, including some parkinsonian phenomena.

Neuroleptic malignant syndrome is an acute reaction that can occur either as a result of treatment with a dopamine-blocking agent [25] or after rapid withdrawal or reduction of one or more dopaminergic drugs in a Parkinson's disease patient, in which case it is referred to as parkinsonism-hyperpyrexia syndrome (PHS) [26]. Although discontinuance of any Parkinson's drug can result in PHS, stopping levodopa is the most common cause. PHS can also occur in other forms of parkinsonism, such as progressive supranuclear palsy or multiple system atrophy (MSA) [27]. The onset of NMS is usually within a month after beginning DRBA therapy or an increase in dosage, but as many as 16% of cases of NMS begin within the first 24 h of therapy and 30% by 2 days [25]. PHS developing in Parkinson's disease patients usually presents shortly after the discontinuance or reduction of a dopaminergic medication [26]. In one series, PHS occurred at a mean of 93 h after medication withdrawal [28]. All neuroleptic drugs can cause NMS, as can all atypical antipsychotic agents [29–32]. The overall incidence of NMS appears to be lower in patients receiving atypical antipsychotic agents, and at least in the case of clozapine [33], olanzapine [34], and risperidone [31], a milder syndrome with less prominent fever or rigidity [35] and less elevation of creatinine kinase may develop. However, in one recent review of the literature [36], 68 reported cases of NMS were related to atypical antipsychotics, and in this survey, clozapine was associated with NMS as often as other atypical agents, suggesting that low extrapyramidal syndrome-inducing potential does not necessarily reduce the occurrence of NMS. Aside from the possible lower incidence of NMS associated with lower-potency neuroleptic agents, one study suggested that NMS mortality may also be lower in cases associated with these less potent agents [206]. Antiemetic DRBAs, such as metoclopramide and prochlorperazine, can also result in NMS [37]. Antidepressants, including tricyclics [38], selective serotonin reuptake inhibitors [39], and lithium [40], either alone or in combination, have all been reported to cause a syndrome resembling NMS, but such cases are uncommon, and often the clinical presentation is atypical or indistinguishable from serotonin syndrome. NMS is more likely to occur in young patients, in males, and in patients who are agitated and dehydrated, who have received large rapidly administered dosages of the offending drug, or who have had previous electroconvulsive therapy [41, 42]. Elevation of serum creatine kinase during a previous psychotic episode unassociated with NMS may be a risk factor for NMS developing during future administration of DRBAs [43].

In addition to dehydration, risk factors for PHS include several characteristics of the underlying parkinsonism. Thus, more severe parkinsonian symptoms, longer disease duration, a history of "wearing off," and a history of an early age of parkinsonism onset are risk factures for PHS [44]. Serious PHS has occurred after perioperative withdrawal of antiparkinsonian medications [45]. PHS has also been reported in Parkinson's patients who abruptly discontinued fava bean ingestion, which was being taken for its levodopa content [46]. The syndrome has also occurred in Parkinson's patients during extreme periods of ambient heat even in the absence of medication withdrawal [47]. Acute akinesia related to levodopa resistance after a surgical procedure resembles PHS [21].

The cardinal clinical manifestations of NMS and PHS are virtually identical and include fever, muscular rigidity, autonomic instability, and confusion or alteration in consciousness [37]. Among autonomic symptoms, tachypnea, tachycardia, labile blood pressure, diaphoresis, and urinary retention are most common [48]. The most frequent movement disorder in NMS is rigidity, which is often preponderantly axial. Other movement disorders are possible, including dystonia and chorea. Fever is typically at least 38 °C and often higher. Creatine kinase levels are usually above 2000 IU/L and often in the range of 15,000–20,000 IU/L [49, 50]. The white blood cell count is often elevated, but usually without a left shift. Milder or atypical forms of the syndrome without one of the classic features, such as muscle rigidity [51] or fever [31, 52], may exist. Cases without rigidity may simply present as a fever of unknown origin [53]. PHS is especially likely to present with fever as the first symptom [27]. An international expert consensus (IEC) panel created a diagnostic score based on a weighted list of these symptoms [207], and the resultant use of this score was shown to have 91% specificity for the diagnosis of NMS [208].

The treatment of NMS and PHS should be considered emergent, especially in cases in which all of the clinical criteria are fulfilled or in patients with extremely high fever and rhabdomyolysis. In these cases, there can be serious morbidity and occasionally a fatal outcome. The most common complications affecting the prognosis are cardiac failure, cerebellar degeneration, respiratory disturbances, and renal failure, the latter of which can be associated with disseminated intravascular coagulation and rhabdomyolysis [54, 55]. The first therapeutic measure that must be taken is discontinuing the offending neuroleptic or another causative dopamine-blocking drug, or in Parkinson's patients with PHS, replacing a recently withdrawn or altered dopaminergic drug. Supportive measures, such as hydration and lowering of fever, must be started early. Anticholinergic drugs should be discontinued in Parkinson's disease patients, since they inhibit heat dissipation. Tapering anticholinergics is advised rather than abrupt cessation to avoid rebound rigidity. Respiratory support may be needed because of severe rigidity of respiratory muscles. Cardiac arrhythmias and blood pressure abnormalities must be treated [56]. In patients with dangerously high body temperature, antipyretics such as aspirin are usually ineffective, but a noninvasive body surface cooling device can be very useful to reverse hyperthermia [57].

The specific first-line medical therapies for NMS include bromocriptine, orally or by nasogastric tube, dantrolene, and amantadine [37]. Bromocriptine is administered in an initial dosage of 2.5 mg every 4 h, being careful to observe for induction or worsening of hypotension. The dose can be increased daily, if required, to as much as 50 mg per day. An alternative dopamine agonist is subcutaneous apomorphine, which can produce a rapid clinical response [58, 59]. Dantrolene can be administered intravenously, if needed, in a dosage of 1–10 mg/kg/day in three divided dosages. Most patients will require dosages in the lower part of this range [60]. Dantrolene is a good choice for initial therapy alone or in combination with bromocriptine when there is severe rigidity and rhabdomyolysis. Carbamazepine is a possible second-line therapy [61]. None of these medical therapies have been proven to be effective by prospective studies but rather derive their reputation for efficacy from case reports and small series culled from the literature. However, a large retrospective review of 734 cases of NMS concluded that treatment with bromocriptine, dantrolene, or amantadine reduced mortality more than supportive care alone [62]. For NMS cases that are refractory to medical therapy, electroconvulsive therapy has been found to be useful in both adults and children [63], as well as in PHS [64].

Recovery from NMS typically occurs over a 1- to 2-week period, but resolution after recovery from the acute phase may be delayed in those having received long-acting depot neuroleptics. Some sequelae, especially neuropsychiatric symptoms, can persist for weeks or months [65]. Pulse methylprednisolone therapy has been reported to significantly shorten the recovery phase in patients with Parkinson's disease [66]. Rechallenge with neuroleptics after recovery results in reoccurrence of NMS in less the 15% of cases. To minimize the likelihood of reoccurrence, rechallenge should be delayed for at least 2 weeks after recovery, and a lower-potency neuroleptic agent or atypical antipsychotic drug should be used.

Serotonin syndrome (*SS*) has become increasingly more common, reflecting the increased number and increased use of serotonergic medications. This pattern of increased use also includes the pediatric population. In a survey of North Carolina Medicaid prescriptions, the prevalence of prescriptions for SSRIs in the 6–14-year-old age group increased sevenfold from 0.2% to 1.5% between 1992 and 1998 [67]. This syndrome, like NMS, includes involuntary abnormal movements, especially myoclonus and tremor, and as such is considered a movement disorder emergency. As the name implies, serotonin syndrome occurs in patients receiving one or more serotonergic drugs. There are two commonly utilized diagnostic criteria for serotonin syndrome, the Sternbach Criteria [68] and the Hunter Serotonin Toxicity Criteria [69]. Using the Sternbach Criteria, there are three requirements:

(a) After the addition of or increase in dosage of a serotonergic agent, at least three of the following clinical features must be present: agitation, mental status changes, myoclonus, hyperreflexia, diaphoresis, shivering, tremor, diarrhea, incoordination, and fever.

(b) Other etiologic causes (infectious, metabolic, substance abuse, or withdrawal) have been ruled out.

(c) An antipsychotic has not been started or increased in dosage before the onset of the symptoms.

To fulfill the Hunter Serotonin Toxicity Criteria, the patient must have taken a serotonergic agent and meet one of the following requirements:

(a) Exhibit spontaneous clonus
(b) Have inducible clonus plus agitation or diaphoresis
(c) Exhibit ocular clonus plus agitation or diaphoresis
(d) Have hypertonia
(e) Have a temperature greater than 38 °C plus ocular clonus or inducible clonus

Both sets of criteria are useful, but a comparison of their utility in patients with an established serotonin syndrome diagnosis suggested that the Hunter Criteria was more sensitive than the Sternbach Criteria (84% vs. 75%) and minimally more specific (97% vs. 96%) [69].

The clinical signs of serotonin syndrome resemble those of NMS, and in many cases the two syndromes appear to overlap in the same patient [70]. For determining proper therapy, distinguishing the two syndromes from one another is very important, since their respective medical therapies are distinct. Both syndromes include mental status changes, fever, autonomic dysfunction, and a variety of movement disorders, but the relative severity of these signs in the two syndromes can be a differentiating factor. Compared to NMS, in serotonin syndrome, fever, elevation of creatine kinase, and alteration in sensorium are generally less prominent, while myoclonus, gastrointestinal symptoms, a shivering-type tremor, hyperreflexia, clonus, and pupillary dilatation are more prominent. Among these differences, hyperreflexia with clonus, the presence of otherwise unexplained myoclonus, and a rapid onset (within hours of the offending pharmacologic event) are among the most useful clues that the patient is suffering from serotonin syndrome

rather than NMS. A comparison of common features of serotonin syndrome, NMS, and features that most accurately discriminate the two syndromes from one another is shown in Table 14.1.

Misdiagnosis, especially early in the course of serotonin syndrome, is common. For example, the presence of hyperreflexia and clonus can lead to the false impression of a pyramidal syndrome, and the presence of diarrhea plus fever can lead to the incorrect diagnosis of an infectious gastroenteritis [71].

The offending therapies that have the potential to contribute to serotonin syndrome fall into one of the following seven pharmacologic categories (Table 14.2). Although serotonin syndrome is thought to result from stimulation of 5-HT_{1A} and 5-HT_{2A} receptors [73], some drugs that stimulate other classes of receptors, such as most triptan agents, probably can contribute to the development of serotonin syndrome.

Although any of these drugs and treatments taken alone can cause serotonin syndrome, the risk is greatest when two or more serotonergic therapies are administered simultaneously [74, 75]. The greatest risk is in those receiving a nonselective MAO inhibitor along with a potent serotonin reuptake inhibitor [76]. Higher dosages of these medications also increase the risk and the

Table 14.1 Serotonin syndrome. Comparison with neuroleptic malignant syndrome

	SS	NMS
Mental status change	+	++
Fever	++	+++
Tachypnea/tachycardia	++	+++
Diarrhea	+++	0
Diaphoresis	++	+++
Rigidity/bradykinesia	0	+++[a]
Stupor	+	+++[a]
Tremor	+++[b]	+
Shivering	+++[b]	0
Myoclonus	+++[b]	+
Hyperreflexia/clonus	+++[b]	0
Elevated CK	+	+++[a]
Pupillary dilation	++	0
Acute onset	+++[b]	+

[a]Important differentiating feature of neuroleptic malignant syndrome (NMS)
[b]Important differentiating feature of serotonin syndrome (SS)

Table 14.2 Agents that can cause serotonin syndrome

1. Inhibitors of serotonin reuptake: all of the SSRIs, SNRIs, several tricyclic antidepressants, dextromethorphan, amphetamine, cocaine, MDMA (ecstasy), St. John's wort, lamotrigine
2. Inhibitors of serotonin metabolism: selective MAO-B inhibitors (selegiline or rasagiline), non-selective MAO inhibitor antidepressants, non-selective MAO inhibitor antibiotic (linezolid), methylene blue
3. Agents that increase serotonin synthesis: L-tryptophan
4. Enhancers of serotonin release: amphetamines, cocaine, fenfluramine, MDMA (ecstasy)
5. Serotonin agonists: buspirone, triptans, ergotamines
6. Nonspecific enhancers of serotonin activity: lithium, electroconvulsive therapy
7. Serotonergic effect, mechanism is uncertain: second-generation antipsychotic agents – quetiapine, olanzapine, clozapine, risperidone, aripiprazole

Adapted from Lane and Baldwin [72]

severity of the syndrome. For example, several cases of serotonin syndrome in children have resulted from accidental ingestion of a large and pharmacologically excessive amount of a parent's medication [77, 78]. Methylenedioxymethamphetamine (MDMA), also known as "ecstasy," is an amphetamine-derived street drug that is commonly used by high school and college students, especially while attending drug-inspired dance gatherings known as "raves" [79] during which there is a high ambient temperature and vigorous physical activity leading to dehydration. This drug has serotonergic properties and either alone or in combination with other serotonergic drugs can produce a syndrome with features of serotonin syndrome [70]. Fatalities have occurred due to MDMA-related serotonin syndrome, often associated with delayed diagnosis in part due to unawareness of the history of illicit drug ingestion. Purposefully combining MDMA with an MAO inhibitor to enhance its effect has proven especially lethal [80]. In the UK, 605 ecstasy-related deaths were reported in a 7-year period [81]. Generally, what contributes to a potential fatal outcome in serotonin syndrome is the development of rhabdomyolysis, myoglobinemia, and renal failure. Acute myocardial infarction has also occurred in the setting of serotonin syndrome [82].

Of interest to neurologists are the risks associated with some serotonin-enhancing drugs that are commonly used in neurologic practice, including antimigraine agents, such as triptans and dihydroergotamine, and the selective MAO-B inhibitors, selegiline and rasagiline, used in Parkinson's disease. Serotonin syndrome was reported in only 11 patients receiving a triptan alone in the FDA adverse event reporting system [83]. However, triptans taken along with other serotonergic agents, especially the commonly used SSRIs, have been reported to cause the serotonin syndrome [84]. In 2006, the FDA issued an alert concerning the potential of serotonin syndrome in patients taking triptans and SSRIs or SNRIs, based on 29 reported cases. Subsequent analysis of these cases has suggested that the risk is very small, and in fact not all of the FDA cases may have met the diagnostic criteria for serotonin syndrome [85, 86]. In regard to selegiline, there is concern that this agent could cause the serotonin syndrome in patients also receiving other serotonergic drugs. Despite this concern, there are very few well documented cases of this interaction, and a similar level of risk seems likely for the newer selective, irreversible MAO-B inhibitor, rasagiline. Recently, it has become apparent that the widely used antibiotic linezolid is an MAO inhibitor that can cause serotonin syndrome when used along with other serotonergic drugs [87]. Another widely used drug with surprising MAO-inhibiting properties is methylene blue which is typically administered after cardiac surgery to combat vasospastic hypotension. Administered along with a serotonergic agent such as an SSRI, methylene blue can result in severe serotonin syndrome, sometimes referred to as "blue coma" [88].

Prevention is very important in the serotonin syndrome. To avoid an interaction leading to serotonin syndrome, there should be a period of at least 2 weeks between stopping an SSRI and starting an MAO inhibitor and approximately 5 weeks after discontinuance of fluoxetine, which has a much longer half-life. Treatment of the acute serotonin syndrome begins with the discontinuation of all serotonergic medications. When the syndrome is relatively mild, consisting only of hyperreflexia, clonus, tachycardia, and anxiety, this strategy alone will often result in resolution of symptoms within 24 h. When symptoms are particularly resistant or severe, consisting of any or all of severe hyperthermia, autonomic instability, rigidity, rhabdomyolysis, and respiratory distress, direct medical therapy should be begun with cyproheptadine. The most commonly recommended dosage plan is 12 mg initially, crushed and by nasogastric tube if necessary, followed by 2 mg every 2 hours while symptoms persist. Once stabilization is achieved, the regimen can be changed to a maintenance dose of 8 mg every 6 hours until symptoms remit [89]. Chlorpromazine has been suggested as a therapy for serotonin syndrome, but its use depends on absolute certainty that the patient does not have NMS instead, which might be worsened by this therapeutic approach [72]. Rehydration and control of fever are important in the presence of severe hyperthermia. A noninvasive cooling device can be used to lower body temperature similar to its use in NMS [57]. Antipyretic agents, such as aspirin and acetaminophen, are not effective for lowering fever since the fever is not of hypothalamic origin in this condition. In the presence of severe muscle rigidity, dantrolene can be used. In patients with such severe autonomic, respiratory and organ failure symptoms, treatment in an intensive care unit is required.

Drug-induced parkinsonism Administration of dopamine-blocking drugs, including typical antipsychotic agents, atypical antipsychotic agents, and dopamine-blocking antiemetics, can all cause rapid-onset parkinsonism, especially when administered in high dosages [24]. A large number of other drugs that are not primary dopamine-blocking agents, such as selective serotonin uptake inhibitors, valproic acid, amiodarone, and certain chemotherapeutic agents, rarely cause severe de novo parkinsonism and can also occasionally significantly exacerbate parkinsonian symptoms in a known PD patient [90]. The calcium channel blockers, cinnarizine and flunarizine, neither marketed in the USA, can cause parkinsonism due to their significant dopamine-blocking capacity. VMAT2 inhibitors such as tet-rabenazine and valbenazine [209], especially the former, can cause parkinsonism. Drug-induced parkinsonism can resemble ordinary Parkinson's disease, although there is a tendency for less tremor and more symmetry in the drug-induced syndrome. Some patients with drug-induced parkinsonism actually have Parkinson's disease that has been uncovered by the administration of the offending drug. These patients may be even more susceptible to drugs that are less obvious dopamine blockers such as selective serotonin uptake inhibitors [91]. SPECT imaging of the dopamine transporter can be used to help determine whether a drug has caused transient parkinsonism or has uncovered latent Parkinson's disease [91]. The initial treatment of drug-induced parkinsonism is to discontinue the offending drug, if medically feasible. Discontinuance may not always be possible in the case of effective antipsychotic agents used to treat a serious psychiatric condition. Even with discontinuance, improvement in drug-induced parkinsonism cannot be expected for days to weeks, occasionally several months, and even, less occasionally, 2 years or more. Once the offending drug has been discontinued, immediate medical therapy can begin with anticholinergic agents or amantadine, although there is uneven evidence that these agents have a major effect. If these are not effective, then a course of levodopa can be considered with appropriate caution regarding the exacerbation of psychosis that this treatment can cause. Identifying patients who might respond to levodopa is greatly enhanced by utilizing a SPECT scan, since most such responders are found to have at least some small component of idiopathic Parkinson's disease [92].

Infection

Any intermittent infection, whether viral or bacterial, can exacerbate ongoing parkinsonian symptoms, especially in moderately or severely advanced PD patients. A recent survey of PD patients admitted to the hospital confirmed that infection was the most common reason for admission, and among infections, pneumonia and urinary tract infection were most common [93].

Occult infection, especially pneumonia or urinary tract infection, should always be considered in PD patients presenting with unexplained worsening of symptoms.

Acute or subacute parkinsonism has been reported as a complication of several different forms of viral encephalitis including encephalitis due to herpes simplex virus-1, West Nile virus, Coxsackieviruses, St. Louis encephalitis virus, and HIV [94–96]. A major clue to this etiology of acute parkinsonism is the recent history or concurrent presence of seizures, fever, or extreme somnolence. Standard antiparkinsonian drugs, such as trihexyphenidyl and carbidopa/levodopa, may improve parkinsonian symptoms during the acute phase of a viral illness [95]. Encephalitis lethargica, which occurred as a pandemic in the early twentieth century, is a well-accepted cause of parkinsonism and, although rare, still does occur [97]. The presence of antineuronal antibodies and the absence of positive viral PCR in parkinsonian patients with encephalitis lethargica suggest that parkinsonism is due to an autoimmune condition rather than an acute viral illness and may require immunomodulatory therapy [98]. Another form of infection that can lead to autoimmune akinesia is parkinsonism after streptococcal infection with associated anti-basal ganglia antibodies [99].

The treatment of infection-related forms of parkinsonism is to first treat the underlying viral or bacterial infection with appropriate antiviral agents or antibiotics. For the parkinsonian features themselves, standard antiparkinsonian therapy such as levodopa is often effective [95, 100]. Those infections associated with anti-basal ganglia antibodies may respond to immunomodulatory therapy, such as corticosteroids [99].

Surgery

Parkinson's disease patients undergoing major surgery commonly note worsening of their symptoms in the postoperative period. Most often, the degree of worsening is mild or moderate, but occasionally it can be severe and associated with profound akinesia [21]. While any type of surgery can have this effect, joint surgery is one of the more common precipitants of postoperative PD worsening. This syndrome appears to be independent of abnormalities of levodopa absorption and, in its most severe form, is associated with refractoriness to all dopaminergic agents [21]. Despite concern for refractoriness to dopaminergic agents, therapy with oral levodopa or nonoral dopaminergic agents, such as subcutaneous apomorphine or transdermal rotigotine, should be attempted if either is available. Should there be no benefit from these agents, supportive care for the immobilized patient is paramount until responsiveness to medication resumes, often in 2–7 days. It is wise to forewarn PD patients undergoing elective surgery that some worsening is likely to occur in the postoperative period in order to minimize personal and family anxiety over this occurrence.

Another potential cause of acute akinesia in the postoperative period is enteral nutrition [101]. This phenomenon is largely the result of persistent interference with levodopa absorption by the high protein content of continuous tube feedings. It can be combated by changing from continuous to intermittent bolus enteral feedings and staging levodopa dosages in between and temporally distant from boluses of tube feedings.

For PD patients undergoing planned or elective operations, the surgical team should be forewarned to avoid administering dopamine-blocking antiemetics or antipsychotic drugs in the postoperative period, if at all possible, since these agents can further exacerbate postoperative parkinsonism. In place of the dopamine-blocking anti-nausea drugs such as droperidol, prochlorperazine, metoclopramide, or domperidone (not available in the USA), trimethobenzamide should be used instead.

Acute Genetic Parkinsonism

There is one form of degenerative parkinsonism that typically has an acute or subacute onset. Rapid-onset dystonia-parkinsonism (RDP) is an autosomal dominant condition related to a mutation in the *ATP1A3* gene in in which both dystonia and parkinsonism develop as rapidly as over a few minutes to as long as 30 days [102]. In this condition, parkinsonian symptoms, such as bradykinesia and hypophonia, often, but not invariably, pursue a rostral-caudal pattern of progression. RDP can be differentiated from idiopathic PD by its sudden onset, its initial rapid progression, the rostral-caudal progression, the association with dystonia, and the absence of tremor. Family history, if present, is useful, but the autosomal dominant gene in this condition displays variable penetrance. Another somewhat helpful differentiating feature from PD is that the great majority of patients with RDP are under the age of 30, and in fact, almost half are under the age of 20 [102]. A variety of triggers leading to the initial clinical presentation have been reported in this condition including running, stress, alcohol consumption, fever, trauma, and psychiatric events, the latter sometimes falsely raising the possibility of psychogenic parkinsonism or autoimmune encephalitis. Typically, these patients' parkinsonian symptoms are refractory to dopaminergic therapy. Atypical forms with slower progression and a less apparent rostral-caudal pattern of onset are not uncommon [103]. While pharmacologic therapy of this form of acute parkinsonism is not very effective, patients can be reassured that in the majority of cases most of the symptoms are minimally progressive after the initial presentation, with only a small number of patients experiencing a second later episode of abrupt worsening.

Severe or Acute Levodopa-Induced Dyskinesias

Parkinson's disease patients are susceptible to severe medication-induced dyskinesias that can be choreic, dystonic, or both. These involuntary movements are usually a complication of dopaminergic medications and can be further exacerbated by levodopa enhancing preparations such as COMT inhibitors or MAO inhibitors. Dyskinesias related to levodopa and/or dopamine

agonist medications typically remit spontaneously given sufficient time, but if the involuntary movements are of extremely high amplitude or involve many body parts simultaneously, they can prove to be frightening and/or exhausting to the patient and to family members, resulting in an emergency department visit. For example, these movements can be sufficiently prolonged and severe to result in rhabdomyolysis and a significant elevation of plasma creatine kinase [104]. Rarely, involvement of the respiratory muscles can lead to a patient's perception of respiratory distress.

Under these circumstances, the causative medication(s) should be temporarily suspended with a plan to reintroduce them at a slightly lower dosage once the dyskinesias have remitted. It is probably unwise to entirely discontinue chronically administered dopaminergic medicines for any sustained period of time for fear of inducing PHS and to avoid producing severe prolonged akinesia. If there is not an immediate reduction in the severity of the dyskinetic movements, then medical therapy will be required in the emergency room setting. Benzodiazepine preparations such as diazepam, lorazepam, or clonazepam can be very helpful, both in relieving the severity of the dyskinesias and diminishing the associated anxiety that accompany them. Often a parenteral route of administration provides more rapid relief. If swallowing is intact and the patient has already ingested a controlled release levodopa preparation, administration of a high-protein snack can be attempted in the hope of limiting further gastrointestinal absorption of levodopa and inhibiting its passage across the blood-brain barrier through competition for the active transport system for large neutral amino acids [105]. If it is necessary to restart dopaminergic medications at the same dosage to control parkinsonian symptoms, strategies to reduce the potential for recurrent severe dyskinesias should be employed including adding amantadine for its antidyskinesia effect and replacing levodopa partially or completely with a dopamine agonist, since this class of agents has a lower potential to cause dyskinesias.

Acute Behavioral Change in Parkinsonism: Psychosis, Delirium, and Panic Attack

A variety of behavioral abnormalities can occur in PD. The most common, dementia, is gradual in evolution and is not typically viewed as an emergency, but many other behaviors can appear suddenly, especially in the chronically demented PD patient. These conditions can result in emergency room visits, emergency inpatient consultations, or involvement by security or law enforcement officials.

Psychosis

Psychosis in PD commonly results in visual hallucinations, delusional thoughts, and illusory phenomena. Auditory and tactile hallucinations can occur but are much less common. Psychosis typically appears in PD patients with cognitive impairment but can also occasionally be seen in nondemented patients. Psychotic symptoms can be rapid in appearance or escalation, suddenly reaching a critical point in severity and resulting in an emergency presentation. The most common emergency presentations are hallucinations that are frightening to the patient or delusions that are threatening. Both have the potential to result in a state of agitation. In these circumstances, reassurance may be somewhat helpful but in the most severe cases is inadequate. Delusions of harm from family or friends or hallucinations of intruders in the home may result in calls from the patient to police or other emergency responders. Recognizing that medications are often a contributing cause of acute psychosis, the most recent additions or dosage increases in antiparkinsonian drugs, or other medications, particularly those with anticholinergic properties, should be evaluated and at least temporarily discontinued if needed. Pharmacologic therapy will often be required for more immediate relief of psychotic symptoms, especially in the emergency room setting. The atypical antipsychotic agents are useful in reversing psychotic symptoms in PD. Clozapine is the most useful but has potentially serious adverse effects, including agranulocytosis, and should not be administered emergently without a thorough review of possible previous administration and adverse effects, a process that cannot be easily accomplished quickly in the emergency room setting [106]. The next most useful and commonly used atypical antipsychotic agent is quetiapine [107]. Although some studies have questioned its efficacy [108], common experience supports its benefit. The only atypical antipsychotic agents readily available in parenteral form for acute administration are olanzapine and ziprasidone. Pimavanserin, a relatively new novel atypical antipsychotic agent with no dopamine-blocking effect, has been shown to be effective in treating Parkinson's disease psychosis [109] with little risk of worsening motor function [110]. The use of atypical antipsychotic agents should be tempered by the "black box" warning of a slight increased risk of death when used to treat elderly patients with dementia [111].

Panic

Anxiety is common in PD. Most forms such as generalized anxiety or social phobia seldom present as an emergency, but panic attacks, which are not uncommon in Parkinson's disease, may result in an emergency room visit. A study of anxiety disorders in PD found a lifetime prevalence of 49% of all forms of anxiety, whereas the specific prevalence of panic disorders in PD patients was 10% [112]. Panic disorder is more likely to appear in patients with an earlier age of PD onset and in those with a family history of parkinsonism [112].

Typical panic attack symptoms include an intense discomfort or fear with sudden onset of associated symptoms such as a sense of impending death, choking, breathlessness, palpitations, or chest pain. A panic attack sometimes is associated with the "off" state in PD. In that circumstance, pharmacologic measures to reverse the parkinsonian "off" state will also improve the sense of panic. When readjustment of antiparkinsonian medications to correct the off state does not reverse a panic attack, anxiolytic therapy will be required. A short-acting, rapid-onset benzodiazepine, such as alprazolam, is useful for reducing the intensity of panic-associated symptoms. Selective serotonin reuptake inhibitors are also useful for panic disorders, but the absence of a rapid-onset formulation makes them less useful for acute panic attacks in the emergency setting than for the treatment of an ongoing persistent panic disorder.

Delirium

The most common causes of acute delirium in PD are intercurrent illness (especially infection), or the postoperative state. When an identifiable infection is present, appropriate antibiotic therapy will aid reversal of delirium. Any form of surgery, especially orthopedic procedures, may result in postoperative delirium. The greatest risk for postoperative delirium is preexistent dementia. In anticipation of the possibility that delirium may develop postoperatively in such patients, certain preventative measures are useful. Thus, in PD patients with known dementia, the use of regional rather than general anesthesia and employing less deep levels of sedation, if possible, are useful strategies that can lessen the risk of delirium after surgery [113, 114].

In addition to treating concurrent illnesses, such as infection, environmental methods to reestablish normal day, night, place, and time orientation should be employed. Encouraging a family member to sit with the patient and provide a focus of orientation can be useful in this regard. In the severely agitated patient, pharmaceutical management will more likely be required. Whereas haloperidol is often considered standard therapy for delirium, it cannot be used in PD patients without severely worsening their parkinsonism. An atypical antipsychotic agent, preferably quetiapine, should be used instead [115–117]. Benzodiazepines are not recommended except in the face of alcohol or other substance withdrawal.

Suicide

One final behavioral emergency in PD is suicidal ideation [118], which has been estimated to occur in as many as one third of PD patients [119]. In some studies the suicide rate was found to be especially high in PD patients having undergone deep brain stimulation of the subthalamic nucleus (STN) [120]. A meta-analysis found that suicide attempts were observed in 1% of STN DBS patients, and successful suicides were documented in 0.5% [121]. A large study, however, found that suicidal ideation and behaviors were not elevated in the 6 months post-DBS period, and furthermore there was no difference in these symptoms between STN and globus pallidus DBS patients [211]. On balance, these data do point out that suicidal thoughts, gestures, and attempts can occur in PD patients, possibly more so in DBS patients, and are true emergencies requiring appropriate psychiatric consultation with consideration of admission to the hospital.

Inspiratory Stridor in Multiple System Atrophy

Multiple system atrophy (MSA) can be associated with inspiratory stridor. Whether stridor in this clinical condition is due to laryngeal abductor weakness or adductor dystonia is uncertain, several, but not all, studies suggest that its appearance increases the potential of an earlier fatal outcome. While stridor is more common in moderately or severely advanced MSA patients, it can occasionally be among the presenting signs of this condition [122]. An early clue to the presence of stridor may be peculiar high-pitched, nonposition-dependent snoring during sleep. Family members should be alerted to the presence of this sound which is clearly different from ordinary snoring. In many patients, this may be the exclusive time of day that stridor occurs. Laryngoscopy is the definitive diagnostic technique for identifying laryngeal abductor dysfunction, and in patients with stridor that occurs exclusively at night, the procedure may have to be performed during sleep to identify the problem. Some patients experience stridor during the daytime as well as at night, which is even more ominous in terms of the potential for serious respiratory embarrassment. One study suggested that MSA patients who develop daytime stridor have a mean survival of less than 1 year [123]. A recent meta-analysis and consensus statement by an international panel of experts noted that not all previous studies found a relationship between the presence of stridor and survival in MSA, yet they noted that those studies not confirming this correlation used less sensitive measures of identifying the presence of stridor [212]. Since stridor has been associated with sudden death in some MSA patients, it is truly an emergency that requires immediate therapeutic attention. Rarely, stridor can be seen in other movement disorders, including Parkinson's disease, Creutzfeldt-Jakob disease, and Machado-Joseph disease [124].

The simplest therapy for stridor associated with MSA is CPAP [125]. Nocturnal video laryngoscopy has documented that CPAP is capable of producing separation of the adducted vocal cords and improvement of stridor [126]. In more advanced patients, where there may also be central hypoventilation, BIPAP has been suggested as the preferred therapy instead [127]. Should none of these approaches be practical or successful, or if there is daytime stridor, tracheostomy, the most definitive therapy, is required [125]. Precipitation or exacerbation of central sleep apnea has been reported to occur after institution of tracheostomy in some MSA patients, occasionally with a fatal outcome [128]. Some deaths during sleep have also been reported in MSA patients despite adequate CPAP therapy, and in these cases concurrent autonomic dysfunction is suspected to have resulted in a cardiac demise [129].

Acute Dystonic Reaction

Acute dystonic reactions (ADR) typically occur after exposure to DRBA. Neuroleptic agents such as haloperidol, or antiemetic agents such as prochlorperazine, are the most common offending agents, though the newer atypical neuroleptics can also potentially lead to development of ADRs [213]. Over 50% of ADRs occur within 24 h after DRBA exposure and approximately 90% occur within 5 days [130]. In the typical clinical presentation, the muscles of the mouth, face, eyes, and neck are involved resulting in one or more dystonic manifestations such as retrocollis, back arching, lateral flexion of the trunk (Pisa syndrome), trismus, tongue protrusion, or deviation of the eyes [131]. Trismus can be severe enough to dislocate the jaw. A potentially fatal form of ADR is dystonic laryngospasm with compromise of the airway [130, 132]. This must be correctly identified and distinguished from an anaphylactic reaction as the therapy of the two conditions is entirely different. The presence of stridor is an important marker of laryngeal dystonia.

Risk factors for ADR include young age, male gender, a primary psychotic disorder, and prior drug-induced dystonic reactions. Patients with homozygous mutations in the CYPZD6 gene that results in slow DRBA drug metabolism are also at greater risk for ADRs [133]. Drug dosage does not seem to be a risk factor. Children have a greater risk for this adverse effect compared to adults. The incidence of ADR seems to be higher after administration of very potent DRBAs, such as haloperidol [132], but milder DRBA such as metoclopramide [134] and drugs with little effect on dopaminergic transmission, such as selective serotonin reuptake inhibitors [135], are also capable of inducing the same syndrome. Rare cases of ADR have been reported after administration of drugs that have no apparent dopamine-blocking function, and patients with this syndrome exhibit the typical brisk response to anticholinergic therapy [136] discussed below. As an example of this phenomenon, both the antiviral drug foscarnet [137] and the commonly used antihistamine agent cetirizine [137] have been associated with ADR. ADR have also been reported with "ecstasy" (MDMA) use [138]. Although atypical antipsychotic agents have been associated with ADR [139], the incidence is lower than that associated with older neuroleptic agents [140, 141]. For example, a 25% incidence of ADR was reported in autistic children being treated with haloperidol [142], while a more recent trial of autistic children being treated with risperidone reported that none of 49 children developed ADR [141]. Cocaine used together with a DRBA predisposes to the development of ADR, and cocaine can cause ADR even when used alone [143]. Prophylactic pretreatment with anticholinergic drugs can reduce the incidence of ADR in susceptible individuals [132]. Interestingly, although having significant effects on the dopaminergic system, there are only limited reports of ADR in patients taking tetrabenazine and no reports of ADRs in patients taking the newer VMAT2 inhibitors, valbenazine or deutetrabenazine [214].

Children are not only at risk for ADR as a result of administration of prescribed DRBA but also from secretive (parent's medication) or unwise (excessive dose) ingestion of these agents [144]. In one example, several teenagers and one younger child developed ADR after ingesting a medication they believed was "street Xanax" but actually contained haloperidol instead [145].

The treatment of ADR consists of administering intravenous diphenhydramine (25–50 mg) or benztropine (1–2 mg). Intravenous diazepam, a second-line therapy, is also usually effective. These therapies are extremely effective, and the prompt benefit they produce helps confirm the diagnosis of ADR and, in the case of laryngospasm, may be lifesaving. After initial therapy of an ADR, it is wise to continue oral anticholinergic agents for 2 weeks, especially if a long-acting DRBA was used or in those cases where DRBA therapy must be continued. Premature discontinuance can result in recrudescence of symptoms [146]. Discontinuing anticholinergics should be done with a slow taper to avoid rebound worsening. Rarely, ADR can continue to recur over months despite discontinuance of the offending drug, requiring longer-term anticholinergic therapy [147].

Status Dystonicus

Status dystonicus (SD), also known as dystonic storm, is characterized by an acute onset of severe dystonic spasms or acute exacerbation of preex-

isting dystonia such that the patient is in extreme pain and/or at extreme risk for life-threatening complications. Status dystonicus can mimic other neurologic emergencies such as status epilepticus, neuroleptic malignant syndrome, serotonin syndrome, acute parkinsonism, intrathecal baclofen withdrawal, etc. and thus needs to be strongly considered as part of a differential [215]. Status dystonicus can develop in patients with primary dystonia (e.g., DYT1 and DYT6 dystonia) or more commonly in patients with secondary dystonia (e.g., Batten's disease or juvenile cerebral palsy) [216]. Acute onset of dystonia can occur in the setting of initiation of a new drug (especially a dopamine-blocking agent), or withdrawal of drugs in a dystonic patient (especially anticholinergic agents or intrathecal baclofen), or may simply be a severe spontaneous progression of a neurological condition for which dystonia is one possible clinical component (e.g., Wilson's disease). More commonly, SD is an event-related exacerbation of preexisting, generalized dystonia such as that associated with the DYT1 mutation or juvenile cerebral palsy. In patients with long-standing dystonia, an acute exacerbation may have an obvious precipitant, such as an intercurrent infection, recent trauma, or a change in medications. Alternatively, there may be no apparent cause for the sudden exacerbation of dystonia. The potential systemic complications of severe sustained dystonia are the main reason to consider this a medical emergency. Much like the systemic complications of NMS, patients experiencing SD can suffer respiratory embarrassment, rhabdomyolysis, and myoglobinuria, potentially leading to renal failure [148]. Because of these potentially life-threatening developments, these patients are typically managed in an intensive care unit.

The circumstances that have precipitated SD in each individual patient are important to understand since they may dictate the therapeutic approach. Infections at the onset of SD potentially account for greater than 50% of all triggers with the next most common etiology being medication adjustments at roughly 30% [216]. Thus, SD related to intercurrent infection requires urgent initiation of appropriate antibacterial or antiviral therapy. Similarly, withdrawal of an offending medication or reinstitution of a precipitously withdrawn medication will prove to be the most important therapeutic step in other patients. Notably, though, roughly one third of cases may not have an identifiable precipitating trigger [216].

Once the precipitating circumstance has been identified and neutralized, therapy must be initiated to improve the dystonia itself and the systemic complications that have resulted from it. Medical therapy of dystonia may require any or a combination of dopamine-depleting agents (tetrabenazine), anticholinergic drugs (trihexyphenidyl), and/or dopamine-blocking agent (haloperidol), each titrated to an effective or maximally tolerated safe dosage [148, 149]. Anticholinergic agents may be tolerated at higher dosages in those already receiving this class of medication and are also similarly well tolerated in high dosages by adolescents or young adults [150]. A variety of additional agents have been reported in individual cases to have provided benefit in cases of severe and acute dystonia, including dantrolene, baclofen, levodopa, carbamazepine, and various benzodiazepines. Intrathecal baclofen has been reported to be of benefit in a few patients refractory to medical therapy but is not uniformly beneficial [151]. On the other hand, there are cases in which intrathecal baclofen was ultimately of benefit despite lack of efficacy of a test bolus prior to proceeding to an implantable pump [152]. Despite the most aggressive medical therapy, severe dystonic spasms are likely to continue in upward of 90% of patients [216], raising the possibility that therapeutic paralysis, deep sedation, and ventilation may be required in an intensive care setting [153]. Deep sedation can be successfully achieved with propofol [154] or midazolam [155], both short-acting agents with the additional benefit of having gabaergic properties that might contribute to the antidystonic effect.

While in the intensive care unit, supportive measures will be required, including rehydration, control of fever, and careful monitoring of cardiac function and blood pressure. In patients who are still uncontrolled after a period of paralysis, ste-reotactic surgery including pallidotomy or bilateral pallidal deep brain stimulation may ultimately be required and is often the most successful strategy for refractory patients [156, 157, 216].

Stiff Person Syndrome

The stiff person syndrome (SPS) is classically associated with autoantibodies directed against glutamic acid decarboxylase (GAD), although newer antibodies have been detected in recent years including anti-amphiphysin, gephyrin antibodies, and gamma-aminobutyric acid type A receptor-associated protein (GABARAP) antibodies, gamma-aminobutyric acid type A receptor (GABA$_A$R) antibodies, glycine receptor antibodies, glycine transporter 2 antibodies, and dipeptidyl-peptidase-like protein-6 (DPPX) antibodies [217]. Although there is controversy about the role of these antibodies, they presumably act by reducing GABA-mediated inhibition of spinal interneurons with resultant axial and limb rigidity [158]. GAD antibodies are also found in patients with type 1 diabetes, but typically at much lower titers. The clinical syndrome consists of profound rigidity of predominantly axial and proximal limb muscles with superimposed, often stimulus sensitive, muscle spasms that can be severe enough to produce long bone fractures. These spasms, and the ongoing rigidity, can occasionally be life threatening, in that they can result in respiratory compromise, autonomic dysfunction, or both [159]. The clinician should be aware that any combination of one, two or three, or all four limbs can be involved separately, giving rise to a variant of the condition termed "stiff limb" syndrome [160].

There is also a paraneoplastic form of SPS, related to anti-amphiphysin antibodies. Unlike ordinary SPS which has a male predominance, the paraneoplastic form, most common in breast cancer, has a female predominance. In SPS the legs and axial muscles, especially the lower paraspinal muscles, are most commonly affected, whereas in amphiphysin antibody SPS, the arms and neck muscles are often most prominently affected [161]. A still more serious, although rarer, form is progressive encephalomyelitis with rigidity and myoclonus (PERM) which has a mortality rate up to 40% with 25% requiring mechanical ventilation [161]. The autoimmune form of SPS is associated with a high incidence of other autoimmune conditions, such as thyroiditis and systemic lupus and in fact may be the initial manifestation of a systemic autoimmune conditions such as lupus [162]. Similarly, paraneoplastic SPS can be the presenting symptoms of an occult carcinoma [163]. The clinician who is unfamiliar with this syndrome can easily conclude that a patient with SPS is hysterical, as sensory, long tract, cognitive, and coordination deficits are typically absent [164], and on occasion, only one, two, or three limbs are affected.

Symptomatic therapy of the rigidity in this condition consists of administration of gabaergic agents, such as clonazepam, diazepam, and baclofen. A variety of antiepileptic drugs, including vigabatrin, tiagabine, gabapentin, and levetiracetam, are considered to be somewhat beneficial [165]. Recommendations for treatment of the underlying autoimmune condition include IVIg [166], corticosteroids [167], and rituximab [168]. IVIG is the best studied immunosuppressive therapy and is generally considered the preferred agent in this category [164], although newer immunotherapies including rituximab have been shown to be potentially beneficial as well [218]. Although immunosuppressive therapy may be effective, it cannot be expected to have an immediate effect in an emergency room setting. Intrathecal baclofen can result in more rapid clinical improvement [169], but paradoxically any dysfunction in the baclofen pump system, such as pump failure or catheter leakage, can cause a baclofen withdrawal syndrome with an even more severe exacerbation of rigidity [170], making it imperative that both the clinician and the patient be aware of this possibility. Recently, the GABA receptor potentiator, propofol, in modest intravenous dosages, has been used with significant benefit to provide immediate relief of SPS spasms without attendant sedation [171]. In this circumstance it can be used as a therapeutic bridge pending the placement of a baclofen pump or until potent immunotherapy takes effect.

Hemiballism and Hemichorea

Large amplitude, proximally predominant flinging movements are characteristic of ballism. These movements are thought to exist on a clinical continuum with the smaller amplitude, more distally predominant movements of chorea. The fact that these two different types of abnormal involuntary movements are pathophysiologically related is supported by the observation that both may exist in the same individual at the same time, and ballism, as it improves, may evolve into chorea. In those cases in which chorea and ballism coexist or the abnormal movement is in an indeterminate zone between the two, the term hemichorea/hemiballism is often used. Ballistic movements are anatomically classified as monoballism (involving one limb), hemiballism (involving one side of the body), biballism (involvement of both sides of the body), or paraballism (involvement of both lower extremities). In those cases in which hemiballism is due to involvement of the STN, the somatotopic organization of this structure may account for the selective involvement of only one limb on one side of the body [172], and the same could be said of patients with a cortical lesion. Although the STN is a common location of structural pathology associated with hemiballism, modern neuroimaging has proven that it may not be the structure involved in the majority of cases. Other structures in the STN afferent or efferent pathways such as the striatum, thalamus, globus pallidus, and cerebral cortex may also be the locus of pathology [173]. In one of the largest series in the literature with poststroke hemichorea/hemiballism, only 4 of 27 patients had lesions confined to the STN, while 6 of them were in the stratum or cortex, with other isolated lesions being found in the putamen, caudate, or globus pallidus [173].

Ischemic and hemorrhagic strokes are the most common causes of hemiballism. In some cases of apparent vascular hemiballism, neuroimaging is totally normal, and in others, the CT scan is normal but MRI reveals a lacunar infarction in the STN or elsewhere [174]. Hemichorea/hemiballism develops on the day of stroke onset in the vast majority of cases, but in up to 10%, it may develop a day later and in rare cases as long as 5 days later [173]. Vascular hemichorea can also appear in the form of a TIA, so-called limb-shaking TIAs [175]. Although the prognosis for survival in those with vascular hemiballism was once thought to be worse than other stroke patients, especially in the preneuroleptic era, recent studies suggest that vascular hemiballism patients, many of whom have had lacunar strokes, have a risk of stroke recurrence and death that is similar to stroke patients in general [176]. As in the case with other stroke syndromes, surgical or neurointerventional procedures that improve cerebral circulation may have a salutary effect on vascular hemiballism [177], as discussed below.

A variety of other pathologies including encephalitis, systemic lupus erythematosus, multiple sclerosis, basal ganglia calcification, and nonketotic hyperglycemia can also result in hemiballism [178]. Structural pathologies such as bacterial or tuberculosis abscess, neoplasm, moyamoya disease, HIV-related toxoplasmosis, or arteriovenous malformation have also been associated with hemiballism. Stereotactic ablation of the STN for the treatment of Parkinson's disease can result in hemiballistic movements that are transient and improve in a matter of weeks [179] but can also rarely result in permanent hemiballism [180]. Similarly, therapeutic stimulation of the STN for Parkinson's disease can produce hemiballism that resolves when the stimulation is adjusted below a given threshold voltage [181].

The syndrome of hemiballism-hemichorea and magnetic resonance striatal hyperintensity associated with nonketotic hyperglycemia has been reported increasingly more frequently in recent years [182] and now represents the second most common cause of hemiballism, stroke being the most common. This syndrome appears to be much more common in patients of Asian descent [182]. In these cases, CT scan of the brain typically reveals hyperintensity in the contralateral striatum corresponding to MRI scans that show increased signal intensity on T1-weighted images and a decreased signal on T2-weighted scans. A high signal is occasionally seen on diffusion-weighted imaging [183]. After metabolic correc-tion of the hyperglycemic state, the abnormal involuntary movement usually disappears along with the CT and MRI abnormalities. In some cases, however, hemiballism persists despite disappearance of the MRI abnormality [184, 185]. Interestingly, the same CT and MRI findings have been seen in some hyperglycemic patients with no involuntary movements [186]. The exact nature of the striatal pathology remains unclear. The finding of normal gradient-echo MR images in hyperglycemic hemiballism along with striatal high signal intensity on a diffusion-weighted scan has suggested to some authors that hyperviscosity with associated cytotoxic edema may play a role in this syndrome [183]. However, autopsy and biopsy evaluation of the striatal tissue demonstrating MRI hyperintensity have revealed evidence of multiple foci of recent infarcts and/or gliosis [187, 188]. PET scans performed in the acute and subacute phases have suggested glucose hypometabolism in the affected regions of the brain [189].

The first therapeutic measure in treating hemiballism is to correct the underlying metabolic, infectious, or vascular abnormality to the extent possible. In the circumstance of nonketotic hyperglycemia and ischemic stroke, the two most common causes of hemiballism, this means correcting the hyperglycemia in the former condition and reversing the ischemia in the second condition through methods such as supporting blood pressure, thrombolytic therapy, and endovascular procedures. Acutely reversing ischemia can be effective in hemiballism due to transient ischemia or stroke [175, 177]. Hemiballism related to hyperglycemia may reverse within hours of correcting the metabolic abnormality, but up to 20% of patients continue to have ballism for months. Vascular hemiballism due to a completed stroke improves spontaneously in the majority of patients. In a series of 25 such patients followed for up to 3 years, hemiballism completely disappeared in 56% of cases after a mean duration of 15 days [173]. In another series of the same size, full recovery was noted after 3–15 days in 56% of patients [176].

In the absence of spontaneous or therapeutic reversal of hemiballism, it must then be treated symptomatically. For control of the abnormal involuntary movement itself, dopamine (DA)-blocking or DA-depleting drugs are the most effective symptomatic therapy. Traditionally, typical neuroleptics such as haloperidol have been used for this purpose, and more recently low-dose clozapine, olanzapine, and other atypical antipsychotic agents have also been found to be effective [190, 191]. Reserpine is an older therapy [192] that has been replaced by recently developed medications. The vascular mono-amine transporter 2 inhibitors tetrabenazine [193], valbenazine [209], and deutetrabenazine [210] can improve ballism. Caution must be exercised with any of these agents not to induce hypotension in patients whose hemiballism is due to stroke. This is especially true of tetrabenazine which has the highest side effect profile among these three drugs. Anticonvulsants can occasionally be beneficial, including valproic acid [194], topiramate [195], and levetiracetam [196]. Sertraline (Zoloft) has been reported to result in a prompt and nearly complete improvement of hemiballism in a single case [197]. In vascular hemichorea, physical therapy may speed improvement in the movement disorder [198]. If all these therapies fail and the amplitude of ballism threatens to produce physical injury, extreme exhaustion, or cardiac symptoms, stereotactic surgery consisting of contralateral GPi DBS for hyperglycemic [199] or vascular [200] hemiballism has been shown to be a useful therapy.

References

1. Curran T, Lang AE. Parkinsonian syndromes associated with hydrocephalus: case reports, a review of the literature, and pathophysiological hypotheses. Mov Disord. 1994;9(5):508–20.
2. Yomo S, Hongo K, Kuroyanagi T, Kobayashi S. Parkinsonism and midbrain dysfunction after shunt placement for obstructive hydrocephalus. J Clin Neurosci. 2006;13(3):373–8.
3. Prashantha DK, Netravathi M, Ravishankar S, Panda S, Pal PK. Reversible parkinsonism following ventriculoperitoneal shunt in a patient with obstructive hydrocephalus secondary to intraven-tricular neurocysticercosis. Clin Neurol Neurosurg. 2008;110(7):718–21.
4. Kim MJ, Chung SJ, Sung YH, Lee MC, Im JH. Levodopa-responsive parkinsonism associated with hydrocephalus. Mov Disord. 2006;21(8):1279–81.
5. Racette BA, Esper GJ, Antenor J, Black KJ, Burkey A, Moerlein SM, et al. Pathophysiology of parkinsonism due to hydrocephalus. J Neurol Neurosurg Psychiatry. 2004;75(11):1617–9.
6. Kinugawa K, Itti E, Lepeintre JF, Mari I, Czernecki V, Heran F, et al. Subacute dopa-responsive Parkinsonism after successful surgical treatment of aqueductal stenosis. Mov Disord. 2009;24(16):2438–40.
7. Vaamonde J, Flores JM, Gallardo MJ, Ibanez R. Subacute hemicorporal parkinsonism in 5 patients with infarcts of the basal ganglia. J Neural Transm. 2007;114(11):1463–7.
8. Peralta C, Werner P, Holl B, Kiechl S, Willeit J, Seppi K, et al. Parkinsonism following striatal infarcts: incidence in a prospective stroke unit cohort. J Neural Transm. 2004;111(10–11):1473–83.
9. Orta Daniel SJ, Ulises RO. Stroke of the substance nigra and parkinsonism as first manifestation of systemic lupus erythematosus. Parkinsonism Relat Disord. 2008;14(4):367–9.
10. Kuo SH, Kenney C, Jankovic J. Bilateral pedunculopontine nuclei strokes presenting as freezing of gait. Mov Disord. 2008;23(4):616–9.
11. Zijlmans JC, Katzenschlager R, Daniel SE, Lees AJ. The L-dopa response in vascular parkinsonism. J Neurol Neurosurg Psychiatry. 2004;75(4):545–7.
12. Choi SM, Lee SH, Park MS, Kim BC, Kim MK, Cho KH. Disappearance of resting tremor after thalamic stroke involving the territory of the tuberothalamic artery. Parkinsonism Relat Disord. 2008;14(4):373–5.
13. Bhatt MH, Elias MA, Mankodi AK. Acute and reversible parkinsonism due to organophosphate pesticide intoxication: five cases. Neurology. 1999;52(7):1467–71.
14. Shahar E, Bentur Y, Bar-Joseph G, Cahana A, Hershman E. Extrapyramidal parkinsonism complicating acute organophosphate insecticide poisoning. Pediatr Neurol. 2005;33(5):378–82.
15. Arima H, Sobue K, So M, Morishima T, Ando H, Katsuya H. Transient and reversible parkinsonism after acute organophosphate poisoning. J Toxicol Clin Toxicol. 2003;41(1):67–70.
16. Choi IS. Parkinsonism after carbon monoxide poisoning. Eur Neurol. 2002;48(1):30–3.
17. Lo CP, Chen SY, Lee KW, Chen WL, Chen CY, Hsueh CJ, et al. Brain injury after acute carbon monoxide poisoning: early and late complications. Am J Roentgenol. 2007;189(4):W205–11.
18. Weaver LK. Clinical practice. Carbon monoxide poisoning. N Engl J Med. 2009;360(12):1217–25.

19. Reddy NJ, Lewis LD, Gardner TB, Osterling W, Eskey CJ, Nierenberg DW. Two cases of rapid onset Parkinson's syndrome following toxic ingestion of ethylene glycol and methanol. Clin Pharmacol Ther. 2007;81(1):114–21.

20. Soykan I, Sivri B, Sarosiek I, Kiernan B, McCallum RW. Demography, clinical characteristics, psychological and abuse profiles, treatment, and long-term follow-up of patients with gastroparesis. Dig Dis Sci. 1998;43(11):2398–404.

21. Onofrj M, Thomas A. Acute akinesia in Parkinson disease. Neurology. 2005;64(7):1162–9.

22. Dafotakis M, Sparing R, Juzek A, Block F, Kosinski CM. Transdermal dopaminergic stimulation with rotigotine in Parkinsonian akinetic crisis. J Clin Neurosci. 2009;16(2):335–7.

23. Galvez-Jimenez N, Lang AE. The perioperative management of Parkinson's disease revisited. Neurol Clin. 2004;22(2):367–77.

24. Rodnitzky RL. Drug-induced movement disorders. Clin Neuropharmacol. 2002;25(3):142–52.

25. Caroff SN, Mann SC. Neuroleptic malignant syndrome. Psychopharmacol Bull. 1988;24(1):25–9.

26. Keyser DL, Rodnitzky RL. Neuroleptic malignant syndrome in Parkinson's disease after withdrawal or alteration of dopaminergic therapy. Arch Intern Med. 1991;151(4):794–6.

27. Takubo H, Harada T, Hashimoto T, Inaba Y, Kanazawa I, Kuno S, et al. A collaborative study on the malignant syndrome in Parkinson's disease and related disorders. Parkinsonism Relat Disord. 2003;9(Suppl 1):S31–41.

28. Serrano-Duenas M. Neuroleptic malignant syndrome-like, or–dopaminergic malignant syndrome–due to levodopa therapy withdrawal. Clinical features in 11 patients. Parkinsonism Relat Disord. 2003;9(3):175–8.

29. Dalkılıc A, Grosch WN. Neuroleptic malignant syndrome following initiation of clozapine therapy. Am J Psychiatry. 1997;154(6):881–2.

30. Filice GA, McDougall BC, Ercan-Fang N, Billington CJ. Neuroleptic malignant syndrome associated with olanzapine. Ann Pharmacother. 1998;32(11):1158–9.

31. Norris B, Angeles V, Eisenstein R, Seale JP. Neuroleptic malignant syndrome with delayed onset of fever following risperidone administration. Ann Pharmacother. 2006;40(12):2260–4.

32. Gray NS. Ziprasidone-related neuroleptic malignant syndrome in a patient with Parkinson's disease: a diagnostic challenge. Hum Psychopharmacol. 2004;19(3):205–7.

33. Karagianis JL, Phillips LC, Hogan KP, LeDrew KK. Clozapine-associated neuroleptic malignant syndrome: two new cases and a review of the literature. Ann Pharmacother. 1999;33(5):623–30.

34. Nielsen J, Bruhn AM. Atypical neuroleptic malignant syndrome caused by olanzapine. Acta Psychiatr Scand. 2005;112(3):238–40.

35. Ferioli V, Manes A, Melloni C, Nanni S, Boncompagni G. Atypical neuroleptic malignant syndrome caused by clozapine and venlafaxine: early brief treatment with dantrolene. Can J Psychiatr. 2004;49(7):497–8.

36. Ananth J, Parameswaran S, Gunatilake S, Burgoyne K, Sidhom T. Neuroleptic malignant syndrome and atypical antipsychotic drugs. J Clin Psychiatry. 2004;65(4):464–70.

37. Rodnitzky RL, Keyser DL. Neurologic complications of drugs. Tardive dyskinesias, neuroleptic malignant syndrome, and cocaine-related syndromes. Psychiatr Clin North Am. 1992;15(2):491–510.

38. Baca L, Martinelli L. Neuroleptic malignant syndrome: a unique association with a tricyclic antidepressant. Neurology. 1990;40(11):1797–8.

39. Halman M, Goldbloom DS. Fluoxetine and neuroleptic malignant syndrome. Biol Psychiatry. 1990;28(6):518–21.

40. Fava S, Galizia AC. Neuroleptic malignant syndrome and lithium carbonate. J Psychiatry Neurosci. 1995;20(4):305–6.

41. Sachdev P, Mason C, Hadzi-Pavlovic D. Case–control study of neuroleptic malignant syndrome. Am J Psychiatry. 1997;154(8):1156–8.

42. Naganuma H, Fujii I. Incidence and risk factors in neuroleptic malignant syndrome. Acta Psychiatr Scand. 1994;90(6):424–6.

43. Hermesh H, Manor I, Shiloh R, Aizenberg D, Benjamini Y, Munitz II, et al. High serum creatinine kinase level: possible risk factor for neuroleptic malignant syndrome. J Clin Psychopharmacol. 2002;22(3):252–6.

44. Harada T, Mitsuoka K, Kumagai R, Murata Y, Kaseda Y, Kamei H, et al. Clinical features of malignant syndrome in Parkinson's disease and related neurological disorders. Parkinsonism Relat Disord. 2003;9(Suppl 1).S15–23.

45. Stotz M, Thummler D, Schurch M, Renggli JC, Urwyler A, Pargger H. Fulminant neuroleptic malignant syndrome after perioperative withdrawal of antiParkinsonian medication. Br J Anaesth. 2004;93(6):868–71.

46. Ladha SS, Walker R, Shill HA. Case of neuroleptic malignant-like syndrome precipitated by abrupt fava bean discontinuance. Mov Disord. 2005;20(5):630–1.

47. Gaig C, Marti MJ, Tolosa E, Gomez-Choco MJ, Amaro S. Parkinsonism-hyperpyrexia syndrome not related to antiparkinsonian treatment withdrawal during the 2003 summer heat wave. J Neurol. 2005;252(9):1116–9.

48. Kurlan R, Hamill R, Shoulson I. Neuroleptic malignant syndrome. Clin Neuropharmacol. 1984;7(2):109–20.

49. Caroff SN. The neuroleptic malignant syndrome. J Clin Psychiatry. 1980;41(3):79–83.

50. Balzan MV. The neuroleptic malignant syndrome: a logical approach to the patient with tempera-

ture and rigidity. Postgrad Med J. 1998;74(868): 72–6.

51. Wong MM. Neuroleptic malignant syndrome: two cases without muscle rigidity. Aust N Z J Psychiatry. 1996;30(3):415–8.

52. Peiris DT, Kuruppuarachchi K, Weerasena LP, Seneviratne SL, Tilakaratna YT, De Silva HJ, et al. Neuroleptic malignant syndrome without fever: a report of three cases. J Neurol Neurosurg Psychiatry. 2000;69(2):277–8.

53. Hall RC, Appleby B, Hall RC. Atypical neuroleptic malignant syndrome presenting as fever of unknown origin in the elderly. South Med J. 2005;98(1):114–7.

54. Taniguchi N, Tanii H, Nishikawa T, Miyamae Y, Shinozaki K, Inoue Y, et al. Classification system of complications in neuroleptic malignant syndrome. Methods Find Exp Clin Pharmacol. 1997;19(3):193–9.

55. Naramoto A, Koizumi N, Itoh N, Shigematsu H. An autopsy case of cerebellar degeneration following lithium intoxication with neuroleptic malignant syndrome. Acta Pathol Jpn. 1993;43(1–2):55–8.

56. Sakkas P, Davis JM, Janicak PG, Wang ZY. Drug treatment of the neuroleptic malignant syndrome. Psychopharmacol Bull. 1991;27(3):381–4.

57. Storm C, Gebker R, Kruger A, Nibbe L, Schefold JC, Martens F, et al. A rare case of neuroleptic malignant syndrome presenting with serious hyperthermia treated with a non-invasive cooling device: a case report. J Med Case Rep. 2009;3:6170.

58. Wang HC, Hsieh Y. Treatment of neuroleptic malignant syndrome with subcutaneous apomorphine monotherapy. Mov Disord. 2001;16(4):765–7.

59. Lattanzi L, Mungai F, Romano A, Bonuccelli U, Cassano GB, Fagiolini A. Subcutaneous apomorphine for neuroleptic malignant syndrome. Am J Psychiatry. 2006;163(8):1450–1.

60. Tsutsumi Y, Yamamoto K, Matsuura S, Hata S, Sakai M, Shirakura K. The treatment of neuroleptic malignant syndrome using dantrolene sodium. Psychiatry Clin Neurosci. 1998;52(4):433–8.

61. Thomas P, Maron M, Rascle C, Cottencin O, Vaiva G, Goudemand M. Carbamazepine in the treatment of neuroleptic malignant syndrome. Biol Psychiatry. 1998;43(4):303–5.

62. Rosebush PI, Stewart T, Mazurek MF. The treatment of neuroleptic malignant syndrome. Are dantrolene and bromocriptine useful adjuncts to supportive care? Br J Psychiatry. 1991;159:709–12.

63. Davis JM, Janicak PG, Sakkas P, Gilmore C, Wang Z. Electroconvulsive therapy in the treatment of the neuroleptic malignant syndrome. Convuls Ther. 1991;7(2):111–20.

64. Meagher LJ, McKay D, Herkes GK, Needham M. Parkinsonism-hyperpyrexia syndrome: the role of electroconvulsive therapy. J Clin Neurosci. 2006;13(8):857–9.

65. Adityanjee SM, Munshi KR. Neuropsychiatric sequelae of neuroleptic malignant syndrome. Clin Neuropharmacol. 2005;28(4):197–204.

66. Sato Y, Asoh T, Metoki N, Satoh K. Efficacy of methylprednisolone pulse therapy on neuroleptic malignant syndrome in Parkinson's disease. J Neurol Neurosurg Psychiatry. 2003;74(5):574–6.

67. Rushton JL, Whitmire JT. Pediatric stimulant and selective serotonin reuptake inhibitor prescription trends—1992 to 1998. Arch Pediatr Adolesc Med. 2001;155(5):560–5.

68. Sternbach H. The serotonin syndrome. Am J Psychiatry. 1991;148(6):705–13.

69. Dunkley EJ, Isbister GK, Sibbritt D, Dawson AH, Whyte IM. The Hunter Serotonin Toxicity Criteria: simple and accurate diagnostic decision rules for serotonin toxicity. QJM. 2003;96(9):635–42.

70. Demirkiran M, Jankovic J, Dean JM. Ecstasy intoxication: an overlap between serotonin syndrome and neuroleptic malignant syndrome. Clin Neuropharmacol. 1996;19(2):157–64.

71. Attar-Herzberg D, Apel A, Gang N, Dvir D, Mayan H. The serotonin syndrome: initial misdiagnosis. Isr Med Assoc J. 2009;11(6):367–70.

72. Lane R, Baldwin D. Selective serotonin reuptake inhibitor-induced serotonin syndrome: review. J Clin Psychopharmacol. 1997;17(3):208–21.

73. Isbister GK, Buckley NA. The pathophysiology of serotonin toxicity in animals and humans: implications for diagnosis and treatment. Clin Neuropharmacol. 2005;28(5):205–14.

74. Mekler G, Woggon B. A case of serotonin syndrome caused by venlafaxine and lithium. Pharmacopsychiatry. 1997;30:272–3.

75. Nisijima K, Shimizu M, Abe T, Ishiguro T. A case of serotonin syndrome induced by concomitant treatment with low-dose trazodone and amitriptyline and lithium. Int Clin Psychopharmacol. 1996;11(4):289–90.

76. Gillman PK. Serotonin syndrome: history and risk. Fundam Clin Pharmacol. 1998;12:482–91.

77. Kaminski CA, Robbins MS, Weibley RE. Sertraline intoxication in a child. Ann Emerg Med. 1994;23:1371–4.

78. Horowitz BZ, Mullins ME. Cyproheptadine for serotonin syndrome in an accidental pediatric sertraline ingestion. Pediatr Emerg Care. 1999;15(5):325–7.

79. Schwartz RH, Miller NS. MDMA (Ecstasy) and the rave: a review. Pediatrics. 1997;100(4):705–8.

80. Vuori E, Henry JA, Ojanpera I, Nieminen R, Savolainen T, Wahlsten P, et al. Death following ingestion of MDMA (ecstasy) and moclobemide. Addiction. 2003;98(3):365–8.

81. Schifano F, Corkery J, Naidoo V, Oyefeso A, Ghodse H. Overview of amphetamine-type stimulant mortality data–UK, 1997–2007. Neuropsychobiology. 2010;61(3):122–30.

82. Ganetsky M, Bird SB, Liang IE. Acute myocardial infarction associated with the serotonin syndrome. Ann Intern Med. 2006;144(10):782–3.

83. Soldin OP, Tonning JM. Serotonin syndrome associated with triptan monotherapy. N Engl J Med. 2008;358(20):2185–6.

84. Wooltorton E. Triptan migraine treatments and anti-depressants: risk of serotonin syndrome. Can Med Assoc J. 2006;175(8):874–5.

85. Evans RW, The FDA. Alert on serotonin syndrome with combined use of SSRIs or SNRIs and Triptans: an analysis of the 29 case reports. MedGenMed. 2007;9(3):48.

86. Orloya Y, Rizzoli P, Loder E. Association of coprescription of triptan antimigraine drugs and selective serotonin uptake inhibitor antidepressants with serotonin syndrome. JAMA Neurol. 2018;75(5):566–72.

87. Huang V, Gortney JS. Risk of serotonin syndrome with concomitant administration of linezolid and serotonin agonists. Pharmacotherapy. 2006;26(12):1784–93.

88. Martino EA, Winterton D, Nardelli P, Pasin L, Calabro MG, Bove T, et al. The blue coma: the role of methylene blue in unexplained coma after cardiac surgery. J Cardiovasc Anesth. 2016;30(2):423–7.

89. Frye JR, Poggemiller AM, Andrew M, McGonagill PW, Pape KO, Galet C, et al. Use of cyproheptadine for the treatment of serotonin syndrome: a case series. J Clin Psychopharmacol. 2020;40(1):95–9.

90. Van Gerpen JA. Drug-induced parkinsonism. Neurologist. 2002;8(6):363–70.

91. Diaz-Corrales FJ, Sanz-Viedma S, Garcia-Solis D, Escobar-Delgado T, Mir P. Clinical features and 123I-FP-CIT SPECT imaging in drug-induced parkinsonism and Parkinson's disease. Eur J Nucl Med Mol Imaging. 2010;37(3):556–64.

92. Tinazzi M, Morgante F, Matinella A, Bovi T, Cannas A, Solla P, et al. Imaging of the dopamine transporter predicts pattern of disease and response to levodopa in patients with schizophrenia and parkinsonism; a 2 year follow-up multicenter study. Schizophr Res. 2014;152(2–3):344–9.

93. Okunoye O, Kojima G, Marston L, Walters K, Schrag A. Factors associated with hospitalisation among people with Parkinson's disease-A systemic review and meta-analysis. Pakinsonism Relat Disord. 2020;71(2):66–72.

94. Jang H, Boltz DA, Webster RG, Smeyne RJ. Viral parkinsonism. Biochim Biophys Acta. 2009;1792(7):714–21.

95. Solbrig MV, Nashef L. Acute parkinsonism in suspected herpes simplex encephalitis. Mov Disord. 1993;8(2):233–4.

96. Robinson RL, Shahida S, Madan N, Rao S, Khardori N. Transient parkinsonism in West Nile virus encephalitis. Am J Med. 2003;115(3):252–3.

97. Lopez-Alberola R, Georgiou M, Sfakianakis GN, Singer C, Papapetropoulos S. Contemporary Encephalitis Lethargica: phenotype, laboratory findings and treatment outcomes. J Neurol. 2009;256(3):396–404.

98. Dale RC, Church AJ, Surtees RA, Lees AJ, Adcock JE, Harding B, et al. Encephalitis lethargica syndrome: 20 new cases and evidence of basal ganglia autoimmunity. Brain. 2004;127(Pt 1):21–33.

99. McKee DH, Sussman JD. Case report: severe acute Parkinsonism associated with streptococcal infection and antibasal ganglia antibodies. Mov Disord. 2005;20(12):1661–3.

100. Dimova PS, Bojinova V, Georgiev D, Milanov I. Acute reversible parkinsonism in Epstein-Barr virus-related encephalitis lethargica-like illness. Mov Disord. 2006;21(4):564–6.

101. Cooper MK, Brock DG, McDaniel CM. Interaction between levodopa and enteral nutrition. Ann Pharmacother. 2008;42(3):439–42.

102. Brashear A, Dobyns WB, de Carvalho AP, Borg M, Frijns CJ, Gollamudi S, et al. The phenotypic spectrum of rapid-onset dystonia-parkinsonism (RDP) and mutations in the ATP1A3 gene. Brain. 2007;130(Pt 3):828–35.

103. Haq IU, Snively BM, Sweadner KJ, Soerken CK, Cook JF, Ozelius LJ, et al. Revising rapid-onset dystonia-parkinsonism: broadening indications for ATP1A3 testing. Mov Disord. 2019;34(10):1528–36.

104. Factor SA, Molho ES. Emergency department presentations of patients with Parkinson's disease. Am J Emerg Med. 2000;18(2):209–15.

105. Karstaedt PJ, Pincus JH. Protein redistribution diet remains effective in patients with fluctuating parkinsonism. Arch Neurol. 1992;49(2):149–51.

106. Thomas AA, Friedman JH. Current use of clozapine in parkinson disease and related disorders. Clin Neuropharmacol. 2010;33(1):14–6.

107. Mcrims D, Balas M, Peretz C, Shabtai H, Giladi N. Rater-blinded, prospective comparison: quetiapine versus clozapine for Parkinson's disease psychosis. Clin Neuropharmacol. 2006;29(6):331–7.

108. Ondo WG, Tintner R, Voung KD, Lai D, Ringholz G. Double-blind, placebo-controlled, unforced titration parallel trial of quetiapine for dopaminergic-induced hallucinations in Parkinson's disease. Mov Disord. 2005;20(8):958–63.

109. Sellers J, Darby RR, Farooque, Claasen DO. Pimavanserin for psychosis in Parkinson's disease-related disorders; a retrospective chart review. Drugs Aging. 2019;36(7):647–53.

110. Kitten KA, Hallowell SA, Saklad SR, Evoy KE. Pimavanserin: a novel drug approved to treat Parkinson's disease psychosis. Innov Clin Neurosci. 2018;15(1–2):16–22.

111. Schneider LS, Dagerman KS, Insel P. Risk of death with atypical antipsychotic drug treatment for dementia: meta-analysis of randomized placebo-controlled trials. JAMA. 2005;294(15):1934–43.

112. Pontone GM, Williams JR, Anderson KE, Chase G, Goldstein SA, Grill S, et al. Prevalence of anxiety disorders and anxiety subtypes in patients with Parkinson's disease. Mov Disord. 2009;24(9):1333–8.

113. Sieber FE, Zakriya KJ, Gottschalk A, Blute MR, Lee HB, Rosenberg PB, et al. Sedation depth during spinal anesthesia and the development of postoperative delirium in elderly patients undergoing hip fracture repair. Mayo Clin Proc. 2010;85(1):18–26.

114. Crosby G, Culley DJ, Marcantonio ER. Delirium: a cognitive cost of the comfort of procedural sedation in elderly patients? Mayo Clin Proc. 2010;85(1):12–4.

115. Devlin JW, Roberts RJ, Fong JJ, Skrobik Y, Riker RR, Hill NS, et al. Efficacy and safety of quetiapine in critically ill patients with delirium: a prospective, multicenter, randomized, double-blind, placebo-controlled pilot study. Crit Care Med. 2010;38(2):419–27.

116. Khouzam HR. Quetiapine in the treatment of postoperative delirium. A report of three cases. Compr Ther. 2008;34(3–4):207–17.

117. Marcantonio ER. Delirium in hospitalized older adults. N Engl J Med. 2017;377(15):1456–66.

118. Shepard MD, Perepezeko K, Broen M, Hinkle JT, Batula,A, Mills KA, et al.Suicide in parkinson's disease. J Neurol Neurosurg Psychiatry. 2019;90(7):822–9.

119. Nazem S, Siderowf AD, Duda JE, Brown GK, Ten Have T, Stern MB, et al. Suicidal and death ideation in Parkinson's disease. Mov Disord. 2008;23(11):1573–9.

120. Xu Y, Yang B, Zhou C, Gu M, Long J, Wang F, et al. Suicide and suicide attempts after subthalamic nucleus stimulation in Parkinson's disease: a systemic review and meta-analysis. Neurol Sci. 2021;42(1):267–74.

121. Voon V, Krack P, Lang AE, Lozano AM, Dujardin K, Schupbach M, et al. A multicentre study on suicide outcomes following subthalamic stimulation for Parkinson's disease. Brain. 2008;131(Pt 10):2720–8.

122. Glass GA, Josephs KA, Ahlskog JE. Respiratory insufficiency as the primary presenting symptom of multiple-system atrophy. Arch Neurol. 2006;63(7):978–81.

123. Silber MH, Levine S. Stridor and death in multiple system atrophy. Mov Disord. 2000;15(4):699–704.

124. Li L, Saigusa H, Nagayama H, Nakamura T, Aino I, Komachi T, et al. A case of Creutzfeldt-Jacob disease with bilateral vocal fold abductor paralysis. J Voice. 2009;23(5):635–8.

125. Isozaki E, Naito A, Horiguchi S, Kawamura R, Hayashida T, Tanabe H. Early diagnosis and stage classification of vocal cord abductor paralysis in patients with multiple system atrophy. J Neurol Neurosurg Psychiatry. 1996;60(4):399–402.

126. Kuzniar TJ, Morgenthaler TI, Prakash UB, Pallanch JF, Silber MH, Tippmann-Peikert M. Effects of continuous positive airway pressure on stridor in multiple system atrophy-sleep laryngoscopy. J Clin Sleep Med. 2009;5(1):65–7.

127. Nonaka M, Imai T, Shintani T, Kawamata M, Chiba S, Matsumoto H. Non-invasive positive pressure ventilation for laryngeal contraction disorder during sleep in multiple system atrophy. J Neurol Sci. 2006;247(1):53–8.

128. Jin K, Okabe S, Chida K, Abe N, Kimpara T, Ohnuma A, et al. Tracheostomy can fatally exacer-bate sleep-disordered breathing in multiple system atrophy. Neurology. 2007;68(19):1618–21.

129. Munschauer FE, Loh L, Bannister R, Newsom-Davis J. Abnormal respiration and sudden death during sleep in multiple system atrophy with autonomic failure. Neurology. 1990;40(4):677–9.

130. Garver DL, Davis DM, Dekirmenjian H, Ericksen S, Gosenfeld L, Haraszti J. Dystonic reactions following neuroleptics: time course and proposed mechanisms. Psychopharmacologia. 1976;47(2):199–201.

131. Cossu G, Colosimo C. Hyperkinetic Movement Disorder Emergencies. Curr Neuro Neurosci Rep. 2017;17(1):6.

132. Aguilar EJ, Keshavan MS, Martinez-Quiles MD, Hernandez J, Gomez-Beneyto M, Schooler NR. Predictors of acute dystonia in first-episode psychotic patients. Am J Psychiatry. 1994;151(12):1819–21.

133. der van PA, Van Schaik RH, Sonneveld P. Acute dystonic reaction to metoclopramide in patients carrying homozygous cytochrome P450 2D6 genetic polymorphisms. Neth J Med. 2006;64(5):160–2.

134. Tait PA. Supraglottic dystonic reaction to metoclopramide in a child. Med J Aust. 2001;174(11):607–8.

135. Najjar F, Price LH. Citalopram and dystonia. J Am Acad Child Adolesc Psychiatry. 2004;43(1):8–9.

136. Dubow JS, Panush SR, Rezak M, Leikin J. Acute dystonic reaction associated with foscarnet administration. Am J Ther. 2008;15(2):184–6.

137. Esen I, Demirpence S, Yis U, Kurul S. Cetirizine-induced dystonic reaction in a 6-year-old boy. Pediatr Emerg Care. 2008;24(9):627–8.

138. Priori A, Bertolasi L, Berardelli A, Manfredi M. Acute dystonic reaction to ecstasy. Mov Disord. 1995;10(3):353.

139. Mason MN, Johnson CE, Piasecki M. Ziprasidone-induced acute dystonia. Am J Psychiatry. 2005;162(3):625–6.

140. Ramos AE, Shytle RD, Silver AA, Sanberg PR. Ziprasidone-induced oculogyric crisis. J Am Acad Child Adolesc Psychiatry. 2003;42(9):1013–4.

141. McCracken JT, McGough J, Shah B, Cronin P, Hong D, Aman MG, et al. Risperidone in children with autism and serious behavioral problems. N Engl J Med. 2002;347(5):314–21.

142. Anderson LT, Campbell M, Grega DM, Perry R, Small AM, Green WH. Haloperidol in the treatment of infantile autism: effects on learning and behavioral symptoms. Am J Psychiatry. 1984;141(10):1195–202.

143. Fines RE, Brady WJ, DeBehnke DJ. Cocaine-associated dystonic reaction. Am J Emerg Med. 1997;15(5):513–5.

144. Russell SA, Hennes HM, Herson KJ, Stremski ES. Upper airway compromise in acute chlorpromazine ingestion. Am J Emerg Med. 1996;14(5):467–8.

145. Hendrickson RG, Morocco AP, Greenberg MI. Acute dystonic reactions to "street Xanax". N Engl J Med. 2002;346(22):1753.

146. Roberge RJ. Antiemetic-related dystonic reaction unmasked by removal of a scopolamine transdermal patch. J Emerg Med. 2006;30(3):299–302.
147. Schneider SA, Udani V, Sankhla CS, Bhatia KP. Recurrent acute dystonic reaction and oculogyric crisis despite withdrawal of dopamine receptor blocking drugs. Mov Disord. 2009;24(8):1226–9.
148. Allen NM, Lin JP, Lynch T, et al. Status Dystonicus: a practice guide. Dev Med Child Neurol. 2014;56(2):105–12.
149. Marsden CD, Marion MH, Quinn N. The treatment of severe dystonia in children and adults. J Neurol Neurosurg Psychiatry. 1984;47(11):1166–73.
150. Fahn S. High-dosage anticholinergic therapy in dystonia. Adv Neurol. 1983;37:177–88.
151. Walker RH, Danisi FO, Swope DM, Goodman RR, Germano IM, Brin MF. Intrathecal baclofen for dystonia: benefits and complications during six years of experience. Mov Disord. 2000;15(6):1242–7.
152. Hou JG, Ondo W, Jankovic J. Intrathecal baclofen for dystonia. Mov Disord. 2001;16(6):1201–2.
153. Vaamonde J, Narbona J, Weiser R, Garcia MA, Brannan T, Obeso JA. Dystonic storms: a practical management problem. Clin Neuropharmacol. 1994;17(4):344–7.
154. Teive HA, Munhoz RP, Souza MM, Antoniuk SA, Santos ML, Teixeira MJ, et al. Status Dystonicus: study of five cases. Arq Neuropsiquiatr. 2005;63(1):26–9.
155. Mariotti P, Fasano A, Contarino MF, Della MG, Piastra M, Genovese O, et al. Management of status dystonicus: our experience and review of the literature. Mov Disord. 2007;22(7):963–8.
156. Elkay M, Silver K, Penn RD, Dalvi A. Dystonic storm due to Batten's disease treated with pallidotomy and deep brain stimulation. Mov Disord. 2009;24(7):1048–53.
157. Apetaucrova D, Schirmer CM, Shils JL, Zani J, Arle JE. Successful bilateral deep brain stimulation of the globus pallidus internus for persistent status dystonicus and generalized chorea. J Neurosurg. 2010;113(3):634–8.
158. Levy LM, Dalakas MC, Floeter MK. The stiff-person syndrome: an autoimmune disorder affecting neurotransmission of gamma-aminobutyric acid. Ann Intern Med. 1999;131(7):522–30.
159. Mitsumoto H, Schwartzman MJ, Estes ML, Chou SM, La Franchise EF, De Camilli P, et al. Sudden death and paroxysmal autonomic dysfunction in stiff-man syndrome. J Neurol. 1991;238(2):91–6.
160. Teive HA, Munhoz RP, Cardoso J, Amaral VC, Werneck LC. Stiff-three limbs syndrome. Mov Disord. 2009;24(2):311–2.
161. Baizabal-Carvallo JF, Jankovic J. Stiff-person syndrome: insights into a complex autoimmune disorder. J Neurol Neurosurg Psychiatry. 2015;86(8):840–8.
162. Munhoz RP, Fameli H, Teive HA. Stiff person syndrome as the initial manifestation of systemic lupus erythematosus. Mov Disord. 2010;25(4):516–7.
163. Liu YL, Lo WC, Tseng CH, Tsai CH, Yang YW. Reversible stiff person syndrome presenting as an initial symptom in a patient with colon adenocarcinoma. Acta Oncol. 2010;49(2):271–2.
164. Fleischman D, Madan G, Zesiewicz TA, Fleischman M. Stiff-person syndrome: commonly mistaken for hysterical paralysis. Clin Neurol Neurosurg. 2009;111(7):644.
165. Dalakas MC. Stiff person syndrome: advances in pathogenesis and therapeutic interventions. Curr Treat Options Neurol. 2009;11(2):102–10.
166. Dalakas MC. The role of IVIg in the treatment of patients with stiff person syndrome and other neurological diseases associated with anti-GAD antibodies. J Neurol. 2005;252(Suppl 1):I19–25.
167. Kim JY, Chung EJ, Kim JH, Jung KY, Lee WY. Response to steroid treatment in anti-glutamic acid decarboxylase antibody-associated cerebellar ataxia, stiff person syndrome and polyendocrinopathy. Mov Disord. 2006;21(12):2263–4.
168. Baker MR, Das M, Isaacs J, Fawcett PR, Bates D. Treatment of stiff person syndrome with rituximab. J Neurol Neurosurg Psychiatry. 2005;76(7):999–1001.
169. Seitz RJ, Blank B, Kiwit JC, Benecke R. Stiff-person syndrome with anti-glutamic acid decarboxylase autoantibodies: complete remission of symptoms after intrathecal baclofen administration. J Neurol. 1995;242(10):618–22.
170. Bardutzky J, Tronnier V, Schwab S, Meinck HM. Intrathecal baclofen for stiff-person syndrome: life-threatening intermittent catheter leakage. Neurology. 2003;60(12):1976–8.
171. Vernino S, McEvoy K. Propofol for stiff-person syndrome: learning new tricks from an old dog. Neurology. 2008;70(18):1584–5.
172. Nambu A, Takada M, Inase M, Tokuno H. Dual somatotopical representations in the primate subthalamic nucleus: evidence for ordered but reversed body-map transformations from the primary motor cortex and the supplementary motor area. J Neurosci. 1996;16(8):2671–83.
173. Chung SJ, Im JH, Lee MC, Kim JS. Hemichorea after stroke: clinical-radiological correlation. J Neurol. 2004;251(6):725–9.
174. Biller J, Graff-Radford NR, Smoker WR, Adams HP Jr, Johnston P. MR imaging in "lacunar" hemiballismus. J Comput Assist Tomogr. 1986;10(5):793–7.
175. Leira EC, Ajax T, Adams HP Jr. Limb-shaking carotid transient ischemic attacks successfully treated with modification of the antihypertensive regimen. Arch Neurol. 1997;54(7):904–5.
176. Ristic A, Marinkovic J, Dragasevic N, Stanisavljevic D, Kostic V. Long-term prognosis of vascular hemiballismus. Stroke. 2002;33(8):2109–11.
177. Mohebati A, Brevetti LS, Graham AM. Resolution of hemiballism after carotid endarterectomy: case report. Ann Vasc Surg. 2005;19(5):737–9.

178. Vidakovic A, Dragasevic N, Kostic VS. Hemiballism: report of 25 cases. J Neurol Neurosurg Psychiatry. 1994;57(8):945–9.

179. Barlas O, Hanagasi HA, Imer M, Sahin HA, Sencer S, Emre M. Do unilateral ablative lesions of the subthalamic nuclei in parkinsonian patients lead to hemiballism? Mov Disord. 2001;16(2):306–10.

180. Chen CC, Lee ST, Wu T, Chen CJ, Huang CC, Lu CS. Hemiballism after subthalamotomy in patients with Parkinson's disease: report of 2 cases. Mov Disord. 2002;17(6):1367–71.

181. Limousin P, Pollak P, Hoffmann D, Benazzouz A, Perret JE, Benabid AL. Abnormal involuntary movements induced by subthalamic nucleus stimulation in parkinsonian patients. Mov Disord. 1996;11(3):231–5.

182. Lin JJ, Lin GY, Shih C, Shen WC. Presentation of striatal hyperintensity on T1-weighted MRI in patients with hemiballism-hemichorea caused by non-ketotic hyperglycemia: report of seven new cases and a review of literature. J Neurol. 2001;248(9):750–5.

183. Chu K, Kang DW, Kim DE, Park SH, Roh JK. Diffusion-weighted and gradient echo magnetic resonance findings of hemichorea-hemiballismus associated with diabetic hyperglycemia: a hyperviscosity syndrome? Arch Neurol. 2002;59(3):448–52.

184. Ahlskog JE, Nishino H, Evidente VG, Tulloch JW, Forbes GS, Caviness JN, et al. Persistent chorea triggered by hyperglycemic crisis in diabetics. Mov Disord. 2001;16(5):890–8.

185. Hashimoto T, Hanyu N, Yahikozawa H, Yanagisawa N. Persistent hemiballism with striatal hyperintensity on T1-weighted MRI in a diabetic patient: a 6-year follow-up study. J Neurol Sci. 1999;165(2):178–81.

186. Sorimachi T, Fujii Y, Tsuchiya N, Saito M. Striatal hyperintensity on T1-weighted magnetic resonance images and high-density signal on CT scans obtained in patients with hyperglycemia and no involuntary movement. Report of two cases. J Neurosurg. 2004;101(2):343–6.

187. Shan DE, Ho DM, Chang C, Pan HC, Teng MM. Hemichorea-hemiballism: an explanation for MR signal changes. Am J Neuroradiol. 1998;19(5):863–70.

188. Ohara S. Dressing and constructional apraxia in a patient with dentato-rubro-pallido-luysian atrophy. J Neurol. 2001;248(12):1106–8.

189. Hsu JL, Wang HC, Hsu WC. Hyperglycemia-induced unilateral basal ganglion lesions with and without hemichorea. A PET study. J Neurol. 2004;251(12):1486–90.

190. Stojanovic M, Sternic N, Kostic VS. Clozapine in hemiballismus: report of two cases. Clin Neuropharmacol. 1997;20(2):171–4.

191. Safirstein B, Shulman LM, Weiner WJ. Successful treatment of hemichorea with olanzapine. Mov Disord. 1999;14(3):532–3.

192. Obeso JA, Marti-Masso JF, Astudillo W, De la PE, Carrera N. Treatment with hemiballism with reserpine. Ann Neurol. 1978;4(6):581.

193. Sitburana O, Ondo WG. Tetrabenazine for hyperglycemic-induced hemichorea-hemiballismus. Mov Disord. 2006;21(11):2023–5.

194. Sethi KD, Patel BP. Inconsistent response to divalproex sodium in hemichorea/hemiballism. Neurology. 1990;40(10):1630–1.

195. Driver-Dunckley E, Evidente VG. Hemichorea-hemiballismus may respond to topiramate. Clin Neuropharmacol. 2005;28(3):142–4.

196. D'Amelio M, Callari G, Gammino M, Saia V, Lupo I, Salemi G, et al. Levetiracetam in the treatment of vascular chorea: a case report. Eur J Clin Pharmacol. 2005;60(11):835–6.

197. Okun MS, Riestra AR, Nadeau SE. Treatment of ballism and pseudobulbar affect with sertraline. Arch Neurol. 2001;58(10):1682–4.

198. Mark VW, Oberheu AM, Henderson C, Woods AJ. Ballism after stroke responds to standard physical therapeutic interventions. Arch Phys Med Rehabil. 2005;86(6):1226–33.

199. Son BC, Choi JG, Ko HC. Globus pallidus internus deep brain stimulation for disabling diabetic hemiballism/hemichorea. Case Rep Neurol Med. 2017;2017:2165905.

200. Ganapa SV, Ramani MD, Ebunlomo OO, Rahman RK, Herscman Y. Treatment of persistent hemiballism with deep brain stimulation of the globus pallidus internus: case report and literature review. World Neurosurg. 2019;132:368–70.

New References

201. Hsieh CY, Chen CH, Sung SF, Hwang WJ. Parkinsonism or other movement disorders presenting as stroke mimics. Acta Neurol Taiwanica. 2016;25(4):124–8.

202. Hu CY, Fang Y, Li FL, Dong B, Hua XG, Jiang W. Association between ambient air pollution and Parkinson's disease: systematic review and meta-analysis. Environ Res. 2019;168:448–59.

203. Mukherjee A, Biswas A, Das SK. Gut dysfunction in Parkinson's disease. World J Gastroenterol. 2016;22(25):5742–52.

204. Triadafilopoulos G, Gandhy R, Barlow C. Pilot cohort of endoscopic botulinum neurotoxin injection in Parkinson's disease. Parkinsonism Relat Disord. 2017;44:33–7.

205. Tomita A, Satoh H, Satoh A, Seto M, Tsujihata M, Yoshimura T. Extrapontine myelinolysis presenting with parkinsonism as a sequel of rapid correction of hyponatremia. J Neeurol Neurosurg Psychiatr. 1997;62(4):422–3.

206. Nakamura M, Yasunaga H, Miyata H, Shimada T, Horigichi H, Matsuda S. Mortality of neuroleptic malignant syndrrome induced by typical and atypical antipsychotic drugs:a propensity- matched analysis from the Japanese procedure combination database. J Clin Psychiatry. 2012;73(4):427–30.

207. Guerra RJ, Caroff SN, Cohen A, Caroll B, De Roos TF, Francis A. An international consensus study of neuroleptic malignant syndrome diagnostic criteria using the Delphi method. J Clin Psychiatry. 2011;72(9):1222–8.

208. Gurrera RJ, Mortllaro G, Velamoor V, Caroff SN. A validation study of the international consensus diagnostic criteria for neuroleptic malignant syndrome. J Clin Psychopharmacol. 2017;37(1):67–71.

209. Akbar U, Kim DS, Friedman JH. Valbenazine-induced parkinsonism. Parkinsonism Relat Disord. 2020;70(1):13–4.

210. Jimenez-Shahed J, Jankovic J. Tetrabenazine for treatment of chorea associated with Huntington's disease and other potential indications. Expert Opin Orphan Drugs. 2013;1:423–36.

211. Weintraub, Duda JE, Carlson K, et al. Suicide ideation and behaviours after STN and GPi DBS surgery for Parkinson's disease: results from a randomised, controlled trial. J Neurol Neurosurg Psychiatry. 2013;84:1113–8.

212. Cortelli P, Calandra-Buonaura G, Benarroch EE, Giannini G, Wenning G, Iranzo A. Stridor in multiple system atrophy. Consensus statement on diagnosis, prognosis and treatment. Neurology. 2019;93(14):630–9.

213. Raja M, Azzoni A. Novel antipsychotics and acute dystonic reactions. Int J Neuropsychopharmacol. 2001 Dec;4(4):393–7.

214. Piotr J, Figura M. Tetrabenazine-induced oculogyric crisis- a rare complication in the treatment of Gilles De La Tourette syndrome. Neuropsychiatr Dis Treat. 2016;12:497–9.

215. Ruiz-Lopez M, Fasano A. Rethinking status Dystonicus. Mov Disord. 2017;32(12):1667–76.

216. Fasano A, Ricciardi L, Bentivoglio AR, et al. Status dystonicus: predictors of outcome and progression patterns of underlying disease. Mov Disord. 2012;27:783–8.

217. Balint B, Bhatia K. Stiff person syndrome and other immune-mediated movement disorders-new insights. Curr Opin Neurol. 2016;29(4):496–506.

218. Fekete R, Jankovic J. Case Rep Neurol. 2012;4(2):92–6.

Encephalopathy

15

Steven L. Lewis

Introduction

Encephalopathy is the term used to describe a general alteration in brain function, manifesting as an attentional disorder anywhere within the continuum between a hyperalert agitated state and coma. In clinical practice, the diagnosis of encephalopathy is usually reserved for the diffuse brain dysfunction felt to be due to a systemic, metabolic, or toxic derangement, rather than, for example, a multifocal structural process; therefore the adjectives "metabolic" or "toxic-metabolic" are usually implied when the diagnosis of encephalopathy is made. The syndrome of toxic-metabolic encephalopathy is essentially synonymous with *delirium*, the term favored by most nonneurologists. Autoimmune encephalopathies are another important mechanism of diffuse brain dysfunction; these syndromes—technically more consistent with "encephalitides" than "encephalopathies"—are characterized by suggestive clinical and laboratory features and response to immune-based therapies (and sometimes removal of an underlying neoplasm), distinguishing them from the toxic-metabolic encephalopathies discussed in this chapter.

Neurologists are frequently asked to evaluate patients with alteration in consciousness from a toxic-metabolic encephalopathy. The consulting physician likely requests the neurologic consultation because of concern for a structural, ischemic, epileptic, or other focal primary neurologic causes of the patient's encephalopathic symptoms. The neurologic diagnosis of a toxic-metabolic encephalopathy is typically made by finding characteristic diffuse clinical symptoms and (mostly) nonlocalizing findings within the appropriate clinical context, usually with exclusion of other processes through imaging and other studies. The diagnosis of toxic-metabolic encephalopathy may lead to the generic and appropriate recommendation to correct any metabolic abnormalities, treat any underlying acute systemic illness, and discontinue or limit the use of sedatives or other medications with central nervous system side effects. In many cases, though, a more specific diagnosis can be made, and prompt recognition of the causative systemic process or medication can lead to a more rapid neurologic recovery, or in some cases, prevention of irreversible neurologic injury [1].

The purpose of this chapter is to discuss an approach to the emergency evaluation of patients with encephalopathy, with an emphasis on those causes of toxic-metabolic encephalopathy that will lead to irreversible neurological dysfunction if not recognized and treated urgently, as well as the encephalopathies whose recognition—by clinical or neuroimaging findings—might lead to

S. L. Lewis (✉)
Division of Neurology, Lehigh Valley Health Network, Allentown, PA, USA
e-mail: Steven_L.Lewis@lvhn.org

more prompt diagnosis and treatment of the causative medical illness.

Epidemiology of Toxic-Metabolic Encephalopathy

The evaluation of encephalopathy is a common aspect of day-to-day neurologic practice, and encephalopathy can occur in any patient at any age with a severe systemic illness or with exposure to a metabolic or toxic derangement causing cerebral dysfunction. The epidemiology of toxic-metabolic encephalopathy, however, is best characterized for hospitalized older adults. Approximately one-third of general medical patients 70 years of age or over have delirium, which may be present on admission or after; in addition, delirium is common after surgery (up to 50% after high-risk procedures) and is most common in patients in the intensive care unit (with a prevalence of over 75%) and at the end of life [2]. Delirium is also associated with an increased risk of mortality; a 2010 meta-analysis found a nearly twofold increased risk of death after an average follow-up of 22.7 months in elderly patients with delirium compared to those without delirium [3]. These statistics underscore both the ubiquity of this clinical syndrome and the fact that encephalopathies are usually reflective of severe underlying acute systemic disease and dysfunction.

Pathophysiology of Toxic-Metabolic Encephalopathy

A detailed discussion of the underlying pathophysiology of each of the many causes of toxic-metabolic encephalopathy is outside the scope of this chapter. However, among the many mechanisms of global neuronal and glial dysfunction that can occur due to metabolic or toxic derangements, general pathophysiologic mechanisms that underlie many of these clinical syndromes include creation of an energy deficit through a decrease in the level of basic metabolic substrates necessary for neuronal survival; oxidative stress; and functional alterations of neurotransmitter

systems, including alterations in neurotransmitter synthesis and release [4].

From an emergency management perspective, brain survival is the primary goal, so it is particularly critical to recognize and immediately treat those pathophysiologic causes of metabolic encephalopathy that may directly result in cell death due to loss of neuronal energy substrates (e.g., glucose, oxygen, and thiamine) in order to prevent irreversible neuronal death and to increase the likelihood of clinical neurologic recovery. It is also critical to immediately recognize those systemic processes that can secondarily cause irreversible neuronal injury, for example, by causing increased intracranial pressure (ICP) and potential cerebral herniation (e.g., acute hepatic encephalopathy from fulminant hepatic dysfunction). On the other hand, all causes of toxic-metabolic encephalopathy share the underlying pathophysiology of usually severe and often life-threatening systemic illness and dysfunction, underscoring the importance of accurate diagnosis and medical or surgical treatment no matter what the underlying systemic process is.

Although the basic underlying cellular pathophysiology of metabolic encephalopathies may differ, they share a common mechanism of generalized, rather than focal, alteration in hemispheric and brainstem dysfunction, leading clinically to a diffuse alteration in attention and arousal. Some encephalopathic syndromes, however, preferentially affect certain vulnerable brain regions specific to the underlying cause of the encephalopathy, such as the medial thalami and periaqueductal gray matter in thiamine deficiency.

Clinical Features of Toxic-Metabolic Encephalopathy

Patients with toxic-metabolic encephalopathy typically present with a global alteration in level of alertness, varying between and within patients, from obtundation and coma to an agitated delirium. The time course of development of the encephalopathy can vary from rapid (e.g., from acute hypoglycemia, hypoxia, or drug overdose) to the more common subacute presentation from insidiously developing systemic disease processes.

On clinical examination, patients with encephalopathy are often lethargic, confused, or agitated, typically without obvious focal localizing neurologic features. Many patients with toxic-metabolic encephalopathies exhibit asterixis, elicited by asking the patient to hold his or her arms outstretched. Asterixis is manifested by a very brief loss of postural tone of the outstretched arms. It is not necessary for the wrists to be dorsiflexed to evaluate for asterixis; however, if the patient is able to perform this, the classic "flap" of brief downward wrist flexion may be observed. The finding of bilateral asterixis is rather specific, but not sensitive, for the presence of a toxic-metabolic encephalopathy from a number of potential processes but is not pathognomonic for any particular cause of the encephalopathy. In clinical practice, though, asterixis is commonly associated with uremic or hepatic encephalopathies.

Although the hallmark of toxic-metabolic encephalopathies is disordered attention, seizures can occur in some syndromes as well, particularly when severe; these include disorders such as hypoglycemia and hyperglycemia, some electrolyte disorders, acute hepatic failure, and various medication-related encephalopathies (see the Section "Encephalopathic Syndromes").

Diagnosis of Toxic-Metabolic Encephalopathy

As when taking any neurologic history, the physician should delineate the clinical neurologic symptoms and their time course (especially from witnesses if the patient is unable to provide a history), carefully detailing the current systemic context, other medical comorbidities, and all current and recent medications. Examination should focus not only on the mental status (especially level of consciousness) and generalized neurologic findings expected in a diffuse encephalopathy, including assessment for asterixis, but should also focus on assessing vital signs; signs of men-

Table 15.1 Examination of the patient with encephalopathy

Level of consciousness
Vital signs
Passive flexion of the neck for meningismus
Funduscopic examination for papilledema
Language (looking for aphasia)
Neurological examination for cranial nerve or focal motor deficits and asterixis

ingeal irritation; observation for aphasia (especially the fluent kind as a mimic of a confusional state); funduscopic examination for signs of increased intracranial pressure; and exclusion of obvious motor or other asymmetries for which an alternative diagnosis may be more likely (Table 15.1).

Despite the diffuse neurologic presentation of patients with a probable toxic-metabolic encephalopathy, diagnostic evaluation often necessitates brain imaging studies (CT or MRI) to rule out causative focal structural or ischemic lesions, especially if there is any uncertainty as to the diagnosis. Although these imaging studies are typically performed to exclude focal structural or ischemic processes, and should therefore not demonstrate a focal structural lesion in the patient ultimately diagnosed with a diffuse encephalopathy, some toxic-metabolic processes are themselves associated with abnormal imaging features that may be helpful in diagnosis [5] and are discussed further in the Section "Encephalopathic Syndromes".

EEG can be helpful in the evaluation of the patient with encephalopathy, particularly when subclinical status epilepticus is a diagnostic consideration. Diffuse slowing on the EEG is a nonspecific and nearly ubiquitous finding in these patients, simply paralleling the clinical syndrome of a diffuse cerebral process. The EEG finding of triphasic waves is rather specific, but not sensitive, for a toxic-metabolic encephalopathic process but is not diagnostic as to the actual cause; however, like asterixis, in clinical practice triphasic waves are often seen in patients with hepatic and uremic encephalopathies.

Laboratory testing is the mainstay of investigation of the etiology of toxic-metabolic

Table 15.2 Diagnostic studies for the patient with an encephalopathy

Blood pressure, serum glucose, and O_2 saturation
Comprehensive metabolic panel and ammonia level
Complete blood cell count with differential
Urinalysis and culture, urine tox screen
Blood cultures
Brain MRI or CT
EEG
Spinal fluid analysis if indicated

encephalopathy. Serum glucose testing (including rapid finger stick determination as well as laboratory analysis of a drawn blood sample) and pulse oximetry should be immediately assessed in all patients because of the potentially irreversible nature of hypoglycemic and hypoxic brain dysfunction unless rapidly diagnosed and treated. A complete metabolic profile (including serum electrolytes and liver and kidney function tests) will quickly assess for the most common metabolic and systemic abnormalities, and a complete blood cell count will quickly exclude profound anemia and an elevated white blood cell count while also looking for clues to an underlying systemic infectious process.

Lumbar puncture (LP) will show only nonspecific, if any, cerebrospinal fluid (CSF) abnormalities in a patient with a toxic-metabolic encephalopathy; however, this should be performed when there is any clinical concern for meningoencephalitis (including autoimmune encephalitis) or subarachnoid hemorrhage. Lumbar puncture in the encephalopathic patient typically should be performed only after screening emergent neuroimaging (most commonly a noncontrast head CT) has excluded a focal cerebral mass lesion (e.g., abscess or hematoma) which might be a contraindication to this procedure. Table 15.2 lists the diagnostic studies for the patient with an encephalopathy.

Encephalopathic Syndromes

Patients with diffuse toxic-metabolic encephalopathies are medically, and secondarily neurologically, ill. Therefore, despite the ubiquity of these clinical syndromes in typical inpatient neurological consultative practice, evaluation of patients with diffuse encephalopathies represents a unique and critically important opportunity for the neurologist to positively impact the medical management, and both the neurological and medical recovery, of these severely systemically ill patients.

This section outlines four common and distinct (but overlapping) presentations the clinician is likely to encounter in clinical practice: encephalopathy from a basic metabolic disorder or deficiency, encephalopathy due to a severe systemic illness or organ failure, encephalopathy due to medication-related toxicity, and encephalopathies diagnosable primarily by findings on brain imaging.

Encephalopathy from Basic Metabolic Disorder or Deficiency

Oxygen, Glucose, and Electrolytes

As stated earlier, hypoxemia and hypoglycemia are critical to consider and be quickly excluded in any encephalopathic patient, as deficiencies of these basic and critical neuronal energy substrates will lead to irreversible neuronal death unless recognized and reversed quickly; most other metabolic disorders are less likely to directly lead (or lead quickly) to neuronal cell death and irreversible injury. Likewise, profound hypotension or anemia can lead to loss of energy supply to neurons and should be excluded quickly via immediate assessment of vital signs, oxygen saturation, and hemoglobin concentration; careful therapeutic attention should be placed on these basic emergency resuscitation parameters in all encephalopathic patients as in any critically ill patient.

In addition to hypoxemia and hypoglycemia, encephalopathy frequently occurs in the setting of hyperglycemia and of certain electrolyte abnormalities, especially hyponatremia, hypernatremia, and hypercalcemia. Though hyperkalemia and hypokalemia are well-known causes of neuromuscular dysfunction (and of cardiac dysfunction which can secondarily cause hypoxic-ischemic encephalopathy), these common abnormalities of potassium concentration are not typically associated with encephalopathy.

Thiamine Deficiency (Wernicke's Encephalopathy)

Thiamine (vitamin B1), in the form of its active phosphorylated derivatives (especially thiamine diphosphate, also called thiamine pyrophosphate), is an important coenzyme in a number of intracellular enzymatic activities, including energy production and various biosynthetic pathways. Deficiency of thiamine causes Wernicke's encephalopathy, characterized classically by the clinical triad of ophthalmoplegia, mental status changes, and ataxia. This is a very important cause of encephalopathy due to the potential irreversibility of clinical findings and especially because of the development of an irreversible amnestic state if thiamine deficiency is not recognized and treated emergently [6, 7]. Although commonly thought of as a disease of patients with alcohol dependence, Wernicke's encephalopathy can occur due to any process that leads to inadequate absorption or intake of thiamine, including hyperemesis states such as hyperemesis gravidarum, malnutrition from any cause, bariatric surgery, chronic diarrheal illnesses, and in the course of many systemic illnesses [7, 8].

Despite the commonly memorized clinical triad, the clinical symptoms and signs in patients with Wernicke's encephalopathy vary, and the full triad is usually not present in an individual patient. The most common symptom is mental status change, manifesting as agitation and confusion or apathy, and can progress to coma. Eye findings, if present, most commonly include nystagmus and sometimes sixth nerve palsies; complete "ophthalmoplegia," as listed in the classic triad, is actually rare. Ataxia of gait is often present. Other signs and symptoms that may be seen in patients with Wernicke's encephalopathy include hypothermia, hypotension, and tachycardia [7].

Brain regions commonly involved in Wernicke's encephalopathy include the mammillary bodies, periaqueductal gray matter, and medial thalami; changes in these regions may be seen on diffusion-weighted and T2-weighted MRI in some patients with Wernicke's encephalopathy. These particularly vulnerable brain regions explain the characteristically severe, and potentially irreversible, amnestic state (called *Korsakoff's syndrome*) that occurs in patients with Wernicke's disease if prompt treatment is not initiated.

Because of the treatable aspect of this condition, and its neurological irreversibility if not treated in a timely fashion, neurologists need to keep this diagnosis in mind in all patients presenting with encephalopathy, whether or not other features of the syndrome (e.g., nystagmus or gait ataxia) are present. The diagnosis is typically entirely clinical; thiamine levels are not useful in practice, especially due to delay in obtaining these results. Although MRI findings can be seen in some patients with Wernicke's encephalopathy, these findings are insensitive for the diagnosis; importantly, one of the priorities is to try to make the clinical diagnosis and begin treatment before the development of any of the characteristic imaging findings.

Treatment with parenteral thiamine should be initiated emergently in any patient in whom the diagnosis is a reasonable consideration and must be given prior to any glucose administration due to the risk of glucose precipitating or worsening Wernicke's encephalopathy. Although the optimal evidence-based dose of thiamine is uncertain, expert recommendations suggest that initial parenteral thiamine dosing should be >500 mg daily, given as a once- or divided-daily regimen, for 3–5 days [7, 9].

Encephalopathy Due to Severe Systemic Illness or Organ Failure

Severe Systemic Illness and Septic Encephalopathy

As discussed in the preceding sections (and inherent in the diagnosis of the clinical syndrome of a toxic-metabolic encephalopathy), encephalopathies commonly occur in the setting of a severe underlying systemic illness.

Encephalopathy is especially common in patients in the medical ICU [10, 11] and in patients whose illness may be severe enough to warrant transfer to a medical ICU setting. Any medical illness of sufficient severity can lead to the clinical syndrome of a toxic-metabolic encephalopathy; in addition, the common finding of encephalopathy in the specific clinical setting of systemic sepsis, with or without multiorgan failure, has led to the designation of the term *septic encephalopathy* [12]. The pathophysiology of septic encephalopathy is unclear, although theoretical mechanisms include the effects of inflammatory mediators, blood-brain barrier dysfunction, and other possible metabolic effects of the severe systemic dysfunction [12]. As in any severe systemic infectious illness, encephalopathy has been reported to be common in patients hospitalized with SARS-CoV-2, with one recent multicenter report finding that of 817 older adults with SARS-CoV-2, delirium was seen on presentation in 28% of patients, and was associated with an increased risk of poor hospital outcomes and death [13]. In another study, encephalopathy was found to be present during the disease course in 31.8% of a consecutive series of 509 patients admitted with confirmed SARS-CoV-2 to a hospital network; these researchers found that encephalopathy was associated with worse functional outcome and higher mortality within 30 days of discharge, independent of the severity of respiratory disease [14].

Although sepsis or severe acute medical (including infectious) illnesses of any cause are common etiologies of encephalopathy, encephalopathies also occur due to single-organ dysfunction or failure. In each of these clinical scenarios, the neurologist is important in diagnosing the causative medical illness, which may have a direct impact on systemic treatment and the course of neurologic improvement. The specific single-organ causes of encephalopathy discussed below include hepatic encephalopathy, uremic encephalopathy, pancreatic encephalopathy, and the fat embolus syndrome.

Hepatic Encephalopathy

Hepatic encephalopathy can occur in patients with either chronic liver disease (cirrhosis) or acute liver failure [15]. Encephalopathy due to chronic liver disease typically progresses slowly, with the clinical features defined in stages, or grades; minimal hepatic encephalopathy is characterized by subtle findings detectable mainly by formal neuropsychological testing: grade I is characterized by psychomotor slowing and lack of attention; grade II is characterized by disorientation, lethargy, and unusual behavior; grade III is characterized by somnolence and stupor; and patients in grade IV hepatic encephalopathy are in coma [16].

Asterixis is most commonly associated with grade II hepatic encephalopathy but can also be seen in other stages. Chronic liver diseases in some patients present as a slowly progressive parkinsonian syndrome, sometimes referred to as acquired (non-Wilsonian) hepatolenticular (or hepatocerebral) degeneration consisting of bradykinesia, rigidity, tremor, dysarthria, and ataxia [17]. Seizures are uncommon in patients with hepatic encephalopathy due to chronic liver disease.

The diagnosis of hepatic encephalopathy due to cirrhosis is made by observing the characteristic neurological clinical features in the appropriate clinical context. Ammonia levels remain helpful in the clinical diagnosis of hepatic encephalopathy, although these levels do not correlate well with the various stages of encephalopathy and a normal serum ammonia level does not exclude the diagnosis of hepatic encephalopathy. As mentioned in the earlier Section "Diagnosis of Toxic-Metabolic Encephalopathy," triphasic waves may be seen on EEG in some patients with hepatic encephalopathy, but this finding is neither sensitive nor specific for this condition. The MRI finding of high signal in the bilateral globus pallidus on noncontrast T1-weighted images has been attributed to manganese deposition in the brain due to reduced biliary manganese excretion; this MRI finding, however, is common in patients with chronic liver disease, whether or not a clinical encephalopathy is present [17].

Treatment of hepatic encephalopathy is aimed at reducing ammonia absorption through the use of nonabsorbable disaccharides, such as lactulose, and reducing ammonia production through the use of antibiotics such as rifaximin [18].

In contrast to patients with chronic cirrhosis and portosystemic shunting, acute liver failure commonly presents as rapidly progressive neurologic deterioration leading to life-threatening cerebral edema, with coma and seizures [19]. The neurologic assessment and treatment of patients with acute hepatic encephalopathy consist of ICP monitoring with aggressive reduction of increased ICP and management of any associated seizures.

Uremic Encephalopathy

Encephalopathy can occur due to either acute or chronic renal failure and typically develops more rapidly in patients with acute kidney dysfunction [20]. Symptoms of uremic encephalopathy include asterixis, myoclonus (uremic twitching), and coarse tremor; seizures may also be seen. The clinical symptoms and signs, including the EEG finding of triphasic waves in severe uremic encephalopathy, mimic those of many other metabolic encephalopathies; however, the tremulousness and twitching seen in many patients with uremic encephalopathy may be somewhat more suggestive of this cause of encephalopathy compared to other systemic processes.

The diagnosis of uremic encephalopathy is clinical, supported by appropriate laboratory studies showing severe kidney dysfunction, along with the reasonable exclusion of other potentially causative systemic, or other, processes. Other systemic causes of encephalopathy that especially need to be considered in the uremic patient include drug toxicities (especially those that are renally metabolized or excreted), electrolyte disturbances, and thiamine deficiency [21]. Treatment of uremic encephalopathy is based on improvement of the uremic state and appropriate adjustment, if possible, of renally metabolized/excreted medications.

Pancreatic Encephalopathy

The term "pancreatic encephalopathy" was coined in 1941 to describe the known association between acute pancreatitis and a severe diffuse encephalopathy [22]. Since then a number of reports further defined this syndrome [23–25].

Pancreatic encephalopathy typically occurs within 2 weeks of pancreatitis onset, especially between the second and fifth days, with varying incidences (up to as high as 35%) reported [1].

The diagnosis of pancreatic encephalopathy should be considered in any patient with a diffuse encephalopathy occurring in the setting of acute pancreatitis. Other than the laboratory findings diagnostic of pancreatitis, no specific laboratory or imaging feature is diagnostic of pancreatic encephalopathy; however, one report described severe diffuse white matter abnormalities on MRI in a patient with this syndrome [26].

Treatment consists solely of management of the pancreatitis; there is no specific neurologic treatment beyond supportive care and avoidance of benzodiazepines, which may worsen the encephalopathy. Neurologic improvement typically parallels the patient's systemic recovery; however, the mortality rate for patients with pancreatic encephalopathy is high [1].

The pathogenesis of pancreatic encephalopathy is unknown but has been proposed to relate to blood-brain barrier breakdown as a consequence of activation of phospholipase A and conversion of lecithin into its hemolytic form [23], although fat embolism (described below) is another putative mechanism. Patients with pancreatitis are also at risk for the development of Wernicke's encephalopathy, which should strongly be considered in the differential diagnosis or as an additional comorbidity in these patients [27].

Fat Embolism

Fat embolism should be considered among the potential emergent diagnoses of any patient presenting with a diffuse encephalopathy in characteristic clinical settings, such as after recent orthopedic procedures or trauma. The fat embolism syndrome is characterized by the classic clinical triad of encephalopathy, pulmonary dysfunction, and a petechial rash [28]. Although most commonly associated with long-bone trauma, fat embolism also occurs in a variety of other scenarios, including acute pancreatitis, diabetes mellitus, burns, joint reconstruction, liposuction, cardiopulmonary bypass, decompression sickness, and parenteral lipid infusion [29].

Clinical symptoms of fat embolism typically, though not invariably, occur 24–48 h after the inciting event [28].

The primary neurologic manifestation of fat embolism is a diffuse encephalopathy, although focal neurologic signs and seizures can occur. In some patients, the neurologic manifestations may be the sole clinical feature; however, pulmonary symptoms are typically present, and these symptoms may range from mild dyspnea to tachypnea to respiratory failure [30]. The finding of petechiae on the skin completes the clinical triad, but this is seen in only about 50% of patients with the syndrome. MRI in some patients has shown multifocal punctate DWI-positive white matter lesions consistent with multifocal embolic lesions and sometimes described as a *starfield pattern* [31, 32].

Two major mechanisms have been proposed to explain fat embolism syndrome. The mechanical theory proposes that bone marrow contents enter the lungs via the venous system, where they may also gain access to the systemic circulation and enter the brain via pulmonary arteriovenous shunts or a patent foramen ovale. The biochemical theory proposes that pulmonary abnormalities result from a toxic effect of circulating free fatty acids on lung cells; these theories are not mutually exclusive, and both mechanisms may be responsible for various aspects of the clinical syndrome [29].

The possibility of fat embolism should be considered in any patient with encephalopathy occurring in the appropriate clinical context, especially if other causes have been excluded. Treatment is currently supportive and focused on pulmonary management [28, 33].

Medication-Related Encephalopathy

Encephalopathy due to medications with central nervous system effects, including sedatives, analgesics, anticholinergics, anticonvulsants, anxiolytics, and any of the wide variety of CNS-active drugs, is well recognized. However, several medications in clinical use are particularly associated with specific and distinctive toxic encephalopathic syndromes and will be discussed here.

These medications are not uncommonly used, and neurologists in clinical practice are likely to be asked to consult on patients with encephalopathy due to one of these agents. Recognition of these unusual encephalopathic syndromes is important in the management of these patients to avoid unnecessary interventions (other than discontinuation or reduction of the offending agent) and possibly for consideration of specific antidotal therapy, such as for ifosfamide encephalopathy. Metronidazole, a commonly used antibiotic, which is also associated with an encephalopathic syndrome, is discussed in the next section on encephalopathies associated with distinctive imaging findings.

Ifosfamide

Ifosfamide, a chemotherapeutic agent used in the treatment of a variety of solid tumors, has been associated with the development of a severe encephalopathy [34]. Ifosfamide encephalopathy typically develops 24–48 h after infusion but may occur later. Encephalopathic symptoms due to ifosfamide may range from mild to severe and progress to coma and death. In addition, a distinctive catatonic-like, severely abulic state with mutism can be seen in patients with ifosfamide encephalopathy. Risk factors for ifosfamide encephalopathy include previous exposure to cisplatin, and concomitant opioids and CYP2B6 inhibitors, as well as abnormal laboratory findings, including low serum albumin, increased serum creatinine, and increased hemoglobin [35]. Due to theoretical considerations regarding the presumptive mechanism of ifosfamide encephalopathy from its metabolite chloroacetaldehyde, methylene blue, an electron acceptor, emerged as antidotal (and anecdotal) intravenous treatment of severe cases of this syndrome [36–38] although not based on controlled trials. Mild cases, however, typically resolve within days after stopping the agent. Due to similarities to Wernicke's encephalopathy, thiamine treatment has also been advocated for management of this syndrome [39, 40].

Cefepime

Many antibiotics have been associated with the development of an encephalopathy [41]; however, cefepime, a fourth-generation cephalosporin used to treat a variety of severe bacterial infections, is much more commonly associated with an encephalopathy than the other cephalosporins [42], manifested by progressive confusion and agitation which can progress to coma [43, 44]. Although cefepime encephalopathy was initially reported in patients with renal failure causing reduced clearance of the drug, cefepime encephalopathy also occurs in patients with normal renal function [45, 46]. In some patients with cefepime encephalopathy, EEG has shown nonconvulsive status epilepticus [47, 48].

Management involves discontinuation of cefepime if possible, which leads to gradual resolution of the encephalopathy. In patients with nonconvulsive status epilepticus due to cefepime (or other cephalosporins) neurotoxicity, several reports have described short-term use of anticonvulsants in addition to discontinuation of the cephalosporin [47, 48], although it is unclear as to whether anticonvulsant therapy contributed to improvement.

Encephalopathies Diagnosed Primarily by Brain Imaging Findings

Findings on neuroimaging play an integral role in the timely recognition of several specific encephalopathic conditions, including the posterior reversible encephalopathy syndrome (PRES) and metronidazole encephalopathy; in addition, the finding of a splenial lesion on MRI, although nonspecific, has been associated with various causes of encephalopathy. The imaging findings and clinical syndromes discussed in this section are in distinction to some of the encephalopathic syndromes discussed earlier, where the imaging findings are not specific or sensitive for an encephalopathy (e.g., T1 high signal in the basal ganglia in patients with chronic hepatic disease with or without encephalopathy) or they represent late findings that play little if any role in clinical diagnosis and emergent empiric therapy (e.g., the MRI findings in Wernicke's encephalopathy).

Posterior Reversible Encephalopathy Syndrome

Posterior reversible encephalopathy syndrome is a very common clinical syndrome, although despite its descriptive name it does not always involve posterior brain regions and is not always completely reversible. Posterior reversible encephalopathy syndrome typically presents clinically with encephalopathy and visual disturbances (due to cortical visual dysfunction), and often also with seizures, and usually in association with elevated systemic blood pressure. The classic imaging finding is hyperintensity on T2-weighted and fluid attenuated inversion recovery (FLAIR) MRI consistent with vasogenic edema, typically predominantly involving the posterior occipital white matter; however, more diffuse involvement (including the brainstem and anterior hemispheres) can also be seen [49]. The predisposing conditions for the development of this syndrome are multiple, although common underlying systemic factors include eclampsia, hypertension with acute kidney disease, and exposure to various chemotherapeutic and immunosuppressive medications. The cause of PRES remains unclear, but the two main putative mechanisms include vascular leakage and vasogenic edema due to (1) elevated blood pressure above the autoregulatory limit and/or (2) as a result of toxin-related endothelial dysfunction [50]. Treatment includes blood pressure control, withdrawal or reduction of the potentially offending agent, and management of seizures if present. Prompt recognition and management of this syndrome should decrease the likelihood of permanent sequelae of this usually reversible condition [51].

Metronidazole Encephalopathy

Metronidazole is a commonly utilized antibiotic that is associated with an uncommon but characteristic toxic encephalopathy manifested primarily by confusion, dysarthria, and ataxia. MRI findings typical of metronidazole encephalopathy include T2 and FLAIR high-signal lesions involving the dentate nuclei [52]; additional involvement of the corpus callosum and deep hemispheric white matter and hypertrophy of the inferior olives have also been described [53, 54]. The clinical and radiographic findings of metronidazole-induced encephalopathy are usually reversible with discontinuation of the antibiotic, although severe persistent sequelae can occur [55]. The syndrome of metronidazole encephalopathy may be more common in patients with hepatic or renal disease [56].

Splenial High-Signal Lesion

The MRI finding of an ovoid or round lesion within the splenium of the corpus callosum (high signal on FLAIR/T2 and often also on DWI) has been described as a nonspecific finding associated with a variety of encephalopathic syndromes, including those due to various metabolic disorders, viral infections (termed "encephalitis/encephalopathy"), and the use of, or withdrawal from, antiepileptic agents [57, 58]. This nonspecific clinical/imaging syndrome has come to be known as *mild encephalitis/encephalopathy with reversible splenial lesion* and has been divided into Type 1, characterized by the classic single lesion in the splenium of the corpus callosum, and Type 2, which includes lesions elsewhere in the white matter or anterior corpus callosum [59].

Patients with this imaging finding may have nonspecific encephalopathic symptoms including drowsiness, confusion, and agitation. Splenial high-signal lesions typically resolve on follow-up imaging in parallel with the patient's clinical resolution. Although nonspecific, this MRI finding can nonetheless be a useful finding supportive of a probable reversible metabolic (or viral) encephalopathic syndrome and, despite its usual DWI positivity, should not be confused with an ischemic process affecting the corpus callosum.

Treatment of Patients with Encephalopathy

Treatment of some of the various specific encephalopathic syndromes has been discussed within the individual sections above. A general approach to management of the encephalopathic patient is, however, reviewed here.

As discussed at the beginning of this chapter, initial evaluation and treatment of the encephalopathic patient should focus on keeping a strong clinical suspicion for those causes of encephalopathy that will lead to irreversible neurologic dysfunction if not recognized and reversed immediately. Therefore, the immediate approach to treatment of any encephalopathic patient includes correction of any circulatory deficiency and replacement of any potentially deficient metabolic substrate (e.g., oxygen, thiamine, or glucose). This should be followed by correction of any other potentially causative metabolic abnormality, management of any underlying causative acute systemic illness or complication of organ failure, and attempt at discontinuation or removal of any likely offending medication or toxin.

Since toxic-metabolic encephalopathies are due, by definition, to an underlying systemic process or medication (even if not yet diagnosed in the individual patient), management should focus on diagnosis and treatment of systemic dysfunction and removal of potential offending agents while attempting to minimize any CNS-active or sedating medications which might complicate or worsen the encephalopathy. For the same reason, it should not be surprising that a 2016 meta-analysis found that the use of antipsychotics in patients with delirium was not associated with change in duration or severity of delirium or hospital or ICU length of stay [60].

Conclusion

Neurologists are frequently asked to evaluate patients with encephalopathies. As reviewed in this chapter, in many cases a specific etiological diagnosis can be made through history, examination, laboratory studies, and, in some cases, imaging, which may lead to a specific medical intervention and more rapid clinical resolution and help prevent irreversible neurologic dysfunction. Physicians should approach each patient with encephalopathy with an especially high level of suspicion for those causes which may lead to incomplete neurologic recovery if not specifically and expeditiously diagnosed and treated. Clinicians should also recognize that patients with toxic-metabolic encephalopathy are inherently systemically critically ill and require emergent diagnosis and management of the underlying medical disorder or reduction or removal of the potentially offending substance.

References

1. Weathers AL, Lewis SL. Rare and unusual…or are they? Less commonly diagnosed encephalopathies associated with systemic disease. Semin Neurol. 2009;29:136–53.
2. Marcantonio ER. Delirium in hospitalized older adults. N Engl J Med. 2017;377:1456–66.
3. Witlox J, Eurelings LS, de Jonghe JF, Kalisvaart KJ, Eikelenboom P, van Gool WA. Delirium in elderly patients and the risk of postdischarge mortality, institutionalization, and dementia: a meta-analysis. JAMA. 2010;304:443–51.
4. Butterworth RF. Metabolic encephalopathies. In: Siegel GJ, Albers RW, Brady ST, Price DL, editors. Basic neurochemistry: molecular, cellular and medical aspects. 7th ed. Burlington, MA: Elsevier; 2006.
5. Sharma P, Eesa M, Scott JN. Toxic and acquired metabolic encephalopathies: MRI appearance. Am J Roentgenol. 2009;193:879–86.
6. Pearce JMS. Wernicke-Korsakoff encephalopathy. Eur Neurol. 2008;59:101–4.
7. Sechi GP, Serra A. Wernicke's encephalopathy: new clinical settings and recent advances in diagnosis and management. Lancet Neurol. 2007;6:442–55.
8. Juhasz-Pocsine K, Rudnicki SA, Archer RL, Harik SI. Neurological complications of gastric bypass surgery for morbid obesity. Neurology. 2007;68:1843–50.
9. Thomson AD, Cook CCH, Touquet R, Henry JA. The Royal College of Physicians report on alcohol: guidelines for managing Wernicke's encephalopathy in the accident and emergency department. Alcohol Alcohol. 2002;37:513–21.
10. Stevens RD, Pronovost PJ. The spectrum of encephalopathy in critical illness. Semin Neurol. 2006;26:440–51.
11. Bolton CF, Young CB, Zochodne DW. The neurological complications of sepsis. Ann Neurol. 1993;33:94–100.
12. Papadoulos MC, Ceri Davies D, Moss RF, Tighe D, Bennett ED. Pathophysiology of septic encephalopathy: a review. Crit Care Med. 2000;28:3019–24.
13. Kennedy M, Helfand BKI, Gou RY, et al. Delirium in older patients with COVID-19 presenting to the Emergency Department. JAMA Netw Open. 2020;3:e2029540.
14. Liotta EM, Batra A, Clark JR, et al. Frequent neurologic manifestations and encephalopathy-associated morbidity in Covid-19 patients. Ann Clin Transl Neurol. 2020;7:2221–30.
15. Ferenci P, Lockwood A, Mullen K, et al. Hepatic encephalopathy—definition, nomenclature, diagnosis, and quantification: final report of the working party at the 11th world congresses of gastroenterology, Vienna, 1998. Hepatology. 2002;35:716–21.
16. Weissenborn K. Hepatic encephalopathy: definition, clinical grading and diagnostic principles. Drugs. 2019;79(Suppl 1):S5–9.
17. Weissenborn K. Neurologic manifestations of liver disease. Contin Lifelong Learn Neurol. 2008;14:165–80.
18. Vilstrup H, Amodio P, Bajaj J, Cordoba J, et al. Hepatic encephalopathy in chronic liver disease: 2014 practice guideline by the American Association for the Study of Liver Diseases and the European Association for the Study of the liver. Hepatology. 2014;60:715–35.
19. Ostapowicz GA, Fontana RJ, Schiodt FV, et al. Results of a prospective study of acute liver failure at 17 tertiary care centers in the United States. Ann Intern Med. 2002;137:947–54.
20. Brouns R, De Deyn PP. Neurological complications in renal failure: a review. Clin Neurol Neurosurg. 2004;107:1–16.
21. Barrett KM. Neurologic manifestations of acute and chronic renal disease. Contin Lifelong Learn Neurol. 2011;17:45–55.
22. Rothermich NO, von Haam E. Pancreatic encephalopathy. J Clin Endocrinol. 1941;1:872–81.
23. Ding X, Liu CA, Gong JP, Li SW. Pancreatic encephalopathy in 24 patients with severe acute pancreatitis. Hepatobiliary Pancreat Dis Int. 2004;3:608–11.
24. Ruggieri RM, Lupo I, Piccoli F. Pancreatic encephalopathy: a 7-year follow-up case report and review of the literature. Neurol Sci. 2002;23:203–5.
25. Bartha P, Shifrin E, Levy Y. Pancreatic encephalopathy—a rare complication of a common disease. Eur J Intern Med. 2006;17:382.
26. Ohkubo T, Shiojiri T, Matsunaga T. Severe diffuse white matter lesions in a patient with pancreatic encephalopathy. J Neurol. 2004;251:476–8.
27. Sun GH, Yang YS, Lui QS, Cheng LF, Huang XS. Pancreatic encephalopathy and Wernicke encephalopathy in association with acute pancreatitis: a clinical study. World J Gastroenterol. 2006;12:4224–7.
28. Parisi DM, Koval K, Egol K. Fat embolism syndrome. Am J Orthop. 2002;31:507–12.
29. Fabian TC. Unraveling the fat embolism syndrome. N Engl J Med. 1993;329:961–3.
30. Jacobson DM, Terrence CF, Reinmuth OM. The neurologic manifestations of fat embolism. Neurology. 1986;36(6):847–51.
31. Hüfner K, Holtmannspötter M, Bürkle H, et al. Fat embolism syndrome as a neurologic emergency. Arch Neurol. 2008;65(8):1124–5.
32. Parizel PM, Demey HE, Veeckmans G, et al. Early diagnosis of cerebral fat embolism syndrome by diffusion-weighted MRI (starfield pattern). Stroke. 2001;32:2942–4.
33. Kwiatt ME, Seamon MJ. Fat embolism syndrome. Int J Crit Illn Inj Sci. 2013;3:64–8.
34. David KA, Picus J. Evaluating risk factors for the development of ifosfamide encephalopathy. Am J Clin Oncol. 2005;28(3):277–80.
35. Szabatura AH, Cirrone F, Harris C, et al. An assessment of risk factors associated with ifosfamide-induced encephalopathy in a large academic cancer center. J Oncol Pharm Pract. 2015;21:188–93.
36. Patel PN. Methylene blue for management of ifosfamide-induced encephalopathy. Ann Pharmacother. 2006;40:299–303.
37. Pelgrims J, De Vos J, Van den Brande J, Schrijvers D, Prové A, Vermorken JB. Methylene blue in the

treatment and prevention of ifosfamide-induced encephalopathy: report of 12 cases and a review of the literature. Br J Cancer. 2000;82(2):291–4.
38. Ajithkumar T, Parkinson C, Shamshad F, Murray P. Ifosfamide encephalopathy. Clin Oncol. 2007;19:108–14.
39. Hamadani M, Awan F. Role of thiamine in managing ifosfamide-induced encephalopathy. J Oncol Pharm Pract. 2006;12:237–9.
40. Lin JK, Chow DS, Sheu L. Rehani B Wernicke-Like encephalopathy associated with Ifosfamide. Neurohospitalist. 2017;7(1):49–50.
41. Bhattacharyya S, Darby R, Rajbagkar P, et al. Antibiotic-associated encephalopathy. Neurology. 2016;86:963–71.
42. Bhattacharyya S, Berkowitz A. Cephalosporin neurotoxicity: an overlooked cause of toxic-metabolic encephalopathy. J Neurol Sci. 2019;398:194–5.
43. Fishbain JT, Monahan TP, Canonica MM. Cerebral manifestations of cefepime toxicity in a dialysis patient. Neurology. 2000;55(1):1756–7.
44. Barbey F, Bugnon D, Wauters JP. Severe neurotoxicity of cefepime in uremic patients. Ann Intern Med. 2001;135(11):1011.
45. Capparelli FJ, Wainsztein NA, Leiguarda R. Cefepime- and cefixime-induced encephalopathy in a patient with normal renal function. Neurol. 2005;65:1840.
46. Maganti R, Jolin D, Rishi D, Biswas A. Nonconvulsive status epilepticus due to cefepime in a patient with normal renal function. Epilepsy Behav. 2006;8:312–214.
47. Dixit S, Kurle P, Buyan-Dent L, Sheth RD. Status epilepticus associated with cefepime. Neurology. 2000;54:2153–5.
48. Fernádez-Torre JL, Martínez-Martínez M, González-Rato J, et al. Cephalosporin-induced nonconvulsive status epilepticus: clinical and electroencephalographic features. Epilepsia. 2005;46(9):1550–2.
49. Fugate JE, Claason DO, Cloft HJ, et al. Posterior reversible encephalopathy syndrome: associated clinical and radiologic findings. Mayo Clin Proc. 2010;85:427–32.
50. Fischer M, Schmutzhard E. Posterior reversible encephalopathy syndrome. J Neurol. 2017;264:1608–16.
51. Staykov D, Schwab S. Posterior reversible encephalopathy syndrome. J Intensive Care Med. 2011; (Epub ahead of print).
52. Bonkowski JL, Sondrup C, Benedict SL. Acute reversible cerebellar lesions associated with Metronidazole therapy. Neurology. 2007;68:180.
53. Seok JI, Yi H, Song YM, Lee WY. Metronidazole-induced encephalopathy and inferior olivary hypertrophy: lesion analysis with diffusion-weighted imaging and apparent diffusion coefficient maps. Arch Neurol. 2003;60:1796–800.
54. Heaney CJ, Campeau NG, Lindell EP. MR imaging and diffusion-weighted imaging changes in metronidazole (flagyl)-induced cerebellar toxicity. Am J Neurorad. 2003;24:1615–7.
55. Kim DW, Park J-M, Yoon B-W, Back MJ, et al. Metronidazole-induced encephalopathy. J Neurol Sci. 2004;224:107–11.
56. Sørensen CG, Karlsson WK, Amin FM, Lindelof M. Metronidazole-induced encephalopathy: a systematic review. J Neurol. 2020 Jan;267:1–13.
57. Tada H, Takanashi J, Barkovich AJ, et al. Clinically mild encephalitis/encephalopathy with a reversible splenial lesion. Neurology. 2004;63:1854–8.
58. Garcia-Monco JC, Martinez A, Brochado AP, et al. Isolated and reversible lesions of the corpus callosum: a distinct entity. J Neuroimaging. 2010;20:1–2.
59. Yuan J, Yang S, Wang S, Qin W, Yang L, Hu W. Mild encephalitis/encephalopathy with reversible splenial lesion (MERS) in adults-a case report and literature review. BMC Neurol. 2017;17:103.
60. Neufeld KJ, Yue J, Robinson TN, Inouye SK, Needham DM. Antipsychotic medication for prevention and treatment of delirium in hospitalized adults: a systematic review and meta-analysis. J Am Geriatr Soc. 2016;64:705–14.

Acute Respiratory Failure in Neuromuscular Disorders

16

Cynthia Bodkin

Overview

Respiratory failure is a common cause of mortality and morbidity in patients with neuromuscular disorders. Respiratory failure can be the presenting symptom of the neuromuscular disorder. Other times there will be a known neuromuscular disorder. Timely recognition and treatment of acute respiratory failure are important in preventing complications and improving outcomes. Adequate monitoring and use of preventive measures in patients with known neuromuscular disorders is as equally important. This chapter will review the pathophysiology, clinical presentation, diagnosis, differential diagnosis, treatment, and prevention of acute respiratory failure in neuromuscular disorders.

Epidemiology

The two most common causes of acute respiratory failure secondary to neuromuscular disorders presenting to the emergency department are myasthenia gravis (MG) and Guillain-Barré syndrome (GBS) [1]. Approximately 30% of patients with GBS will require mechanical ventilation [2]. Patients with GBS who require mechanical ventilation have a mortality rate of 20% [3]. Of 2014 patients admitted for myasthenia crisis between 2000 and 2005 in a nationwide study, 21.5% required endotracheal intubation and 6.5% required noninvasive positive airway pressure [4]. Age, diagnosis of MG crisis, and respiratory failure requiring endotracheal intubation were major predictors of death. Overall hospital mortality rate for all myasthenia gravis admissions was 2.2% and 4.4% among patients admitted for myasthenia crisis.

Pathophysiology

The mechanisms of breathing consist of two primary components: the respiratory motor unit and the central network of neurons coordinating breathing. Neuromuscular disorders affect the respirator motor unit, while strokes, tumors, and degenerative brain diseases affect the central network. The central network includes the pontine respiratory group, the dorsal respiratory group (DRG), and the ventral respiratory group (VRG) [5].

The initiation of breathing starts when carotid chemoreceptors detect a change in O2. A decrease in O2 stimulates the DRG, which is located in the nucleus of the solitary tract. The DRG also receives excitation from central CO_2 chemoreceptors in the medulla [5, 6]. In addition, the nucleus of the solitary tract receives input from baroreceptors and cardiac receptors. The VRG

C. Bodkin (✉)
Indiana University School of Medicine, Indiana University Health, Indianapolis, IN, USA
e-mail: cbodkin@iu.edu

consists of a group of neurons that contain expiratory and inspiratory neurons. The Bötzinger complex, the most rostral portion of the VRG, inhibits inspiratory neurons in the VRG and projects to expiratory neurons in the spinal cord. Just caudal to the Bötzinger complex is the pre-Bötzinger complex, which plays an important role in respiratory rhythm generation [5, 7, 8]. Caudal to the pre-Bötzinger complex are inspiratory bulbospinal neurons of the VRG. The most caudal portion of the VRG contains expiratory bulbospinal neurons [5]. The VRG extends from ventrolateral medulla to C1 cervical cord. Respiratory phase timing, integration of reflexes from pulmonary mechanoreceptors, and relay station from medullary respiratory neurons to the hypothalamus, amygdala, and other suprapontine structures occur in the pontine respiratory group [5]. Descending neurons from the respiratory centers are located in the anterolateral white matter and connect to respiratory motor neurons in the spinal cord [5]. Autonomic respiratory neurons travel closely to the spinothalamic tract, while voluntary respiratory neurons travel near the corticospinal tracts [5].

The respiratory motor unit includes the anterior horn cell, axon, neuromuscular junction, and muscle fibers the motor neuron innervate. Inspiratory nerves and muscles include the phrenic nerve to the diaphragm, intercostal nerves to the external intercostal muscles, cervical spinal nerves to the scalene muscles, and spinal accessory nerve (cranial nerve XI) to the sternocleidomastoid. Expiratory nerves and muscles include intercostal nerves to the internal intercostal muscles and lower thoracic and lumbar spinal nerves to the rectus abdominis, obliques, and transversus abdominis muscles. In a healthy individual, expiratory muscles are generally not needed and are more important for generating adequate cough.

Respiratory muscles require enough strength to overcome the elastic load, which encompasses upper airway resistance, abdominal pressure, and chest wall and lung compliance. Obesity and weakness of oropharyngeal muscles increase upper airway resistance. Abdominal pressure will rise with distension (i.e., constipation). Lung compliance decreases secondary to microatelectasis [9]. Microatelectasis also contributes to ventilation-perfusion mismatch and further restriction of pulmonary compliance [10–12]. Chest wall compliance is increased in children with neuromuscular disorders 3 months to 4 years of age, which can lead to chest wall deformities and possibly reduced lung growth [9, 13]. As adults, chest wall compliance decreases secondary to deformities, scoliosis, and increased stiffness of the ribcage [9, 14, 15]. A change to any one of these will increase demand on the respiratory muscles.

Respiratory failure in neuromuscular patients can occur from three main mechanisms: (1) aspiration secondary to oropharyngeal weakness, (2) fatigue of respiratory muscles, and (3) weak cough. Weakness in oropharyngeal muscles will impair the ability to swallow and protect the airway, placing the patient at increased risk for aspiration. This can lead to recurrent pneumonias and parenchymal disease.

Fatigue of respiratory muscles occurs when strength has fallen below 25–30% of normal [11]. Of all the inspiratory muscles, the diaphragm performs the majority of the work and accounts for about 70% of the inspiratory effort at rest [11]. Therefore diaphragmatic fatigue plays a major role in respiratory failure in neuromuscular patients. Diaphragmatic fatigue will occur in less than 60 min when the pressure it must produce (Pdi) is greater than 40% of the maximum pressure it can generate (Pdi_{max}) or when the ratio of time the diaphragm must contract (Ti) to total respiratory cycle (T_{tot}) is 0.5 [9, 16]. Decreased lung and wall compliance will increase Pdi, while muscle weakness will decrease the Pdi_{max}. However, the Ti/T_{tot} also plays an important role in diaphragmatic fatigue. Endurance time (T_{lim}) is inversely related to Ti/T_{tot} [17]. An increase in respiratory rate (RR) secondary to fever and illness or to compensate for hypercapnia and an increase in upper airway resistance secondary to oropharyngeal weakness will increase the Ti/T_{tot} ratio and lead to fatigue sooner. Tension-time index of the diaphragm (TTdi), which is the time integral of diaphragmatic tension per breath, may be a better indicator for predicting respiratory failure because it takes into consideration Ti/T_{tot} and Pdi/Pdi_{max}. TTdi is calculated by multiplying Ti/T_{tot} by Pdi/Pdi_{max}. A TTdi above 0.15 was found to have T_{lim} less than 45 minutes and therefore $TTdi_{crit}$ is 0.15 [17]. Tension-time index of the ribcage muscles (TTrc) has also been calculated with a higher critical value of 0.30 [18]. However, the importance of TTrc in the clinical setting is unclear.

Normal response to parenchymal disease and/or hypercapnia is to increase minute ventilation. Patients with neuromuscular disease have a normal central drive response to hypercapnia and hypoxemia as controls; however, the mechanism of increasing minute ventilation is different [9, 19, 20]. Healthy individuals increase tidal volume more than RR, while neuromuscular patients increase RR [9, 20]. This may in part relate to neuromuscular patients having a decreased Pdi_{max}.

An adequate cough is also important in maintaining respiratory function. Without an adequate cough, secretions cannot be cleared leading to atelectasis, mucus plugs, and pneumonias. An adequate cough requires good inspiratory effort (60–90% of total lung capacity), glottic closure, and good expiratory effort [9]. An abnormality in any one of these will lead to an impaired cough.

Clinical Presentation

Clinical signs of respiratory failure can be different depending on the rate of respiratory failure. Patients with chronic neuromuscular disease will usually develop sleep complaints first and are less likely to complain of dyspnea. Patients with a more rapid progression will notice dyspnea, orthopnea, and staccato speech (needing to take breaths between words) [11]. Preceding infection or illness can often be a precipitating factor to respiratory failure.

Sleep difficulties can be the first presenting sign of respiratory muscle involvement in chronic neuromuscular diseases. Sleep difficulties can be a result of obstructive sleep apnea (OSA) or nocturnal sleep-related hypoventilation [21, 22]. Patients with oropharyngeal weakness are at risk

of developing OSA. Symptoms can include snoring, fragmented sleep, excessive daytime sleepiness, frequent urination, non-restorative sleep, hypertension, congestive heart failure, and pulmonary hypertension. Although snoring can often be heard in OSA, OSA can occur without the presence of snoring. A more common sleep-related breathing disorder among neuromuscular disorders is nocturnal hypoventilation. As the diaphragm becomes weaker, patients rely more on accessory respiratory muscles. Normally, during rapid eye movement (REM) sleep, the body is paralyzed except for the diaphragm. Therefore, patients with diaphragm weakness, who rely on accessory muscles to maintain adequate ventilation, will usually develop hypoventilation during REM sleep initially. As the weakness progresses, hypoventilation can be seen in all stages of sleep. Symptoms of nocturnal hypoventilation are similar to OSA; however, nocturnal hypoventilation is more likely to result in nocturnal confusion, morning confusion, and morning headaches secondary to hypercapnia. Insidious onset of orthopnea can also make sleeping difficult. As sleep complaints are often the first sign of chronic respiratory insufficiency, a detailed sleep history is important when evaluating a patient with a neuromuscular disease.

Independent of time and course of respiratory insufficiency, signs of impending failure include dyspnea at rest, tachypnea, orthopnea, staccato speech, use of accessory muscles, forehead sweating, profound neck flexion weakness, paradoxical breathing, and vague sense of anxiety or discomfort [10]. One exception to orthopnea would be a patient with primarily intercostal and accessory muscle weakness, such as in patients with spinal muscular atrophy (SMA). These patients rely heavily on the diaphragm and have more difficulty with exhalation rather than inhalation. In the supine position, the diaphragm has an increased mechanical advantage to assist with exhalation. Therefore, patients with SMA may benefit from placement in the Trendelenburg position [23].

Other signs of impending respiratory failure can be related to oropharyngeal weakness or weak cough. These patients are at risk for aspiration and/or pneumonia. Coughing after drinking or eating can be a sign of aspiration. Trouble with increased oral secretions is a sign of difficulty swallowing, while a weak cough increases the difficulty in getting secretions up. Therefore, it is important to be aware of the wide range of symptoms of respiratory insufficiency in neuromuscular patients, from trouble sleeping, coughing after meals, to severe dyspnea, orthopnea, and tachypnea.

Diagnosis

Diagnosis of respiratory failure in neuromuscular diseases can be broken down into diagnosing a neuromuscular cause of respiratory failure compared to other causes of respiratory failure and diagnosing the type of neuromuscular disease. In the acute emergent situation, diagnosis of the type of respiratory failure is imperative. Early diagnosis of the type of neuromuscular disease is also essential when initiating treatment and for prognosis.

The majority of patients with neuromuscular diseases that cause respiratory failure will have findings of other muscle involvements on physical examination, specifically weakness of neck flexion, proximal muscles, and bulbar muscles. However, there are a few exceptions, such as Pompe's disease, that can present with isolated respiratory muscle weakness. A detailed history and examination can provide evidence of a neuromuscular cause of respiratory failure. For example, paradoxical breathing in the supine position suggests diaphragm weakness. In addition to history and physical examination, the diagnosis of neuromuscular weakness as the cause of respiratory failure may require ancillary tests.

Objective tests to aid in the diagnosis of respiratory failure secondary to neuromuscular weakness include arterial blood gas (ABG), pulmonary function tests (PFTs), chest imaging, electrocardiogram (ECG), and blood tests. In a hypoxic patient, an ABG should demonstrate elevations of $PaCO_2$. One should question respiratory muscle weakness as a cause of hypoxemia without hypercapnia. Hypoxemia can be seen without hypercapnia in a neuromuscular patient when the hypoxemia is secondary to pneumonia or aspiration. With acute respiratory failure due to respiratory muscle weakness, the ABG should demonstrate a decrease in pH, elevation in $PaCO_2$, minimal rise in bicarbonate level, and, depending on the severity, a decrease in PaO_2. With chronic respiratory failure, there is a greater bicarbonate rise and a less significant decrease in pH. However, in patients with only sleep-related hypoventilation, the ABG may demonstrate a normal $PaCO_2$, PaO_2, and pH with a mildly elevated bicarbonate level. Although an ABG is extremely helpful, specifically in a hypoxic patient, the ABG may be normal in the early stages of the disease. Therefore, an ABG alone is not enough to diagnose or monitor a patient with respiratory muscle weakness. Elevated serum bicarbonate level is a marker of chronic hypoventilation in neuromuscular patients and warrants further evaluation.

Pulmonary function tests are an extremely important tool in diagnosing and monitoring patients with neuromuscular disease. Although full PFTs usually demonstrate a restrictive pattern, their value in the acute setting is limited. However, forced vital capacity (FVC), maximal inspiratory pressure (MIP), maximal expiratory pressure (MEP), and peak cough flows (PCFs) can be performed at the bedside. Healthy, nonobese controls have less than a 10% drop in FVC in the supine position compared to the sitting position [24]. A drop of more than 15–20% in the supine position is a strong indicator of diaphragm weakness [11, 12]. An absolute decrease in FVC is not specific to neuromuscular weakness; however a FVC of less than 20 mL/kg is a strong predictor for mechanical ventilation [12]. The MIP reflects the strength of all inspiratory muscles. A normal MIP (< −80 cm H_2O in males and < −70cm H_2O in females) excludes significant respiratory muscle weakness [11]. While the MEP reflects the strength of expiratory muscles, the MEP differs from PCFs in that the MEP measures the peak pressure and PCFs measure the peak flow.

Adults require PCFs of >160 L/min to clear secretions [25–27]. Major limitations of PFTs are that they require a good oral seal, which patients with bulbar weakness may not be able to obtain and are effort dependent.

A single breath count can also be a useful tool in assessing FVC. The patient counts out loud with one breath. Normally one should reach 50. A count less than 15 suggests severe decrease in FVC; however, it is not specific for a neuromuscular cause of decreased FVC [12]. In general, if the patient can count to 10 with a single breath, the FVC is about one liter, and counting to 25 suggests a FVC of approximately two liters. This method can be helpful when bedside PFTs are not available or when seeing a patient through a video telehealth visit.

Chest imaging cannot only assist with the diagnosis of respiratory muscle weakness but can also aid in ruling out other causes of respiratory failure. An upright chest X-ray can demonstrate an elevated diaphragm with diaphragmatic weakness, which is most useful in unilateral diaphragmatic paralysis. Chest X-ray can also aid in the evaluation of pneumonia, congestive heart failure, and mass lesions. The sniff test evaluates diaphragmatic movement under fluoroscopy, which can be extremely valuable. CT of the chest aids in evaluation of pneumonia, parenchymal lung disease, mass lesions, and pulmonary emboli (PE). Non-ambulatory patients are at an increased risk for developing a PE, and therefore a PE needs to be considered in any unexpected acute respiratory failure.

It is also important to rule out other causes of respiratory failure. ECG and cardiac enzymes should be considered to evaluate for a cardiac cause of symptoms, especially as many neuromuscular disorders also have significant cardiac abnormalities, e.g., Pompe's disease, Duchene's muscular dystrophy, myotonic dystrophy, and mitochondria myopathies. Severe electrolyte abnormalities can cause neuromuscular weakness; therefore, chemistries, including calcium, phosphorus, and magnesium, are important and crucial to the evaluation. Creatine kinase (CK) can be elevated in myopathies as well as mildly elevated in severe neurogenic disorders, such as amyotrophic lateral sclerosis (ALS). In the presence of altered mental status, a complete metabolic workup, including urine toxicology, is indicated.

Electromyography (EMG) with nerve conduction studies (NCS) can be essential to the diagnosis of a neuromuscular disease. However, the utility of EMG/NCV in the acute setting can be limited for a number of reasons. First, quality studies require an electrically quite environment. Intensive care units and emergency rooms have electrical beds, IV pumps, monitors, ventilators, and compression stockings. All of these devices contribute to the 60 Hz artifact, consequently affecting the ability to record quality wave forms. Secondly, depending on the time since onset of symptoms, it may take 2 weeks or more to find significant abnormalities on EMG.

Polysomnography (PSG) is useful in diagnosing sleep-related hypoventilation and obstructive sleep apnea (OSA) in patients with neuromuscular diseases without significant daytime breathing difficulties, either clinically or by PFTs. The first abnormality in sleep-related hypoventilation is a rise in CO_2, defined by 10 minutes or more above 55 mmHg or rise of more than 10 mmHg while asleep with more than 10 minutes above 50 mmHg, most often during REM sleep. CO_2 can be monitored during PSG by either transcutaneous CO_2 or end-tidal CO_2. However, a "routine" PSG does not usually record CO_2. Therefore, it is important to specify the type of PSG requested on a neuromuscular patient. Due to comorbid diseases, or when CO_2 increases significantly, O_2 saturations will decrease. The decrease in O_2 is a continuous drop rather than repeated dips as seen with OSA. The hypoxemia will usually first occur during REM sleep. Routine overnight oximetry can detect hypoxemia but cannot detect hypercapnia and OSA without desaturations. PSG is important in the titration of positive airway pressure, either in the form of continuous positive airway pressure (CPAP) or bi-level positive airway pressure for the treatment of sleep-related hypoventilation.

Differential Diagnosis of Neuromuscular Disorder

Once there is a diagnosis of respiratory failure secondary to neuromuscular weakness, the next step is to determine the cause of neuromuscular weakness. Often the patient will already have a history of a neuromuscular disease. However, in some cases the first presenting symptom will be respiratory failure. Differentiating the cause of weakness involves a detailed history and detailed neurological examination, followed by the appropriate ancillary test to confirm or narrow the number of disorders in the differential diagnosis.

The first step in diagnosing the etiology of the symptoms involves a detailed history. Is there a history of a neurological disorder? Many patients with ALS, muscular dystrophy, myotonic dystrophy, and myasthenia gravis already have a diagnosis. However, this is not always the case, although there may be clues of a progressive neuromuscular disorder, e.g., falls, trouble swallowing, talking, weakness, weight loss, and dyspnea. In patients with a known risk of developing respiratory failure, investigate the possibilities of what may have triggered the respiratory failure, such as infection, aspiration, medication, or expected progression of the underlying disease. Does the patient have weakness other than in the respiratory muscles? Where did the weakness start? Weakness beginning in the legs and ascending up to the arms is typical of Guillain-Barré syndrome, while prominent bulbar or cranial nerve weakness is suggestive of MG or botulism. Inquire about other neurological symptoms, such as numbness, double vision, cognitive disturbance, cramps, pain, fasciculations, or seizures. Numbness and sensory loss suggest a neurogenic disorder rather than a myopathy or disorder of the neuromuscular junction. Recent medications, drugs, or toxin exposures are important to ascertain, as is a history of an insect or snake bite. Systemic symptoms or disorders including lung cancer may suggest a vasculitic neuropathy or Lambert-Eaton myasthenic syndrome (LEMS). Abdominal pain may suggest porphyria. At times in the emergency setting, the history may be incomplete especially if the patient is unresponsive. However, family and/or friends can be extremely helpful in providing significant details in the history of a neurological patient.

The second step in determining the etiology involves localizing the neurological problem. Neuromuscular weakness can localize to the anterior horn cell, nerve root, plexus, nerve, neuromuscular junction, or muscle. The neurological examination is fundamental to localization. Increased reflexes and spasticity suggest an upper motor neuron disorder. Decreased reflexes, fasciculations, decreased tone, and atrophy are signs of a lower motor neuron disorder. The presence of both upper and lower motor neuron signs suggests ALS. The distribution of weakness can assist in localization. Symmetrical proximal weakness suggests a myopathy, while distal weakness is more common in polyneuropathies. Variable or fluctuating weakness is indicative of a disorder of the neuromuscular junction, while sensory abnormalities favor a peripheral neuropathy as opposed to a disorder of muscle or neuromuscular junction. Despite a detailed neurological examination, there are times it is still difficult to localize the process with complete certainty. Electromyography (EMG) and nerve conduction studies (NCS) are an extremely useful adjunct to the neurological examination in localizing lower motor neuron abnormalities.

An EMG can provide information on pathophysiology, severity, evolution, and chronicity. It may confirm or exclude a diagnosis or identify an unrecognized disease. The muscles involved in a neurogenic process can assist in localizing the abnormality. The NCS not only evaluates motor nerves but large fiber sensory nerves as well. Conduction velocities, presence of conduction block, or dispersion on NCS provides information on the myelination of the nerve.

Further ancillary testing will depend on the differential diagnosis. For disorders localizing to the muscle, see Table 16.1 for differential diagnosis. The majority of myopathies will have small complex motor unit potentials (MUPs) on EMG. However, the definitive diagnosis will usually require a muscle biopsy or genetic testing. For disorders localizing to the neuromuscular junction, see Table 16.2. Decrement on

Table 16.1 Disorders causing neuromuscular respiratory weakness localizing to the muscle

Disorder	Key clinical findings	Key test
Acid maltase deficiency (Pompe's disease) [28]	Significant respiratory muscle involvement Cardiac involvement prominent in children Adults slow course with early diaphragm involvement Axial/paraspinal weakness Scapular winging	EMG: myopathic findings with myotonic discharges; findings may only be in paraspinal muscles Alpha-glucosidase deficiency in leukocytes, fibroblasts, or muscle Genetic testing
Congenital muscular dystrophy [29]	Hypotonia and weakness at birth Almost always fatal during childhood or adolescents	Normal to increased CK Muscle biopsy
Congenital myopathy [5, 11, 30]	Hypotonia and weakness as infant Respiratory failure most likely in nemaline myopathy, multiminicore disease, and myotubular myopathy and less likely in central core disease	Muscle biopsy
Idiopathic nemaline myopathy [31]	Proximal to generalized weakness Complication of HIV [32], monoclonal gammopathy [33, 34], or hypothyroidism [35]	HIV UPEP TSH Muscle biopsy
Dystrophinopathy	Progressive weakness starting in childhood Cardiomyopathy Calf pseudohypertrophy X-linked	Marked increased CK (50–100 × normal) Dystrophin gene testing
Myofibrillar myopathy [5]	Distal myopathy Usually adult onset Cardiac abnormalities	Muscle biopsy
Bethlem myopathy [36]	Muscle cramps and weakness Contractures common Autosomal dominant	Muscle biopsy
Myotonic dystrophy	Distal and bulbar weakness more prominent Male pattern baldness Cardiac abnormalities Myotonia on exam Autosomal dominant	Myotonic discharges on EMG Mutation in DMPK gene (type 1) Mutation in CNBP (type 2)
Mitochondrial myopathy [37]	Ophthalmoparesis indolent Generalized weakness Hearing loss Cardiomyopathy	Increased lactic acid level Muscle biopsy may show ragged red fibers
Limb girdle muscular dystrophy (especially 2C-2F, 2L) [5, 11]	Pelvic and should girdle weakness Usually present in adults	Muscle biopsy Normal to increased CK
Inflammatory myopathy	Proximal muscle weakness Muscle pain Skin rash with dermatomyositis	Increased CK Muscle biopsy Screen for possible malignancy
Inclusion Body Myositis [38–40]	Significant flinger flexor weakness Onset typically over age 50 Years of slow progression Disproportionate quad weakness/atrophy	Muscle biopsy Mild increased CK
Toxic [41, 42]	Muscle pain Generalized weakness Alcohol, cholesterol-lowering agents, colchicine, chloroquine, cyclosporine, and L-tryptophan, zidovudine	Marked increased CK Phosphate level Liver function test

(continued)

Table 16.1 (continued)

Disorder	Key clinical findings	Key test
Metabolic myopathy with myoglobinuria [43]	Muscle pain Swelling Rhabdomyolysis Carnitine palmitoyl transferase deficiency Glycolytic enzyme defects	Marked increased CK following exercise Myoglobinuria Monitor renal function Ischemic exercise test
Periodic paralysis	Hereditary Associated with thyrotoxicosis [44] Episodic weakness Andersen-Tawil syndrome (prolonged QT)	Check K level ECG Normal or increased CK TSH
Trichinosis myositis [45]	Cardiomyopathy Severe weakness Periorbital and facial edema	Increased CK Eosinophilia Muscle biopsy demonstrated larvae of *Trichinella spiralis*
Critical illness myopathy [46]	History of multi-organ failure Steroid or neuromuscular-blocking agents Failure to wean off ventilator	Usually normal CK EMG may be normal Muscle biopsy

Table 16.2 Disorders causing neuromuscular respiratory weakness localizing to the neuromuscular junction

Disorder	Key clinical findings	Key test
Myasthenia gravis	Ocular muscle weakness Bulbar weakness Fatigable weakness Normal pupil function	Acetylcholine receptor antibodies Anti-muscle-specific kinase (MuSK) antibody [47] Decrement on 2 Hz repetitive stimulation Increase Jitter on single fiber
Lambert-Eaton myasthenic syndrome (LEMS)	Limb weakness Autonomic symptoms Strength gets better with brief exercise	Anti-VGCC Decrement on 1–5 Hz repetitive stimulation Facilitation on 30–50 Hz repetitive stimulation Screen for possible malignancy
Organophosphate poisoning [48]	Weakness proximal >distal Diarrhea and cramping Increase salvation	Spontaneous repetitive firing of compound muscle action potential after single stimulation
Botulism	Ophthalmoplegia Pupil affected Nausea, vomiting, abdominal pain Generalize weakness Autonomic symptoms	EMG similar to LEMS Detection of botulinum toxin in blood or stool
Hypermagnesemia [49]	Renal failure History of magnesium intake	Mg level Bun, Cr, urinalysis

1–5 Hz repetitive stimulation suggests a disorder of the neuromuscular junction. Postsynaptic disorders usually demonstrate a greater decrement than pre-synaptic disorders. Facilitation, defined as an increase in more than two times the baseline amplitude of the compound muscle action potential (CMAP), can be demonstrated with 10 seconds of exercise or 30–50 Hz repetitive stimulation in presynaptic disorders. Increased jitter on single-fiber EMG can be seen in all types of neuromuscular junction disorders. For disorders localizing to the peripheral nerve, see Table 16.3. Sensory abnormalities on NCS are key findings to localize the abnormality to the peripheral nerve or plexus. Slowed conduction velocities and conduction block suggest a demyelinating neuropathy as can be seen with acute inflammatory demyelinating neuropathy

Table 16.3 Disorders causing neuromuscular respiratory weakness localizing to the peripheral nerve

Disorder	Key clinical findings	Key test
Guillain-Barré syndrome	Progressive weakness, usually ascending Peak weakness by 2–3 weeks Dysesthesias in feet and hands Areflexia Autonomic symptoms	CSF elevated protein Anti-GM1 seen with *Campylobacter jejuni* infection Anti-GQ1b seen in Miller-Fisher variant NCS demonstrate slowed conduction velocities, prolonged F-waves, and reduced CMAP
Porphyria [50]	Abdominal pain Weakness (arms > legs) Autonomic symptoms Triggered by infection, alcohol, stress, smoking, and P450-inducing drugs	Urine porphyrin, porphobilinogen, and δ-aminolevulinic acid levels EMG demonstrates primarily motor axonal neuropathy
Neuralgic amyotrophy [51]	Severe shoulder and arm pain Weakness and numbness in arm follows pain Can have isolated phrenic nerve involvement	EMG consistent with a brachial plexus lesion
Vasculitic neuropathy [52]	Multiple mononeuropathies or asymmetric polyneuropathy Painful Sensory loss May have symptoms of systemic vasculitis	ESR CBC ANA RF ANCA Urinalysis Complement levels Hepatitis screen HIV Cryoglobulins Nerve biopsy
Critical illness polyneuropathy [46]	History of multi-organ failure or sepsis Steroid or neuromuscular blocking agents Failure to wean off ventilator	EMG: axonal sensorimotor polyneuropathy
Poems syndrome [53]	Polyneuropathy Organomegaly Endocrinopathy M-protein spike Skin changes	SPEP UPEP EMG: sensorimotor polyneuropathy
Multifocal motor neuropathy with conduction block [54]	Asymmetrical limb weakness Upper extremities > lower extremities	Anti-GM1 NCS demonstrate conduction block
Arsenic poisoning [55]	Encephalopathy Symmetrical neuropathy Painful	EMG shows primarily axonal, sensorimotor neuropathy Urine arsenic level
Diphtheria [56]	History of sore throat CN involvement Pupil abnormalities	Throat culture for *C. diphtheriae* CSF elevated protein and pleocytosis NCS similar to GBS

(AIDP), while decreased CMAP amplitudes, with normal-to-mild slowing of conduction velocities, suggest axonal neuropathy. Disorders localizing to the motor neuron (Table 16.4) will spare sensory NCS. There are some disorders, specifically neurotoxins, which can affect the motor neuron, neuromuscular junction, and/or muscle (Table 16.5). These disorders can demonstrate a combination of findings on NCS and EMG.

Table 16.4 Disorders causing neuromuscular respiratory weakness localizing to the motor neuron

Disorder	Key clinical findings	Key test
Amyotrophic lateral sclerosis	Upper and lower motor findings Progressive weakness without significant pain or sensory symptoms Fasciculations	EMG: diffuse fibrillation potentials, fasciculation potentials, and neurogenic MUPs
Poliomyelitis and postpolio syndrome [57]	Asymmetrical weakness Fever and meningismus History of poliomyelitis usually affecting bulbar or respiratory muscles	CSF: elevated protein and pleocytosis EMG: neurogenic MUPs
Spinal muscular atrophy (types 1 > 2 > 3) [23]	Proximal > distal weakness Decrease deep-tendon reflexes Intercostal muscle weakness >> diaphragm weakness	Gene testing for SMN1 EMG: neurogenic MUPs, normal sensory NCS

Table 16.5 Disorders causing neuromuscular respiratory weakness affecting multiple locations

Disorder	Key clinical findings	Key test
Scorpion venom [58, 59]	History of sting Muscle jerks and restlessness Tachycardia and tachypnea Hyperpyrexia Excessive salivation	Elevated WBC
Tick paralysis [60]	Ascending flaccid paralysis (hours to few days) Ataxia	Search and remove tick
Seafood toxins [43, 61] (ciguatera and saxitoxin)	History of recent seafood ingestion Nausea, vomiting, and diarrhea Paresthesia face and mouth Generalized weakness	Diagnosis made clinically Commercially available toxin assays are currently not available

Treatment

The initial priority in the treatment of neuromuscular respiratory failure includes ventilation, protecting the airway, and clearing secretions. The second priority involves treating the underlining disease, if treatment is available, or treating precipitating factors (i.e., pneumonia). The third priority in treatment involves implementation of preventative strategies in patients with known neuromuscular disorders.

Ventilation is the primary treatment for respiratory failure secondary to neuromuscular weakness. The optimal method of ventilation will depend on the condition of the patient and the type of neuromuscular disease. In general (and contrary to common practice for patients with respiratory insufficiency), neuromuscular patients should not be put on oxygen without some mode of secure or enhanced ventilation. Patients with chronic hypoventilation may have a chronic elevation of pCO_2 leading to a "hypoxic drive" of respiration. Treatment with supplemental oxygen raises the pO_2 resulting in loss of the "hypoxic drive." Subsequently the patient further hypoventilates leading to increasing levels of CO_2. Such patients often appear "more comfortable," in part because of the sedating effects of hypercapnia. As such sedation becomes increasingly profound over the next few hours, the patient follows a vicious cycle of increased sedation leading to reduced ventilation, which in turn raises the pCO_2 even further, producing increasing sedation and ultimately a respiratory arrest. In patients with hypoxemia secondary to aspiration or pneumonia without any respiratory muscle weakness or elevated CO_2, oxygen alone may be appropriate. However, CO_2 levels need to be monitored very closely in these patients to ensure adequate ventilation.

Invasive ventilation is generally recommended for reversible neuromuscular weakness and acute respiratory failure. A forced vital capacity of less than 15 mL/kg, oropharyngeal weakness with aspiration, or PO_2 less than 70 mm Hg are the accepted absolute criteria for intubation in patients with GBS [62]. Impaired consciousness, respiratory or cardiac arrest, shock, arrhythmias, and blood-gas abnormalities are also accepted absolute criteria for intubation in all patients [12]. In patients who do not meet the absolute criteria for intubation, the decision to intubate is more difficult. Patients to be considered for intubation include those having dyspnea at rest, tachypnea, orthopnea, staccato speech, tachycardia, accessory muscle use, weak cough, cough after swallowing, markedly weakened neck muscles, bulbar dysfunction, or dysautonomia [10, 12, 63]. These patients need to be monitored very closely, ideally in the ICU, and elective intubation should be performed prior to complications from respiratory failure and abnormalities on ABG. Monitoring should include vital signs, bedside PFTs, clinical symptoms, and bulbar, neck, and extremity weakness. Patients with rapidly progressive GBS are also at an increased risk for acute respiratory failure [63]. Bedside pulmonary function tests can assist in predicting those patients at risk for acute respiratory failure. A FVC less than 20 mL/kg, MIP worse than −30 cm H_2O, MEP less than 40 cm H_2O, or 30% drop in FVC, MIP, or MEP indicates a risk for respiratory failure in GBS [64]. The clinician must be cautious when interpreting bedside spirometry (FVC, MIP, and MEP) in neuromuscular patients. Often when patients have severe weakness of facial muscles, they will be unable to maintain a seal around the mouthpiece resulting in falsely low values. Also those patients with corticobulbar tract upper motor neuron disease (as is seen with ALS) may be unable to volitionally integrate the necessary components for a reliable measurement (similar to an apraxia) resulting in unreliably low values. It behooves the clinician to conduct a bedside assessment to assure that the spirometry measurements are consistent with the patient's clinical status. In patients with MG, repetitive measurements of FVC correlate less well with the need for mechanical ventilation [65]. When intubating a neuromuscular patient, depolarizing neuromuscular blocking agents should be avoided secondary to potentially life-threatening hyperkalemia [66, 67]. It is recommended to use topical anesthesia, short-acting benzodiaze-pines, and if needed atropine when intubating a neuromuscular patient [12].

Noninvasive positive pressure ventilation (NPPV) may be an alternative to mechanical ventilation for those patients without oropharyngeal weakness and/or without expected prolonged need for mechanical ventilation. However the use of NPPV in the acute respiratory weakness setting has not been well studied [68] [1]. Bi-level positive airway pressure allows for establishing the expiratory pressure (EPAP) and inspiratory pressure (IPAP), with IPAP being high enough over EPAP to effectively ventilate the patient. The differential of IPAP to EPAP needed to ventilate a patient will depend on the elastic load of the lungs and chest wall. If the patient's weakness is severe enough where the patient cannot trigger the pressure-support breaths or the patient has central apnea, then a spontaneous/timed (S/T) mode is indicated and will provide a minimum respiratory rate. When bi-level positive airway pressure cannot adequately ventilate a patient or the patient cannot tolerate bi-level positive airway pressure, there must be consideration for mechanical ventilation either with volume-cycle mask ventilation (close circuit vs. the open circuit with bi-level) or invasive ventilation. However, in an emergent situation, invasive ventilation is more appropriate, especially if there is a risk for aspiration secondary to bulbar weakness or decreased level of consciousness.

Noninvasive positive pressure ventilation may limit complications from invasive ventilation. Mortality, ICU stay, and complication rates were lower in a small retrospective series of chronic progressive neuromuscular patients with acute respiratory failure treated with NPPV compared to historical controls treated with invasive ventilation [69]. Those patients with difficulty clearing secretions using NPPV received a cricothyroid "mini-tracheostomy" (CM). The CM allows tracheal access to suction secretions. Benefits of NPPV include enabling the patient to eat and speak. Preservation of communication is an obvious priority in patients with progressive neuromuscular diseases. Patients on NPPV have the ability to participate in medical decision-making, while a patient with endotracheal intubation will require sedation limiting their ability to make important medical choices. Occasional patients with progressive neuromuscular disorders, who undergo tracheostomy without their consent, would have chosen not to have the tracheostomy if given the opportunity to make their own medical decisions [70]. Noninvasive positive pressure ventilation also spares some patients with MG from intubation [71]. However, hypercapnia greater than 50 mm Hg predicts failure of NPPV.

Cough augmentation devices, either manual or mechanical, can help with clearing the airway when patients have a weak cough. Manual cough augmentation encompasses manual hyperinflation of the lungs. If expiratory muscles are weak, an abdominal thrust maneuver may increase peak cough flows [72]. Mechanical cough augmentation has preset insufflation and exsufflation pressures. Consider cough augmentation in patients with early respiratory infections to prevent further respiratory failure. Cough augmentation can be used as often as necessary and should be considered when there is a rapid drop in O_2 with the intent to enhance clearing of secretions.

Sialorrhea is common in patients with neuromuscular disorders with bulbar weakness. This can lead to increased risk of aspiration and intolerance to NPPV. Anticholinergic medications are commonly used to block the cholinergic input to the salivary glands. Common medications used include glycopyrrolate, topical atropine, amitriptyline, and scopolamine patch.

Treatment of underlying neurological disease is the next step in treating the patient with respiratory failure. Treatment may include replacing electrolyte abnormalities, discontinuing triggering or exacerbating drugs, treating underlying infections, and supportive care. Intravenous immunoglobulin (IVIG) or plasmapheresis may be indicated, specifically for AIDP (see Chap. 12) and MG (discussed later), while corticosteroids can be considered for inflammatory myositis or vasculitis. Avoid dehydration, fasting, and fever, each of which can increase metabolic demand and increase RR. In patients where the acute respiratory failure is secondary to progression of a non-curable disease without any exacerbating factors, decisions on long-term ventilation need to be addressed. If the patient does not wish to have long-term ventilation, comfort care is indicated. Ideally, these discussions should occur prior to acute respiratory failure.

Prevention

Prevention of acute respiratory failure is important in patients with known neuromuscular weakness. Close surveillance with PFTs, use of NPPV when appropriate, and airway clearance with mechanical cough assist devices are important in preventing acute respiratory failure. High-frequency chest wall compression is typically not as helpful given that most neuromuscular patients do not have difficulty with mucociliary clearance.

Routine PFTs can help anticipate patients who are at risk for respiratory failure. Recommendations for the management of respiratory care in the patient with Duchenne's muscular dystrophy include monitoring FVC, MIP, and PCF [66, 73]. Nocturnal NPPV should be considered in patients with decreased FVC, MIP, or MEP. In some patients, PFTs may be relatively unremarkable, but they may still suffer from significant sleep-related breathing disorders. In these patients, a polysomnogram should be considered.

Nocturnal NPPV has been demonstrated to improve quality of life, decrease hypercarbia, and increase survival rates in patients with neuromuscular disease [73–77]. Nocturnal NPPV is thought to improve respiratory function by resting muscles at night, improving microatelectasis, and possible altering the CO_2 set point [78–80]. In young children with spinal muscular atrophy, NPPV improves lung development and helps prevent chest wall deformities [13, 23, 81]. Bi-level machines with volume-assured pressure allows the tidal volume to be set and the IPAP pressure titrated to meet the target volume. This method may theoretically be beneficial for neuromuscular disorders with a faster progression. It ensures an adequate tidal volume without having to re-titrate the IPAP pressure needed to adequately ventilate a patient.

Peak cough flows can help identify those patients who are risk for pneumonia. Adults require PCFs of >160 L/min to clear secretions [25–27]. Patients with PCFs less than 270 L/min are at risk of dropping below 160 L/min when ill, and therefore patients with PCFs less than 270 L/min are felt to be at an increased risk for recurrent pneumonias [9, 26, 82]. Patients with PCFs below 270 L/min should be monitored closely and be considered for training with cough augmentation devices. A more aggressive protocol using frequent monitoring of PFTs, home oximetry monitoring, air stacking, assisted coughing, and intermittent NPPV has been shown to decrease hospitalization in patients with neuromuscular diseases, specifically due to upper respiratory tract infections [26, 82].

Preventive measures need to be taken for elective procedures requiring sedation or anesthesia in neuromuscular patients. Depolarizing muscle relaxants and neuromuscular blockers are absolutely contraindicated because of rhabdomyolysis and fatal hyperkalemia [66, 67]. Malignant hyperthermia-like reactions can occur with inhalational anesthetics, especially in central core myopathy. Patients with decreased FVC < 50% are at a higher risk for respiratory failure with anesthesia and may need prolonged ventilation with either NPPV or invasive ventilation. These patients should be monitored closely post-op and may need to be empirically placed on NPPV with a backup rate. Those patients already using NPPV should, at minimum, be using their NPPV. Supplemental O2 should not be used without some form of ventilation. Lastly, mechanical cough augmentation devices can be helpful in preventing atelectasis and post-op pneumonia. Mechanical cough augmentation devices are recommended for post-op patients with Duchenne's muscular dystrophy with MEP <60cmH2O or PCF <270 l/minute [66].

Specific Neuromuscular Conditions Commonly Associated with Respiratory Failure

Late-Onset or Adult-Onset Acid Maltase Deficiency

Late-onset or adult-onset acid maltase deficiency should be considered in adults who present with a chronic myopathy associated with early or disproportionate diaphragm weakness. Late-onset acid maltase deficiency is a lysosomal glycogen storage disorder caused by mutations in the gene that encodes α-glucosidase (GAA) whose deficiency results in accumulation of glycogen in lysosomal structures in muscle fibers and other tissues. Symptoms can begin in childhood or in adulthood, and respiratory symptoms may be the initial presentation in a third of patients. Muscle enzymes can be mildly elevated but not uncommonly are normal. The EMG shows small myopathic motor units and myotonic discharges in the paraspinal muscles. Muscle biopsy results are variable. In the classic case, there is positive staining for acid-phosphatase vacuoles and increase in glycogen. Diagnosis is made by assay of GAA activity in dried blood spot and can be confirmed with a genetic test.

The distribution of weakness can be variable with a third presenting with respiratory weakness. Proximal and paraspinal weakness, difficulty with posture, and scapular winging should suggest this diagnosis, including those with floppy head syndrome and bent spine syndrome. The disorder has become the focus of heightened interest given the development of enzyme replacement therapy. Replacement therapy in infants prolongs survival and improves motor outcomes. Adults appeared to receive a stabilizing benefit – in an 18-month, randomized, placebo-controlled study of 90 patients. An increased walking distance and stabilization of pulmonary function were observed in the treated patients compared with those receiving placebo [83–86].

Myasthenia Gravis

Myasthenia gravis (MG) is an autoimmune disorder of neuromuscular transmission involving the production of autoantibodies directed against the nicotinic acetylcholine receptor. Acetylcholine receptor antibodies (AChR) are detectable in the serum of 80–90% of patients with MG. The prevalence of MG is about 1 in 10–20,000. Women are affected about twice as often as men. Symptoms may begin at virtually any age with a peak in women in the second and third decades, while the peak in men occurs in the fifth and sixth decades. Associated autoimmune diseases, such as rheumatoid arthritis, lupus, and pernicious anemia, are present in about 5% of patients. Thyroid disease occurs in about 10%, often in association with antithyroid antibodies. About 10–15% of MG patients have a thymoma, while thymic lymphoid hyperplasia with proliferation of germinal centers occurs in 50–70% of cases. In most patients the cause of autoimmune MG is unknown. However, there are iatrogenic causes for autoimmune MG. D-penicillamine (used in the treatment of Wilson's disease and rheumatoid arthritis), checkpoint inhibitors, and alfa-interferon therapy are capable of inducing MG. In addition, bone marrow transplantation is associated with the development of MG as part of the chronic graft versus host disease.

Clinical Features

The hallmark of myasthenia gravis is fluctuating or fatigable weakness. The presenting symptoms are ocular in half of all patients (25% of patients initially present with diplopia, 25% with ptosis), and by 1 month into the course of illness, 80% of patients have some degree of ocular involvement. Presenting symptoms are bulbar (dysarthria or dysphagia) in 10%, leg weakness (impaired walking) in 10%, and generalized weakness in 10%. Respiratory failure is the presenting symptom in 1% of cases. Patients usually complain of symptoms from focal muscle dysfunction, such as diplopia, ptosis, dysarthria, dysphagia, inability to work with arms raised over the head, or disturbance of gait. In contrast, patients with MG tend not to complain of "generalized weakness,"

"generalized fatigue," "sleepiness," or muscle pain. In the classic case, fluctuating weakness is worse with exercise and improved with rest. Symptoms tend to progress later in the day. Many different factors can precipitate or aggravate weakness, such as physical stress, emotional stress, infection, or exposure to medications that impair neuromuscular transmission (perioperative succinylcholine, aminoglycoside antibiotics, quinine, quinidine, botulinum toxin).

Diagnosis

The diagnosis is based on a history of fluctuating weakness with corroborating findings on examination. There are several different ways to validate or confirm the clinical diagnosis.

Antibodies

The standard assay for receptor binding antibodies is an immunoprecipitation assay using human limb muscle for acetylcholine receptor antigen. In addition, assays for receptor modulating and blocking antibodies are available. Binding antibodies are present in about 80% of all myasthenia patients (50% of patients with pure ocular MG, 80% of those with mild generalized MG, 90% of patients with moderate to severe generalized MG, and 70% of those in clinical remission). By also testing for modulating and blocking antibodies, the sensitivity improves to 90% overall. Specificity is outstanding with false positives exceedingly rare in reliable labs. If blood is sent to a reference lab, the test results are usually available within a week

About 25–47% of patients seronegative for acetylcholine receptor antibodies have been shown to have muscle-specific kinase (MuSK) antibodies. The clinical features of MuSK-positive patients may differ from non-MuSK MG patients. MuSK antibody-positive patients tend to be younger women (under age 40) and have lower likelihood of abnormal repetitive stimulation and edrophonium test results. Bulbar symptoms are significantly more common at onset of disease in MuSK antibody-positive patients. MuSK antibodies may also be more commonly associated with patients having weakness of neck extensor, shoulders, or respiratory muscles.

In patients who are double negative (lack AChR or MuSK antibody), LRP4 antibodies may be found in about 1–2% of autoimmune MG. Patients with LRP4 MG tend to be younger and female and often have mild disease [87].

EMG (Electrophysiological Testing)

Repetitive stimulation testing is widely available and has variable sensitivity depending on number and selection of muscles studied and various provocative maneuvers. However, in most labs this technique has a sensitivity of about 50% in all patients with MG (lower in patients with mild or pure ocular disease). In general, the yield from repetitive stimulation is higher when testing muscle groups having clinically significant weakness. Single-fiber EMG is a highly specialized technique, usually available in major academic centers, with a sensitivity of about 90%. Abnormal single-fiber results are common in other neuromuscular diseases, and therefore the test must be used in the correct clinical context. The specificity of single-fiber EMG is an important issue in that mild abnormalities can clearly be present with a variety of other diseases of the motor unit including motor neuron disease, peripheral neuropathy, and myopathy. Disorders of neuromuscular transmission other than MG can have substantial abnormalities on SFEMG. In contrast, acetylcholine receptor antibodies (and MuSK antibodies) are not found in non-MG patients. However, a normal SFEMG in a clinically weak muscle rules out MG as the cause of that weakness. In summary, the two highly sensitive laboratory studies are single-fiber EMG and acetylcholine receptor antibodies; nonetheless, neither test is 100% sensitive.

Prognosis

Management of the patient with autoimmune MG requires understanding of the natural course of the disease. The long-term natural course of MG is not clearly established other than being highly variable. Several generalizations can be made. About half of MG patients present with ocular symptoms and by 1 month 80% have eye findings. By 1 month, symptoms remain purely ocular in 40%, generalized in 40%, limited to the

limbs in 10%, and limited to bulbar muscles in 10%. Weakness remains restricted to the ocular muscles on a long-term basis in about 15–20% (pure ocular MG). Most patients with initial ocular involvement tend to develop generalized weakness within the first year of the disease (90% of those who generalize do so within the initial 12 months). Maximal weakness occurs within the initial 3 years in 70% of patients. In the modem era, death from MG is rare. Spontaneous long-lasting remission occurs in about 10–15%, usually in the first year or two of the disease. Most MG patients develop progression of clinical symptoms during the initial 2–3 years. However, progression is not uniform, as illustrated by 15–20% of patients whose symptoms remain purely ocular and those who have spontaneous remission.

Treatment

The course of MG is variable for each patient; it is therefore important to know when to hospitalize the patient. Approximately one-fifth of patients will develop a myasthenic crisis during the course of their disease [88]. Myasthenic crisis (Table 16.6) is a medical emergency characterized by respiratory failure from diaphragm weak-

Table 16.6 The acutely deteriorating myasthenic patient

Myasthenic crisis
Respiratory distress
Respiratory arrest
Cyanosis
Increased pulse and blood pressure
Diaphoresis
Poor cough
Inability to handle oral secretions
Dysphagia
Weakness
Improves with edrophonium
Cholinergic crisis
Abdominal cramps
Diarrhea
Nausea and vomiting
Excessive secretions
Miosis
Fasciculations
Diaphoresis
Weakness
Worse with edrophonium

ness or severe oropharyngeal weakness leading to aspiration. Crisis can occur in the setting of surgery (post-op), acute infection, and change in medication or following rapid withdrawal of corticosteroids, although some patients have no precipitating factors. Therefore, those having dyspnea should be hospitalized immediately in a constant observation or an intensive care setting. Patients with moderate or severe dysphagia, weight loss, as well as those with rapidly progressive or severe weakness should be admitted urgently. This will allow close monitoring and early intervention in the case of respiratory failure and will also expedite the diagnostic workup and initiation of therapy. Patients in myasthenic crisis should be placed in an ICU setting and have FVC checked every 2 hours. Changes in arterial blood gases occur relatively late in neuromuscular respiratory failure. There should be a low threshold for initiation of NPPV or intubation and mechanical ventilation. Criteria for intubation include a drop in the FVC below 15 ml/kg (or below one liter in an average-sized adult), severe aspiration from oropharyngeal weakness, or labored breathing regardless of the measurements. If the diagnosis is not clear-cut, it is advisable to secure the airway with intubation and stabilize ventilation and only then address the question of the underlying diagnosis. If the patient has been taking cholinesterase inhibitors (CEIs), the drug should be temporarily discontinued in order to rule out the possibility of "cholinergic crisis." Patient should be screened for and have any underlying medical problems corrected, such as systemic infection, metabolic problems (i.e., diabetes), and thyroid disease, as these can exacerbate MG. In patients with MG exacerbation, plasma exchange or IVIG can hasten recovery.

Plasma Exchange

Plasma exchange (plasmapheresis) removes acetylcholine receptor antibodies and results in rapid clinical improvement. The standard course involves removal of 2–3 liters of plasma every other day or three times per week until the patient improves (usually a total of 3–5 exchanges). Improvement begins after the first few exchanges and reaches maximum within 2–3 weeks. The improvement is moderate to marked in nearly all patients but usually wears off after 4–8 weeks due to the re-accumulation of pathogenic antibodies. Vascular access may require placement of a central line. Complications include hypotension, bradycardia, electrolyte imbalance, hemolysis, infection, and access problems (such as pneumothorax from placement of a central line). Indications for plasma exchange include any patient in whom a rapid temporary clinical improvement is needed. There are occasional patients who have severe dysfunction and do poorly on medication such that weekly plasma exchange eventually becomes the mainstay of their long-term management.

High-Dose IVIg

High-dose intravenous immunoglobulin (IVIg) administration is associated with rapid improvement in MG symptoms in a timeframe similar to plasma exchange. The mechanism is unclear but may relate to downregulation of acetylcholine receptor antibody production or to the effect of anti-idiotype antibodies. The usual protocol is 2 grams/kg administered over 5 consecutive days (0.4 g/kg/day). Different IVIg preparations are administered intravenously at different rates (contact the pharmacy for guidelines). The majority of MG patients improve, usually within 1 week of starting IVIg. The degree of response is variable and the duration of response is limited similar to plasma exchange, to about 4–8 weeks. Complications include fever, chills, and headache, which respond to slowing down the rate of the infusion and giving diphenhydramine. Occasional cases of aseptic meningitis, renal failure, nephrotic syndrome, and stroke have been reported. Also, patients with selective IgA deficiency can have anaphylaxis best avoided by screening for IgA deficiency ahead of time. The treatment is relatively expensive, comparable to plasma exchange. In a randomized, placebo-controlled trial, 51 patients with severe MG weakness were assigned to receive an infusion with 2 g/kg of intravenous immunoglobulin or an equivalent volume of 5% intravenous dextrose in water. In patients treated with intravenous immu-noglobulin, a clinically meaningful improvement in QMG score was observed at day 14 and per-sisted at day 28. The greatest improvement occurred in patients with more severe disease. The study provides level 1 evidence for the effec-tiveness of IVIg in patients with worsening weak-ness due to myasthenia gravis [89]. Occasional patients do poorly on alternative therapy and rely on scheduled periodic IVIg for their long-term maintenance therapy.

Corticosteroids

There are no controlled trials documenting the benefit of corticosteroids in MG. However, nearly all authorities have personal experience attesting to the virtues (and complications) of corticosteroid use in MG patients. In general, corticosteroids are used in patients with moder-ate to severe, disabling symptoms which are refractory to cholinesterase inhibitors (CEIs). Patients are commonly hospitalized to initiate therapy due to the risk of early exacerbation. Opinions differ regarding the best method of administration. For patients with severe MG, it is best to begin with high-dose therapy of 60–80 mg/day orally. Early exacerbation occurs in about half of patients usually within the first few days of therapy and typically lasts 3–4 days. In 10% of cases, the exacerbation is severe requiring mechanical ventilation or a feeding tube (thus the need to initiate therapy in the hos-pital). Overall about 80% of patient show a favorable response to steroids (with 30% attain-ing remission and 50% marked improvement). Mild to moderate improvement occurs in 15%, and 5% have no response. Improvement begins as early as 12 hours and as late as 60 days after beginning prednisone, but usually the patient begins to improve within the first week or two. Improvement is gradual, with marked improve-ment occurring at a mean of 3 months and maxi-mal improvement at a mean of 9 months. Of those patients having a favorable response, most maintain their improvement with gradual dosage reduction at a rate of 10 mg every 1–2 months. More rapid reduction is usually associated with a flare-up of the disease. While many patients can

eventually be weaned off of steroids and main-tain their response, the majority cannot. They require a minimum dose (5–30 mg alternate day) in order to maintain their improvement. Complications of long-term high-dose predni-sone therapy are substantial, including Cushingoid appearance, hypertension, osteopo-rosis, cataracts, aseptic necrosis, and the other well-known complications of chronic steroid therapy. Older patients tend to respond more favorably to prednisone. An alternative predni-sone regimen involves low-dose alternate day, gradually increasing schedule in an attempt to avoid the early exacerbation. Patients receive prednisone 25 mg on alternate days with an increase of 12.5 mg every third dose (about every fifth day) to a maximum dose of 100 mg on alternate days or until sufficient improvement occurs. Clinical improvement usually begins within 1 month of treatment. The frequency and severity of early exacerbation is less than that associated with high-dose daily regimens. High-dose intravenous methylprednisolone (1000 mg IV daily for 3–5 days) can provide improvement within 1–2 weeks, but the clinical improvement is temporary.

Cholinesterase Inhibitors

Cholinesterase inhibitors are safe, effective, and first-line therapy in all stable patients. Inhibition of acetylcholinesterase (AChE) reduces the hydrolysis of acetylcholine (ACh), increasing the accumulation of ACh at the nicotinic postsynap-tic membrane. The CEIs used in MG bind revers-ibly (as opposed to organophosphate CEIs, which bind irreversibly) to AChE. These drugs cross the blood-brain barrier poorly and tend not to cause central nervous system side effects. Absorption from the gastrointestinal tract is inefficient and variable, with oral bioavailability of about 10%. Muscarinic autonomic side effects of gastroin-testinal cramping, diarrhea, salivation, lacrimation, diaphoresis, and, when severe, bradycardia may occur with all of the CEI preparations. A feared potential complication of excessive CEI use is skeletal muscle weakness (cholinergic weak-ness). Patients receiving parenteral CEI are at the greatest risk to have cholinergic weakness. It is uncommon for patients receiving oral CEI to develop significant cholinergic weakness even while experiencing muscarinic cholinergic side effects.

Pyridostigmine (Mestinon) is the most widely used CEI for long-term oral therapy. Onset of effect is within 15–30 minutes of an oral dose, with peak effect within 1–2 hours, and wearing off gradually at 3–4 hours post-dose. The starting dose is 30–60 mg three to four times per day depending on symptoms. Optimal benefit usually occurs with a dose of 60 mg every 4 hours. Muscarinic cholinergic side effects are common with larger doses. Occasional patients require and tolerate over 1000 mg per day, dosing as frequently as every 2–3 hours. Patients with significant bulbar weakness will often time their dose about 1 hour before meals in order to maximize chewing and swallowing. Of all the CEI preparations, pyridostigmine has the least muscarinic side effects. Pyridostigmine may be used in a number of alternative forms to the 60 mg tablet. The syrup may be necessary for children or for patients with difficulty swallowing pills. Sustained release pyridostigmine 180 mg (Mestinon timespan) is sometimes preferred for nighttime use. Unpredictable release and absorption limit its use. Patients with severe dysphagia or those undergoing surgical procedures may need parenteral CEI. Intravenous pyridostigmine should be given at about 1/30 of the oral dose. Neostigmine (prostigmine) has a slightly shorter duration of action and slightly greater muscarinic side effects.

For patients with intolerable muscarinic side effects at CEI doses required for optimal power, a concomitant anticholinergic drug such as atropine sulfate (0.4–0.5 mg p.o.) or glycopyrrolate (Robinul) (I-2 mg po) on an as needed basis or with each dose of CEI may be helpful. Patients with mild disease can often be managed adequately with CEIs. However, patients with moderate, severe, or progressive disease will usually require more effective therapy.

Thymectomy

The association of the thymus gland with myasthenia gravis was first noted around 1900, and thymectomy has been standard therapy for over 50 years. All patients with suspected thymoma undergo surgery. Thymectomy for patients without a thymoma has been controversial until a large randomized international multicenter controlled trial indicated clear benefit in patients having acetylcholine receptor-positive generalized non-thymoma MG [90].

The MGTX Clinical Trial randomized 126 AChR-positive patients to trans-sternal thymectomy plus prednisone or prednisone alone. Patients had a Myasthenia Gravis Foundation of America (MGFA) Class II–IV clinical involvement. Follow-up was 3 years. Patients in both groups received oral prednisone titrated up to 100 mg alternate day until acquiring a clinical status of minimal manifestations. Patients randomized to thymectomy had significant improvement in MG symptoms, and lower dose of prednisone was needed to maintain optimal clinical status.

An American Academy of Neurology Practice Advisory: Thymectomy for Myasthenia Gravis (Practice Parameter Update) guidelines listed two level B recommendations:

1. "Clinicians should discuss thymectomy with patients who have AChR ab+ generalized MG and are 18−65 years of age. The discussion should clearly indicate the anticipated benefits and risks of the procedures and uncertainties surrounding the magnitude of these benefits and risks"
2. Clinicians should counsel patients with AChR ab+ generalized MG considering minimally invasive thymectomy techniques that it is uncertain whether the benefit attained by extended transsternal thymectomy will also be attained by minimally invasive approaches [91].

The international consensus guidance for management of myasthenia gravis also provides consensus opinion regarding other clinically relevant questions with respect to thymectomy. "Thymectomy may be considered in patients with generalized MG without detectable AChR antibodies if they fail to respond adequately to IS therapy, or to avoid/minimize intolerable adverse effects from IS therapy." "Current evidence does not support an indication for thymectomy in patients with MuSK, LRP4, or agrin antibodies" [92].

Alternative Immunosuppressive Drug Therapy

Steroid-sparing immunosuppressive medication is often required for patients who have contraindication to steroids or who experience relapse in symptoms when tapering steroids. Historically azathioprine, mycophenolate mofetil, and cyclosporine have been used as steroid-sparing agents. However, cyclosporine is the only medication with double-blinded controlled studies that demonstrated improvement in strength and symptoms [93]. Trials with mycophenolate mofetil failed to show improvement in 3 months; however it is suggested that it may take 6–12 months to demonstrate improvement and a 3-month study is too short [94–95].

Complement Inhibitors

Complement inhibitors are a new class of drugs used in AChR MG. Eculizumab is the first complement inhibitor approved for MG. It binds to human terminal complement protein C5 and inhibits enzymatic cleavage of C5 to C5a and C5b, preventing C5a-induced attraction of proinflammatory cells and related lysis of the postsynaptic membrane. The REGAIN study demonstrated clinical benefit in the treatment of myasthenia gravis [96]. Eculizumab was well-tolerated and associated with improvement in quality of life, muscle power, and activities of daily living. The meningococcal vaccination is recommended prior to the first infusion to limit the risk of meningococcal meningitis. MuSK MG is not believed to involve complement; therefore complement inhibitors would not be indicated in Musk + patients.

Rituximab

Rituximab has been reported to be effective in treating MG in selected patients. The anecdotal reports tend to involve relatively refractory patients who have done poorly with alternative treatment options. The rituximab benefits in

MuSK patients are particularly notable given the disproportionate tendency for such patients to be refractory to many other immunosuppressive agents.

Drugs to Avoid

Avoid using d-penicillamine, alfa-interferon, chloroquine, quinine, quinidine, procainamide, and botulinum toxin. Aminoglycoside antibiotics should be avoided unless needed for a life-threatening infection. Fluoroquinolones (ciprofloxacin) and erythromycin have significant neuromuscular-blocking effects. Telithromycin (Ketek), a ketolide antibiotic, has been reported to cause life-threatening weakness in patients with MG and should not be used. Neuromuscular-blocking drugs, such as pancuronium and D-tubocurarine, can produce marked and prolonged paralysis in MG patients. Depolarizing drugs, such as succinylcholine, can also have a prolonged effect and should be used by a skilled anesthesiologist who is well aware of the patient's MG. Recent reports suggest that in some patients statin drugs may aggravate MG [97].

Miscellaneous Myasthenia Issues

Transient neonatal myasthenia occurs in 10–15% of babies born to mothers with autoimmune MG. Within the first few days after delivery, the baby has a weak cry or suck, appears floppy, and, on occasion, requires mechanical ventilation. The condition is caused by maternal antibodies that cross the placenta late in pregnancy. As these maternal antibodies are replaced by the baby's own antibodies, the symptoms gradually disappear, usually within a few weeks, and the baby is normal thereafter. Infants with severe weakness are treated with oral pyridostigmine 1–2 mg/kg every 4 hours.

Congenital myasthenia represents a group of rare hereditary disorders of the neuromuscular junction. Patients tend to have life-long relatively stable symptoms of generalized fatigable weakness. These disorders are non-immunologic, without acetylcholine receptor antibodies, and, therefore, patients do not respond to immune therapy (steroids, thymectomy, and plasma exchange). Most of these patients improve on cholinesterase inhibitors. While there are many established subtypes of congenital myasthenia, several are worth noting due in part to specific therapeutic implications. The fast channel congenital myasthenic syndrome tends to be static or slowly progressive but usually very responsive to combination therapy with 3,4-diaminopyridine (enhances release of acetylcholine) and pyridostigmine (reduces metabolism of acetylcholine). In congenital slow channel myasthenic syndrome, the disease typically worsens over the years as the endplate myopathy progresses. Although cholinesterase inhibitors typically worsen symptoms, quinidine and fluoxetine, which reduce the duration of acetylcholine receptor channel openings, are both effective treatments for slow channel syndrome. The congenital myasthenic syndrome associated with acetylcholine receptor deficiency tends to be relatively nonprogressive and may even improve slightly as the patient ages. The disorder typically responds to symptomatic therapy with pyridostigmine and/or 3,4-diaminopyridine. Ephedrine produces benefit in some cases. Patients with congenital endplate acetylcholinesterase deficiency usually present in infancy or early childhood with generalized weakness, underdevelopment of muscles, slowed pupillary responses to light, and either no response or worsening with cholinesterase inhibitors. No effective long treatment has been described for congenital endplate acetylcholinesterase deficiency.

Lambert-Eaton Syndrome

Lambert-Eaton syndrome (LES) (the myasthenic syndrome) is a presynaptic disease characterized by chronic fluctuating weakness of proximal limb muscles. Symptoms include difficulty walking, climbing stairs, or rising from a chair (Table 16.7). In LES there may be some improvement in power with sustained or repeated exercise. In contrast, the myasthenia gravis ptosis, diplopia, dysphagia, and respiratory failure are far less common but can occur. In addition, LES patients often complain of myalgias, muscle stiffness of the back and legs, distal paresthesias,

Table 16.7 Lambert-Eaton syndrome (LES) symptoms

Proximal limb weakness
Legs > arms
Fatigue or fluctuating symptoms
Difficulty rising from a sitting position, climbing stairs
Metallic taste in mouth
Autonomic dysfunction
Dry mouth
Constipation
Blurred vision
Impaired sweating
Signs
Proximal limb weakness
Legs > arms
Weakness on exam is less compared to patient's level of disability
Hypoactive or absent muscle stretch reflexes
Lambert's sign (grip becomes more powerful over several seconds)

metallic taste, dry mouth, impotence, and other autonomic symptoms of muscarinic cholinergic insufficiency. Lambert-Eaton syndrome is rare compared to myasthenia gravis, which is about 100 times more common. About half of LES patients have an underlying malignancy, which is usually small cell carcinoma of the lung. In patients without malignancy, LES is an autoimmune disease and can be associated with other autoimmune phenomena. In general, patients with Lambert-Eaton syndrome over age of 40 are more likely to be men and have an associated malignancy, whereas younger patients are more likely to be women and have no malignancy. Lambert-Eaton syndrome symptoms can precede detection of the malignancy by 1–2 years.

The examination of a LES patient typically shows proximal lower extremity weakness, although the objective bedside assessment may suggest relatively mild weakness relative to the patient's history. The muscle stretch reflexes are absent. On testing sustained maximal grip, there can be a gradual increase in power over the initial 2–3 seconds (Lambert's sign).

The diagnosis is confirmed with EMG studies, which typically show low amplitude of the compound muscle action potentials and a decrement to slow rates or repetitive stimulation. Following brief exercise, there is marked facilitation of the CMAP amplitude. At high rates of repetitive stimulation, there may be an incremental response. Single-fiber EMG is markedly abnormal in virtually all patients with LES. The pathogenesis involves auto-antibodies directed against voltage-gated calcium channels at cholinergic nerve terminals. These IgG antibodies also inhibit cholinergic synapses of the autonomic nervous system. Antibodies to voltage-gated calcium channels are present in serum in over 75% of LES patients, providing another important diagnostic test.

In patients with associated malignancy, successful treatment of the tumor can lead to improvement in the LES symptoms. Symptomatic improvement in neuromuscular transmission may occur with the use of cholinesterase inhibitors, such as pyridostigmine. Guanidine has shown some benefit, but its use has been limited by bone marrow, renal, and hepatic toxicity. Guanidine increases the release of ACh by increasing the duration of the action potential at the motor nerve terminal. 3,4-Diaminopyridine (DAP) increases ACh release by blocking voltage-dependent potassium conductance and thereby prolonging depolarization at the nerve terminal and enhancing the voltage-dependent calcium influx. 3,4-DAP has been shown to clearly improve symptoms in most patients with LES with relatively mild toxicity and is becoming increasingly available, such that it represents first-line symptomatic therapy for LES. The typical beginning dose is 10 mg every 4–6 hours with gradual increase as needed up to a maximum of 80–100 mg per day. Immunosuppressive therapy is used in patients with disabling symptoms. Long-term high-dose corticosteroids, plasma exchange, and IVIg have all been used with moderate success. In general, the use of these therapies should be tailored to the severity of patient's symptoms.

Amyotrophic Lateral Sclerosis

As most ALS patients die from complications of respiratory failure, the clinician should anticipate the signs and symptoms of hypoventilation. Whether the goal is prolonged survival or maximal comfort or both, the management of respira-

tory failure in the ALS patient should be a high priority. Often the earliest signs of respiratory weakness are those associated with disturbed sleep. Daytime spirometry and blood gases may appear stable, and yet at night the patient may experience severe hypoventilation. In general, the pCO_2 will not begin to rise until the forced vital capacity falls below 50% of predicted. As respiratory function deteriorates, the patient develops CO_2 retention from hypoventilation, and the serum bicarbonate levels become elevated as compensation for the respiratory acidosis. Significant hypercapnia typically develops when the forced vital capacity is <30% of predicted, at which time the patient is at major risk for acute respiratory decompensation. As the forced vital capacity falls to 50–60%, the ALS patient begins to develop symptoms of hypoventilation, and the use of NPPV will improve symptoms (quality of life). Early initiation of NPPV has been associated with improved survival; therefore multiple measures along with patients symptoms should be considered when deciding to initiate NPPV [98].

Botulism

Consumption of sausage spoiled by *Clostridium botulinum* resulted in an outbreak of a paralytic illness in the 1700s in Germany, leading to the name botulism, derived from the Latin term for sausage, "botulus." Botulinum toxin blocks ACh release at the presynaptic motor nerve terminal and causes dysautonomia by blocking muscarinic autonomic cholinergic function as well. The intracellular target of botulinum toxin appears to be a protein of the ACh vesicle membrane. The toxin is a zinc-dependent protease that cleaves protein components of the neuroexocytosis apparatus.

Classic Botulism
Classic botulism occurs after ingestion of food contaminated by botulinum toxin. Eight different toxins have been identified, but disease in humans is caused by A, B, and E. Type E is associated with contaminated seafood. All types produce a

similar clinical picture, although type A may produce more severe and enduring symptoms. In all three types, the condition is potentially fatal. Most cases result from ingestion of bottled or canned foods that have not been properly sterilized during preparation, especially "home-canned foods." Today's tomatoes used in home canning may have a lower acid content as compared to the "good old days" and therefore may be more vulnerable for contamination. Foods cooked on an outdoor grill and then wrapped in foil for a day or two, creating an anaerobic environment, can lead to toxin production. Home-bottled oils and honey may be contaminated.

Clinical Features

Clinical features begin 12–48 hours after ingestion of tainted food. Bulbar symptoms including diplopia, ptosis, blurred vision, dysarthria, and dysphagia occur initially and are followed by weakness in the upper limbs and then in the lower limbs. In contrast to the typical patient with Guillain-Barré syndrome, botulism is sometimes said to produce an acute "descending paralysis." Severe cases result in respiratory failure requiring mechanical ventilation. Botulism produces autonomic dysfunction, including constipation, ileus, dry mouth, and dilated pupils (note: some of these signs are seen in most but not all patients; normal pupils do not "rule out" the diagnosis of botulism).

Diagnosis

The compound motor action potential (CMAP) amplitudes are typically low on the motor nerve conduction studies (NCS). Repetitive stimulation studies before and following exercise may show a decrement to low rates of repetitive stimulation and post-exercise facilitation of the CMAP amplitude. Send both stool and serum specimens to the lab for detection of the toxin. The specimen is injected into the peritoneum of a mouse, while a neutralized or inactivated specimen is injected as the control. If the mouse becomes paralyzed and dies, the diagnosis is botulism. Toxin is found in blood samples 30–40% of the time, while stool samples have a somewhat higher yield (thus the

need to send both). Newer PCR tests for the organism have been used to screen for the bacteria in food.

Management

Management involves placement of the patient in the intensive care unit and assiduous monitoring of pulmonary function every few hours. When the FVC falls below 15 ml/kg or below 1 liter, or if the patient appears to be having respiratory difficulty, intubation and mechanical ventilation are necessary. There is a trivalent botulinum antitoxin, but its use is controversial, in part because of adverse side effects that occur in about 20% of patients. There is some evidence that the antitoxin shortens the course of the illness, especially that associated with type E. If the diagnosis is made early, it is reasonable to treat with antitoxin.

Clinical Course

With aggressive support, the overall mortality remains about 5–10%, usually the result of respiratory or septic complications. Improvement occurs over a period of several weeks to several months. In those who survive, the eventual level of recovery is usually near complete. Several years after the illness, some patients have subjective fatigue and autonomic symptoms, including constipation, impotence, and dry mouth. Clinical recovery results from brisk sprouting of new motor axons from the nerve terminal with reinnervation of denervated muscle fibers.

Infant Botulism

Infant botulism is probably the most frequent form of botulism. The infant ingests the spores of *Clostridium botulinum*, which lodge in the intestinal tract, germinate there, and produce botulinum toxin in the gut. Honey has often been implicated as the contaminated food in infant disease. In adults, the small amount of *C. botulinum* in honey appears inadequate to colonize the GI tract. The typical presentation is an infant between the ages of 6 weeks and 6 months who exhibits generalized weakness and constipation. The weakness may start in the cranial muscles and then descend, causing a weak suck, a poor cry, and reduced spontaneous movement. The cranial muscles are weak, with poor extraocular movements, reduced gag reflex, and drooling. Finding *C. botulinum* in feces validates the diagnosis. The toxin is usually not detectable in the serum. EMG studies are helpful in the diagnosis in 80–90% of cases. Infantile botulism can range from mild to severe. Management centers on observation and general support (including respiratory stability). The recovery is usually excellent and runs a course of several weeks to several months.

Wound Botulism

Wound botulism occurs when toxin is produced from *C. botulinum* infection of a wound. The symptoms are similar to those of classic botulism except that the onset may be delayed for up to 2 weeks after contamination of the wound. The diagnosis is supported by EMG studies, demonstration of toxin in the patient's blood or finding the organism in the patient's wound. Wounds at risk for botulism include direct trauma, surgical wounds, and wounds associated with drug use (such as intravenous and intranasal cocaine).

Hypokalemic Periodic Paralysis

Hypokalemic periodic paralysis should be considered in the differential diagnosis of patients presenting with acute quadriparesis. The majority of such patients do not experience significant respiratory failure (Table 16.8).

Thyrotoxic Periodic Paralysis (TPP)

Screen every patient with hypokalemic periodic paralysis for hyperthyroidism. TPP is more common in Asians. Even though hyperthyroidism is more common in women than men, TPP is 70 times more common in men than women. Often, they do not have the typical systemic features of hyperthyroidism (they look clinically euthyroid). The disorder is usually sporadic (there is no family history), and the attacks stop when the patient becomes euthyroid.

Table 16.8 Hypokalemic periodic paralysis

"Primary" – hereditary (autosomal dominant)
Genetic defect on chromosome 1 gene code for the dihydropyridine receptor
Presents in teenage years or in 20s
Upon awakening the patient is weak (can be mild or quadriplegia)
Limbs are hypotonic
Muscle stretch reflexes are absent
Cranial and respiratory muscles are usually spared
Serum potassium is low during the attack
Recovery occurs gradually over several hours
Precipitating factors include physical or emotional stress, high carbohydrate load
Most patients recover completely from an acute attack of paralysis, but some patients acquire mild fixed proximal weakness after many years of attacks
Preferred treatment of the hypokalemia 0.25 mEq/kg potassium chloride by mouth – in an unsweetened 10–25% solution – may be repeated every 30 minutes until strength returns
Forms of secondary hypokalemic periodic paralysis
Urinary or gastrointestinal loss of potassium
Primary hyperaldosteronism
Thiazide diuretic therapy
Excessive mineralocorticoid therapy for Addison's disease
Laxative abuse
Prolonged GI suction
Prolonged vomiting
Sprue
Villous adenoma of the rectum

Tick Paralysis

Clinical Features

Tick paralysis is one of the eight most common tick-mediated diseases. While it can affect a variety of species and any age group, it is most often reported in children. Usually the tick bite occurs 5–7 days before the onset of symptoms. The female tick then feeds and becomes engorged (such engorgement is facilitated by mating with the male tick), eggs become fertilized, and the female tick produces a neurotoxin – often referred to as ixobotoxin. The natural course of the tick encounter is that engorgement of the female tick reaches an end point at which point the female tick releases and eventually deposits its eggs. Children tend to present with a day or two of progressive paresthesias and leg weakness with a tendency to fall. Usually, there is no fever. Over the next day or two, the weakness tends to ascend and involve axial as well as limb muscles. There is truncal instability. The patient has difficulty with sitting, cannot walk, and becomes areflexic. As the disease progresses over the next day or two, the patient may develop bulbar weakness and involvement of respiratory muscles. Some patients appear encephalopathic. The initial erroneous diagnosis is often Guillain-Barré syndrome.

Diagnostic Studies

One of the best diagnostic tests in the literature is an electroencephalogram, in that an astute EEG technician may first spot the tick in the scalp while placing the electrodes. The nerve conduction studies may suggest a peripheral neuropathy with prolonged distal latencies on the motor nerve conduction studies, reduced nerve conduction velocity, and some reduction in amplitude of the sensory and motor responses. Repetitive stimulation studies are often unhelpful.

Treatment

If a tick is detected and removed (and usually it is in the hair or scalp), patients typically demonstrate dramatic resolution of their weakness over hours to several days. Otherwise, treatment involves general intensive care monitoring and support.

Subtypes of Tick Paralysis

In Australia the *Ixodes holocyclus* tick produces a toxin which seems to act similar to botulinum toxin in impairing the release of acetylcholine at motor nerve terminals. Patients in Australia with exposure to this tick classically have a more severe and fulminant paralytic illness than those exposed to the North American ticks. In addition, over the first 1–2 days after removal of the tick, clinical symptoms often become more pronounced, and the clinical recovery tends to be slower. In Australia it is generally recommended that *Ixodes holocyclus* antitoxin be given to the patient prior to removing the tick and that patients be monitored for an extended period of time following tick removal.

In North America *Dermacentor* sp. ticks (*Dermacentor andersoni*, the North American wood tick) and *Dermacentor variabilis* (the common dog tick) are those that of concern for causing paralysis in adults, even though many other tick species can cause tick paralysis in animals. The *Dermacentor* sp. ticks are fairly easy to spot when they are engorged. Tick paralysis is somewhat more common in the spring and summer in the southeast and northwestern United States.

Conclusion

Neuromuscular disorders can present with acute respiratory failure either as the presenting symptom or as a complication of the known neuromuscular disorder [99]. However, patients with neuromuscular disorders can also present with other common causes of acute respiratory distress, e.g., pulmonary embolism. Therefore, an accurate diagnosis of respiratory failure is extremely important in initiating treatment. The method of ventilation should be determined based on the severity of respiratory insufficiency or failure, type of neuromuscular disease, and patient's wishes. The decision to intubate should be done early before acute respiratory arrest, mental status changes, or cardiac abnormalities develop. Patients who do not acutely need intubation should be monitored extremely vigilantly. Diagnosis of the neuromuscular disorder itself is not only valuable in initiating appropriate treatment but for prognosis as well. In patients with known neuromuscular disorders, preventive measures, such as nocturnal NPPV and cough augmentation, should be offered. Lastly, discussions on long-term ventilation wishes need to occur in all patients with known progressive neurological disorders prior to acute respiratory failure.

References

1. Rabinstein AA. Update on respiratory management of critically ill neurologic patients. Curr Neurol Neurosci Rep. 2005;5(6):476–82.

2. Orlikowski D, et al. Respiratory dysfunction in Guillain-Barre Syndrome. Neurocrit Care. 2004;1(4):415–22.
3. Fletcher DD, et al. Long-term outcome in patients with Guillain-Barre syndrome requiring mechanical ventilation. Neurology. 2000;54(12):2311–5.
4. Alshekhlee A, et al. Incidence and mortality rates of myasthenia gravis and myasthenic crisis in US hospitals. Neurology. 2009;72(18):1548–54.
5. Nogues MA, Benarroch E. Abnormalities of respiratory control and the respiratory motor unit. Neurologist. 2008;14(5):273–88.
6. Putnam RW, Filosa JA, Ritucci NA. Cellular mechanisms involved in CO(2) and acid signaling in chemosensitive neurons. Am J Physiol Cell Physiol. 2004;287(6):C1493–526.
7. Richter DW, Spyer KM. Studying rhythmogenesis of breathing: comparison of in vivo and in vitro models. Trends Neurosci. 2001;24(8):464–72.
8. Gray PA, et al. Normal breathing requires preBotzinger complex neurokinin-1 receptor-expressing neurons. Nat Neurosci. 2001;4(9):927–30.
9. Panitch HB. The pathophysiology of respiratory impairment in pediatric neuromuscular diseases. Pediatrics. 2009;123 Suppl 4:S215–8.
10. Rabinstein AA, Wijdicks EF. Warning signs of imminent respiratory failure in neurological patients. Semin Neurol. 2003;23(1):97–104.
11. Hutchinson D, Whyte K. Neuromuscular disease and respiratory failure. Pract Neurol. 2008,8(4).229–37.
12. Mehta S. Neuromuscular disease causing acute respiratory failure. Respir Care. 2006;51(9):1016–21; discussion 1021–3.
13. Bach JR, Bianchi C. Prevention of pectus excavatum for children with spinal muscular atrophy type 1. Am J Phys Med Rehabil. 2003;82(10):815–9.
14. Estenne M, De Troyer A. The effects of tetraplegia on chest wall statics. Am Rev Respir Dis. 1986;134(1):121–4.
15. Estenne M, et al. Chest wall stiffness in patients with chronic respiratory muscle weakness. Am Rev Respir Dis. 1983;128(6):1002–7.
16. Roussos CS, Macklem PT. Diaphragmatic fatigue in man. J Appl Physiol. 1977;43(2):189–97.
17. Bellemare F, Grassino A. Effect of pressure and timing of contraction on human diaphragm fatigue. J Appl Physiol. 1982;53(5):1190–5.
18. Zocchi L, et al. Effect of pressure and timing of contraction on human rib cage muscle fatigue. Am Rev Respir Dis. 1993;147(4):857–64.
19. Perrin C, et al. Pulmonary complications of chronic neuromuscular diseases and their management. Muscle Nerve. 2004;29(1):5–27.
20. Begin R, et al. Control of breathing in Duchenne's muscular dystrophy. Am J Med. 1980;69(2):227–34.
21. Alves RS, et al. Sleep and neuromuscular disorders in children. Sleep Med Rev. 2009;13(2):133–48.
22. Steljes DG, et al. Sleep in postpolio syndrome. Chest. 1990;98(1):133–40.
23. Schroth MK. Special considerations in the respiratory management of spinal muscular atrophy. Pediatrics. 2009;123 Suppl 4:S245–9.
24. Vilke GM, et al. Spirometry in normal subjects in sitting, prone, and supine positions. Respir Care. 2000;45(4):407–10.
25. Bach JR. Amyotrophic lateral sclerosis: predictors for prolongation of life by noninvasive respiratory aids. Arch Phys Med Rehabil. 1995;76(9):828–32.
26. Tzeng AC, Bach JR. Prevention of pulmonary morbidity for patients with neuromuscular disease. Chest. 2000;118(5):1390–6.
27. Bach JR, Saporito LR. Criteria for extubation and tracheostomy tube removal for patients with ventilatory failure. A different approach to weaning. Chest. 1996;110(6):1566–71.
28. Winkel LP, et al. The natural course of non-classic Pompe's disease; a review of 225 published cases. J Neurol. 2005;252(8):875–84.
29. Shahrizaila N, Kinnear WJ, Wills AJ. Respiratory involvement in inherited primary muscle conditions. J Neurol Neurosurg Psychiatry. 2006;77(10):1108–15.
30. Rowe PW, et al. Multicore myopathy: respiratory failure and paraspinal muscle contractures are important complications. Dev Med Child Neurol. 2000;42(5):340–3.
31. Whitaker J, et al. Idiopathic adult-onset nemaline myopathy presenting with isolated respiratory failure. Muscle Nerve. 2009;39(3):406–8.
32. Dwyer BA, Mayer RF, Lee SC. Progressive nemaline (rod) myopathy as a presentation of human immunodeficiency virus infection. Arch Neurol. 1992;49(5):440.
33. Chahin N, Selcen D, Engel AG. Sporadic late onset nemaline myopathy. Neurology. 2005;65(8):1158–64.
34. Keller CE, et al. Adult-onset nemaline myopathy and monoclonal gammopathy. Arch Neurol. 2006;63(1):132–4.
35. Reyes MG, et al. Nemaline myopathy in an adult with primary hypothyroidism. Can J Neurol Sci. 1986;13(2):117–9.
36. Haq RU, et al. Respiratory muscle involvement in Bethlem myopathy. Neurology. 1999;52(1):174–6.
37. Cros D, et al. Respiratory failure revealing mitochondrial myopathy in adults. Chest. 1992;101(3):824–8.
38. Voermans NC, et al. Primary respiratory failure in inclusion body myositis. Neurology. 2004;63(11):2191–2.
39. Cohen R, Lipper S, Dantzker DR. Inclusion body myositis as a cause of respiratory failure. Chest. 1993;104(3):975–7.
40. Littleton ET, et al. Human T cell leukaemia virus type I associated neuromuscular disease causing respiratory failure. J Neurol Neurosurg Psychiatry. 2002;72(5):650–2.
41. Kuncl RW, George EB. Toxic neuropathies and myopathies. Curr Opin Neurol. 1993;6(5):695–704.
42. Kuncl RW, Wiggins WW. Toxic myopathies. Neurol Clin. 1988;6(3):593–619.

43. Bella I, Chad DA. Neuromuscular disorders and acute respiratory failure. Neurol Clin. 1998;16(2):391–417.
44. Ober KP. Thyrotoxic periodic paralysis in the United States. Report of 7 cases and review of the literature. Medicine (Baltimore). 1992;71(3):109–20.
45. Compton SJ, et al. Trichinosis with ventilatory failure and persistent myocarditis. Clin Infect Dis. 1993;16(4):500–4.
46. De Jonghe B, et al. Critical illness neuromuscular syndromes. Neurol Clin. 2008;26(2):507–20, ix.
47. Evoli A, et al. Clinical correlates with anti-MuSK antibodies in generalized seronegative myasthenia gravis. Brain. 2003;126(Pt 10):2304–11.
48. Besser R, et al. End-plate dysfunction in acute organophosphate intoxication. Neurology. 1989;39(4):561–7.
49. Schelling JR. Fatal hypermagnesemia. Clin Nephrol. 2000;53(1):61–5.
50. Asselbergs FW, et al. Acute intermittent porphyria as a cause of respiratory failure: case report. Am J Crit Care. 2009;18(2):180. 178-9
51. Rubin DI. Neuralgic amyotrophy: clinical features and diagnostic evaluation. Neurologist. 2001;7(6):350–6.
52. Kissel JT, Mendell JR. Vasculitic neuropathy. Neurol Clin. 1992;10(3):761–81.
53. Mokhlesi B, Jain M. Pulmonary manifestations of POEMS syndrome: case report and literature review. Chest. 1999;115(6):1740–2.
54. Boonyapisit K, Katirji B. Multifocal motor neuropathy presenting with respiratory failure. Muscle Nerve. 2000;23(12):1887–90.
55. Vahidnia A, van der Voet GB, de Wolff FA. Arsenic neurotoxicity–a review. Hum Exp Toxicol. 2007;26(10):823–32.
56. Logina I, Donaghy M. Diphtheritic polyneuropathy: a clinical study and comparison with Guillain-Barre syndrome. J Neurol Neurosurg Psychiatry. 1999;67(4):433–8.
57. Thorsteinsson G. Management of postpolio syndrome. Mayo Clin Proc. 1997;72(7):627–38.
58. Berg RA, Tarantino MD. Envenomation by the scorpion Centruroides exilicauda (C sculpturatus): severe and unusual manifestations. Pediatrics. 1991;87(6):930–3.
59. Boyer LV, et al. Antivenom for critically ill children with neurotoxicity from scorpion stings. N Engl J Med. 2009;360(20):2090–8.
60. Li Z, Turner RP. Pediatric tick paralysis: discussion of two cases and literature review. Pediatr Neurol. 2004;31(4):304–7.
61. Friedman MA, et al. Ciguatera fish poisoning: treatment, prevention and management. Mar Drugs. 2008;6(3):456–79.
62. Ropper AH, Kehne SM. Guillain-Barre syndrome: management of respiratory failure. Neurology. 1985;35(11):1662–5.
63. Sharshar T, et al. Early predictors of mechanical ventilation in Guillain-Barre syndrome. Crit Care Med. 2003;31(1):278–83.
64. Lawn ND, et al. Anticipating mechanical ventilation in Guillain-Barre syndrome. Arch Neurol. 2001;58(6):893–8.
65. Rieder P, et al. The repeated measurement of vital capacity is a poor predictor of the need for mechanical ventilation in myasthenia gravis. Intensive Care Med. 1995;21(8):663–8.
66. Birnkrant DJ. The American College of Chest Physicians consensus statement on the respiratory and related management of patients with Duchenne muscular dystrophy undergoing anesthesia or sedation. Pediatrics. 2009;123 Suppl 4:S242–4.
67. Larsen UT, et al. Complications during anaesthesia in patients with Duchenne's muscular dystrophy (a retrospective study). Can J Anaesth. 1989;36(4):418–22.
68. Luo F, Annane D, Orlikowski D, He L, Yang M, Zhou M, Liu GJ. Invasive versus non-invasive ventilation for acute respiratory failure in neuromuscular disease and chest wall disorders. Cochrane Database Syst Rev. 2017;12:CD008380.
69. Vianello A, et al. Non-invasive ventilatory approach to treatment of acute respiratory failure in neuromuscular disorders. A comparison with endotracheal intubation. Intensive Care Med. 2000;26(4):384–90.
70. Moss AH, et al. Patients with amyotrophic lateral sclerosis receiving long-term mechanical ventilation. Advance care planning and outcomes. Chest. 1996;110(1):249–55.
71. Rabinstein A, Wijdicks EF. BiPAP in acute respiratory failure due to myasthenic crisis may prevent intubation. Neurology. 2002;59(10):1647–9.
72. Boitano LJ. Equipment options for cough augmentation, ventilation, and noninvasive interfaces in neuromuscular respiratory management. Pediatrics. 2009;123 Suppl 4:S226–30.
73. Finder JD. A 2009 perspective on the 2004 American Thoracic Society statement, "respiratory care of the patient with Duchenne muscular dystrophy". Pediatrics. 2009;123 Suppl 4:S239–41.
74. Bourke SC, et al. Noninvasive ventilation in ALS: indications and effect on quality of life. Neurology. 2003;61(2):171–7.
75. Lechtzin N, et al. Early use of non-invasive ventilation prolongs survival in subjects with ALS. Amyotroph Lateral Scler. 2007;8(3):185–8.
76. Bach JR, Campagnolo DI, Hoeman S. Life satisfaction of individuals with Duchenne muscular dystrophy using long-term mechanical ventilatory support. Am J Phys Med Rehabil. 1991;70(3):129–35.
77. Simonds AK, et al. Impact of nasal ventilation on survival in hypercapnic Duchenne muscular dystrophy. Thorax. 1998;53(11):949–52.
78. Schonhofer B, et al. Daytime mechanical ventilation in chronic respiratory insufficiency. Eur Respir J. 1997;10(12):2840–6.
79. Piper AJ, Sullivan CE. Effects of long-term nocturnal nasal ventilation on spontaneous breathing during sleep in neuromuscular and chest wall disorders. Eur Respir J. 1996;9(7):1515–22.

80. Mehta S, Hill NS. Noninvasive ventilation. Am J Respir Crit Care Med. 2001;163(2):540–77.
81. Perez A, et al. Thoracoabdominal pattern of breathing in neuromuscular disorders. Chest. 1996;110(2):454–61.
82. Bach JR, Ishikawa Y, Kim H. Prevention of pulmonary morbidity for patients with Duchenne muscular dystrophy. Chest. 1997;112(4):1024–8.
83. Winkel, et al. Enzyme replacement therapy in late-onset Pompe's disease a three year follow-up. Ann Neurol. 2004;55:495–502.
84. Kishnani PS, et al. Recombinant human acid [alpha]-glucosidase: major clinical benefits in infantile-onset Pompe disease. Neurology. 2007;68:99–109.
85. van der Ploeg AT, et al. A randomized study of alglucosidase alfa in late-onset Pompe's disease. N Engl J Med. 2010;362:1396–406.
86. Van Capelle CI, van der Beek NAME, Hagemans MLC, et al. Effect of enzyme therapy in juvenile patients with Pompe disease: a three-year open-label study. Neuromuscul Disord. 2010;20:775–82.
87. Bacchi S, Kramer P, Chalk C. Autoantibodies to low-density lipoprotein receptor-related protein 4 in double seronegative myasthenia gravis: a systematic review. Can J Neurol Sci. 2018;45:62–7.
88. Thomas CE, Mayer SA, Gungor Y, Swarup R, Webster EA, Chang I, Brannagan TH, Fink ME, Rowland LP. Myasthenic crisis: clinical features, mortality, complications, and risk factors for prolonged intubation. Neurology. 1997;48:1253–60.
89. Zinman L, Ng E, Bril V. IV immunoglobulin in patients with myasthenia gravis: a randomized controlled trial. Neurology. 2007;68(11):837–41.
90. Wolfe GI, Kaminski HJ, Aban IB, Minisman G, Kuo HC, Marx A, Strobel P, Mazia C, Oger J, Cea JG, et al. Randomized trial of thymectomy in myasthenia gravis. N Engl J Med. 2016;375:511–22.
91. Gronseth GS, Barohn R, Narayanaswami P. Practice advisory: thymectomy for myasthenia gravis (practice parameter update): report of the guideline development, dissemination, and implementation subcommittee of the American Academy of Neurology. Neurology. 2020;94:705–9.
92. Sanders DB, Wolfe GI, Benatar M, Evoli A, Gilhus NE, Illa I, Kuntz N, Massey JM, Melms A, Murai H, et al. International consensus guidance for management of myasthenia gravis: executive summary. Neurology. 2016;87:419–25.
93. Tindall RS, Phillips JT, Rollins A, Wells L, Hall K. A clinical therapeutic trial of cyclosporine in myasthenia gravis. Ann N Y Acad Sci. 1993;681:539–51.
94. Sanders DB, Hart IK, Richman DP, et al. An international, phase III, randomized trial of mycophenolate mofetil in myasthenia gravis. Neurology. 2008;71:400–6.
95. Cahoon WD Jr, Kockler DR. Mycophenolate mofetil treatment of myasthenia gravis. Ann Pharmacother. 2006;40:295–8.
96. Howard JF Jr, Utsugisawa K, Benatar M, Murai H, Barohn RJ, Illa I, Jacob S, Vissing J, Burns TM, Kissel JT, et al. Safety and efficacy of eculizumab in anti-acetylcholine receptor antibody-positive refractory generalised myasthenia gravis (REGAIN): a phase 3, randomised, double-blind, placebo-controlled, multicentre study. Lancet Neurol. 2017;16:976–86.
97. WWW.myasthenia.org (the web page for the Myasthenia Gravis Foundation of America- contains an up to date review of adverse drug effects in myasthenia gravis).
98. Lechtzin N, Scott Y, Busse A, Clawson L, Kimball R, Wiener C. Early use of non-invasive ventilation prolongs survival in subjects with ALS. Amyotroph Lateral Scler. 2007;8:185–8.
99. Cabrera Serrano M, Rabinstein AA. Causes and outcomes of acute neuromuscular respiratory failure. Arch Neurol. 2010;67:1089–94.

Coma, Disorders of Consciousness, and Brain Death

17

Rohan Mathur, Clotilde Balucani, Amjad Elmashala, and Romergyko Geocadin

Introduction

Consciousness is the state of full awareness of the self and one's relationship to the environment [1]. Classical neurological thought makes a distinction between the content of consciousness and the level of consciousness. The content of consciousness includes specific modalities, such as symbolic language, or memory. The level of consciousness is the degree to which a person can maintain a waking state, termed arousal, and their awareness of the environment. It is these disorders of the level of consciousness that is the focus of this chapter.

Historically, clinicians have classified and organized disorders of the level of consciousness based on clinical findings at the bedside. Clinical syndromes include encephalopathy, minimally conscious states, unresponsive wakefulness syndrome, and coma (Table 17.1). Physicians in emergent and critical care settings are required to assess and manage patients with various disorders of consciousness, ranging from encephalopathy to coma, and to distinguish these living patients from those with brain death. The adept physician is able to use the neurological exam in conjunction with a variety of diagnostic modalities to define the specific syndrome and cause of their patient's presentation. Accurate and competent assessment of these disorders, and an understanding of the neuroanatomical and neurophysiological mechanisms underlying them, is crucial for guiding treatment plans and prognostication.

On the extreme end of the disorders of consciousness is coma. Coma is defined as a state of complete unresponsiveness to external or internal stimuli. It is characterized by a failure of arousal and consciousness: patients in coma have no spontaneous eye opening, do not arouse to sensory stimuli, have no sleep-wake cycles, and do not follow any commands. However, they do have at least one brainstem reflex preserved. In some cases, there may be preservation of complex brain-derived reflexes with inputs from the cortical and subcortical structures of the brain. Coma results from severe damage to the brainstem, thalamus, and/or both cerebral hemispheres simultaneously. Unresponsive wakefulness syndrome (UWS), previously known as the persistent vegetative state, is a syndrome where patients are awake (eyes open, or other evidence of a sleep-wake cycle such as EEG patterns) but remain otherwise unresponsive, showing only reflexive movements [2]. Minimally conscious state is a syndrome where the patient is awake but in which there is only evidence of a minimal

R. Mathur (✉) · C. Balucani · R. Geocadin
Division of Neurocritical Care, The Johns Hopkins School of Medicine, Baltimore, MD, USA
e-mail: rmathur2@jhmi.edu; cbaluca1@jhmi.edu; rgeocadi@jhmi.edu

A. Elmashala
The University of Iowa Carver College of Medicine, Iowa City, IA, USA
e-mail: amjad-elmashala@uiowa.edu

© The Author(s), under exclusive license to Springer Nature Switzerland AG 2021
K. L. Roos (ed.), *Emergency Neurology*, https://doi.org/10.1007/978-3-030-75778-6_17

Table 17.1 Level of consciousness

	Sleep-wake cycles	Episodes of awareness	Ability to track a visual stimulus;	Ability to follow commands
Disorder of consciousness				
Coma	Absent	Absent	Absent	Absent
Unresponsive Wakefulness syndrome	Present	Absent	Absent	Absent
Minimally conscious state	Present	Present but frequency can vary from rare to frequent	Present	Can vary in degree
Normal Consciousness	Present	Present	Present	Intact
Mimics of consciousness				
Locked-in state	Present	Present	Can track using vertical eye movements	Can only be detected at the bedside using vertical eye movements
Covert Consciousness	Present	Present	Absent	Can only be detected with tasked-based MRI or EEG

awareness of self or environment [3]. Recently, there has been a further subclassification of minimally conscious state based on the presence of language: MCS− and MCS+. Patients with MCS+ have at least one of the following features: command following, intelligible verbalization, or intentional communication [4]. This distinction was made to facilitate research in prognostication.

Akinetic mutism is a rare form of arousal failure, characterized by an emotionless, frequently motionless state with intact visual tracking, and occurs commonly due to lesions in the bilateral anterior cingulate gyri. Encephalopathy is characterized by failure of normal arousal, in which the level of arousal fluctuates. Patients with encephalopathy have an abnormal level of consciousness and arouse inconsistently to internal and sensory stimuli in contrast to patients in coma who arouse to neither internal nor external stimuli. Encephalopathy, like coma, results from damage to the brainstem, thalamus, or both cerebral hemispheres, but the damage is less severe. The neuroanatomical localization of arousal failure to the brainstem, thalamus, or both cerebral hemispheres is the most important principle to consider in the approach to a comatose or encephalopathic patient. Localization of the brain injury producing the arousal failure leads to efficient and timely treatment of the disease.

Mimics of Disorders of Consciousness

Great care must be taken by the clinician to distinguish true disorders of consciousness with mimics such as the locked-in syndrome and covert consciousness. The locked-in syndrome is where a patient with intact consciousness is only able to communicate with an observer through vertical eye movements or blinking. This occurs due to pontine injury that prevents motor signals from controlling any other movements in the body. Since 2005, further studies have identified syndromes of covert consciousness. These patients are conscious in that they are alert and aware but lack the ability to communicate with an observer. Evidence of their consciousness is gathered using task-based functional MRI which shows evidence of activity in specific brain regions when patients are presented with a task [5] or using resting and task-based continuous EEG which can identify patterns of activity associated with conscious states. From an ethical perspective, there is an imperative to identify these patients because there is the potential to discover and provide a possible means of reliable communication which can dramatically impact the patient's quality of life, as well as to possibly restore at least some element of the patient's autonomy and capacity for decision-making [6, 7]. Furthermore, patients with covert consciousness, as identified by EEG analysis, have a significantly better prognosis compared to those patients truly in comatose states. For instance, in a study of 104 unresponsive patients, assessed to be comatose at the bedside, 16 were detected to have brain activation by EEG after a median of 4 days after injury, and those patients had a four and a half times greater odds of achieving a state where they could function independently for 8 h on a 12-month follow-up [8]. Appropriate identification of these patients can thereby significantly change prognosis and guide decision-making by proxy decision-makers and clinicians. At the time of writing this chapter, the use of these advanced functional diagnostic tests and analysis to identify covert consciousness is not widespread and is usually done as part of research protocols at certain centers. More research is likely needed to incorporate the use of these technologies in the ICU and clinical setting.

Finally care must be taken to distinguish between brain death and coma. Brain death is not a disorder of consciousness because the person is no longer alive. Brain death is characterized by the irreversible absence of all clinical brain activity after exclusion of toxic or metabolic confounders, such as drug overdose, general anesthesia, or hypothermia. The specific criteria and variation in determining brain death are discussed in the Brain Death section of this chapter.

Anatomy and Pathophysiology of Disorders of Consciousness

As a general rule, disorders of arousal and consciousness result from significant injury to the upper brainstem, thalamus, thalamocortical projections, or bilateral cortices. The anatomy and physiology of these structures as they pertain to arousal are described below. Figure 17.1 schematically approximates these arousal systems neuroanatomically. Table 17.2 summarizes the components of each of the arousal systems.

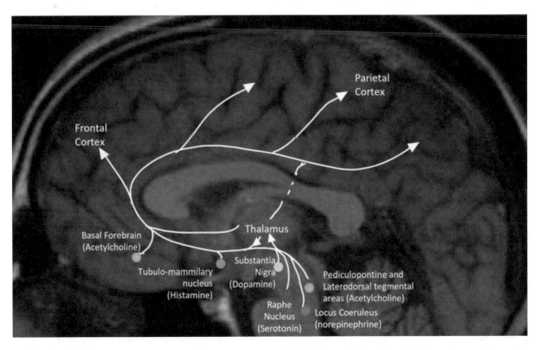

Fig. 17.1 Some of the key areas of the brain important to maintaining arousal are shown overlayed on a sagittal MRI image of the brain. Neurons from different brainstem nuclei send excitatory signals, using different neurotransmitters, to the targets in the thalamus, cortex, and subcortical white matter that ultimately lead to arousal. The arousal nuclei that are in the brainstem are in turn innervated by orexin neurons in the lateral hypothalamus for further modulation. Cholinergic neurons from the pedun-culopontine and laterodorsal tegmental area (shown in green) activate targets in the thalamus as well as the forebrain. Serotonergic neurons from the dorsal raphe nuclei (red), histaminergic neurons in the tuberomammillary nucleus (orange), dopaminergic neurons from the substantia nigra and ventral tegmental area (yellow), and adrenergic neurons from the locus coeruleus (blue) send excitatory inputs to many cortical and subcortical targets

Table 17.2 Arousal systems

Brainstem arousal systems
Reticular activating system (RAS)
Pedunculopontine tegmental and laterodorsal nuclei (PPT/LDT)
Locus coeruleus (LC)
Substantia nigra pars compacta and ventral tegmental area (SNPC-VTA)
Raphe nucleus (RN)
Thalamic arousal systems
Specific thalamocortical system
Nonspecific thalamocortical system
Basal forebrain arousal systems
Substantia innominata
Nucleus basalis of Meynert
Diagonal band of Broca
Magnocellular preoptic nucleus
Median septum
Globus pallidus
Hypothalamic arousal system
Posterior hypothalamus
Anterior hypothalamus

Arousal Systems

Arousal or vigilance is mediated by a complex interaction of cortical and subcortical networks. Cortical activation is required for arousal and awareness, but anatomic and physiological data suggest that the cortex does not contain an intrinsic mechanism for the generation and maintenance of arousal [9, 10]. As such, a number of subcortical networks participate in the generation of arousal [11]. These networks include arousal systems located in the brainstem, thalamus, basal forebrain, and hypothalamus. Signals from peripheral sensory organs, such as the eyes, ears, or skin, are detected by sentinel arousal systems within the brainstem, which in turn excite thalamocortical neurons. Sensory transmission within the thalamus also directly excites thalamocortical neurons. Thalamocortical neuron excitation promotes cortical excitation, which is supportive of arousal. The hypothalamus and basal forebrain are also important in arousal, although the precise identification of their role is still under investigation. These systems are summarized in the sections that follow.

Brainstem Arousal Systems

The brainstem arousal systems comprise the reticular activating system (RAS), the pedunculopon-tine tegmental and laterodorsal (PPT/LDT) nuclei, the locus coeruleus, the substantia nigra pars compacta, and the midline raphe nuclei. These nuclei are located in disparate anatomical sites in the brainstem, but each is optimally positioned to broadly send and receive information. Because of their anatomical positioning and broad rostral projections, these nuclei may serve as sentries for the arousal system. The RAS is the best studied of these nuclei and is representative of the structure and function of these systems. The RAS comprises neurons in core nuclei located near the cerebral aqueduct of the midbrain and near the fourth ventricle in the pons [12, 13]. These neurons are interspersed in a web-like reticulum between the ascending and descending fibers, which comprise the motor and sensory tracts as they traverse the brainstem. The RAS neurons have long dendrites that interdigitate those fibers and are thus optimally situated to integrate information from a wide variety of sources, including sensory input from visual, somatosensory, auditory, and vestibular systems, as well as sensory and motor output from the cerebral cortex, thalamus, and basal ganglia [14, 15]. Ascending arousal signals from the reticular formation to the forebrain are conveyed through two systems: the dorsal system that traverses the thalamus and transmits diffusely to the cortex through thalamocortical projections and the ventral system, which comprises the basal forebrain and hypothalamus, that acts as key relay components.

Thalamic Arousal Systems

The thalamus is crucial for achieving and maintaining arousal through its connections with the cortex. The thalamus receives and sends data to and from virtually all central nervous system structures. Functionally, thalamic nuclei have been classified into "specific" and "nonspecific" thalamocortical systems through which the thalamus projects to the cortex [16]. "Specific" thalamocortical projections convey information within the sensory, visual, auditory, or motor systems, which have precise neuroanatomical localizations within the cortex and thalamus, and include such thalamic nuclei as the medial and lateral geniculate nuclei and the group of ventral nuclei. In contrast, "nonspecific" thalamocortical projections transmit information from multiple subcortical nuclei, including the reticular nuclei, dorsal raphe, PPT/LDT nuclei, locus coeruleus, basal forebrain, and hypothalamus, to multiple cortical regions. Nonspecific thalamocortical projections originate from midline, medial, and intralaminar groups of thalamic nuclei, which are located in the central thalamus. Contrary to initial reports, these central thalamic nuclei actually have a specific neuroanatomical localization, which has drawn into question their identification as "nonspecific" [17]. Because of their connection with the cortex, each of the thalamocortical projection systems can play a role in cortical activation.

Hypothalamic and Basal Forebrain Arousal Systems

The hypothalamus plays a vital role in both arousal and sleep generation. Based on studies in cats, the posterior hypothalamus appears to be the most important hypothalamic center for arousal behaviors, whereas the anterior hypothalamus and hypothalamic–mesencephalic junction promote sleep [18]. Studies of the cellular physiology mediating the influence of the hypothalamus on arousal and vigilance are ongoing. Hypothalamic nuclei comprise many types of neurons, including histaminergic and peptidergic neurons, which produce orexins. Histaminergic neurons are found primarily in the tuberomammillary nucleus and posterior hypothalamus and can influence arousal via projections to the anterior hypothalamus, the dorsal raphe nuclei, the mesopontine tegmentum, the thalamus, the substantia innominata, and directly to the cortex [19]. Histaminergic neurons can influence the firing mode of thalamocortical neurons depending on the relative distribution and activation of distinct histamine receptors (H1R and H2R), which each has different mechanisms of postsynaptic activity [20]. Orexins (hypocretins) are neuropeptides that promote arousal; they project to almost every brain region involved in the regulation of wakefulness; and they fire most strongly during active wakefulness, high motor activation, and sustained attention [21]. Orexin-producing neurons, located within the

posterior and lateral hypothalamic areas in the region of the fornix, are known to have widespread excitatory CNS projections, with densest projections to the locus coeruleus, in addition to other regions of the hypothalamus, the basal forebrain, the thalamocortical system, and to multiple brainstem nuclei [22, 23].

Basal forebrain structures include the substantia innominata, the nucleus basalis of Meynert, the diagonal band of Broca, the magnocellular preoptic nucleus, the medial septum, and the globus pallidus [24]. Neurons in the basal forebrain are a major source of acetylcholine release throughout the brain and thus play a major excitatory role in cortical activation and arousal [25]. However, unlike thalamocortical neurons, intact basal forebrain activity is not required for arousal: destruction of the basal forebrain in cats does not abolish cortical activation [26]. The basal forebrain's exact contribution to arousal is still under investigation.

Approach to Patient Presenting with Acute Coma

A patient presenting with an acutely unresponsive state is treated as a medical emergency. The etiologies of an acute unresponsive state are broad. Some are rapidly reversible; others require emergent management to prevent or minimize permanent injury to the brain. A structured systematic approach can help guide the clinician to determine the cause and emergently treat their patient. In this section, we will discuss the differential diagnosis for a patient presenting with acute coma; describe a systematic step-by-step approach to diagnosis; and then describe the emergent management of these patients with an emphasis on the "brain code," which is the management of cerebral herniation.

Etiologies of Acute Coma

Disruption or dysfunction in the pathways of consciousness are the final common pathway for the syndrome of coma. This can happen either through structural lesions that disrupt the pathways of consciousness or nonstructural dysfunction that prevents the pathways from working. A helpful mnemonic for considering all possible etiologies in neurological disorders, especially for neurological disorders such as coma with a myriad of potential etiologies, is "VITAMINS C/D," which stands for vascular, infection, trauma, tumor, autoimmune/inflammatory, metabolic, medications, intracranial pressure (high or low), neoplasms, seizures, cerebrospinal fluid disorders (hydrocephalus), and developmental/congenital anomalies. For coma, there are etiologies in each of these categories. Etiologies classified using this classification are summarized in Table 17.3.

Vascular injuries, such as focal cerebral ischemia due to ischemic stroke, global cerebral ischemia due to cardiac arrest, intracerebral hemorrhage, subarachnoid hemorrhage, or vasculitis, can cause disorders of arousal by directly damaging the brainstem or thalamus. Also, mass effect caused by cerebral edema after vascular injuries can lead to elevated intracranial pressure, obstructive hydrocephalus, and herniation, which can in turn damage the arousal system through direct compression. Vascular injuries tend to occur abruptly and, in the case of ischemic stroke and intracerebral hemorrhage, are likely to present with neurological dysfunction localizable to brainstem or thalamic injury when they also affect the level of consciousness. Basilar migraine, a rare migraine subtype, is an unusual cause of acute coma and may be suspected based on a history of headaches, but it is usually a diagnosis of exclusion after ruling out other more sinister diagnoses including basilar artery stroke. Posterior reversible encephalopathy syndrome (PRES) is an acute neurotoxic syndrome that may present with disorders of consciousness including coma and is also associated with seizures, visual disturbances, and focal neurological deficits [27, 28]. Common triggers include blood pressure fluctuations, renal failure, eclampsia, exposure to immunosuppressive or cytotoxic agents, and autoimmune disorders, and PRES is typically diagnosed through classic radiographical findings that show subcortical vasogenic edema [29].

Infections, such as meningitis, encephalitis, or abscess, can affect the level of consciousness through at least two mechanisms. The infectious process and associated inflammatory process can impair cortical activity diffusely through changes in blood flow, altered CSF dynamics, and cerebral edema. Alternatively, the infection itself may directly involve the cells in the arousal system. Infections can present acutely, subacutely, or chronically, may be associated with fever and leukocytosis, and usually cause an abnormal cerebrospinal fluid. The differential diagnosis for the various organisms that cause meningitis/encephalitis is beyond the scope of this chapter.

Trauma frequently causes failure of arousal either by direct traumatic injury to the arousal system or through compression of the arousal system due to concomitant cerebral edema. Diffuse axonal injury can also lead to slowed or decreased signal transmission throughout the subcortical white matter and may result in a variety of disorders of consciousness. Trauma can also cause subdural hematomas, typically through shearing of the dural bridging veins, which over time can cause compression, high ICP, and resultant coma. Trauma can also cause epidural hematomas, typically caused by damage to a meningeal artery, presenting with initial loss of consciousness, followed by a lucid period, and then subsequent rapid decline. Trauma is usually suggested by the history and presentation and evidence of trauma on physical examination.

Autoimmune or inflammatory etiologies can cause failure of arousal through mechanisms similar to infection. The clinical presentation may be identical to infection, except that there is no evidence of an infectious etiology on cultures. Numerous new antibodies associated with distinct syndromes of autoimmune encephalitis have been characterized, and this continues to be an ongoing research endeavor. Paraneoplastic autoimmune encephalitis is part of this subset, and investigation for neoplasm should occur if a noninfectious encephalitis is high on the differential. In addition to primary autoimmune encephalitis, systemic autoimmune diseases can also have CNS manifestations with presentations of coma through a variety of mechanisms such as

Table 17.3 Non-exhaustive summary of causes of acute coma, sorted using the VITAMINS C mnemonic

Vascular	Ischemic stroke/hypoperfusion
	Intracerebral hemorrhage
	Subarachnoid hemorrhage
	Cardiac arrest
	Vasculitis
	Posterior reversible encephalopathy syndrome [48]
	Basilar migraine
Infection	Meningitis
	Encephalitis
	Abscess
Trauma	Direct damage to key structures from trauma
	Diffuse axonal injury
	Subdural hematoma
	Epidural hematoma
Autoimmune/inflammatory	Autoimmune meningitis
	Autoimmune encephalitis
	Systemic autoimmune diseases with CNS involvement
	Posterior reversible leukoencephalopathy syndrome
Metabolic derangements	Hypoxia
	Hypoglycemia
	Hyperglycemia (diabetic ketoacidosis, hyperosmolar nonketotic hyperglycemia)
	Hyponatremia
	Osmotic demyelination syndrome (from rapid correction of hyponatremia)
	Thyroid dysfunction: myxedema coma, thyrotoxicosis
	Pituitary apoplexy
	Adrenal crisis
	Uremia
	Hypercarbia
	Hyperammonemia
	Hypo- and hypercalcemia
Medications/drug toxicities	Opioid intoxication/overdose
	Gabapentinoids
	Propofol
	Sedative hypnotics (alcohol, benzodiazepines, barbiturates, baclofen, and clonidine)
	Cocaine washout syndrome
	Carbon monoxide (CO) poisoning
	Tricyclic antidepressant overdose
	Organophosphate poisoning
	Cefepime neurotoxicity [48]
	Serotonin syndrome
	Neuroleptic malignant syndrome
	Antiepileptic drugs
Intracranial pressure	High ICP
Neoplasm	Benign and malignant cranial tumors causing mass effect/edema
	Carcinomatous meningitis
Seizures	Nonconvulsive status epilepticus from various causes
	Post-ictal state
CSF disorders	Hydrocephalus (communicating or non-communicating)
Developmental/congenital anomalies	

inflammation of cerebral tissue, mass lesions in the CNS, meningitis and encephalitis, and vasculitis. In these diseases, serum markers of inflammation are elevated, such as ESR, ANA, or ANCA.

Metabolic derangements and medications are among the most common causes of arousal failure and can be diagnosed by history or laboratory testing. Common metabolic derangements that can alter consciousness are hypo- and hyperglycemia (in the case of diabetic ketoacidosis or hyperosmolar nonketotic hyperglycemic syndrome), hypo- or hypernatremia, hyperuremia, hypercarbia, hypoxia, hyperammonemia, and hypercalcemia. Endocrine disorders can also present with coma. This includes thyroid disorders such as myxedema coma (severe untreated hypothyroidism) and thyrotoxic storm; pituitary apoplexy which is characterized by sudden hemorrhage or infarction of the pituitary gland; acute adrenal crisis either from primary Addison's disease, a secondary disorder or glucocorticoid-induced [30]. Osmotic demyelination syndrome, which includes central pontine myelinolysis, is typically caused by rapid correction of hyponatremia and can cause damage to different parts of the brain but most typically causes pontine dysfunction. This can lead to locked-in-syndrome, a mimic of coma, that is discussed in more detail in the Chronic Coma section, and should be screened for on neurological assessment.

Medications and toxins that can lead to a depressed level of consciousness include, but are not limited to, opioids, gabapentinoids, antiepileptic medications, sedative hypnotics (including alcohol, benzodiazepines, barbiturates, baclofen, and clonidine), stimulant washout syndromes (such as cocaine), carbon monoxide (CO) poisoning, and toxin-induced brain-death mimickers (such as tricyclic antidepressant overdose, organophosphate poisoning, and cefepime neurotoxicity) [31]. The elderly and patients with preexisting brain injuries are particularly sensitive to both metabolic derangements and medications which alter the level of consciousness [32]. Serotonin syndrome is a potentially life-threatening syndrome caused by overdose of serotoninergic drugs and can present with coma, along with autonomic hyperactivity including tachycardia and hyperthermia and neuromuscular abnormalities such as clonus, hyperreflexia, and rigidity. A wide range of drug classes can contribute to serotonin syndrome, including but not limited to a broad range of antidepressant classes, anxiolytics, amphetamines, cocaine, tramadol, L-dopa, and lithium [33]. Neuroleptic malignant syndrome is another classic drug toxicity syndrome that can present with coma. It is characterized by altered mental status (including coma), generalized rigidity, hyperpyrexia, and dysautonomia and is typically caused by antipsychotic agent use [34]. The prompt identification of serotonin syndrome and neuroleptic malignant syndrome as distinct causes of coma is important because removal of the provoking drug and appropriate supportive care can dramatically alter the prognosis.

High intracranial pressure is often heralded by arousal failure and is most frequently caused by vascular lesions, infections, neoplasms, and hydrocephalus. High intracranial pressure can cause arousal failure through at least two mechanisms (1) cerebral herniation, where the pressure due to a lesion in a neighboring brain region forces brain tissue into the arousal system, and (2) diffusely elevated pressure causing diffuse cortical dysfunction.

Neoplasms can cause arousal failure if they grow directly into the arousal system, by compression of the arousal system after growth from a nearby focus or through derangement of the arousal system by vasogenic edema.

Seizures cause arousal failure through several mechanisms: (1) status epilepticus (convulsive or nonconvulsive) is associated with poor arousal; (2) during a single seizure or cluster of seizures, patients may be poorly arousable, depending on the size of the seizure focus; and (3) patients may fail to arouse reliably during the postictal period and after administration of sedating antiepileptic medications. Seizure as a cause of arousal failure is suggested by a history of epilepsy, witnessed tonic-clonic activity, or other seizure-related signs, such as tongue biting, and by an electroencephalogram with evidence of ongoing or recent seizure.

Cerebrospinal fluid disorders, mainly hydrocephalus, can compress and cause dysfunction in the thalamus and midbrain and can also lead to diffuse dysfunction of bilateral cortical projections. Hydrocephalus can be congenital or develop as a sequela of neoplasm, CNS infection, inflammatory disease, hemorrhage, or ischemic stroke. In patients with congenital hydrocephalus, failure of a shunt device should also be considered a possible cause of arousal failure.

A Systematic Clinical Approach to the Patient Presenting with Acute Coma

Clinicians must have an organized and expedient approach involving time-sensitive diagnostic and therapeutic actions that often occur simultaneously. In order to codify and organize the approach to an acutely unresponsive patient in a stepwise manner, the Neurocritical Care Society first created the Emergency Neurological Life Support Recommendations in 2012 and have since revised them as of 2019. Figure 17.2, from the ENLS guidelines, offers a step-by-step approach for any emergent practitioner to follow when treating an acutely comatose patient [35].

In practice, multiple diagnostic tests and interventions occur simultaneously as new information is made available and as assessments continue. Nevertheless, clinicians should use an organized approach, as much as is feasible, in evaluating and treating patients with acute coma.

ACLS and ATLS Evaluation As per the algorithm above, the initial assessment of all patients with critical illness should focus on the ABCDs (airway, breathing, circulation, and defibrillation) of Advanced Cardiac Life Support (ACLS) and Advanced Trauma Life Support (ATLS). A full description of ACLS and ATLS guidelines is beyond the scope of this chapter. Relevant materials can be obtained from their respective sponsoring organizations with the American Heart Association for the ACLS and the American College of Surgeons for the ATLS. If trauma or c-spine injury cannot be ruled out, stabilization of the c-spine should occur early so as to prevent any exacerbation of spinal cord or nerve injury.

Rapid Neurological Assessment The next step is to perform a rapid neurological assessment. The purpose of this rapid screen is to identify potential neurological catastrophes which must

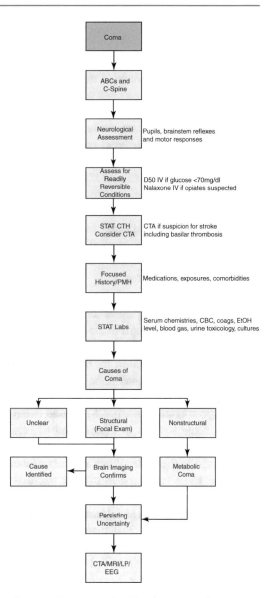

Fig. 17.2 Suggested algorithm from ENLS for approach to acute coma. (Reproduced from Venkatasubramanian et al. [35], with permission from Springer Nature)

be intervened upon emergently, such as cerebral herniation or a stroke syndrome. A rapid neurological assessment includes determination of level of consciousness, evaluation for pupil asymmetry and light reactivity, brainstem reflexes, and evaluation of motor function. If the rapid neurological assessment suggests cerebral herniation, impending herniation, or intracranial hypertension, then medications to reduce intracranial pressure should be emergently initiated ("brain code"; see "Emergent Therapies for Arousal Failure" section). Concurrent presence of hypertension, bradycardia, and hyperventilation comprises the "Cushing's reflex," which is also seen frequently in patients with intracranial hypertension. This triad is a physiological response that can maintain cerebral perfusion in the setting of high intracranial pressure through systemic hypertension, increased cardiac filling time, and decreased cerebral blood volume (through hyperventilation-induced arteriolar vasoconstriction) [36]. Other helpful observations in the neurological exam include observation for any rhythmic movements of the body or of the eyes, or gaze deviation, that may be suspicious for ongoing seizures.

Standardized scoring scales for consciousness such as the Glasgow Coma Scale and the FOUR Score (Tables 17.4 and 17.5) are commonly used in emergent settings to allow for rapid communication of the patient's status among providers and allow for efficient algorithmic decision-making. The Glasgow Coma Scale (GCS) is used extensively in acute settings to assess level of consciousness. The table below shows how points are assigned in the scale. When patients cannot speak due to an endotracheal tube or tracheostomy, the GCS score is annotated with a "T." For instance, a patient with endotracheal intubation, no eye opening, and a best motor response of extensor posturing to pain will have a GCS score of 4 T. The GCS is limited as it does not account for brainstem dysfunction, hemiparesis, or aphasia. This means that patients with the same GCS score could have varying clinical presentations from very different etiologies. The Full Outline of UnResponsiveness (FOUR) Score includes eye responses, motor responses, brainstem reflexes, and respiratory pattern and therefore incorporates more detailed information that could be extremely clinically useful [37]. For example, using the FOUR score, one can identify a patient who has locked-in syndrome, and is actually conscious but only able to communicate through eye movements. The FOUR score has been validated in a variety of clinical settings, including the ICU setting [38].

Table 17.4 Glasgow Coma Scale

Eye examination
4 – Eyes open spontaneously
3 – Eyes open to voice
2 – Eyes open to pain
1 – No eye opening
Verbal response
5 – Oriented
4 – Confused
3 – Inappropriate words
2 – Incomprehensible sounds
1 – No verbal response
Motor examination
6 – Obeys commands
5 – Localizing pain stimuli
4 – Withdrawal from painful stimuli
3 – Flexor posturing to painful stimuli
2 – Extensor posturing to painful stimuli
1 – No motor response
Total score: 3 (lowest) to 15 (highest)

Table 17.5 Four score scale

Eye response
4 – Eyelids open or opened, tracking or blinking to command
3 – Eyelids open spontaneously, but not tracking nor blinking to command
2 – Eyelids closed but open to loud voice
1 – Eyelids closed but open to pain
0 – Eyelids remain closed even with pain
Motor response
4 – Thumbs up, fist or peace sign (to command)
3 – Localizes to pain
2 –Flexion response to pain
1 – Extension response to pain
0 – No response to pain or generalized myoclonus
Brainstem reflexes
4 – Pupillary light reflex and corneal reflexes present
3 – One pupil wide and fixed
2 – Either the pupillary light reflex or the corneal reflex is absent
1 – Both the pupillary light reflex and corneal reflex are absent
0 – Absent pupil, corneal, and cough reflex
Respiration
4 – Regular breathing pattern
3 – Cheyne–Stokes breathing pattern
2 – Irregular breathing
1 – Triggers ventilator or breathes above the set ventilator rate
0 – Apnea or breathing at the set ventilator rate only
Total score: 0 (lowest) to 16 (highest)

Although the ENLS algorithm makes a distinction between the steps of emergent medical and emergent neurological assessments, there are a number of special considerations in patients with emergently critical neurological illness that interplay between the two.

Comatose patients (GCS <9) are often thought to have lost the ability to "protect their airway." On examination, comatose or encephalopathic patients are often snoring loudly or "gurgling." This is because their neurological injury decreases their normal upper airway muscular tone and increases upper airway resistance. This makes spontaneous ventilation more difficult and increases the risk of aspiration. In general, comatose patients (GCS <9) undergo emergent endotracheal intubation for airway protection to facilitate ventilation and minimize the risk of aspiration and pulmonary complications. Until intubation and mechanical ventilation are achieved, patients should be supported for both ventilation and oxygenation using bag mask ventilation with adequate FiO2 and, if needed, an oral or nasopharyngeal airway to maintain airway patency. During bag mask ventilation and after endotracheal intubation, initial goals of normocapnia ($PaCO_2$ 35–39 mmHg) and normal oxygenation (SaO_2 95–100% or $PaO_2 > 80$ mmHg) should be set. After identification of the neurological insult, these goals may be modified.

Patients with critical neurological illness can present with a wide range of cardiac rhythms and blood pressures. Again, standard ACLS guidelines take immediate precedence in the emergent assessment of a comatose patient. Therefore, unstable cardiac rhythms and very low blood pressures (SBP <80 mmHg) should be assessed using the ACLS guidelines. At this stage in the emergent assessment, the precise etiology of the neurological injury may still not be known, although the history and examination may point to a likely cause. In the comatose patient who does not require ACLS resuscitation, blood pressure should be initially evaluated with consideration of all possible etiologies of critical neurological illness. Blood pressure goals are normally set to a fairly broad range until the etiology of the neurological injury is identified (usually in parallel to establishing adequate ventilation). At this stage in the assessment, the clinician should initially employ a broad blood pressure goal range in order to seek a balance between treating the neurological injury and avoiding iatrogenic exacerbation of the injury. For example, patients with acute ischemic stroke may require higher blood pressures to maintain perfusion of ischemic brain territories, whereas patients with intracerebral or subarachnoid hemorrhages will ultimately require lower blood pressures to prevent worsening of the hemorrhage [39, 40]. A broad blood pressure range also helps guide the use of anesthetic agents during endotracheal intubation, which may result in precipitous swings in blood pressure.

Evaluation for Hypoglycemia and Drug Toxicity All acutely comatose patients should have a rapid glucose test, either in the field or on arrival to the emergent setting, as hypoglycemia can cause coma and can result in permanent brain injury if not rapidly corrected. If blood glucose is less than 70 mg/dL, dextrose should ideally be administered intravenously. If the patient's history is suspicious for someone with malnutrition (history of alcohol dependence, cancer, bariatric surgery, eating disorders), if their appearance is cachectic, or if the relative history is unknown, then intravenous thiamine should be given prior to dextrose. These patients are at a higher risk for thiamine deficiency, and starting an intravenous glucose infusion without first replenishing thiamine can result in acceleration of damage to structures in the brain. If the patient's history or exam is suspicious for opioid toxicity, administer naloxone intravenously or intranasally and repeat as needed. Clinical signs suspicious of opiate toxicity include depressed respirations (apnea or bradypnea) and small pupils. As part of the initial survey, making note of any marks in the extremities or torso suspicious for intravenous injection should also be done. If patients have taken a longer acting opioid such as hydromorphone, repeated doses of naloxone may be needed.

Initial Diagnostic Tests

After initial stabilization of ABCs, securement of the c-spine, and intervening for emergencies such as cerebral herniation or status epilepticus, the next step is to get an emergent noncontrast computed tomography (CT) scan of the head, possibly along with a CT angiogram (CTA) of the head and neck and a CT perfusion (CTP) scan, to look for any structural causes of coma that may need emergent intervention. A CT head without contrast can help identify intracranial hemorrhage, evolving ischemic strokes with edema, mass effect from edema or lesions, hydrocephalus, extra-axial fluid collections, and subarachnoid hemorrhage among other structural causes. The need for a rapid CT is evident from the fact that further management does change significantly based on what is found on the head CT. For instance, identification of hydrocephalus makes CSF decompression through the placement of an intraventricular catheter of paramount importance. Similarly, identification of an aneurysmal subarachnoid hemorrhage triggers the need for stricter BP control, a neurovascular workup, and ultimate procedural securement of the aneurysm either through clipping, coiling, or a flow diverter device. A CTA head/neck along with a CT perfusion scan can help identify possible basilar occlusion and/or other large vessel occlusions that may be amenable to intravenous tissue plasminogen activator treatment (iv tPA) or intraarterial thrombolysis. A CTA head/neck could also identify possible vascular malformations or aneurysms in the setting of intracranial hemorrhage.

The next step in the ENLS prescribed algorithm is to pursue lab work. As discussed previously in this section, there are a variety of metabolic and toxic etiologies that can cause coma. Unless a readily reversible cause has been identified and reversed, such as hypoglycemia, additional laboratory testing should be obtained. Initial testing typically involves serum chemistries, basic hematological panel, blood gas analysis, ethanol level, and toxicology screen.

Further Testing

If no structural cause has been identified, and the workup described above is unclear, further diagnostic testing should include an electroencephalogram (EEG) to evaluate for nonconvulsive status epilepticus or post-ictal state, as well as any signs that may suggest particular metabolic or toxic derangements. Lab workup can be expanded to include thyroid function panel to evaluate for hypothyroidism, thyrotoxicosis, and myxedema coma; hepatic panel and ammonia testing to evaluate for hepatic encephalopathy; and acetaminophen levels and other drug levels based on history obtained. If there is no significant risk for downward herniation identified on imaging, and no clinical signs of high ICP, then a lumbar puncture should be pursued to evaluate for signs of inflammation and infection within the CNS.

Management of Cerebral Herniation

The first step is securement of the "ABCs" – airway, breathing, and circulation – using the ACLS and ATLS algorithms. However, once this is done, other emergent treatment considerations should also be pursued while the cause of the coma is still under investigation. This involves assessing for and treating cerebral herniation syndromes. This section describes the management of cerebral herniation. As the etiology of the coma becomes evident, disease-specific treatments should be implemented, and these are described in the disease-specific chapters of this textbook.

If the patient exhibits clinical evidence of intracranial hypertension (e.g., coma, pupillary abnormalities, Cushing's triad), a "brain code" should be performed. A "brain code" is the systematic administration of therapies to lower intracranial pressure.

The algorithm below summarizes the steps involved in a brain code

1. Position head of bed to at least 30°, make sure the neck is straight and that the sides of the neck are not being compressed.
2. Hyperventilate the patient to a goal PaCO2 of 28–32.
3. Review, access, and administer one of the following:
   (a) 1 g/kg mannitol [can be given through a peripheral IV, IO, or central line]
   (b) 23.4% Hypertonic saline push (colloquially known as a saline bullet) [can be given through an IO or central line]

4. If unsuccessful with either of the above, administer the other therapy.
5. If still unsuccessful, start hypertonic saline with a bolus and then infusion.
6. Consider placement of an intraventricular catheter – extraventricular drain system (IVC or EVD). This requires a noncontrast head CT to guide placement.

When cerebral herniation is first identified at the bedside, usually in the form of a dilated pupil, the most rapid intervention is to ensure that venous drainage is not being impaired through positioning. This involves setting the head of the patient's bed up at an angle greater than 30° and making sure the jugular veins are not being compressed by external devices.

Next, hyperventilate the patient with a goal $PaCO2$ of 28–32. If the patient is intubated and on mechanical ventilation, this can be accomplished by increasing the set respiratory rate up to approximately 25–30 breaths per minute. If the patient is not on mechanical ventilation, the same effect can be achieved through adequate bag mask ventilation. End-tidal carbon dioxide monitors should be used where possible to guide hyperventilation therapy. Hyperventilation works by inducing cerebral vasoconstriction, thereby decreasing the amount of blood in the intracranial compartment and creating more space and alleviating the downward cerebral herniation.

The next step in treatment is to administer an agent that would pull fluid out of the cerebral interstitial fluid and tissue and into the blood vessels, so as to deliver it out of the cranium, thereby decompressing the brain. Mannitol (20% or 25%) and hypertonic saline are the agents of choice. Mannitol creates an osmotic gradient allowing water to flow out of both the edematous and normal brain, which decreases cerebral volume and, consequently, intracranial pressure. Mannitol can be easily administered through a peripheral intravenous line. Hypertonic saline comes in different concentrations. A 23.4% hypertonic saline push, colloquially known as a "saline bullet" is preferred in the emergent herniation setting. Historically, it required the placement of a central venous catheter to administer, but recent evidence has shown that it can be safely administered using an intraosseous line, which can be placed quickly in emergency settings [41]. No matter which you start with, mannitol or hypertonic saline, if you are unsuccessful in restoring pupillary reactivity, administer the other agent as well. 2% saline can be administered safely through a peripheral intravenous line, and 3% saline use through peripheral intravenous lines tends to be institution specific based on available nursing safety protocols.

Finally, if these medical interventions are unsuccessful, CSF diversion out of the cranium using an IVC/EVD may be a possible solution. This does however require at least a recent noncontrast head CT to help the proceduralist plan and place the device.

While the mortality of acute intracranial hypertension is high, with frequent progression to brain death, there is significant potential for good neurological outcomes. In a prospective study of 28 patients with acute intracranial hypertension and cerebral herniation, 16 (~60%) patients died, including the 13 patients who progressed to brain death. However, with aggressive medical therapy as described in the preceding paragraphs, seven (25%) of these patients were functionally independent in approximately 1 year [42]. In a retrospective study of the efficacy of 23.4% NaCl in the reversal of cerebral herniation, 5 of 68 patients (7.4%) had mild or moderate disability at discharge [43]. Both of these studies indicate that despite the high risk of severe disability and death due to intracranial hypertension and cerebral edema, prompt recognition and initiation of a "brain code" can lead to good neurological outcomes in up to 25% of affected patients.

Complete Neurological Assessment of the Comatose Patient

The purpose of a complete neurological examination in comatose patients is to localize the lesion responsible for failure of arousal. This more comprehensive evaluation should be performed after emergent assessment and stabilization of an acutely comatose patient. Neurological examination and anatomical localization allow for an accurate assessment of the condition of the patient as an important guide for immediate and future investigation and therapy. The neurological examination in the comatose patient is performed with the same format as in conscious patients, except that the approach is modified for performance in a patient who cannot cooperate or follow commands [44]. The standard format of the general neurological examination proceeds through each of the following neurological systems: mental status and/or level of consciousness; cranial nerves; motor system; sensory system; reflexes; coordination; and gait. In a poorly arousable patient, assessment of the level of consciousness is paramount and takes precedence over the standard mental status examination, in which the content of consciousness is assessed. In fact, further assessment of the content of consciousness (e.g., language, calculation, memory) is not possible or reliable without an adequate level of arousal. Cranial nerves, motor and sensory systems, and reflexes are also examined in detail. Examination of coordination and gait is more difficult in an uncooperative patient and does not usually contribute to neuroanatomical localization in disorders of arousal.

In disorders of arousal, accurate assessment of the level of consciousness is imperative. The approach to examination of a patient's level of consciousness is to ascertain the degree of wakefulness, orientation, and attention. The first step in examining an unresponsive patient (after the rapid neurological assessment) is to observe the patient for a period of time to assess whether the patient arouses spontaneously (to internal stimuli). The next step is to assess the patient's responsiveness to external (examiner-induced) stimuli. These stimuli should be applied in a graded fashion from least to most noxious. Common stimuli include the following: voice or loud sound, especially calling of the patient's name; painful stimulus (pinch or rub) applied to arm, leg, trapezius muscle, chest, or orbit; nasopharyngeal stimulation with a cotton swab; and in-line suctioning of endotracheal or tracheostomy tube. Attention should be paid to the amount of stimulation needed for arousal, the level of arousal achieved with stimulation, and how long the patient remains aroused after discontinuation of the stimulus. If the patient arouses reliably, then the level of attention and orientation can be assessed by performing a limited mental status exam or a Folstein Mini-Mental Status Exam (MMSE). The patient should be asked to follow commands or verbalize if not intubated. If verbal, the patient should be asked to state his name, the location, the date or year, season, and reason for hospitalization. Cues can be given, but the use of cues should be accounted for when assessing level of arousal, i.e., reliance on cues suggests less orientation and more abnormal arousal. Patients should also be asked to follow commands. Midline commands (e.g., eye opening and closing, sticking out the tongue) should be tested first, followed by appendicular commands (e.g., showing two fingers or thumbs up). An ability to follow appendicular commands belies more complex processing and higher level of arousal than obeying midline commands alone. A patient in coma will not follow commands, open eyes, arouse to any painful or noxious stimuli, or respond in any meaningful way. An encephalopathic patient will arouse, open eyes, and follow commands inconsistently.

The cranial nerve examination is important for localization of the lesion responsible for the altered level of consciousness and to monitor for disease progression. The RAS, which controls cortical activation and arousal, traverses the brainstem longitudinally and is anatomically proximate to many cranial nerves and their nuclei, especially those from the mid-pons and more rostrally. Examination of the cranial nerves proceeds in the numerical order of the nerves, with exclusion of the olfactory nerve (first cranial nerve). The function of the optic nerve (second cranial nerve) can be examined through several approaches. In an unresponsive patient, the integrity of optic nerve function is examined by testing for pupillary function, blink reflex to a threat stimulus, and the ability to track visual stimuli. When testing pupils, light from the examiner is directed onto the retina, and pupil constriction (miosis) is triggered. Miosis requires an intact optic nerve, midbrain, oculomotor nerve (third cranial nerve), and parasympathetic nervous system. Furthermore, in normal patients, when light is directed into one eye, both pupils constrict consensually. Pupillary constriction and the consensual response in the contralateral eye are dependent on the Edinger–Westphal nucleus, which is located in the midbrain. To activate this pathway, an examiner's light stimulates retinal ganglion cells located in the retina. Most of the retinal ganglion cells project via the optic nerves and tracts to the lateral geniculate nucleus and ultimately the visual cortex to encode visual information. However, a number of neurons project to the pretectal nucleus of the midbrain and thus form the afferent limb of the pupillary light reflex. From the pretectal nucleus, the pathway projects to the Edinger–Westphal nucleus, which gives rise to the pupil-constricting fibers of the oculomotor nerve. A lesion along these pathways could cause an inability of one or both pupils to constrict, depending on the precise location of the lesion and the structures affected. A lesion involving the optic nerve will lead to an inability of both pupils to constrict consensually to light directed into the affected eye because the afferent limb of the pupillary light reflex is dysfunctional. This type of lesion can be highlighted using the swinging flashlight test, where the examiner's light is directed into each eye alternately. During this test, when the light is directed into the affected eye, both pupils dilate. In contrast, when the light is directed into the normal eye, both pupils constrict appropriately. Lesions affecting the optic nerve in isolation rarely affect the level of consciousness. The most common location for lesions affecting both the pupillary light reflex and the level of consciousness is in or near the midbrain, and such lesions usually result in oculomotor nerve or nucleus dysfunction. Examination of oculomotor nerve function will be discussed below.

A test for reflexive blink to visual threat is another way to test the optic nerve in an unresponsive patient. The examiner can move his fingers or hand toward the patient's eye in a brisk, "threatening" manner and can even present the stimulus within quadrants of confrontational visual field testing. Reflexive blink to a visual threat requires an intact optic nerve, which serves as the afferent limb of the reflex pathway, and an intact facial nerve, which serves as the efferent limb of the pathway producing a blink response. However, an absent reflexive blink to visual threat is nonlocalizing because lesions producing a failure to blink to threat have been postulated in multiple disparate locations, including the striate cortex, higher-order visual processing centers, frontal eye fields, and mid- to upper brainstem [45]. Reflexive visual stimulus tracking can also be examined in an unresponsive patient. Like the blink-to-threat pathway, tracking of visual stimuli is also controlled through a complex neurological pathway. Nonetheless, the afferent limb is also the optic nerve. To test for the ability to track visual stimuli, various items and objects can be moved through the visual fields. Most directly, the patient can be asked to follow fingers or a face with his eyes. Several powerful stimuli to test the ability to track are the human face, paper money, and photographs of loved ones. Another tracking stimulus is the optokinetic nystagmus (OKN) strip or wheel, in which a strip of paper or wheel with alternating colors is moved across the patient's visual fields. OKN strips or wheels trigger nystagmus in normal patients. In order to have a normal response to OKN testing, patients must have intact optic nerves in addition to intact higher-order cerebral processing centers, such as in the occipital and parietal cortices [46]. OKN testing can be used to test for normal optic nerve and visual function in an unresponsive patient, but absent OKN is difficult to localize.

The oculomotor nerve (third cranial nerve) has two principal functions (1) control of pupillary constrictors and (2) extraocular eye movements. Again, bilateral symmetrical pupillary constriction requires intact optic nerves (second cranial nerve), midbrain, oculomotor nerves (third cranial nerve), and parasympathetic nervous system function. The efferent limb of the pupillary light reflex begins at the Edinger–Westphal nucleus, which gives rise to parasympathetic fibers that travel within the medial aspect of the midbrain before joining onto the surface of the oculomotor nerve. The nuclei of the oculomotor nerve also are located in the medial aspect of the midbrain and give rise to the fibers that control eye movements. The eye movements controlled by the oculomotor nerve include all of the cardinal directions (upward, downward, medially) in the ipsilateral eye, except lateral and the combination of downward and medial. The lateral and downward/medial movements are controlled by the lateral rectus nerve (sixth cranial nerve) and trochlear nerve (fourth cranial nerve), respectively.

Integrity of the oculomotor nerve and its nuclei is tested by testing pupillary function and eye movements. In the case of the oculomotor nerve, derangement of the parasympathetic fibers causes marked pupillary dilation ("blown pupil"). Damage to Edinger–Westphal and oculomotor nuclei within the midbrain causes bilateral failure of pupillary constriction and pupils that are midsized (2–4 mm) and unreactive. In contrast, damage to the pons can lead to pupils that are pinpoint and poorly reactive, due to interruption of descending sympathetic pathways and consequently unopposed parasympathetic activity produced by the midbrain. Because of the close proximity of the oculomotor nerve and nuclei to the cerebral aqueduct and the RAS, lesions affecting pupil reaction often are accompanied by arousal failure. Pupil size and reactivity, in addition to other exam findings, can help identify the precise neuroanatomical location of the responsible lesion. For example, bilaterally midsized pupils and loss of consciousness would be attributable to a medial midbrain lesion. In contrast, a fixed and dilated pupil without alteration in consciousness would likely be attributable to ipsilateral oculomotor nerve compression without impingement on the midbrain. A fixed and dilated pupil with an alteration in consciousness suggests oculomotor nerve dysfunction in or near the midbrain. Small, unreactive ("pinpoint") pupils bilaterally and arousal failure are attributable to a lesion in the upper pons.

In the unresponsive patient, extraocular movements are observed for the oculomotor and abducens nerves (third and sixth cranial nerves, respectively). Trochlear nerve (fourth cranial nerve) function is difficult to test in unconscious patients. In the unresponsive patient, spontane-ous eye movements and passive eye positioning should first be observed to determine any obvious weakness. Weakness with gaze in any direction might be observed in the patient's spontaneous eye movements. The patient can be asked to track a visual stimulus or a powerful tracking stimulus, which can be moved across the patient's visual fields. As described, examples of powerful tracking stimuli include a human face, high denomination paper money, or an OKN strip or drum. In an unresponsive or uncooperative patient, eye movements can be tested using the oculocephalic reflex, also sometimes referred to as testing for doll's eyes. For this test, the examiner moves the patient's head laterally from side to side and observes the patient's lateral eye movements. Normally, tonic activity bilaterally within the vestibular systems drives the eyes to the contralateral side. This activity is balanced unless the head is moved. When the head is moved laterally, activity increases in the vestibular system ipsilateral to the direction of head movement and decreases in the vestibular system contralateral to the head movement. *Thus, in a patient with normal eye movements, the eyes move in the opposite direction to the head turn.* This test can also be performed using vertical head movements. A normal oculocephalic reflex requires a normal vestibular apparatus, vestibulocochlear nerve (afferent limb, eighth cranial nerve), brainstem, oculomotor nerve (efferent limb, medial eye movement), and abducens nerve (efferent limb, lateral eye movement). An absence of eye movements with oculocephalic testing can be due to diffusely abnormal brainstem activity or no brain activity at all. However, this test should be interpreted with caution because conscious patients can suppress the oculocephalic reflex with gaze fixation on a distant object. If the oculocephalic reflex is present in some directions but not others, then the test should be interpreted to determine which particular extraocular muscles are weak and ultimately which nerves or their nuclei have failed: the oculomotor nerves control medial eye movements, and the abducens nerves control lateral eye movements.

If the oculocephalic reflex is absent, then a stronger test to confirm absent eye movements is the vestibulo-ocular reflex or cold caloric test. For this test, water that has been cooled for 5 min with ice is instilled continuously into one external auditory meatus for 2 min. The eyes are observed for movement during and several minutes after the infusion. After several minutes to allow rewarming, cold water should be infused into the contralateral ear. Like the oculocephalic reflex, a normal cold caloric response requires a normal vestibular apparatus, vestibulocochlear nerve (afferent limb, eighth cranial nerve), brainstem, oculomotor nerve (efferent limb, medial eye movement), and abducens nerve (efferent limb, lateral eye movement). As mentioned, normally tonic activity bilaterally within the vestibular system drives the eyes to the contralateral side. Cooling of the tympanic membrane disrupts this balance. *Thus, in a patient with normal pons and midbrain activity, inhibition of tonic activity by tympanic membrane cooling causes the eyes to move toward the cooled ear.* The lateral and medial eye movements are mediated by the abducens and oculomotor nerves, respectively. If the patient also has intact cortical activity, a corrective saccade away from the cooled ear will also be present. The classic mnemonic "COWS: *c*old *o*pposite, *w*arm *s*ame" refers to the corrective saccade produced by the different water temperatures used in caloric testing. This mnemonic has little clinical utility in the comatose patient because cortical activity is usually absent or markedly abnormal. In patients where the cold caloric response is asymmetrical or absent on one side, the other clinical and neurological examination data should be interpreted to determine the location of the lesion. In a patient with absent pons and midbrain activity, the eyes will remain in the midline during cold caloric testing on both sides. Eye motion abnormalities often accompany loss of consciousness because of the close proximity of extraocular movement nuclei to the RAS, especially in the midbrain.

Brain injury that produces arousal failure can often produce certain patterns of eye movements, which can aid in localization. Ocular bobbing is produced by pontine lesions and is defined by a rapid downbeat and slow upward phase. Midbrain lesions can produce retraction nystagmus, con-

version nystagmus, and sunsetting eyes with forced downgaze. Ping pong eyes and periodic alternating gaze are induced by injuries to both hemispheres, cerebellar vermis, or the midbrain. Though rare, when present with coma or encephalopathy, these eye movement abnormalities can portend neurological catastrophe.

In the unresponsive patient, the corneal reflex is the most reliable way to test the trigeminal nerve (fifth cranial nerve) function. In this test, the cornea is stimulated, which causes a blink reflex in both eyes. This reflex requires a normal ipsilateral trigeminal nerve, pons, and bilateral facial nerves. Like the pupillary light response, there is a consensual blink response to corneal stimulation. A component of the corneal reflex is also controlled by the contralateral parietal lobe. The trigeminal nerve is the afferent limb of this reflex and can be stimulated using techniques of graded intensity. The most benign form of stimulation is to gently touch or move the patient's eyelashes. If the patient blinks symmetrically, then the corneal reflex is intact and no further corneal stimulation is needed. Corneal stimulation techniques of greater intensity include placing drops of normal saline in the eye and touching a tapered cotton swab to the cornea. The cotton swab provides the highest level of corneal stimulation. Care should be taken with repeated corneal reflex testing to avoid the region directly in the front of the lens because a corneal abrasion in this location could affect vision. It is advisable to test the corneal reflex as distal from the lens as possible, such as where the sclera and the cornea intersect.

The facial nerve (seventh cranial nerve) can be tested by observing passive face posture, such as palpebral fissure width and the nasolabial fold. As mentioned above, the efferent limbs of the blink and corneal reflexes are controlled by the facial nerve. Facial weakness should be interpreted in conjunction with other clinical variables as it relates to an altered level of consciousness. The vestibulocochlear nerve (eighth cranial nerve) is tested as described above, using the oculocephalic and vestibulo-ocular reflexes. The glossopharyngeal and vagus nerves (ninth and tenth cranial nerves, respectively) are tested via gag and cough. Patients with a severely diminished level of consciousness often have weaker or more poorly coordinated gag and cough. The exact etiology of this poor coordination is not clear as the glossopharyngeal and vagal nuclei are often spared by lesions that affect the level of consciousness. Comatose patients are usually intubated for airway protection because even with a present gag and cough, there is a high risk of poor ventilation, aspiration, and pneumonia. The spinal accessory nerve and hypoglossal nerves are not commonly tested in the unresponsive patient.

The brainstem is responsible for control of the pattern of breathing. Lesions within the brainstem can cause pathologic breathing patterns that are typified by the location of the lesion. Cheyne–Stokes breathing is defined by short periods of hyperpnea followed by short periods of apnea and may be associated with other signs of heightened arousal, such as improved motor exam or eye opening. Cheyne–Stokes breathing usually results from bilateral thalamic injury, injury to widespread bilateral cortical projections, or metabolic derangements and is therefore frequently associated with arousal failure. Apneustic breathing is associated with pontine injury and is characterized by long inspiratory pauses. Central neurogenic hyperventilation is characterized by sustained hyperventilation with respiratory rates >40 breaths per minute. This pattern localizes injuries to both cerebral hemispheres, the pons, or the midbrain. Cluster breathing is defined by irregular clusters of breaths, followed by pauses of irregular duration. Injuries to both hemispheres, the pons, or rostral medulla can result in cluster breathing. Ataxic breathing results from medullary lesions, is defined by a completely irregular pattern (the "atrial fibrillation" of respiratory patterns), and can signal impending respiratory failure.

As in the examination of the cranial nerves, the motor system is examined first by passive observation. The examiner should note whether the patient is moving symmetrically, briskly, and spontaneously and whether the patient is posturing any extremities. Next the examiner should ask the patient to follow commands in the midline and with all four of his extremities. If the patient is conscious, confrontational power testing can be performed as in the classic neurological examination. Similarly, if the patient is awake and lucid, the sensory system can be tested in detail. However, in the unresponsive patient, the motor and sensory systems are tested together as the patient responds to painful stimuli delivered centrally and peripherally. When a painful stimulus is applied, if the patient moves any extremities or grimaces, then there is evidence that a sensory signal is being processed. If the patient moves his extremity in a complex way in response to a painful stimulus, especially against gravity, then the patient has localized. Localization is not stereotyped: the patient may perform a different or very purposeful action with each painful stimulus, which belies higher cortical processing. In contrast, withdrawal of the extremity to a painful stimulus can be stereotyped and is often within the plane of gravity. Posturing of the extremities or absent extremity movement portends severe neurologic injury. There are two types of posturing: extensor (decerebrate) and flexor (decorticate) posturing. Extensor posturing is associated with poorer clinical outcomes and usually results from injuries to larger brain territories, including the pons and midbrain. With extensor posturing, painful stimuli trigger a very stereotyped response in which the patient extends and pronates one or both arms to his side, extends both wrists, extends both legs, and plantar flexes the feet. In contrast, with flexor posturing, painful stimuli also trigger a stereotyped response except that the arms flex at the wrist and elbow. Flexor posturing is also associated with poor neurological outcomes but is caused by injury to less brain territory than extensor posturing, usually involving the regions rostral to the upper midbrain. Because of the uncertainly regarding the precise localization of these posturing reflexes, it is advised to use the terms extensor and flexor instead of decerebrate or decorticate posturing. To determine with certainty whether the patient's movement is a withdrawal or posture, the patient's hand should be placed on his abdomen and a painful stimulus applied to the upper arm. With localization or withdrawal, the patient will move the arm away from the painful stimulus. With a posture, the arm will move in a stereotyped manner irrespective of the stimulus location. Applying a painful stimulus to the lower extremities may also trigger a triple flexion response, in which the hip and knee flex and the ankle dorsiflexes. This finding is a spinal cord reflex and is consistent with severe neurological dysfunction. While flexor and extensor posturing are associated with poor neurological outcomes, both require brain activity. The triple flexion reflex may persist in the absence of brain activity and in the setting of brain death.

Tendon reflexes play a diminished role in the examination of the comatose patient, as compared to the traditional neurological examination. The jaw jerk reflex is a reflex that tests the integrity of the trigeminal nerve and its nuclei. Elevated jaw jerk reflexes can be seen with lesions above the trigeminal nuclei and with diffuse metabolic and toxic processes that can cause altered level of consciousness. Other tendon reflexes can be tested for hyper- or hyporeactivity, which can be seen in the setting of toxic and metabolic derangements, or asymmetry which could help localize the neurological injury in conjunction with other clinical data and the neurological examination as described in the preceding sections.

Prognostication in Chronic Disorders of Consciousness

For patients that persist in a state of disordered consciousness after the acute period, the goal of management shifts toward optimizing treatment and assisting with prognostication. This is an imperfect and uncertain arena, prone to error, and for which research and novel diagnostics continue to provide new information. Furthermore, the underlying cause of injury, whether or not it is active or resolved, the patient's comorbidities, and other confounding factors make it highly difficult to prognosticate in broad groups. Individual prognostication requires expert clinical judgement, a thorough and up-to-date understanding of the current literature, and an ability to apply the relevant literature to the patient at hand. Most of the statistics in the prognosis of disorders of consciousness comes from studies looking at patients with either traumatic brain injury or anoxic-ischemic injury, typically in the setting of a cardiac arrest. Clinicians must be exceptionally careful when trying to apply these statistics to patients with other mechanisms of injury. Clinicians are also cautioned on the limitations and the low quality of the current neurologic prognostication studies for comatose survivors of cardiac arrest [47], especially in the era of targeted temperature management where neurologic findings and drug metabolism are significantly altered.

As alluded earlier in this chapter, emerging evidence suggests that covert consciousness may be present in 15–20% of patients with disorders of consciousness and these patients have a better functional recovery 1 year post-injury. Detection of these patients is currently done through fMRI and task-based EEG studies, and the use of these technologies is not widespread at this time. The JFK Coma Recovery Scale – Revised (CRS-R) is the most widely used behavioral assessment tool for detecting consciousness in subacute and chronic disorders of consciousness [48]. The current literature suggests multiple CRS-R examinations can optimize the detection of volitional behaviors. Ongoing longitudinal research using the CRS-R is attempting to characterize the long-term outcomes of patients in different disorders of consciousness.

Our recommendation for clinicians attempting to prognosticate recovery for patients with disorders of consciousness is to evaluate the specific up-to-date literature for their patients based on the specific etiology of the state, the syndrome seen at bedside, and the timepoint from injury. We discourage the extrapolation of findings to other populations that were not identical to the ones specifically studied. Further useful information from a variety of tests such as MRI imaging, EEG activity, and if possible task-based functional diagnostic studies can help assist the clinician in formulating a reasonable prognosis.

Treatment of Chronic Disorders of Consciousness

The management of patients with disorders of consciousness secondary to catastrophic brain injuries remains a challenging issue particularly in regard to the limited therapeutic options currently available. Different treatments, pharmacological and non-pharmacological, have been investigated for patients with disorders of consciousness including coma (where there is no wakefulness, reflex behaviors only), unresponsive wakefulness syndrome (UWS, previously known as vegetative state, where there is wakefulness but reflex behaviors only), and minimally conscious state (MCS, where there is clinical demonstration of signs of consciousness). Promisingly, new clinical and neuroimaging data have suggested a potential benefit of treatment for prolonged disorder of consciousness even years after the brain injury. However, despite the multitude of treatments tested, only few have been proven of limited efficacy in improving arousal. Extensive reviews of available treatment have been published elsewhere.

Pharmacological Intervention

Various drugs including amantadine (dopamine agonist and NMDA antagonist) [49–54], apomorphine (a nonselective dopamine agonist with a high affinity for D2 receptors) [55–57], intrathecal baclofen (GABA agonist) [58], zolpidem (non-benzodiazepine GABA agonist) [55, 59–63], midazolam (benzodiazepine GABA agonist), and ziconotide (calcium channel blocker) and most recently psychedelics [64, 65] have been used to improve consciousness and functional recovery in patients with disorders of consciousness.

Neurostimulants, like amantadine, are provided to enhance neural transmission by increasing the synaptic concentration of dopamine, serotonin, and noradrenaline in various brain regions. The effects of neurostimulants include enhanced arousal, wakefulness, awareness, attention, memory, mental processing speed, and/or motor processing speed. In a large class II ran-

domized controlled trial, amantadine (up to 200 mg twice a day) accelerated the pace of functional recovery during active treatment in 184 patients with disorders of consciousness secondary to traumatic brain injury (TBI) [51]. Based on these findings, the American Practice Guidelines for patients with disorder of consciousness published in 2018 only recommends amantadine for patients with UWS and MCS between 4 and 16 weeks after a TBI [50]. Few case reports have also reported clinical improvement with amantadine in patients with disorder of consciousness secondary to causes other than TBI. The administration of one or more neurostimulants (i.e., amantadine, bromocriptine, levodopa, methylphenidate, and modafinil) has also been evaluated in a retrospective cohort study of patients with disorders of consciousness of various etiologies; however, it did not result in a meaningful improvement.

Zolpidem has been shown to modulate the thalamocortical connectivity through the disinhibition of the thalamus by acting on the globus pallidus interna and, consequently, promotes the recovery of consciousness. Zolpidem demonstrated improvement of consciousness and functional recovery in around 5% of patients [55, 59–63].

Non-pharmacological Intervention

- Invasive brain stimulation (i.e., deep brain stimulation or vagal nerve stimulation)
- Noninvasive brain stimulation [i.e., transcranial direct current stimulation (TDCS), repeated transcranial magnetic stimulation, transcutaneous auricular vagal nerve stimulation, and low-intensity focused ultrasound pulse]
- Sensory stimulation programs

Of the noninvasive techniques, TDCS has shown the most promising results. TDCS is a neuromodulation technique that can modulate cortical excitability through the application of a weak (usually ≤2 mA) direct current through the brain between two electrodes. It has been suggested that the underlying mechanisms by which TDCS can influence cortical activity and act on neuroplasticity depend on membrane potential changes as well as modulations of NMDA receptor efficacy.

TDCS applied over the dorsolateral prefrontal cortex induced some clinical improvement in five randomized controlled trials (four class III and one class II evidence) in patients in MCS from TBI and non-TBI etiologies [66].

Sensory stimulation programs include, among others, motor-based therapy, auditory-based training, music therapy, and multisensory training programs. Only one double-blind randomized controlled trial has been done on sensory stimulations, showing that auditory stimulations could speed up recovery in patients with prolonged disorders of consciousness [67].

In conclusion, several randomized controlled trials have been done, but only two of them support amantadine as a pharmacological treatment and transcranial direct current stimulation as non-pharmacological treatment with class II evidence of clinical improvement in patients with chronic disorder of consciousness. Large double-blind randomized controlled trials are still needed to confirm possible therapeutic effects of other interventions, particularly to better define the phenotype of potential good candidates to these treatments and to identify a set of biomarkers that correlate with treatment response.

Brain Death

Clinical Determination of Brain Death/Death by Neurological Criteria

The advancement of cardiopulmonary resuscitation techniques has extended "life," and the concept of brain death has emerged – where there is cessation of all brain functions within an artificially maintained cardiorespiratory physiology. Catastrophic brain injuries lead to irreversible compromise of neurological function and consequent brain death. The idea of brain death was first recognized in 1959 as "coma dépassé" and subsequently clinically defined as "brain death" in 1968 by the Harvard Brain Death Criteria [68, 69]. The Uniform Determination of Death Act in 1981 legally established brain death in the United States as "irreversible cessation of all functions of the entire brain, including the brain stem [70]."

Determination of brain death by establishing cessation of neurologic function should be consistent and uniform. In 1995, the American Academy of Neurology Practice Parameter (AANPP) published guidelines on how to determine brain death in the adult patients. These guidelines were subsequently revised in 2010 in order to improve adherence [71]. The brain death standards for adults and children that are widely accepted by the medical profession are the following guidelines, the American Academy of Neurology (AAN)'s 2010 Evidence-Based Guideline Update: Determining Brain Death in Adults and the 2011 Guidelines for the Determination of Brain Death in Infants and Children, published by the Pediatric Section of the Society of Critical Care Medicine, the Sections of Neurology and Critical Care of the American Academy of Pediatrics, and the Child Neurology Society [72].

Most recently, the World Brain Death Project recently formulated a consensus declaration of recommendations on determination of brain death or death by neurological criteria (BD/DNC). These recommendations have been endorsed by international societies to improve consistency in BD/DNC determination within and between countries and to diminish confusion and variability on the worldwide acceptance of BD/DNC as synonym of human death [73–75].

Despite the efforts made in standardizing determination of BD/DNC, research continued to highlight variability in hospital policy and documentation as well as lack of training in healthcare providers when determining brain death. The lack of specificity in most states' laws, coupled with inconsistency among brain death protocols in medical facilities, has contributed to differing interpretations by the courts in a few high-profile cases [76, 77]. Improvement of medical knowledge of brain death determination and the implementation of specific uniform laws, policies, and practices across the country for the determination of brain death are critically important and have been advocated by the scientific community to provide the highest-quality patient-centered neurologic and end-of-life care. To respond to the need for programs that train and credential physicians in the determination of brain death, the Neurocritical Care Society (NCS) recently developed a brain death toolkit [https://www.pathlms.com/ncs-ondemand/courses/1223].

Proposed Brain Death Protocol

Absolute Prerequisites BD/DNC is characterized by the irreversible and complete absence of all brain functions (determined on neurological examination as thoroughly described in the preceding paragraphs). BD/DNC is a clinical diagnosis; because of the implications and consequences of this diagnosis, a conservative approach and criteria are recommended.

(i) It is imperative for a diagnosis of BD/DNC to be considered that such a catastrophic CNS injury is identified, and all possible confounders, metabolic and toxic causes, that may mimic BD/DNC are excluded.
(ii) Neuroimaging findings are consistent with a catastrophic brain injury.
(iii) The person should have a core temperature of ≥36 °C, as defined by esophageal, bladder, rectal, or central venous or arterial catheter temperature measurements that can be achieved with available warming devices as needed.
(iv) Adults should have a systolic blood pressure of at least 100 mm Hg, or a mean arterial pressure of at least 60 mm Hg, that can be achieved with use of vascular volume, vasopressors, and/or inotropes as needed.
(v) Confounders should be eliminated or corrected if possible:
   • Pharmacological paralysis
   • CNS depressant drugs
   • Severe metabolic, acid-base, and endocrine derangements that could affect the examination
(vi) No spontaneous respirations are observed.
(vii) Clinician should be cautions and allow for an adequate observation period before BD/DNC testing. A minimum of 24 h is recommended specifically for anoxic brain injury

after resuscitated cardiac arrest, while no recommended observation time has been established for other etiologies.

Neurological Examination Determination of BD/DNC can be done with a clinical examination that demonstrates coma, brainstem areflexia, and apnea. The number of clinical examinations required to pronounce BD/DNC varies according to age, hospital, state, or country and generally ranges from one to three. A single examination, including apnea testing, is the minimum standard for determination of BD/DNC for adults. Of note, if two examinations are required to declare death, the time of death is the time that the second examination is completed either by neurological examination or with ancillary tests.

The neurological evaluation for determination of BD/DNC includes an assessment for coma and an evaluation for brainstem areflexia to demonstrate that:

(i) Pupils are fixed in a midsize or dilated position and are nonreactive to light.
(ii) The corneal, oculocephalic, and oculovestibular reflexes are absent.
(iii) There is no facial movement to noxious cranial stimulation (stimuli at supraorbital nerve, temporomandibular joint).
(iv) The gag reflex is absent to bilateral posterior pharyngeal stimulation.
(v) The cough reflex is absent to deep tracheal suctioning.
(vi) There is no brain-mediated motor response to noxious stimulation of the limbs (spinally mediated reflexes are permissible).

Only if all the prior points are consistent with BD/DNC it is possible to proceed with the apnea test. If any aspect of the clinical examination cannot be completed, but to the extent completed and is consistent with BD/DNC, ancillary testing is recommended.

Apnea Test The goal of the apnea test is to challenge the medullary drive of respiration. As part of the apnea test, the patient is disconnected from the ventilator, after being preoxygenated with a following increase in serum carbon dioxide and a decrease in the central nervous system pH to levels that would normally maximally stimulate the respiratory centers in a functioning medulla. If the medullary function is absent because permanently injured, there will be no respiratory effort in response to profound hypercarbia and acidosis.

Prior to the initiation of the apnea test, the SBP should be at least 100 mm Hg or the MAP be at least 60 mm Hg in adults (and above age-appropriate targets in pediatrics); temperature should be at least 36 °C. Before disconnecting the ventilator, the person should be preoxygenated with 100% O2 for at least 10 min, and the minute ventilation should be adjusted to establish normocarbia ($PaCO_2$ of 35–45 mm Hg [4.7–6.0 kPa]), confirmed by a pretest arterial blood gas. The use of CPAP/PEEP (continuous positive airway pressure/positive end-expiratory pressure) can help prevent de-recruitment and decrease the risk of cardiopulmonary instability. Oxygen can also be delivered via placement of a tracheal cannula.

An arterial blood gas should be drawn at 8–10 min after the initiation of the test; then the patient should be reconnected to the ventilator. The apnea test, to be positive, targets a pH less than 7.30 and $PaCO_2$ of at least 60 mm Hg (8.0 kPa) unless a patient has preexisting hypercapnia, in which case it should be at least 20 mm Hg (2.7 kPa) above their baseline $PaCO_2$, if known.

The apnea test should be aborted if:

- Spontaneous respirations are observed.
- Systolic blood pressure becomes lower than 100 mm Hg, or mean arterial pressure becomes lower than 60 mm Hg despite titration of fluids/inotropes/vasopressors.
- There is sustained oxygen desaturation below 85%.
- An unstable arrhythmia occurs.

When BD/DNC can be determined by the above-described neurologic examination – without ancillary tests – the time of death is the time the arterial $PaCO_2$ reaches the target during the apnea test as reported by the laboratory.

Ancillary Testing Ancillary tests consist of blood flow studies and electrophysiologic studies, and they are meant to support the clinical diagnosis of BD/DNC. These tests are typically used when any part of the clinical examination, including the apnea test, for any reasons, cannot be completed [78]. Also, ancillary tests should be considered when there are confounding factors that remain of uncertain interpretation (i.e., observed movements likely expression of spinal reflexes). If ancillary tests are performed, the time of death is documented as the time that the ancillary test results are formally interpreted and documented by the attending physician.

Blood Flow Studies
- Digital subtraction angiography/conventional four-vessel angiography remains the reference standard of ancillary testing. Absence of contrast within the intracranial arterial vessels, where the internal carotid and vertebral arteries enter the skull base, with a patent external carotid circulation, is consistent with BD/DNC with the highest diagnostic accuracy (both sensitivity and specificity are 100%). Four-vessel angiography is invasive and requires contrast and patient transport and equipment and operator dependence limit its routine use.
- Radionuclide angiography is another neuroimaging technique where absence of radiologic activity upon imaging of the intracranial vault is consistent with BD/DNC. This test can be done at bedside and does not require contrast; however, it provides limited evaluation of brainstem, is of limited availability, and has low specificity.
- Radionuclide perfusion scintigraphy imaging, of this SPECT (single-photon emission com-

puted tomography), is preferred over perfusion scintigraphy planar imaging as the latter has limited accuracy at the brainstem. These studies should illustrate absence of intracranial isotope in order to make a determination of BD/DNC.

- Transcranial Doppler (TCD) ultrasonography is as an alternative to conventional four-vessel cerebral angiography or scintigraphy. When used it is recommended that at least two examinations are performed at least 30 min apart to make a diagnosis of cerebral circulatory arrest. The examinations should be done bilaterally, anteriorly, and posteriorly to include both internal carotid arteries as well as the vertebrobasilar circulation. Biphasic oscillating flow and systolic spikes with reversal of flow in diastole are consistent with BD/DNC on TCD. Despite the advantage of being easily done at the bedside and being noninvasive, TCD is operator dependent; 10–20% of patients have no acoustic windows. TCD should not be used in pediatrics in the absence of validation studies.
- Computed tomography angiography (CTA) and magnetic resonance angiography (MRA) should not be used to support a diagnosis of cerebral circulatory arrest at present, pending further research that could confirm their diagnostic accuracy.

Electrophysiologic Studies

- Electroencephalogram (EEG). The most recent consensus document on BD/DNC determination suggested EEG to no longer be used routinely as an ancillary test in adults, unless required by regional laws or policy or when other tests may not be reliable (craniovascular impedance has been affected by an open skull fracture, decompressive craniectomy, or an open fontanelle/sutures in infants). EEG is limited by potential confounding factors and has limited brainstem assessment and great interobserver variability. Indeed, given the limitations of EEG for evaluating brainstem function, when used as an ancillary test it should be used in conjunction with somatosensory and brainstem auditory evoked potentials. No detectable electrical activity ($\geq 2\ \mu V$) over a 30-min period of EEG recording is considered consistent with BD/DNC.

- Somatosensory evoked potentials (SSEP). SSEP can be performed noninvasively at bedside. Bilateral absence of any electrical transmission through the brainstem and cerebrum in the setting of an intact signal in the brachial plexus and spinal cord has a limited specificity as an isolated test. SSEP be confounded by cervical spinal cord injury, isolated brainstem lesions, sedation, and hypothermia.

- Auditory and visual evoked potentials. Bilateral absence of waveforms through the brainstem to auditory and visual cortex is consistent with BD/DNC. However, as these evoked potentials are limited to the auditory and visual cortex and as these signals can be possibly confounded in cases of eighth nerve or brainstem lesions or retinal or optic nerve lesions, their utility as an isolated test is somewhat limited [79].

Specific Protocols Different protocols for those receiving therapeutic hypothermia and for those receiving extracorporeal membrane oxygenation (ECMO) have been recommended as these situations can pose specific challenges for the correct execution of the BD/DNC determination.

Therapeutic hypothermia or targeted temperature management (TTM), most commonly used after resuscitated cardiac arrest, can blunt brainstem reflexes and alter pharmacokinetics and pharmacodynamics resulting in delayed drug elimination in sedated patients. This poses a challenge when determining BD/DNC as one of the prerequisites is a core temperature of $\geq 36\ °C$. There is no standard on how long it is necessary to wait after treatment with therapeutic hypothermia before BD/DNC can be determined. Neuroimaging should be obtained after rewarming from TTM if the clinical exam appears consistent with BD/DNC to assess for severe cerebral edema and brainstem herniation. At 24 h after rewarming to a core temperature of $\geq 36\ °C$, recent administration of CNS-depressing medications should be assessed; if absent, BD/DNC testing can be initialed. If present, there are two recommended options:

(a) BD/DNC testing is *initiated*, and if the clinical exam is consistent with brain death, then ancillary tests are obtained.
(b) BD/DNC testing is *delayed* for a certain time for drug levels or drug half-lives to clear in consideration of renal/hepatic dysfunction (≥ 5 half-lives for all CNS-depressing medications).

ECMO is a life-support modality used in patients with refractory cardiac and/or respiratory failure.

Patients requiring ECMO and other forms of extracorporeal support are at high risk of complications leading to irreversible brain injury and BD/DNC, and in these patients BD/DNC determination becomes even more relevant given the artificial circulatory support prevents arrest of circulation. In general, the criteria for BD/DNC determination in patients receiving ECMO are not different from those not on ECMO, and all patients receiving ECMO should meet the absolute prerequisite, undergo the clinical exam and the apnea test, and should have the same apnea testing targets and indications for ancillary tests as previously described. However, veno-arterial ECMO is particularly problematic in this regard because it provides both gas exchange and circulatory support. CO2 elimination by ECMO prevents hypercapnia, which is required to perform an apnea test. Previous literature has shown great variability and inconsistency in determining BD/DNC in patients on ECMO.

The World Brain Death Project Consensus statement has recently provided recommendations on BD/DNC determination in patients receiving veno-arterial ECMO for circulatory and respiratory support. These recommendations are relative to certain specific aspects of BD/DNC determination that in patients receiving ECMO support are specifically challenging and are summarized below.

Recommendations on BD/DNC determination in V-A ECMO:

- The extracorporeal blood flow is maintained at all times during the BD/DNC determination in order to prevent hemodynamic instability and provide a MAP ≥ 60 mm Hg in adults (veno-arterial ECMO flow rates may be increased to support the MAP).
- A period of preoxygenation before the apnea test of at least 10 min should be provided for all patients receiving ECMO by administering 100% inspired oxygen via the mechanical ventilator and increasing the O2 in the membrane lung from the ECMO machine.
- During the apnea test in patients receiving ECMO, 100% oxygen is delivered to the lungs via CPAP on the mechanical ventilator or via a resuscitation bag with a functioning PEEP valve, or as oxygen flow via a tracheal cannula. If the patient being evaluated for BD/DNC is not mechanically ventilated during ECMO to maintain oxygenation during the apnea test, 100% oxygen will be provided in the sweep gas. If oxygenation cannot be maintained, the test should be aborted, and ancillary tests should be performed.
- In cases of veno-arterial ECMO with intrinsic cardiac output, arterial blood gases should be measured simultaneously from the distal arterial line and post-oxygenator ECMO circuit. The apnea test targets for both sampling sites should be pH < 7.30 and PaCO2 of at least 60 mm Hg (20 mm Hg above the patient's baseline PaCO2 for persons with preexisting hypercapnia).
- Oxygen should be maintained in the membrane lung at 100% throughout the duration of the apnea test.
- The sweep gas flow rate can be titrated to 0.5–1.0 L/min while maintaining oxygenation.
- Spontaneous breathing should be observed while targeting traditional apnea test targets via serial blood gases keeping in mind that achieving a pH less than 7.30 and PaCO2 $\geq$ 60 mm Hg (20 mm Hg above the patient's baseline PaCO2 for patients with preexisting hypercapnia) may take longer than in a person without ECMO support.
- The test should be immediately terminated if spontaneous respiratory movements are observed or hemodynamic instability occurs.

- Mechanical ventilation should be restarted with the prior ECMO sweep gas flow rate when the pH reaches less than 7.30 and PaCO2 reaches 60 mm Hg (20 mm Hg above their baseline PaCO2 if there is premorbid hypercapnia).

If the apnea test cannot be safely conducted or completed, an ancillary test should always be considered.

References

1. Posner JB, Plum F. Plum and Posner's diagnosis of stupor and coma. 4th ed. Oxford: Oxford University Press; 2007.
2. Laureys S, Celesia GG, Cohadon F, et al. Unresponsive wakefulness syndrome: a new name for the vegetative state or apallic syndrome. BMC Med. 2010;8:68.
3. Giacino S, Ashwal N, Childs R, Cranford B, Jennett DI, Katz JP, Kelly JH, Rosenberg J, Whyte RD, et al. The minimally conscious state. Neurology. 2002;58(3):349–53.
4. Thibaut A, Bodien YG, Laureys S, Giacino JT. Minimally conscious state "plus": diagnostic criteria and relation to functional recovery. J Neurol. 2020;267:1245–54.
5. Owen AM, Coleman MR, Boly M, Davis MH, Laureys S, Pickard JD. Detecting awareness in the vegetative state. Science. 2006;313:1402.
6. Monti MM, Vanhaudenhuyse A, Coleman MR, Boly M, Pickard JD, Tshibanda L, et al. Willful modulation of brain activity in disorders of consciousness. N Engl J Med. 2010;362:579–89.
7. Edlow BL, Claassen J, Schiff ND, Greer DM. Recovery from disorders of consciousness: mechanisms, prognosis and emerging therapies. Nat Rev Neurol. 2020;14:1–22.
8. Claasen J, Doyle K, Matory Am Couch C, et al. Detection of brain activation in unresponsive patients with acute brain injury. N Engl J Med. 2019;380:2497–505.
9. Steriade M. Corticothalamic resonance, states of vigilance and mentation. Neuroscience. 2000;101(2):243–76.
10. Llinas RR, Steriade M. Bursting of thalamic neurons and states of vigilance. J Neurophysiol. 2006;95(6):3297–308.
11. Hoesch RE, Koenig MA, Geocadin RG. Coma after global ischemic brain injury: pathophysiology and emerging therapies. Crit Care Clin. 2008;24(1):25–44. vii–viii
12. Lindsley DB, Schreiner LH, Knowles WB, Magoun HW. Behavioral and EEG changes following chronic brain stem lesions in the cat. Electroencephalogr Clin Neurophysiol. 1950;2(4):483–98.
13. Jones BE. Arousal systems. Front Biosci. 2003;8:s438–51.
14. Starzl TE, Taylor CW, Magoun HW. Ascending conduction in reticular activating system, with special reference to the diencephalon. J Neurophysiol. 1951;14(6):461–77.
15. Steriade M, Oakson G, Ropert N. Firing rates and patterns of midbrain reticular neurons during steady and transitional states of the sleep-waking cycle. Exp Brain Res. 1982;46(1):37–51.
16. Jones EG. Thalamic circuitry and thalamocortical synchrony. Philos Trans R Soc Lond Ser B Biol Sci. 2002;357(1428):1659–73.
17. Groenewegen HJ, Berendse HW. The specificity of the 'nonspecific' midline and intralaminar thalamic nuclei. Trends Neurosci. 1994;17(2):52–7.
18. Lin JS, Sakai K, Vanni-Mercier G, Jouvet M. A critical role of the posterior hypothalamus in the mechanisms of wakefulness determined by microinjection of muscimol in freely moving cats. Brain Res. 1989;479(2):225–40.
19. Panula P, Yang HY, Costa E. Histamine-containing neurons in the rat hypothalamus. Proc Natl Acad Sci U S A. 1984;81(8):2572–6.
20. Jin CY, Kalimo H, Panula P. The histaminergic system in human thalamus: correlation of innervation to receptor expression. Eur J Neurosci. 2002;15(7):1125–38.
21. Alexandre C, Andermann ML, Scammell TE. Control of arousal by the orexin neurons. Curr Opin Neurobiol. 2013;23(5):752–9.
22. Peyron C, Tighe DK, van den Pol AN, de Lecea L, Heller HC, Sutcliffe JG, Kilduff TS. Neurons containing hypocretin (orexin) project to multiple neuronal systems. J Neurosci. 1998;18:9996–10015.
23. Saper CB, Scammell TE, Lu J. Hypothalamic regulation of sleep and circadian rhythms. Nature. 2005;437:1257–63.
24. Rye DB, Wainer BH, Mesulam MM, Mufson EJ, Saper CB. Cortical projections arising from the basal forebrain: a study of cholinergic and noncholinergic components employing combined retrograde tracing and immunohistochemical localization of choline acetyltransferase. Neuroscience. 1984;13(3):627–43.
25. Buzsaki G, Bickford RG, Ponomareff G, Thal LJ, Mandel R, Gage FH. Nucleus basalis and thalamic control of neocortical activity in the freely moving rat. J Neurosci. 1988;8(11):4007–26.
26. Szymusiak R, McGinty D. Sleep-related neuronal discharge in the basal forebrain of cats. Brain Res. 1986;370(1):82–92.
27. Hinchey J, Chaves C, Appignani B, Breen J, Pao L, Wang A, et al. A reversible posterior leukoencephalopathy syndrome. N Engl J Med. 1996;334(8):494–500.
28. McKinney AM, Jagadeesan BD, Truwit CL. Central-variant posterior reversible encephalopathy syndrome: brainstem or basal ganglia involvement lacking cortical or subcortical cerebral edema. AJR Am J Roentgenol. 2013;201:631–8.

29. Hinduja A. Posterior reversible encephalopathy syndrome: clinical features and outcome. Front Neurol. 2020;11:71.

30. Ishii M. Endocrine emergencies with neurological manifestations. Continuum (Minneap Minn). 2017;23(3):778–801.

31. Krause M, Hocker S. Toxin-induced coma and central nervous system depression. Neurol Clin. 2020;38(4):825–41.

32. McNicoll L, Pisani MA, Zhang Y, Ely EW, Siegel MD, Inouye SK. Delirium in the intensive care unit: occurrence and clinical course in older patients. J Am Geriatr Soc. 2003;51(5):591–8.

33. Volpi-Abadie J, Kaye AM, Kaye AD. Serotonin syndrome. Oschsner J. 2013;13(4):533–40.

34. Oruch R, Pryme IF, Engelsen BA, Lund A. Neuroleptic malignant syndrome; an easily overlooked medical emergency. Neuropsychiatr Dis Treat. 2017;13:161–75.

35. Venkatasubramanian C, Lopez GA, O'Phelan KH, et al. Emergency neurological life support: fourth edition, updates in the approach to early management of a neurological emergency. Neurocrit Care. 2020;32:636–40.

36. Fodstad H, Kelly PJ, Buchfelder M. History of the cushing reflex. Neurosurgery. 2006;59(5):1132–7. discussion 1137

37. Wijdicks EF, Bamlet WR, Maramattom BV, Manno EM, McClelland RL. Validation of a new coma scale: the FOUR score. Ann Neurol. 2005;58(4):585–93.

38. Iyer VN, Mandrekar JN, Danielson RD, Zubkov AY, Elmer JL, Wijdicks EF. Validity of the FOUR score coma scale in the medical intensive care unit. Mayo Clin Proc. 2009;84:694–701.

39. Anderson CS, Heeley E, Huang Y, Wang J, Stapf C, Delcourt C, INTERACT2 Investigators, et al. Rapid blood-pressure lowering in patients with acute intracerebral hemorrhage. N Engl J Med. 2013,368.2355–65.

40. Hemphill JC, Greenberg SM, Anderson CS, Becker K, Bendok BR, Cushman M, et al. American Heart Association Stroke Council; Council on Cardiovascular and Stroke Nursing; Council on Clinical Cardiology. Guidelines for the management of spontaneous intracerebral hemorrhage: a guideline for healthcare professionals from the American Heart Association/American Stroke Association. Stroke. 2015;46:2032–60.

41. Farrokh S, Cho SM, Lefebvre AT, Zink EK, Schiavi A, Puttgen HA. Use of intraosseous hypertonic saline in critically ill patients. J Vasc Access. 2019;20(4):427–32.

42. Qureshi AI, Geocadin RG, Suarez JI, Ulatowski JA. Long-term outcome after medical reversal of transtentorial herniation in patients with supratentorial mass lesions. Crit Care Med. 2000;28(5):1556–64.

43. Koenig MA, Bryan M, Lewin JL, Mirski MA, Geocadin RG, Stevens RD. Reversal of transtentorial herniation with hypertonic saline. Neurology. 2008;70(13):1023–9.

44. Brazis PW, Masdeu JC, Biller J. Localization in clinical neurology. 5th ed. Philadelphia: Lippincott Williams & Wilkins; 2007.

45. Liu GT, Ronthal M. Reflex blink to visual threat. J Clin Neuroophthalmol. 1992;12(1):47–56.

46. Baloh RW, Yee RD, Honrubia V. Optokinetic nystagmus and parietal lobe lesions. Ann Neurol. 1980;7(3):269–76.

47. Geocadin RG, Callaway CW, Fink EL, Golan E, Greer DM, Ko NU, Lang E, Licht DJ, Marino BS, McNair ND, Peberdy MA, Perman SM, Sims DB, Soar J, Sandroni C, American Heart Association Emergency Cardiovascular Care Committee. Standards for studies of neurological prognostication in comatose survivors of cardiac arrest: a scientific statement from the American Heart Association. Circulation. 2019;140(9):e517–42.

48. Giacino JT, Kalmar K, White J. The JFK coma recovery scale – revised: measurement characteristics and diagnostic utility. Arch Phys Med Rehabil. 2004;85(12):2020–9.

49. Thibaut A, Schiff N, Giacino J, Laureys S, Gosseries O. Therapeutic interventions in patients with prolonged disorders of consciousness. Lancet Neurol. 2019;18:600–14.

50. Giacino JT, Katz D, Schiff N, et al. Practice guideline update recommendations summary: disorders of consciousness. Neurology. 2018;91:450–60.

51. Giacino JT, Whyte J, Bagiella E, Kalmar K, Childs N, Khademi A, Eifert B, Long D, Katz DI, Cho S, Yablon SA, Luther M, Hammond FM, Nordenbo A, Novak P, Mercer W, Maurer-Karattup P, Sherer M. Placebo-controlled trial of amantadine for severe traumatic brain injury. N Engl J Med. 2012;366:819–26.

52. Schnakers C, Hustinx R, Vandewalle G, et al. Measuring the effect of amantadine in chronic anoxic minimally conscious state. J Neurol Neurosurg Psychiatry. 2008;79:225–7.

53. Estraneo A, Pascarella A, Moretta P, Loreto V, Trojano L. Clinical and electroencephalographic on–off effect of amantadine in chronic non-traumatic minimally conscious state. J Neurol. 2015;262:1584–6.

54. Herrold AA, Pape TLB, Guernon A, Mallinson T, Collins E, Jordan N. Prescribing multiple neurostimulants during rehabilitation for severe brain injury. Sci World J. 2014;2014:964578.

55. Gosseries O, Charland-Verville V, Thonnard M, Bodart O, Laureys S, Demertzi A. Amantadine, apomorphine and zolpidem in the treatment of disorders of consciousness. Curr Pharm Des. 2014;20:4167–84.

56. Fridman EA, Calvar J, Bonetto M, Gamzu E, Krimchansky BZ, Meli F, et al. Fast awakening from minimally conscious state with apomorphine. Brain Inj. 2009;23:172–7.

57. Fridman EA, Krimchansky BZ, Bonetto M, Galperin T, Gamzu ER, Leiguarda RC, et al. Continuous subcutaneous apomorphine for severe disorders of consciousness after traumatic brain injury. Brain Inj. 2010;24:636–461.

58. Margetis K, Korfias SI, Gatzonis S, et al. Intrathecal baclofen associated with improvement of consciousness disorders in spasticity patients. Neuromodulation. 2014;17:699–704.

59. Whyte J, Rajan R, Rosenbaum A, et al. Zolpidem and restoration of consciousness. Am J Phys Med Rehabil. 2014;93:101–13.

60. Machado C, Estevez M, Rodriguez R, et al. Zolpidem arousing effect in persistent vegetative state patients: autonomic, EEG and behavioral assessment. Curr Pharm Des. 2014;20:4185–202.

61. Calabrò RS, Aricò I, De Salvo S, Conti-Nibali V, Bramanti P. Transient awakening from vegetative state: is high-dose zolpidem more effective? Psychiatry Clin Neurosci. 2015;69:122–3.

62. Thonnard M, Gosseries O, Demertzi A, et al. Effect of zolpidem in chronic disorders of consciousness: a prospective open-label study. Funct Neurol. 2014;28:259–64.

63. Williams ST, Conte MM, Goldfine AM, et al. Common resting brain dynamics indicate a possible mechanism underlying zolpidem response in severe brain injury. elife. 2013;2:e01157.

64. Scott G, Carhart-Harris RL. Psychedelics as a treatment for disorders of consciousness. Neurosci Conscious. 2019;2019:niz003.

65. Varley TF, Carhart-Harris R, Roseman L, Menon DK, Stamatakis EA. Serotonergic psychedelics LSD & psilocybin increase the fractal dimension of cortical brain activity in spatial and temporal domains. NeuroImage. 2020;220:117049. https://doi.org/10.1016/j.neuroimage.2020.117049.

66. Thibaut A, Bruno M-A, Ledoux D, Demertzi A, Laureys S. tDCS in patients with disorders of consciousness: sham-controlled randomized double-blind study. Neurology. 2014;82:1112–8.

67. Pape TL-B, Rosenow JM, Harton B, et al. Preliminary framework for Familiar Auditory Sensory Training (FAST) provided during coma recovery. J Rehabil Res Dev. 2012;49:1137.

68. Mollaret P, Goulon M. Le coma depasse. Rev Neurol (Paris). 1959;101:3–15.

69. A definition of irreversible coma: report of the Ad Hoc Committee of the Harvard Medical School to Examine the Definition of Brain Death. JAMA. 1968;205:337–40.

70. President's Commission for the Study of Ethical Problems in Medicine and Biomedical Behavioral Research. Defining Death: A Report on the Medical, Legal and Ethical Issues in the Determination of Death. President's Council on Bioethics; 1981.

71. The Quality Standards Subcommittee of the American Academy of Neurology. Practice parameters for determining brain death in adults (summary statement). Neurology. 1995;45(5):1012–4.

72. Wijdicks EFM, Varelas PN, Gronseth GS, Greer DM. Evidence-based guideline update: determining brain death in adults—report of the quality standards subcommittee of the American Academy of Neurology. Neurology. 2010;74(23):1911–8.

73. Greer DM, Varelas PN, Haque S, Wijdicks EFM. Variability of brain death determination guidelines in leading US neurologic institutions. Neurology. 2008;70(4):284–9.

74. Greer DM, Shemie SD, Lewis A, Torrance S, Varelas P, Goldenberg FD, Bernat JL, Souter M, Topcuoglu MA, Alexandrov AW, Baldisseri M, Bleck T, Citerio G, Dawson R, Hoppe A, Jacobe S, Manara A, Nakagawa TA, Pope TM, Silvester W, Thomson D, Al Rahma H, Badenes R, Baker AJ, Cerny V, Chang C, Chang TR, Gnedovskaya E, Han MK, Honeybul S, Jimenez E, Kuroda Y, Liu G, Mallick UK, Marquevich V, Mejia-Mantilla J, Piradov M, Quayyum S, Shrestha GS, Su YY, Timmons SD, Teitelbaum J, Videtta W, Zirpe K, Sung G. Determination of brain death/death by neurologic criteria: the world brain death project. JAMA. 2020;324:1078–97.

75. Lewis A, Bakkar A, Kreiger-Benson E, Kumpfbeck A, Liebman J, Shemie SD, Sung G, Torrance S, Greer D. Determination of death by neurologic criteria around the world. Neurology. 2020;95:e299–309.

76. Machado C. Brain death: a reappraisal. New York: Springer Science+Business Media, LLC; 2007.

77. Machado C. Jahi McMath: a new state of disorder of consciousness. J Neurosurg Sci. 2021;65(2):211–3.

78. Walter U, Fernandez-Torre JL, Kirschstein T, Laureys S. When is "brainstem death" brain death? The case for ancillary testing in primary infratentorial brain lesion. Clin Neurophysiol. 2018;129:2451–65.

79. Machado C. Multimodality evoked potentials and electroretinography in a test battery for an early diagnosis of brain death. J Neurosurg Sci. 1993;37:125–31.

18

Laura M. Tormoehlen

Toxin-Induced Hyperthermic Syndromes

General Considerations

Regulation of body temperature is a balance between the production and dissipation of heat. Toxin-induced hyperthermia occurs when heat production is increased or the body's ability to dissipate heat is impaired [1]. The complex process of thermoregulation is regulated by hypothalamic control of the sympathetic nervous system and by mitochondrial oxidative phosphorylation. Serotonin and sympathomimetic syndromes cause hyperthermia via heat generation from increased motor activity, as well as impaired dissipation from vasoconstriction of cutaneous blood vessels [1]. Anticholinergic syndrome causes hyperthermia by muscarinic inhibition, resulting in impaired sweating in the setting of severe agitation and hyperactivity. Severe salicylate toxicity results in hyperthermia via uncoupling of oxidative phosphorylation. Withdrawal of gamma-aminobutyric acid (GABA) agonists, including ethanol, benzodiazepines, barbiturates, baclofen, and gamma-hydroxybutyrate (GHB), can cause hyperthermia via autonomic overstimulation.

L. M. Tormoehlen (✉)
Neurology and Emergency Medicine, Indiana University School of Medicine,
Indianapolis, IN, USA
e-mail: laumjone@iupui.edu

Serotonin Syndrome

Introduction

The serotonin syndrome was first defined by Sternbach in 1991 [2], although the clinical manifestations of the syndrome were described in patients taking monoamine oxidase inhibitors (MAOIs) and tryptophan in 1960 [3]. Serotonin syndrome is typically characterized by mental status changes, autonomic instability, and motor hyperactivity. The practitioner must have a high level of suspicion for this diagnosis, as the altered mental status often precludes a reliable history and many patients present without one or more of the cardinal findings [2]. In addition, symptoms of mild or early serotonin syndrome such as diarrhea, tremor, and irritability may be overlooked, and thus the causative medications may not be discontinued. The severe complications of serotonin syndrome include seizures, rhabdomyolysis, respiratory failure, and cardiac arrhythmia.

Epidemiology

Serotonin syndrome occurs most often when two or more proserotonergic medications are used in combination [2, 4]. It is difficult to determine the true incidence of this syndrome, as the majority of cases remain unrecognized [5]. Symptoms of moderate-to-severe toxicity occur in 17% of patients who overdose on selective serotonin reuptake inhibitors (SSRIs), and death occurs in 0.2% [6]. In a survey of consecutive admissions to an inpatient toxicology unit, serotonin syndrome

K. L. Roos (ed.), *Emergency Neurology*, https://doi.org/10.1007/978-3-030-75778-6_18

occurred in 14% of patients with overdose of a single SSRI [7]. In patients taking nefazodone, the incidence of two or more symptoms of serotonin syndrome is 0.4 cases per 1000 treatment-months [5].While this syndrome more commonly arises from drug-drug interactions of two or more different serotonergic drugs, serotonin syndrome occurred with a single agent in 40% of patients in a pharmacovigilance database [8, 9]. A large number of pharmaceuticals have been reported in association with serotonin syndrome, and caution must be exercised when prescribing a new pro-serotonergic medication to patients already taking another [10]. The major drug categories implicated are SSRI/SNRIs, MAOIs, tricyclic antidepressants (TCAs), antimicrobials, opioid analgesics, antiemetics, migraine rescue therapies, drugs of abuse, and herbal supplements.

Pathophysiology

Serotonin, or 5-hydroxytryptamine (5-HT), is synthesized by hydroxylation and decarboxylation of L-tryptophan. After vesicular release from neurons, serotonin is removed from the synapse by the serotonin reuptake transporter (SERT). The first step in serotonin metabolism is deamination, preferentially performed by monoamine oxidase type A, to 5-hydroxyindoleacetic acid (5-HIAA). There are seven subgroups of serotonin receptors, and serotonin syndrome is likely a combination of effects at several of these individual receptor types. However, activity of $5-HT_{2A}$ receptors is characterized by hyperactivity of both central and peripheral serotonergic neurons. In the central nervous system, serotonergic neurons are located mainly in the midline raphe nuclei of the brainstem [11]. These structures are involved in thermoregulation, wakefulness, muscle tone, and chemoreceptor-mediated emesis. Serotonergic receptors are abundant in the peripheral nervous system and are responsible for gastrointestinal motility and vascular smooth muscle tone [12]. The function of serotonergic neurons in the central and peripheral nervous systems correlates directly with the clinical features of serotonin syndrome: cognitive dysfunction, autonomic instability (hyperthermia, hypertension, diarrhea), and motor hyperactivity.

The possible mechanisms of increased serotonergic activity are (1) increased serotonin synthesis, (2) increased serotonin release, (3) direct serotonin receptor agonism, (4) inhibition of serotonin reuptake, and (5) decreased serotonin metabolism. There are xenobiotics that may cause serotonin syndrome by each of these mechanisms. By example, tryptophan supplementation results in increased serotonin synthesis. Amphetamines cause increased serotonin release [13–15]. The triptans [16] and lysergic acid diethylamide are serotonin receptor agonists. The SSRI/SNRIs, TCAs, trazodone/vilazodone [17, 18], bupropion [19, 20], tramadol [21–26] and cocaine inhibit serotonin reuptake, and the MAOIs, methylene blue [27–37], and linezolid [38–41] decrease serotonin metabolism. Some drugs, such as bromocriptine and lithium, are thought to cause a nonspecific increase in serotonin activity. Some drugs may cause multiple pro-serotonergic effects; for example, fentanyl provokes an increase in serotonin release and also acts as an agonist at some 5-HT receptors [25, 26, 42, 43]. In addition, fentanyl is one of the most common causes of in-hospital development of this syndrome [44]. Serotonin syndrome is caused by an acute increase in intrasynaptic serotonin and is a drug reaction for which all patients taking pro-serotonergic medications are at risk [45]. Very limited autopsy data demonstrates loss of cerebellar Purkinje and granule cells [46].

Clinical Features/Diagnosis

The original diagnostic criteria proposed by Sternbach [2] require the addition or titration of a serotonergic agent, without a recent addition or titration of a neuroleptic (antipsychotic) medication, and three of the following clinical findings: altered mental status, agitation, myoclonus, hyperreflexia, diaphoresis, shivering, tremor, diarrhea, incoordination, and fever. Other possible etiologies, including infection and withdrawal, must be excluded. Similar, revised criteria were proposed by Radomski in 2000 [47].

In 2003, the Hunter Serotonin Toxicity Criteria were published in a comparison study to the Sternbach criteria in a retrospective analysis of prospectively collected data. The Hunter criteria allows the diagnosis of serotonin syndrome with the administration of a serotonergic agent within the past 5 weeks and any one of the following: (1) spontaneous clonus, (2) inducible clonus and agitation or diaphoresis, (3) ocular clonus and agitation or diaphoresis, (4) tremor and hyperreflexia, and (5) muscle rigidity and hyperthermia (>38 °C) and either ocular or inducible clonus. The Hunter criteria were somewhat more sensitive (84% vs. 75%) and nearly identical in specificity (97% vs. 96%) to the Sternbach criteria, although they have not been independently validated [48, 49]. The serotonin syndrome scale was developed to augment the Sternbach criteria by scoring based upon severity of symptoms [50]. Symptoms of motor hyperactivity, manifested by spontaneous, inducible, or ocular clonus, are the hallmark of serotonin toxicity [2, 3, 45, 51, 52]. Mydriasis occurs in more than 30% and tachycardia in 40% of patients with serotonin syndrome [48].

Serotonin syndrome represents a spectrum of symptoms (Fig. 18.1) and usually develops and progresses over a few hours. Individual patients with serotonin toxicity might not meet the Hunter, Radomski or Sternbach criteria for diagnosis. This is most likely to occur early in the course prior to the onset of more severe symptoms [50], or late in the course when muscle rigidity has become severe enough to prevent tremor or clonus [48]. Patients with life-threatening serotonin toxicity are more likely to have muscle rigidity and hyperthermia, and may require intubation if the rigidity causes respiratory compromise [48].

Differential Diagnosis

Neuroleptic malignant syndrome (NMS), malignant hyperthermia, sympathomimetic syndrome, anticholinergic syndrome, strychnine toxicity, tetanus, and salicylate toxicity are other toxicologic diagnoses to consider. Meningoencephalitis, stiff-person syndrome, nonconvulsive status epilepticus, hyperthyroidism, and sepsis also bear consideration in the differential diagnosis.

The symptom onset and progression of NMS is typically slower, occurring over days to weeks instead of hours. In addition, NMS is a hypokinetic syndrome characterized by bradykinesia and rigidity, whereas mild or moderate serotonin syndrome is a hyperkinetic syndrome. The rigidity of severe serotonin syndrome is usually more prominent in the lower extremities than in the upper extremities [53].

Serotonin syndrome, neuroleptic malignant syndrome, and malignant hyperthermia are all hyperthermic syndromes, but the causative medications are different. A comprehensive history regarding recent changes in medications can favor one diagnosis over another. Because of the medications involved in malignant hyperthermia, this syndrome is very unlikely to occur outside of the operating room. There is, unfortunately, no single laboratory test that will definitively and accurately distinguish between serotonin syndrome and NMS. Some basic laboratory studies, including CK, hepatic panel, white blood cell count, and iron levels may help differentiate NMS from serotonin syndrome [54]. There may

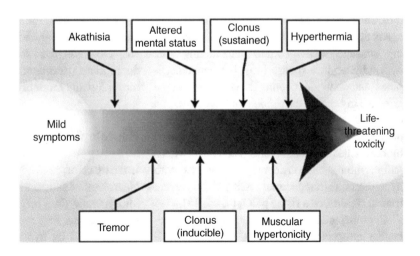

Fig. 18.1 Spectrum of clinical features of serotonin syndrome. (From Boyer and Shannon [4]. Copyright © 2005. Massachusetts Medical Society. Reprinted with permission from the Massachusetts Medical Society)

be differences in the levels of neurotransmitter metabolites in cerebrospinal fluid [55, 56]; however, the results of these specialty labs are often not available in time to be clinically helpful.

Anticholinergic and sympathomimetic syndromes are both associated with agitation, mydriasis, tachycardia, hypertension, and tremor. In contrast to serotonin syndrome, anticholinergic syndrome is characterized by absent bowel sounds, dry skin, and normal reflexes. Those with sympathomimetic syndrome may exhibit excessive neuromuscular activity that can be difficult to differentiate from the tremor and clonus of serotonin syndrome. The key to the diagnosis rests in the history, although a reliable history is not always available. Fortunately, the mainstay of treatment for all of these syndromes is cooling, benzodiazepines for agitation and increased muscle activity, intravenous fluids, and supportive care.

Treatment

The first steps in management of serotonin syndrome are removal of the causative agents and provision of supportive care. Many cases of serotonin syndrome will resolve within 24 hours of treatment initiation. In patients with mild symptoms (tremor and agitation without fever or autonomic instability), intravenous fluids and benzodiazepines may be adequate. However, any clinical deterioration should prompt a rapid, aggressive response [45, 48].

The etiology of hyperthermia in serotonin syndrome is severe, excessive muscle activity; thus, antipyretics may not be effective in its management. Benzodiazepines are useful in decreasing muscle activity and attenuating the hyperadrenergic response [45], but benzodiazepines and external cooling alone may not be effective in treating the rigidity and hyperthermia of severe serotonin syndrome. Paralysis with nondepolarizing agents, immediately followed by orotracheal intubation and mechanical ventilation, should be considered for patients with hyperthermia (temperature >38.5 °C), severe truncal rigidity, or a rising pCO_2 [4, 45, 48].

Cyproheptadine, an antihistamine with nonselective antiserotonergic effects, may be considered in patients with moderate or severe symptoms, typically as adjunctive therapy with GABA-A agonists as first-line therapy with aggressive supportive care. This drug has been shown to prevent the development of serotonin syndrome in animal models [57, 58]. Human case series detail improvement in symptoms after administration of cyproheptadine, but no clear benefit was observed in an 11-year retrospective case series of 288 cases [45, 59–62]. The recommended dosing of cyproheptadine in adults is an initial dose of 12 mg, followed by 2 mg every 2 hours until symptoms improve. Maintenance dosing is 8 mg every 6 hours [4]. Cyproheptadine is available in pill form only, but it may be crushed and administered via a nasogastric tube. Resolution of mydriasis after cyproheptadine administration has been reported [60]. While this finding has not been validated as a diagnostic tool, it may support the diagnosis of serotonin toxicity. In cyproheptadine overdose, some patients developed anticholinergic syndrome [63], so careful consideration should be given before using cyproheptadine for patients with an overdose including anticholinergics.

In the past, some parenteral antipsychotics with antiserotonergic properties have been used for treatment when oral intake was not possible. However, there is some limited emerging evidence that second-generation antipsychotics might contribute to serotonin syndrome in some cases [64], so it would be prudent to eliminate this treatment option in preference to the other treatment strategies outlined above.

Serotonin syndrome can be life-threatening and is underrecognized. A high level of clinical suspicion will lead to accurate diagnosis, and appropriate treatment can prevent significant morbidity and mortality.

Neuroleptic Malignant Syndrome

Introduction

Neuroleptic malignant syndrome (NMS) is an idiosyncratic drug reaction to dopamine antagonists that was first reported in 1960 [65]. It is characterized by hyperthermia, diffuse rigidity, autonomic instability, and encephalopathy. Many patients who are prescribed antipsychotic drugs are also prescribed antidepressants, so NMS and serotonin syndrome must be considered simultaneously. The severe, life-threatening complications of NMS include coma, rhabdomyolysis, acute renal failure, and respiratory failure. Appropriate, prompt consideration of medication effect as a cause of encephalopathy and hyperthermia is critical to avoid these potential complications.

Epidemiology

The reported incidence of NMS with therapeutic use of antipsychotic drugs ranges from 0.02% to 2.4% [66–72]. It is most common with typical (first-generation) antipsychotics but has been reported with the atypical (second-generation) antipsychotics and antiemetics as well [67, 73–79]. It has also been reported with tetrabenazine therapy [80] and withdrawal of dopamine agonists (drug discontinuation as well as interaction with enteral nutrition [81–84]). The mortality rate is around 10% but may be decreasing over time [66, 68, 85]. Risk factors for development of NMS with therapeutic doses of antipsychotic medications are young age [68, 86], use of the depot formulation [70, 87, 88], intramuscular administration [89], presence of intellectual disability [90, 91], higher dose of antipsychotic [90], psychomotor agitation [90, 92, 93], dehydration [93], and male sex [86]. In a retrospective review of the California Poison Center database, the incidence of NMS in acute overdose was 1.2% for typical antipsychotics and 0.3% for atypical antipsychotic drugs [94].

Pathophysiology

The exact pathophysiology of NMS is not yet clear; however, dopamine blockade likely plays a central role in the generation of NMS. Of the drugs known to cause NMS, dopamine blockade is the common mechanism of action. The cerebrospinal fluid of patients with NMS has a lower concentration of the dopamine metabolite homovanillic acid than controls [95]. In additional support of the anti-dopamine hypothesis, withdrawal of dopaminergic medications can produce a syndrome similar to NMS [96, 97], and dopaminergic drugs are useful in the treatment of NMS. Elevation of catecholamines in the plasma and urine [98], as well as the cerebrospinal fluid [95], suggests that the autonomic dysfunction of NMS is related to sympathoadrenal hyperactivity [99].

Clinical Features/Diagnosis

The diagnosis of NMS should be entertained for hyperthermia or rigidity in the setting of neuroleptic/antipsychotic therapy or recent withdrawal of dopaminergic medications. Levenson's criteria allow for diagnosis of NMS in the presence of all three major criteria: fever, rigidity, and elevated serum creatine phosphokinase (CK). If only two of the major criteria are present, the diagnosis may be made in the presence of four of the minor criteria: tachycardia, abnormal blood pressure, tachypnea, altered consciousness, diaphoresis, and leukocytosis [54, 100, 101]. An International Consensus via Delphi method produced criteria of recent exposure to dopamine antagonist or dopamine agonist withdrawal, hyperthermia, rigidity, altered mental status, CK elevation, autonomic instability, and a negative evaluation of alternative etiologies [102, 103].

The onset of NMS is usually insidious and occurs over days, although acute onset within hours of drug administration does occur [104]. Nearly all cases of NMS occur within 1 month of antipsychotic drug initiation. With supportive care and discontinuation of the offending agent, average recovery time is 7–10 days [104]. Complications include rhabdomyolysis, acute kidney injury, and respiratory failure [105]. Acute respiratory failure is the strongest predictor of mortality [105]. A rating scale has been proposed for following the clinical course of NMS [106, 107]. It is based upon severity of extrapyramidal symptoms, altered consciousness, catatonia, hyperthermia, autonomic instability, dehydration, CK elevation, leukocytosis, and other laboratory abnormalities. This rating scale may be used to objectively follow symptom severity over time.

Differential Diagnosis

Because NMS is an idiosyncratic adverse drug reaction, it remains a diagnosis of exclusion. Some laboratory findings (leukocytosis and elevation of CPK) can be supportive; however, no single laboratory abnormality can secure the diagnosis. Therefore, a complete diagnostic evaluation should be performed, including electrolyte panel with calcium and magnesium, renal and hepatic function tests, creatine kinase level, complete blood count, and urinalysis. Neuroimaging and lumbar puncture should be considered, as indicated [108].

The differential diagnosis for NMS is similar to that of serotonin syndrome and includes malignant hyperthermia, central nervous system infection, anticholinergic delirium, nonconvulsive status epilepticus, salicylate poisoning, baclofen withdrawal, thyrotoxicosis, and heat stroke [108, 109]. There are many case reports that propose a clinical spectrum of NMS with malignant catatonia [110–112].

Treatment

Stabilization of vital signs and removal of the offending agent(s) are the primary steps in management of NMS. Severe hyperthermia has been associated with poor outcome [113], so prompt institution of cooling measures is indicated. Aggressive volume resuscitation and repletion of electrolytes are important, as dehydration is a common presenting feature of NMS [108, 109]. Complications of NMS include coma, aspiration pneumonia, respiratory failure, rhabdomyolysis with subsequent renal failure, and coagulopathy [98, 109]. Patients should be carefully monitored for these complications in an intensive care setting.

Supportive care measures may be sufficient treatment in milder cases of NMS; however, in more severe cases, pharmacological treatment may be indicated. Although the efficacy of benzodiazepines is modest [114], they are indicated as first-line therapy for agitation and may result in resolution of mild NMS. A parenteral dose of lorazepam at 2 mg is a reasonable initial treatment [109].

Dantrolene is a peripheral muscle relaxant that attenuates calcium release at the sarcoplasmic reticulum of skeletal muscle via inhibition of the ryanodine receptor [115]. NMS-related hyperthermia is partially due to the heat produced by muscular rigidity. This tonic, diffuse contraction may also cause rhabdomyolysis. Dantrolene should be considered in patients with severe rigidity and hyperthermia. An initial dose of intravenous dantrolene 1–2.5 mg/kg of body weight should be administered, followed by 1 mg/kg every 6 hours (maximum 10 mg/kg/day). Tapering or transition to oral dantrolene may be made after 48–72 hours, although symptoms may return if this change is made prematurely [109, 115]. Dantrolene has been associated with drug-induced hepatitis, so hepatic function should be monitored during treatment [108, 109]. Dopamine agonists and benzodiazepines may be given in combination with dantrolene, but dantrolene should not be given with calcium channel antagonists because of risk of cardiovascular collapse [109].

In addition to the heat produced by rigidity, the hyperthermia of NMS may also be related to dopamine blockade in the anterior hypothalamus, resulting in inhibition of heat-loss pathways [115]. Dopamine agonists have been associated with reduced time to recovery [116] and mortality rates [117]. First-line dopamine agonist therapy is bromocriptine 2.5–5 mg orally every 8 hours or oral amantadine 100 mg orally every 8 hours [109, 118, 119]. Both medications may be given by nasogastric tube if necessary. Bromocriptine may worsen underlying psychosis and may cause hypotension. If a parenteral agent is necessary, L-dopa can be given intravenously at 50–100 mg/day in divided doses, if available [120]. L-dopa [121], bromocriptine [122], and amantadine [123] have all been reported to increase central serotonergic activity, so they should be avoided if serotonin syndrome remains in the differential diagnosis.

Severe NMS that is refractory to dantrolene and dopamine agonists may respond to electroconvulsive therapy (ECT) [124–130]. ECT may also be effective for the underlying condition for which the antipsychotic was prescribed. It is a reasonable treatment of choice for NMS if idiopathic malignant catatonia is a possible alternative diagnosis [109].

Acute withdrawal of dopamine replacement therapy may cause a neuroleptic malignant-like syndrome. Symptom onset usually occurs 3–4 days after discontinuation of dopaminergic medications and is usually characterized by worsening of baseline rigidity followed by hyperthermia and altered consciousness [96]. Treatment of neuroleptic malignant-like syndrome is discontinuation of any medications with dopamine blocking activity and reinstitution of dopamine replacement [96, 97].

Malignant Hyperthermia

Introduction
Malignant hyperthermia is a rare, autosomal dominant pharmacogenetic disorder of calcium regulation in striated muscle that was first described in the 1960s [131]. It manifests as a hypermetabolic response to inhaled volatile anesthetics and the depolarizing muscle relaxant succinylcholine [132–136]. Increased carbon dioxide (CO_2) production, hyperthermia, tachycardia, tachypnea, muscle rigidity, and rhabdomyolysis are the classic characteristics of malignant hyperthermia. Complications of malignant hyperthermia include hyperkalemia-induced arrhythmias, compartment syndrome, congestive heart failure, bowel ischemia, disseminated intravascular coagulation, rhabdomyolysis-induced renal failure, and death. Prompt recognition of the early signs of malignant hyperthermia, which are an increase in end-tidal carbon dioxide, tachycardia, and rigidity, is critical [137].

Epidemiology
Estimates of malignant hyperthermia susceptibility range from 1 in 200 to 1 in 250,000 [138, 139], depending upon geographical location and prevalence of malignant hyperthermia susceptibility genes. For example, in the state of New York, the prevalence rate of malignant hyperthermia was 1 in 100,000 surgeries in 2001–2005 [140]. The risk for developing malignant hyperthermia is higher in males than in females [137, 140]. A successful anesthesia with agents known to trigger malignant hyperthermia does not exclude the possibility of malignant hyperthermia during future anesthesia [136, 137].

Pathophysiology
The clinical effects of malignant hyperthermia are secondary to uncontrolled calcium release from the sarcoplasmic reticulum, resulting in sustained muscle contraction [141]. Anaerobic metabolism is increased, resulting in hypoxia and acidosis. This is followed by rhabdomyolysis, which may produce hyperkalemia and acute renal failure. Uncoupling of oxidative phosphorylation produces heat, manifested as hyperthermia.

Malignant hyperthermia is associated with abnormalities in both the ryanodine (RYR1) and dihydropyridine (CACNA1S) calcium channels and is inherited as an autosomal dominant disease with variable penetrance [141–150]. Many people with a genetic susceptibility to malignant hyperthermia do not exhibit signs of myopathy; however, there are some genetic myopathies that are linked to malignant hyperthermia. These include central core, core-rod, and multiminicore myopathies, as well as King-Denborough syndrome and Brody myopathy [142, 151–155]. It is not yet clear if there is an association between statin-induced myopathy and a tendency for hyperthermia [156]. While not true malignant hyperthermia, inhalational anesthetics and succinylcholine may produce severe hyperkalemia and rhabdomyolysis in patients with Duchenne and Becker muscular dystrophies [142, 153].

Clinical Features/Diagnosis
The initial sign of malignant hyperthermia is an unexplained rise in end-tidal CO_2 during a general anesthetic procedure that involves a triggering agent [141]. This is followed by tachycardia, hypertension, generalized muscle rigidity or masseter spasm, metabolic acidosis, and hyperthermia. Given the causative agents associated with malignant hyperthermia, the diagnosis will nearly always be made in the operating room or post-anesthesia recovery room [136]. Young children may have more severe acidosis [157], but

otherwise pediatric presentations are similar to adults [158]. Those patients with symptoms consistent with malignant hyperthermia should be referred to specialized centers for consideration of genetic and in vitro contracture testing (IVCT) to confirm their malignant hyperthermia susceptibility [137, 159].

Differential Diagnosis

Sepsis, thyrotoxicosis, and iatrogenic overheating may resemble malignant hyperthermia during anesthesia. The measurement of end-tidal CO_2 is helpful in distinguishing malignant hyperthermia from these disorders [137].

Treatment

Discontinuation of the etiologic agent should be followed immediately by hyperventilation with 100% oxygen, administration of dantrolene, external cooling measures, and treatment of hyperkalemia. Dantrolene sodium is an inhibitor of intracellular calcium release and is an effective antidote for malignant hyperthermia [1, 115, 137, 141]. It should be administered immediately, as delays in treatment are associated with a higher complication rate [136]. Dosing of dantrolene is 2 mg/kg as a bolus intravenous dose, repeated at 5–15-minute intervals as needed to a suggested maximum dose of 10 mg/kg [160–162]. Clinical target of treatment is stabilization of cardiac and respiratory signs and symptoms. Maintenance dosing at 1 mg/kg intravenously every 4–6 hours should be continued for at least 24 hours postoperatively, with careful monitoring for return of symptoms [1, 115, 137, 162]. External cooling and cooled IV fluids are also recommended for temperature reduction [162]. Potential side effects of dantrolene include weakness and respiratory failure, dizziness, gastrointestinal discomfort, and hepatic toxicity [115, 163, 164]. Electrolyte, creatinine, transaminase, and CK levels, as well as coagulation profiles, should be followed regularly. Arrhythmias and hypertension should be treated as indicated, with careful avoidance of calcium channel antagonists [137].

Toxin-Induced Cerebrovascular Events

General Considerations

Toxin-induced stroke is uncommon; however, abuse of recreational drugs has become a risk factor for stroke in adolescents and young adults [165]. In addition, environmental toxins and pharmaceutical agents may contribute to cerebrovascular events. Toxic mechanisms of stroke include (1) sympathomimetic vasoconstriction (cocaine, amphetamines, lysergic acid diethylamide, phencyclidine), (2) hypoxia (opioids and carbon monoxide), (3) cardioembolism (drug-induced cardiomyopathy and endocarditis), (4) vasculitis (amphetamines, cocaine, heroin), (5) enhancement of coagulation (cocaine), (6) venous sinus thrombosis (asparaginase), and gas embolism (hydrogen peroxide). In addition, there are an ever-increasing number of immunosuppressant and chemotherapeutic agents that can cause posterior reversible encephalopathy syndrome. Severe cases can result in cerebral infarction. Toxic mechanisms of hemorrhagic stroke include (1) hypertension-induced arterial rupture with or without underlying vascular malformation (cocaine, amphetamines, and phencyclidine), (2) vasculitis (amphetamines, cocaine, heroin), (3) rupture of septic aneurysm (any intravenous drug use), and (4) coagulopathy (snake venom). In 2018, there was an outbreak of long-acting anticoagulant contamination of synthetic cannabinoids, resulting in varying degrees of coagulopathy with intracerebral hemorrhage in a few cases [166]. Synthetic cannabinoids themselves, as well as cannabis (THC), have increasingly become linked to stroke, as the understanding of the effects of these substances improves [167–172]. These are examples of how contaminants, emerging drugs of abuse, and increase in use of a known substance may contribute to stroke, so careful history is required in cases of cryptogenic stroke, especially in the young.

Cocaine

Introduction

Cocaine, or benzoylmethylecgonine, is a weak base that is extracted from the leaves of the *Erythroxylum coca* plant. It is treated with acid to form the water-soluble salt, cocaine hydrochloride. The cocaine is then ground into a fine powder and may be mixed with diluents that contribute bulk (talc, sugar) or mimic the effect of cocaine (lidocaine, procaine, caffeine) [173]. The hydrochloride form of cocaine may be injected, insufflated, or applied directly to oral mucous membranes. The high melting point precludes smoking of cocaine hydrochloride. The alkaloid forms of cocaine (freebase and crack) are prepared from the hydrochloride form. Although extracted by different methods, freebase and crack cocaine are the same chemical compound. Because of a lower melting point, both can be smoked [173].

Cocaine has a half-life of 30–90 minutes. Peak concentrations occur at 30–60 minutes with nasal insufflation of cocaine hydrochloride [174] and at 2–5 minutes with smoking of crack cocaine [175]. The major metabolites of cocaine (ecgonine methyl ester and benzoylecgonine) are pharmacologically inactive. Norcocaine, a minor metabolite produced in the liver, has pharmacologic activity similar to cocaine [173, 176]. Cocaethylene is an active cocaine metabolite that is produced in the presence of ethanol. It prolongs the clinical effect of cocaine and accounts for the frequent simultaneous ingestion of cocaine and alcohol [177].

Epidemiology

Stroke was first reported in association with cocaine use in 1977 [178]. As abuse of stimulants has increased, so has the awareness of cocaine-induced stroke. Cocaine abuse is associated with both hemorrhagic and ischemic stroke [179]. In young adults (aged 15–44 years) with ischemic stroke, 12.1% had a history of recent illicit drug use. In 4.7%, drug use was the probable cause of stroke [180]. In a case-control study of young adults (aged 15–44 years), those admitted for stroke were more likely to abuse drugs than those admitted for other reasons (34% vs. 8%). The risk of stroke in drug abusers was 6.5 times higher than controls. In 22% of stroke patients, drug use was the probable cause of stroke. The drug most frequently used by these patients was cocaine [165].

Pathophysiology

Cocaine is a potent sympathomimetic and causes vasoconstriction via inhibition of presynaptic reuptake of norepinephrine, serotonin, and dopamine. Vasoconstriction has been observed by magnetic resonance angiography after cocaine administration and appears to occur in a dose-dependent fashion [181]. Cocaine also promotes vasoconstriction by increasing intracellular calcium release in smooth muscle cells by direct action on calcium channels, an effect that appears to be independent of cocaine's adrenergic effects [182, 183]. Blockade of fast sodium channels produces the local anesthetic effect of cocaine and is the mechanism by which cocaine causes cardiac dysrhythmias and seizures [184].

The proposed mechanisms by which cocaine produces ischemic stroke include vasospasm, enhanced platelet aggregation, vasculitis, and cardioembolism [185]. Other possible causes of stroke in patients who use cocaine are related to the adulterants of illicit cocaine. Direct toxic effects of contaminants, such as lidocaine, procainamide, and amphetamines, may contribute to clinical effects. Talc and sugar are sometimes added to cocaine to increase the volume, and when administered intravenously these substances can travel as an embolus to the cerebral vasculature. Bacterial endocarditis, as a complication of any intravenous drug use, may cause ischemic stroke via embolism or hemorrhagic stroke via rupture of a septic aneurysm.

Vasospasm has been identified by angiography in patients with cocaine-associated ischemic stroke [186–190]. This appears to be related to a direct toxic effect of cocaine, both by adrenergic stimulation and effect on calcium channels, although acute severe hypertension may contribute to vasospasm as well [184]. Severe vasospasm may cause focal injury to the arterial endothelium [191]. In vitro, cocaine enhances platelet response to arachidonic acid, thus promoting platelet aggregation [192]. The combination of vasospasm-induced endothelial damage and the procoagulant effects of cocaine may result in cerebral arterial thrombosis.

Cocaine use has been associated with cerebral vasculitis by angiographic findings of characteristic narrowing and dilation of arteries [193, 194]. Two cases of biopsy-proven vasculitis have been reported in association with crack cocaine use, although one of the patients had a history of intravenous cocaine use. Angiography was normal in one case and showed multiple large vessel occlusions without characteristic vasculitic findings in the other [195]. Cocaine-associated cerebral vasculitis occurs rarely, and its diagnosis is complicated by the difficulty in differentiating vasculitis from vasospasm on angiography. Vasculitis has been reported more commonly with amphetamine use, and cocaine may cause vasculitis by a similar mechanism. However, it is important to note that cocaine products are frequently adulterated with amphetamines, so determination of etiology can be difficult.

Both acute cocaine toxicity and chronic recurrent cocaine use increase the risk of cardioembolic stroke. Acute cocaine toxicity can induce dysrhythmia or myocardial infarction [196]. Chronic cocaine use predisposes to ischemic cardiomyopathy [197]. Either of these may result in embolic ischemic stroke in the event of left ventricular thrombus formation and subsequent embolism to the cerebral vasculature.

While cocaine-induced ischemic stroke is most likely attributable to vasoconstriction, the principal mechanism of cocaine-induced intracerebral and subarachnoid hemorrhage is acute blood pressure elevation. Cocaine-induced hemorrhagic stroke may occur with or without an underlying vascular abnormality. In the presence of an aneurysm or vascular anomaly, acute hypertension causes rupture of the weak, abnormal vessel wall. In the absence of a predisposing lesion, the effect of cocaine on cerebral autoregulation likely contributes to arterial rupture. Normal cerebral autoregulation allows mainte-nance of constant blood flow over a range of mean arterial pressure. Above the upper limit of autoregulation, vasodilation occurs, and cerebral blood flow increases [198]. Cocaine disrupts autoregulation by lowering the upper limit of this range [199]. Thus, cocaine not only causes systemic hypertension but also shifts the autoregulation curve such that cerebral blood flow increases at a lower mean arterial pressure. This combination increases risk for arterial rupture and intracerebral hemorrhage. This mechanism may also contribute to reperfusion injury and hemorrhagic transformation of cocaine-induced ischemic stroke.

Clinical Features/Diagnosis

The onset of stroke symptoms usually occurs within 3 hours of cocaine use [200]. The type of stroke seems to differ based upon the form of cocaine used. In a comparative study of cerebrovascular events associated with the two different forms of cocaine use, the hydrochloride form was associated predominantly with hemorrhagic stroke (intracerebral or subarachnoid). The alkaloidal form (crack cocaine) was associated with equal numbers of hemorrhagic and ischemic strokes [189]. Cocaine has been associated with ischemic stroke in all vascular territories, as well as the retina and spinal cord. Cerebral hemorrhage may be intraparenchymal, intraventricular, or subarachnoid in location [200]. About half of patients with hemorrhagic stroke associated with cocaine have an underlying vascular abnormality [184, 186]. Therefore, it may be necessary to obtain additional neuroimaging after the acute hemorrhage has resolved.

Differential Diagnosis

As discussed above, the differential diagnosis of toxin-induced stroke includes amphetamines, PCP, LSD, opioids, and carbon monoxide. The etiologic evaluation of stroke in general is beyond the scope of this discussion. However, consideration should be given to obtaining urine cocaine, PCP, and amphetamine screens in addition to the usual laboratory evaluation of stroke in young adults. There are many substances that can produce false-positive results on urine PCP and amphetamine screens, and the presence of a drug or its metabolite does not prove causality. Thus, careful interpretation of urine drug screening is necessary.

Treatment

Management of acute ischemic or hemorrhagic stroke should be performed to the usual standard of care, independent of cocaine use. A retrospective review of cocaine-associated ischemic stroke patients demonstrated similar outcomes in patients who received tissue plasminogen activator (tPA) and those who did not. There were no complications related to tPA in the patients with cocaine-associated stroke [201]. Based upon this small retrospective study, it appears that tPA may be safe for patients with cocaine-associated ischemic stroke.

One exception to the usual care rule pertains to treatment of hypertension in patients with cocaine toxicity. During acute cocaine intoxication, use of beta-blocking antihypertensive agents may produce unopposed alpha stimulation, resulting in paradoxical hypertension [202]. Therefore, it is best to avoid beta-blockers in the acute setting, especially if signs or symptoms of cocaine intoxication remain present. Benzodiazepines are often used as symptomatic management of agitation, and the subsequent decrease in sympathetic outflow results in improvement of hypertension and tachycardia [203]. If the sedating effects are acceptable, benzodiazepines are a reasonable first choice in acute cocaine intoxication [204].

Amphetamines

Introduction

Amphetamine is the generic term for the racemic α(alpha)-methylphenethylamine of the phenylethylamine family. Substitutions on the phenylethylamine structure produce a variety of compounds with similar effects, including dextroamphetamine, ephedrine, methamphetamine, and 3,4-methylenedioxymethamphetamine (MDMA or ecstasy) [205].

Epidemiology

The true incidence of amphetamine-related cerebrovascular events is not known. Both ischemic and hemorrhage stroke have been reported in association with amphetamines, most often in case series of young stroke patients.

Pathophysiology

Amphetamines cause both increased release and decreased reuptake of multiple neurotransmitters, including dopamine and norepinephrine. The mechanism of stroke in the setting of amphetamine use is similar to that of cocaine. Cerebral ischemia is most likely secondary to focal arterial vasoconstriction related to accelerated atherosclerosis or acute vasospasm [206]. Cerebral vasculitis has also been proposed as a mechanism of ischemic and hemorrhagic stroke and may be a response to the amphetamine or to contaminants or diluents admixed with the amphetamine [207]. However, it is not clear if the findings in each of the reported cases represent true inflammatory arteritis, as the angiography results could also be consistent with vasospasm or multifocal stenosis. Hemorrhagic stroke induced by amphetamines is likely related to acute severe hypertension. Those with preexisting vascular malformations may be at increased risk of this complication [205].

Clinical Features/Diagnosis

Both hemorrhagic and ischemic stroke have been reported in association with amphetamines [165, 179, 208–211], methamphetamines [206, 212, 213], and MDMA [214–217]. Over-the-counter ephedra-like compounds (phenylpropanolamine, ephedrine, pseudoephedrine) have all been linked to stroke as well [218–222]. Hemorrhagic stroke may occur as subarachnoid or intraparenchymal hemorrhage with or without an underlying aneurysm or arteriovenous malformation. In ischemic stroke, angiography can demonstrate arterial occlusion, dissection, or vasospasm.

Treatment

The history of amphetamine use is often unavailable at the time of acute stroke care. This may be due to stroke-related deficits as well as lack of voluntary reporting of drug use. In addition, there are no clinical studies aimed at the specific treatment of amphetamine-related strokes. Therefore, the usual standard of stroke care, based upon the mechanism and location of infarct or hemorrhage, should be applied. The preferred treatment of amphetamine-related agitation, or any other sympathomimetic symptoms, is benzodiazepines.

Toxin-Induced Seizures

Introduction

Seizures are a common, serious manifestation of drug and toxin effects. Xenobiotics may contribute to seizures by (1) direct effect on electrocerebral activity, (2) induction of metabolic derangements, (3) decreased threshold in epilepsy patients, (4) withdrawal of drugs or alcohol, or (5) idiosyncratic drug reaction [223, 224]. Most toxin-related seizures are generalized tonic-clonic. The presence of focal or lateralizing features should prompt evaluation for an underlying lesion. The standard treatment algorithm for status epilepticus requires modification in this setting because toxin-related seizures may not respond to phenytoin [223]. Some toxins that cause seizures are associated with distinct clinical features that may guide diagnosis and treatment.

Epidemiology

The exact incidence of drug- and toxin-induced seizures is not known. A retrospective review of the California Poison Control Center database revealed 386 drug-induced seizures in 2003. The leading cause of drug-induced seizures was bupropion (23%), whereas in 1993 the leading cause was tricyclic antidepressants. Other factors commonly associated with seizures include drugs such as stimulants (cocaine and amphetamines), diphenhydramine, tramadol, antidepressants, antipsychotics, and isoniazid and withdrawal from sedatives. In this population, 68.6% had a single seizure, 27.7% had multiple seizures, and 3.6% had status epilepticus [225].

Pathophysiology

The rate of tonic firing in the cerebral cortex is a balance of excitatory and inhibitory stimuli. Excitation occurs by (1) increased sodium influx, (2) decreased chloride influx, or (3) decreased potassium efflux. Inhibition occurs by (1) decreased sodium influx, (2) increased chloride influx, or (3) increased potassium efflux [223]. A general increase in excitatory or decrease in inhibitory stimuli increases the chance of seizure occurrence.

Glutamate and glycine are excitatory neurotransmitters that cause sodium influx, resulting in neuronal depolarization. Gamma-aminobutyric acid (GABA) is the chief inhibitory neurotransmitter in the central nervous system. Its effect on the neuron is to allow chloride influx, resulting in membrane hyperpolarization. Thus, an increase in glutamate activity (e.g., ibotenic acid), a decrease in GABA activity (e.g., cicutoxin), or withdrawal of GABA agonists (e.g., ethanol, benzodiazepines) increases the incidence of seizures [224].

Histamine and adenosine increase GABA and decrease glutamate in the brain; thus, antihistamines (e.g., diphenhydramine) and adenosine antagonists (e.g., theophylline) can cause seizures [223]. Pyridoxine is a cofactor required for synthesis of GABA from glutamate by glutamic acid decarboxylase (GAD). Pyridoxine is converted to its active form by pyridoxal kinase. Inhibitors of this enzyme (isoniazid, gyromitrins, hydrazines) result in decreased GABA synthesis and refractory seizures. Toxins may also produce seizures secondary to severe metabolic derangements, including hyponatremia (MDMA), hypoxia (carbon monoxide, cyanide, hydrogen sulfide), and hypoglycemia (insulin, sulfonylureas). Table 18.1 summarizes the categories of xenobiotics that are known to cause seizures, although this list is ever expanding over time.

Clinical Features/Diagnosis

The associated signs and symptoms at presentation are often helpful in identifying the drug or toxin responsible for the seizure occurrence, as can be the occurrence of status epilepticus as the

Table 18.1 Selected xenobiotics associated with seizures

Category	Xenobiotics
Antidepressants/antipsychotics	Bupropion
	Lithium
	Antipsychotics
	Selective serotonin reuptake inhibitors
	Serotonin-norepinephrine reuptake inhibitors
	Tricyclic antidepressants
Anesthetics/analgesics	Local anesthetics
	Meperidine
	Propoxyphene
	Salicylates
	Tramadol
Anticonvulsants (in overdose)	Carbamazepine
	Lamotrigine
	Phenytoin
	Topiramate
	Valproic acid
Stimulants	Amphetamines/MDMA
	Cocaine
	Phencyclidine
	Synthetic cannabinoids
	Synthetic cathinones
Antimicrobials	Carbapenems
	Cephalosporins/penicillins
	Chloroquine
	Fluoroquinolones
	Isoniazid
Gases	Carbon monoxide
	Cyanide
	Hydrogen sulfide
Fungi/plants	*Amanita muscaria* mushroom (ibotenic acid)
	Gyromitra esculenta mushroom (gyromitrins)
	Tobacco (nicotine)
	Water hemlock (cicutoxin)
Pesticides	Camphor
	Carbamates
	Lindane
	Organophosphates
Methylxanthines	Caffeine
	Theophylline
Withdrawal	Baclofen
	Barbiturates
	Benzodiazepines
	Ethanol
	Gamma-hydroxybutyrate (GHB)
Miscellaneous	Antihistamine/anticholinergics
	Flumazenil
	Iron
	Lead
	Shellfish (domoic acid)

presenting symptom [226]. If the seizure occurs prior to clinical assessment, it can be difficult to differentiate the persistent effect of the seizure itself (the postictal state) with drug-induced delirium. If available, history regarding signs and symptoms prior to the onset of seizure can provide the key to the diagnosis. In addition, recent addition of new medications, including psychoactive and antibiotic medications, can be illustrative [227, 228].

Findings consistent with the sympathomimetic toxidrome, including mydriasis, tachycardia, hypertension, diaphoresis, and agitated delirium, would suggest the involvement of cocaine, amphetamines, MDMA, PCP, synthetic cathinones or cannabinoids, or other stimulant substance [229]. While most toxin-induced seizures are generalized in onset, these sympathomimetics can cause intracerebral hemorrhage or ischemic stroke (as discussed above). These structural brain lesions may produce focal-onset seizures. Therefore, urgent head imaging is indicated if focal-onset seizure is suggested by the history.

Tricyclic antidepressants have multiple mechanisms of action, including inhibition of serotonin reuptake as well as blockade of fast sodium channels and muscarinic receptors. Mild tricyclic antidepressant toxicity may present with predominant anticholinergic symptoms. More severe toxicity is associated with seizures and QRS interval prolongation [230]. In fact, QRS duration longer than 100 milliseconds is associated with increased risk of seizures [231, 232]. Serotonin syndrome may develop, especially if tricyclic antidepressants are taken with other serotonergic medications.

The combination of coma, respiratory depression, and miosis is characteristic of the opioid toxidrome. Propoxyphene causes seizures and, because of sodium channel blockade, can result in QRS prolongation. Normeperidine, a metabolite of meperidine, and tramadol also lower the seizure threshold.

The presence of agitated delirium prior to the seizure should also suggest the possibility of drug or alcohol withdrawal. Abrupt discontinuation of GABA agonists, including ethanol, barbiturates, benzodiazepines, and baclofen, can cause a life-threatening withdrawal syndrome characterized by agitation, tremor, tachycardia, hallucinations, autonomic instability, and seizures. Ethanol withdrawal seizures are usually brief in duration; however, benzodiazepine or baclofen withdrawal is more likely to cause status epilepticus [233, 234].

Isoniazid frequently causes refractory seizures by producing a functional pyridoxine deficiency. The neurotoxin in *Gyromitra esculenta* mushrooms (false morels) is structurally similar to isoniazid and is also associated with status epilepticus. Severe theophylline toxicity also results in refractory seizures [235]. Seizure activity that does not respond to benzodiazepines should prompt consideration of these toxins.

Differential Diagnosis

The consideration of toxin-induced seizures should not preclude an evaluation for structural, infectious, or metabolic causes of seizure. Detailed history should be obtained to determine the circumstances and characteristics of the reported seizure in order to differentiate a generalized (from onset) seizure that may be toxin-induced from a focal-onset seizure, nonepileptic myoclonus, psychogenic nonepileptic event, or acute movement disorder (chorea, tremor, dystonia). Some toxins, including strychnine, tetanus, and black widow spider envenomation, can cause severe muscle spasms that can mimic seizure. Electroencephalogram, head imaging, lumbar puncture, and laboratory studies may be necessary to confirm the diagnosis.

Treatment

A single, self-limited toxin-induced seizure may be managed with careful clinical observation without the need for long-term anticonvulsant therapy. The first step in management of prolonged or recurrent seizures is benzodiazepines [236]. Some toxins so reliably cause seizures that prophylaxis with benzodiazepines or phenobarbital should be considered. A single dose of lorazepam has been shown to decrease the risk of seizure recurrence in ethanol withdrawal [237], whereas phenytoin does not [238]. Bupropion overdose is associated with seizures in about 30% of patients, and seizure onset may be delayed, especially with the extended-release formulation. In one study, tachycardia, agitation, and tremor were more common in patients who developed seizures than those who did not [239]. Use of benzodiazepines to treat these symptoms may prevent the delayed seizure as well. Theophylline toxicity can result in refractory seizures that are associated with increased morbidity [240, 241]. Prophylaxis with a loading dose of phenobarbital (20 mg/kg intravenously) is recommended for altered mental status, agitation, or theophylline levels of greater than 100 μ(mu)g/mL [224], with careful attention to airway management.

A comprehensive treatment algorithm for status epilepticus is discussed in Chap. 10. For drug- and toxin-induced seizures, the first-line therapy is benzodiazepines (lorazepam), followed by barbiturates (phenobarbital) if necessary. While phenytoin is the standard second-line therapy in management of status epilepticus, it is usually not effective and may actually worsen toxin-induced seizures [242]. There are no data for use of valproic acid in this circumstance, and very limited data for levetiracetam [243]. In general, anticonvulsants with GABA agonist properties (benzodiazepines, barbiturates, propofol) are preferred.

As discussed above, many toxins have multiple mechanisms of action and thereby cause a constellation of symptoms that may include seizures. Therefore, it may be necessary to consider additional treatments or antidotes. For example, enhanced elimination by hemodialysis may be indicated for theophylline, salicylate, or lithium toxicity [244–246]. Sodium bicarbonate is indicated for QRS widening in tricyclic antidepressant and cocaine toxicity and for serum and urinary alkalinization in salicylate toxicity. Magnesium supplementation and potassium repletion are indicated for QTc prolongation in olanzapine toxicity. Intravenous dextrose should be administered to correct hypoglycemia secondary to insulin or sulfonylurea toxicity. In sulfonylurea toxicity, octreotide may be indicated for refractory hypoglycemia. Prolonged seizures secondary to isoniazid or gyromitrin toxicity may respond to intravenous pyridoxine supplementation (1 g for every gram of isoniazid ingested or empiric dose of 5 g) after failing to respond to benzodiazepines alone. Baclofen should be restarted, in addition to benzodiazepines, for seizures related to baclofen withdrawal. Multiple-dose activated charcoal may rarely be useful in severe carbamazepine or theophylline toxicity because of the enterohepatic recirculation of these drugs. Atropine or pralidoxime may be necessary for management of organophosphate poisoning. For assistance with management of the poisoned patient, a clinical toxicologist is available for consultation by calling the American Association of Poison Control Centers at (800) 222–1222 [223].

Toxin-Induced Acute Weakness

While toxin-induced weakness is rare, it is important to consider toxins in the differential diagnosis of both spastic and flaccid weakness, especially when the history suggests a possible exposure. Removing the source of exposure (e.g., tick paralysis) and administration of specific antitoxin may be instrumental in management. Cholinergic symptoms with or without seizures should prompt consideration of organophosphate, carbamate, or nicotine toxicity. Descending paralysis is characteristic of botulism, while ascending paralysis is the hallmark of the demyelinating polyneuropathy of diphtheria. Botulism, diphtheria, tick paralysis, and anthracenone toxicity (*Karwinskia humboldtiana*, Fig. 18.2) cause flaccid paralysis. Tetanospasmin, strychnine, and latrotoxin (black widow spider) cause severe muscle spasms. Botulism, scorpion, and *Elapidae* snake venom are associated with cranial nerve palsies. Table 18.2 reviews the pathophysiology, clinical features, and treatment of toxins that can produce acute weakness. Administration of antitoxins may be considered depending upon the species and availability of the antitoxin. Local poison control centers (AAPCC 1-800-222-1222) can be an invaluable resource for timely information and recommendations. Many of the antitoxins used in the treatment of arthropod and snake envenomations are associated with anaphylactoid reactions. Pretreatment with antihistamines with or without epinephrine may be considered, and immediate availability of these medications during the initial infusion is wise [247–249].

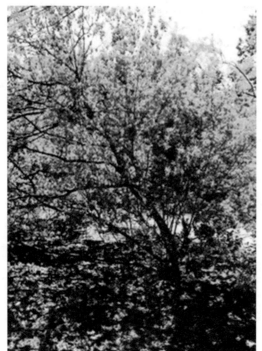

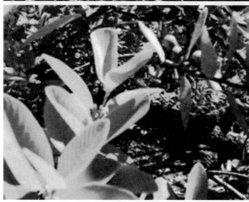

Fig. 18.2 *Karwinskia humboldtiana.* (Photos courtesy of Thomas and Madonna Jones)

Toxin-Induced Acute Encephalopathy

Introduction

Alteration of mental status is a nonspecific finding with a very broad differential diagnosis, including many drugs and toxins. Attention to the characteristic features of the change in mentation, as well as the associated symptoms, is the key to defining possible etiologies. Alteration of cognitive function is a common side effect of many medications, even at therapeutic doses.

This discussion is limited to severe poisoning resulting in agitated delirium and stupor or coma.

Pathophysiology

Because of the complex neurophysiology of the central nervous system, drugs and toxins can cause encephalopathy by a variety of mechanisms. Agents with anticholinergic, sympathomimetic, serotonergic, GABA agonist, opioid agonist, adenosine antagonist, and antihistamine effects cause varying degrees of encephalopathy. Withdrawal of GABA agonists can also produce severe encephalopathy. Environmental toxins that cause hypoxia and drugs that cause respiratory depression, hypoglycemia, or other metabolic derangements can result in central nervous system depression.

Clinical Features/Diagnosis

Recognition of the syndromic presentation of specific drugs and toxins can reveal the diagnosis even in the absence of exposure history. Opioid and sedative-hypnotic toxidromes cause depression of the central nervous system, resulting in stupor and coma. Sympathomimetic, anticholinergic, and withdrawal toxidromes produce agitated delirium. Cholinergic syndrome, characterized by miosis, increased secretions, diarrhea, bradycardia, and weakness, can cause encephalopathy especially when seizures occur.

Opioid poisoning causes miosis, respiratory depression, and coma. Reversal of symptoms with naloxone supports the diagnosis of acute opioid toxicity. Associated prolongation of the QTc interval is suggestive of tramadol or methadone intoxication. Seizures in the setting of the opioid toxidrome suggest propoxyphene, tramadol, or meperidine toxicity, if in the acute phase. In patients who have had prolonged respiratory depression, seizures may be indicative of hypoxic brain injury.

Sedative-hypnotic toxicity from benzodiazepines or ethanol results in somnolence and is usually associated with normal or near-normal vital signs. Respiratory depression can occur when sedatives are ingested with alcohol, opioids, or other sedating medications. Methanol and ethyl-

Table 18.2 Toxin-induced acute weakness

Category	Toxin	Mechanism of action	Source	Clinical presentation	Treatment considerations (in addition to symptomatic and supportive care)
Synthetic compounds	Organophosphates	Inhibit AChE	Pesticides Bioterrorism (VX, sarin gases)	Cholinergic crisis (diarrhea, vomiting, bronchospasm) with fasciculations and paralysis	Atropine for muscarinic symptoms Pralidoxime for nicotinic symptoms Benzodiazepines for seizures
	Carbamates	Inhibit AChE	Pesticides		Atropine for muscarinic symptoms Consider avoiding pralidoxime due to rapid reactivation of carbamylated AChE Benzodiazepines for seizures
Bacteria	Botulinum toxin	Inhibits fusion of presynaptic ACh vesicles, prevents release of Ach	*Clostridium botulinum* Home-canned foods Bioterrorism IV drug use (wound) Botulinum neurotoxin, complication of therapeutic use	Cranial nerve palsies, followed by descending flaccid paralysis	Botulinum antitoxin Notify the health department
	Diphtheria toxin	Inhibits protein synthesis, resulting in demyelination of motor and sensory nerves	*Corynebacterium diphtheriae* Respiratory droplets Direct contact with skin lesions	Tonsillar pseudomembrane, followed within weeks by rapidly ascending flaccid paralysis	Diphtheria antitoxin Antibiotics for bacterial eradication
	Tetanospasmin	Prevents the release of GABA and glycine from spinal interneurons by cleaving synaptobrevin	*Clostridium tetani* Soil contamination of skin wound	Hypertonia, painful generalized muscle contractions, trismus, and increased sympathetic activity	Tetanus immunoglobulin Benzodiazepines Paralytics with ventilatory support for severe muscle spasm

(continued)

Table 18.2 (continued)

Cateory	Toxin	Mechanism of action	Source	Clinical presentation	Treatment considerations (in addition to symptomatic and supportive care)
Plants	Anthracenones	Decrease ATP production, resulting in Schwann cell injury	*Karwinskia* species, including *K. humboldtiana* (coyotillo)	Vomiting and diarrhea followed within weeks by ascending flaccid paralysis	Notify health department
	Aconitine	Increases sodium influx via opening of sodium channels	*Aconitum* species, including monkshood and wolfsbane	Paresthesia, followed by nausea, diarrhea, progressive weakness with bradycardia and/or dysrhythmia	Atropine may be useful for bradycardia or hypersalivation
	Strychnine	Antagonizes glycine	*Strychnos* species	Muscle spasms followed by severe generalized convulsions with intact consciousness	Benzodiazepines or phenobarbital paralytics with ventilatory support for severe muscle spasm
	Nicotine	Activates nicotinic ACh receptors	*Nicotiana* species, including multiple types of tobacco plant	Cholinergic crisis (diarrhea, vomiting, bronchospasm) with fasciculations and paralysis	Atropine for muscarinic symptoms Benzodiazepines for seizures
Shellfish	Saxitoxins	Inhibits sodium, calcium, and potassium channels, resulting in conduction block	*Alexandrium* species of dinoflagellate Ingestion of shellfish	Perioral then generalized paresthesia followed by pain and paralysis with nausea and headache	Notify the health department
	Tetrodotoxin	Inhibits voltage-gated sodium channels	*Vibrionaceae* family of marine bacteria Ingestion of puffer fish or Japanese shellfish Envenomation by blue-ringed octopus	Perioral then generalized paresthesia, followed by nausea, diarrhea, and paralysis	Notify the health department

Category	Toxin	Mechanism of action	Source	Clinical presentation	Treatment considerations (in addition to symptomatic and supportive care)
Arthropods	Latrotoxin	Stimulates neurotransmitter release (including ACh), resulting in vesicle depletion	*Latrodectus* species of spiders, including black widow	Diffuse muscle spasms and rigidity with hypertension, nausea, and diaphoresis	Benzodiazepines for muscle spasm Black widow antivenom for severe cases
	Ixovotoxin	Inhibits ACh release at neuromuscular junction	Ixodid and Argasid families of ticks	Ascending, flaccid paralysis	Tick removal Antitoxin used only in severe illness secondary to high risk of anaphylaxis and serum sickness
	Scorpion venom (multiple components, species specific)	Opening of sodium channels, activation of sympathetic and parasympathetic nerves, causing ACh and catecholamine release	Buthidae family of scorpions, including *Centruroides exilicauda* (bark scorpion)	Pain and paresthesia, followed by neuromuscular excitability, cranial nerve palsies, and weakness	Antivenom
Snakes (Elapidae family)	α-Bungarotoxin	Inhibits binding of ACh at nicotinic receptors			
	β-Bungarotoxin	Inhibits ACh release	*Bungarus* species (krait)	Local swelling and nausea followed by cranial nerve palsies and paralysis	Monovalent antivenom if species is known, polyvalent antivenom if species is unknown
	Cobrotoxin	Inhibits binding of ACh at nicotinic receptors	*Naja* species (cobra)		
	Dendrotoxin	Inhibits potassium channels, facilitating ACh release	*Dendroaspis* species (mamba)		Pressure immobilization of wound
	Fasciculin	Inhibits AChE			

AChE acetylcholinesterase, *ACh* acetylcholine, *GABA* gamma-aminobutyric acid, *ATP* adenosine triphosphate ene glycol ingestion result in central nervous system depression, similar to ethanol toxicity, but are also associated with an anion gap metabolic acidosis. Acidosis in this setting should prompt further laboratory evaluation (serum osmolality, methanol and ethylene glycol levels), treatment with fomepizole, and nephrology consultation for possible renal-replacement therapy. Evaluation for other causes of anion gap metabolic acidosis, including salicylate toxicity, diabetic or alcoholic ketoacidosis, and lactic acidosis, should also be performed.

Sympathomimetic toxicity is characterized by mydriasis, agitated delirium, tachycardia, hypertension, diaphoresis, and hyperthermia. The most common causes of this toxidrome are amphetamines and cocaine. When hallucinations are a prominent feature, especially in the presence of nystagmus, phencyclidine intoxication should be considered. Anticholinergic syndrome also causes an agitated delirium that is similar in presentation to sympathomimetic syndrome. The distinguishing features of anticholinergic toxicity are anhidrosis, decreased bowel sounds, and garbled speech. Patients may also exhibit the picking behaviors that are characteristic of this toxidrome. Tricyclic antidepressants, antipsychotic medications, antihistamines (e.g., diphenhydramine), and cyclobenzaprine are common causes of anticholinergic symptoms. Withdrawal of ethanol and benzodiazepines results in mydriasis, tachycardia, tremor, and agitated delirium. Serotonin syndrome causes an agitated delirium with autonomic instability and motor hyperactivity in the setting of serotonergic medications. These syndromes are also discussed in the hyperthermic syndromes section of this chapter.

Differential Diagnosis

Metabolic derangements, central nervous system or systemic infection, cerebral structural lesions or hemorrhage, and nonconvulsive status epilepticus may all cause a general alteration of mental status. Neuroimaging, lumbar puncture, laboratory testing, and electroencephalography are often necessary for diagnosis. Basic chemistry profile, serum acetaminophen and salicylate levels, and electrocardiogram (ECG) can assist in determining which drugs are most likely to be involved, especially when intentional overdose is suspected, and historical information is unavailable.

Urine drug screening should not be routinely performed because of the high rate of false-positive and false-negative results, although should be considered in cases of undifferentiated encephalopathy. Care should be taken when interpreting data from these screening tests. A positive result does not prove intoxication, and a negative result does not always exclude exposure.

Treatment

Identification and discontinuation of the toxic agent, in addition to supportive care, is the mainstay of therapy for toxin-induced encephalopathy. Benzodiazepines are the recommended treatment for toxin-induced agitated delirium, including sympathomimetic, anticholinergic, withdrawal, and serotonin syndromes. Antidotes exist for opioid, benzodiazepine, and anticholinergic poisoning. The potential side effects of these antidotes should be carefully considered prior to administration.

Naloxone is an opioid antagonist that is used therapeutically and diagnostically in the setting of presumed opiate or opioid toxicity. The initial dose of naloxone is usually 0.4 mg given intravenously; however, because naloxone can precipitate severe withdrawal symptoms, a smaller test dose should be considered when opioid dependence is suspected. Additional doses may be given at 5-minute intervals until neurologic and respiratory status has improved [250]. Higher doses of naloxone may be required for reversal of the synthetic opioids. The clinical effect of naloxone may be as short as 45 minutes [251]. Resedation may occur after naloxone reversal, especially in the setting of toxicity from methadone or sustained release opioid preparations. Patients should be observed closely for 6 hours after naloxone administration. If resedation does occur, a naloxone infusion can be initiated at an hourly rate of two-thirds of the effective bolus dose [252]. Admission to a monitored setting is required to monitor for withdrawal symptoms or resedation.

In general, benzodiazepine withdrawal is more likely to cause complications than benzodiazepine toxicity. Benzodiazepines are not potent respiratory depressants, so reversal is not likely to prevent the need for mechanical ventilation in patients who have ingested multiple sedating medications. In polysubstance overdose or benzodiazepine-dependent patients, reversal of benzodiazepines can precipitate refractory seizures [224]. For this reason, use of the benzodiazepine antagonist, flumazenil, should be limited to pediatric poisonings or iatrogenic toxicity in patients who are not chronic benzodiazepine users.

Physostigmine is an inhibitor of acetylcholinesterase that may be used for severe anticholinergic poisoning. The diagnosis of anticholinergic toxicity should be clinically certain prior to administration of this antidote, although in rare circumstances physostigmine may be used diagnostically. Toxicologists generally prefer to use physostigmine in toxicity from drugs that are primarily anticholinergic rather than from drugs that have multiple actions or polysubstance ingestion [253]. Emerging evidence suggests that physostigmine is safer than previously thought, although benzodiazepines remain the preferred first-line treatment of medical toxicologists [254–259]. Potential complications of physostigmine administration include vomiting, seizures, bronchorrhea, bradycardia, and arrhythmias. ECG evidence of prolongation of the PR, QRS, or QTc intervals contraindicates use of physostigmine [250]. Benzodiazepines are the preferred treatment for undifferentiated agitated delirium and are reasonable in monotherapy of anticholinergic toxicity.

Conclusion

Toxin-induced neurologic emergencies are common but generally require a high level of clinical suspicion to identify. Acute encephalopathy with or without hyperthermia, stroke in young patients, unexplained seizures, and acute weakness should prompt consideration of toxicologic etiologies. Early identification of the causative toxin allows for appropriate diagnostic testing and initiation of definitive treatment.

References

1. Rusyniak DE, Sprague JE. Toxin-induced hyperthermic syndromes. Med Clin N Am. 2005;89(6):1277–96.
2. Sternbach H. The serotonin syndrome. Am J Psychiatr. 1991;148(6):705–13.
3. Oates JA, Sjoerdsma A. Neurologic effects of tryptophan in patients receiving a monoamine oxidase inhibitor. Neurology. 1960;10:1076–8.
4. Boyer EW, Shannon M. The serotonin syndrome. N Engl J Med. 2005;352(11):1112–20.
5. Mackay FJ, Dunn NR, Mann RD. Antidepressants and the serotonin syndrome in general practice. Br J Gen Pract. 1999;49(448):871–4.
6. Watson WA, Litovitz TL, Rodgers GC Jr, Klein-Schwartz W, Reid N, Youniss J, et al. 2004 annual report of the American Association of Poison Control Centers toxic exposure surveillance system. Am J Emerg Med. 2005;23(5):589–666.
7. Isbister GK, Bowe SJ, Dawson A, Whyte IM. Relative toxicity of selective serotonin reuptake inhibitors (SSRIs) in overdose. J Toxicol Clin Toxicol. 2004;42(3):277–85.
8. Abadie D, Rousseau V, Logerot S, Cottin J, Montastruc JL, Montastruc F. Serotonin syndrome: analysis of cases registered in the French pharmacovigilance database. J Clin Psychopharmacol. 2015;35(4):382–8.
9. Culbertson VL, Rahman SE, Bosen GC, Caylor ML, Xu D. Use of a bioinformatics-based toxicity scoring system to assess serotonin burden and predict population-level adverse drug events from concomitant serotonergic drug therapy. Pharmacotherapy. 2019;39(2):171–81.
10. Pilgrim JL, Gerostamoulos D, Drummer OH. Deaths involving serotonergic drugs. Forensic Sci Int. 2010;198(1–3):110–7.
11. Azmitia EC, Whitaker-Azmitia PM. Awakening the sleeping giant: anatomy and plasticity of the brain serotonergic system. J Clin Psychiatry. 1991;52(Suppl):4–16.
12. Cooper JR, Bloom FE, Roth RH. Serotonin, histamine, and adenosine. The biochemical basis of neuropharmacology. 8th ed. Oxford: Oxford University Press; 2003. p. 271–320.
13. Prosser JM, Nelson LS. The toxicology of bath salts: a review of synthetic cathinones. J Med Toxicol. 2012;8(1):33–42.
14. Schep LJ, Slaughter RJ, Vale JA, Beasley DM, Gee P. The clinical toxicology of the designer "party pills" benzylpiperazine and trifluoromethylphenylpiperazine. Clin Toxicol (Philadelphia, Pa). 2011;49(3):131–41.
15. Tang MH, Ching CK, Tsui MS, Chu FK, Mak TW. Two cases of severe intoxication associated with analytically confirmed use of the novel psychoactive substances 25B-NBOMe and 25C-NBOMe. Clin Toxicol (Philadelphia, Pa). 2014;52(5):561–5.

16. Evans RW, Tepper SJ, Shapiro RE, Sun-Edelstein C, Tietjen GE. The FDA alert on serotonin syndrome with use of triptans combined with selective serotonin reuptake inhibitors or selective serotonin-norepinephrine reuptake inhibitors: American Headache Society position paper. Headache. 2010;50(6):1089–99.

17. Acker EC, Sinclair EA, Beardsley AL, Ahmed SS, Froberg BA. Acute vilazodone toxicity in a pediatric patient. J Emerg Med. 2015;49(3):284–6.

18. Heise CW, Malashock H, Brooks DE. A review of vilazodone exposures with focus on serotonin syndrome effects. Clin Toxicol (Philadelphia, Pa). 2017;55(9):1004–7.

19. Thorpe EL, Pizon AF, Lynch MJ, Boyer J. Bupropion induced serotonin syndrome: a case report. J Med Toxicol. 2010;6(2):168–71.

20. Moss MJ, Hendrickson RG. Serotonin toxicity: associated agents and clinical characteristics. J Clin Psychopharmacol. 2019;39(6):628–33.

21. Solhaug V, Molden E. Individual variability in clinical effect and tolerability of opioid analgesics – importance of drug interactions and pharmacogenetics. Scand J Pain. 2017;17:193–200.

22. Tashakori A, Afshari R. Tramadol overdose as a cause of serotonin syndrome: a case series. Clin Toxicol (Philadelphia, Pa). 2010;48(4):337–41.

23. Park J, Chung ME. Botulinum toxin for central neuropathic pain. Toxins. 2018;10(6):224.

24. Ryan NM, Isbister GK. Tramadol overdose causes seizures and respiratory depression but serotonin toxicity appears unlikely. Clin Toxicol (Philadelphia, Pa). 2015;53(6):545–50.

25. Baldo BA, Rose MA. The anaesthetist, opioid analgesic drugs, and serotonin toxicity: a mechanistic and clinical review. Br J Anaesth. 2020;124(1):44–62.

26. Baldo BA. Opioid analgesic drugs and serotonin toxicity (syndrome): mechanisms, animal models, and links to clinical effects. Arch Toxicol. 2018;92(8):2457–73.

27. Chan BS, Becker T, Chiew AL, Abdalla AM, Robertson TA, Liu X, et al. Vasoplegic shock treated with methylene blue complicated by severe serotonin syndrome. J Med Toxicol. 2018;14(1):100–3.

28. Francescangeli J, Vaida S, Bonavia AS. Perioperative diagnosis and treatment of serotonin syndrome following administration of methylene blue. Am J Case Rep. 2016;17:347–51.

29. Hencken L, To L, Ly N, Morgan JA. Serotonin syndrome following methylene blue administration for vasoplegic syndrome. J Card Surg. 2016;31(4):208–10.

30. Martino EA, Winterton D, Nardelli P, Pasin L, Calabro MG, Bove T, et al. The blue coma: the role of methylene blue in unexplained coma after cardiac surgery. J Cardiothorac Vasc Anesth. 2016;30(2):423–7.

31. Ng BK, Cameron AJ. The role of methylene blue in serotonin syndrome: a systematic review. Psychosomatics. 2010;51(3):194–200.

32. Oz M, Isaev D, Lorke DE, Hasan M, Petroianu G, Shippenberg TS. Methylene blue inhibits function of the 5-HT transporter. Br J Pharmacol. 2012;166(1):168–76.

33. Smith CJ, Wang D, Sgambelluri A, Kramer RS, Gagnon DJ. Serotonin syndrome following methylene blue administration during cardiothoracic surgery. J Pharm Pract. 2015;28(2):207–11.

34. Snyder M, Gangadhara S, Brohl AS, Ludlow S, Nanjappa S. Serotonin syndrome complicating treatment of ifosfamide neurotoxicity with methylene blue. Cancer Control J Moffitt Cancer Center. 2017;24(5):1073274817729070.

35. Stanford SC, Stanford BJ, Gillman PK. Risk of severe serotonin toxicity following co-administration of methylene blue and serotonin reuptake inhibitors: an update on a case report of post-operative delirium. J Psychopharmacol (Oxford, England). 2010;24(10):1433–8.

36. Top WM, Gillman PK, de Langen CJ, Kooy A. Fatal methylene blue associated serotonin toxicity. Neth J Med. 2014;72(3):179–81.

37. Zuschlag ZD, Warren MW, Schultz KS. Serotonin toxicity and urinary analgesics: a case report and systematic literature review of methylene blue-induced serotonin syndrome. Psychosomatics. 2018;59(6):539–46.

38. Frykberg RG, Gordon S, Tierney E, Banks J. Linezolid-associated serotonin syndrome. A report of two cases. J Am Podiatr Med Assoc. 2015;105(3):244–8.

39. Karkow DC, Kauer JF, Ernst EJ. Incidence of serotonin syndrome with combined use of linezolid and serotonin reuptake inhibitors compared with linezolid monotherapy. J Clin Psychopharmacol. 2017;37(5):518–23.

40. Ramsey TD, Lau TT, Ensom MH. Serotonergic and adrenergic drug interactions associated with linezolid: a critical review and practical management approach. Ann Pharmacother. 2013;47(4):543–60.

41. Woytowish MR, Maynor LM. Clinical relevance of linezolid-associated serotonin toxicity. Ann Pharmacother. 2013;47(3):388–97.

42. Koury KM, Tsui B, Gulur P. Incidence of serotonin syndrome in patients treated with fentanyl on serotonergic agents. Pain Physician. 2015;18(1):E27–30.

43. Robles LA. Serotonin syndrome induced by fentanyl in a child: case report. Clin Neuropharmacol. 2015;38(5):206–8.

44. Pedavally S, Fugate JE, Rabinstein AA. Serotonin syndrome in the intensive care unit: clinical presentations and precipitating medications. Neurocrit Care. 2014;21(1):108–13.

45. Gillman PK. The serotonin syndrome and its treatment. J Psychopharmacol. 1999;13(1):100–9.

46. Slettedal JK, Nilssen DO, Magelssen M, Loberg EM, Maehlen J. Brain pathology in fatal serotonin syndrome: presentation of two cases. Neuropathology. 2011;31(3):265–70.

47. Radomski J, Dursun S, Reveley M, Kutcher S. An exploratory approach to the serotonin syndrome: an update of clinical phenomenology and revised diagnostic criteria. Med Hypotheses. 2000;55(3):218–24.

48. Dunkley EJC, Isbister GK, Sibbritt D, Dawson AH, Whyte IM. The hunter serotonin toxicity criteria: simple and accurate diagnostic decision rules for serotonin toxicity. QJM. 2003;96(9):635–42.

49. Werneke U, Jamshidi F, Taylor DM, Ott M. Conundrums in neurology: diagnosing serotonin syndrome – a meta-analysis of cases. BMC Neurol. 2016;16:97.

50. Hegerl U, Bottlender R, Gallinat J, Kuss HJ, Ackenheil M, Moller HJ. The serotonin syndrome scale: first results on validity. Eur Arch Psychiatry Clin Neurosci. 1998;248(2):96–103.

51. Hilton SE, Maradit H, Moller HJ. Serotonin syndrome and drug combinations: focus on MAOI and RIMA. Eur Arch Psychiatry Clin Neurosci. 1997;247(3):113–9.

52. Baloh RW, Dietz J, Spooner JW. Myoclonus and ocular oscillations induced by L-tryptophan. Ann Neurol. 1982;11(1):95–7.

53. Mills KC. Serotonin syndrome. A clinical update. Crit Care Clin. 1997;13(4):763–83.

54. Perry PJ, Wilborn CA. Serotonin syndrome vs neuroleptic malignant syndrome: a contrast of causes, diagnoses, and management. Ann Clin Psychiatry. 2012;24(2):155–62.

55. Nisijima K. Abnormal monoamine metabolism in cerebrospinal fluid in a case of serotonin syndrome. J Clin Psychopharmacol. 2000;20(1):107–8.

56. Nisijima K, Nibuya M, Sugiyama H. Abnormal CSF monoamine metabolism in serotonin syndrome. J Clin Psychopharmacol. 2003;23(5):528–31.

57. Stewart RM, Campbell A, Sperk G, Baldessarini RJ. Receptor mechanisms in increased sensitivity to serotonin agonists after dihydroxytryptamine shown by electronic monitoring of muscle twitches in the rat. Psychopharmacology. 1979;60(3):281–9.

58. Gerson SC, Baldessarini RJ. Motor effects of serotonin in the central nervous system. Life Sci. 1980;27(16):1435–51.

59. Graudins A, Stearman A, Chan B. Treatment of the serotonin syndrome with cyproheptadine. J Emerg Med. 1998;16(4):615–9.

60. McDaniel WW. Serotonin syndrome: early management with cyproheptadine. Ann Pharmacother. 2001;35(7–8):870–3.

61. Lappin RI, Auchincloss EL. Treatment of the serotonin syndrome with cyproheptadine. N Engl J Med. 1994;331(15):1021–2.

62. Nguyen H, Pan A, Smollin C, Cantrell LF, Kearney T. An 11-year retrospective review of cyproheptadine use in serotonin syndrome cases reported to the California Poison Control System. J Clin Pharm Ther. 2019;44(2):327–34.

63. Chu FK. Review of the epidemiology and characteristics of intentional cyproheptadine overdose in Hong Kong. Clin Toxicol (Philadelphia, Pa). 2011;49(7):681–3.

64. Racz R, Soldatos TG, Jackson D, Burkhart K. Association between serotonin syndrome and second-generation antipsychotics via pharmacological target-adverse event analysis. Clin Transl Sci. 2018;11(3):322–9.

65. Delay J, Pichot P, Lemperiere T, Elissalde B, Peigne F. A non-phenothiazine and non-reserpine major neuroleptic, haloperidol, in the treatment of psychoses. Ann Med Psychol. 1960;118(1):145–52.

66. Caroff SN, Mann SC. Neuroleptic malignant syndrome. Med Clin N Am. 1993;77(1):185–202.

67. Stubner S, Rustenbeck E, Grohmann R, Wagner G, Engel R, Neundorfer G, et al. Severe and uncommon involuntary movement disorders due to psychotropic drugs. Pharmacopsychiatry. 2004;37(Suppl 1):S54–64.

68. Spivak B, Maline DI, Kozyrev VN, Mester R, Neduva SA, Ravilov RS, et al. Frequency of neuroleptic malignant syndrome in a large psychiatric hospital in Moscow. Eur Psychiatry. 2000;15(5):330–3.

69. Addonizio G, Susman VL, Roth SD. Symptoms of neuroleptic malignant syndrome in 82 consecutive inpatients. Am J Psychiatr. 1986;143(12):1587–90.

70. Deng MZ, Chen GQ, Phillips MR. Neuroleptic malignant syndrome in 12 of 9,792 Chinese inpatients exposed to neuroleptics: a prospective study. Am J Psychiatr. 1990;147(9):1149–55.

71. Keck PE Jr, Pope HG Jr, McElroy SL. Frequency and presentation of neuroleptic malignant syndrome: a prospective study. Am J Psychiatr. 1987;144(10):1344–6.

72. Kimura G, Kadoyama K, Brown JB, Nakamura T, Miki I, Nisiguchi K, et al. Antipsychotics-associated serious adverse events in children: an analysis of the FAERS database. Int J Med Sci. 2015;12(2):135–40.

73. Ananth J, Parameswaran S, Gunatilake S, Burgoyne K, Sidhom T. Neuroleptic malignant syndrome and atypical antipsychotic drugs. J Clin Psychiatry. 2004;65(4):464–70.

74. Anzai T, Takahashi K, Watanabe M. Adverse reaction reports of neuroleptic malignant syndrome induced by atypical antipsychotic agents in the Japanese Adverse Drug Event Report (JADER) database. Psychiatry Clin Neurosci. 2019;73(1):27–33.

75. Belvederi Murri M, Guaglianone A, Bugliani M, Calcagno P, Respino M, Serafini G, et al. Second-generation antipsychotics and neuroleptic malignant syndrome: systematic review and case report analysis. Drugs R&D. 2015;15(1):45–62.

76. Breeden R, Ford H, Chrisman C, Mascioli C. Neuroleptic malignant syndrome secondary to metoclopramide use in an elderly gastroenterologic surgery patient. Gastroenterol Nursing. 2017;40(2):93–100.

77. Lau Moon Lin M, Robinson PD, Flank J, Sung L, Dupuis LL. The safety of metoclopramide in children: a systematic review and meta-analysis. Drug Saf. 2016;39(7):675–87.

78. Lau Moon Lin M, Robinson PD, Flank J, Sung L, Dupuis LL. The safety of prochlorperazine in children: a systematic review and meta-analysis. Drug Saf. 2016;39(6):509–16.

79. Lertxundi U, Ruiz AI, Aspiazu MA, Domingo-Echaburu S, Garcia M, Aguirre C, et al. Adverse reactions to antipsychotics in Parkinson disease: an analysis of the Spanish pharmacovigilance database. Clin Neuropharmacol. 2015;38(3):69–84.

80. Guay DR. Tetrabenazine, a monoamine-depleting drug used in the treatment of hyperkinetic movement disorders. Am J Geriatr Pharmacother. 2010;8(4):331–73.

81. Bonnici A, Ruiner CE, St-Laurent L, Hornstein D. An interaction between levodopa and enteral nutrition resulting in neuroleptic malignant-like syndrome and prolonged ICU stay. Ann Pharmacother. 2010;44(9):1504–7.

82. Fiore S, Persichino L, Anticoli S, De Pandis MF. A neuroleptic malignant-like syndrome (NMLS) in a patient with Parkinson's disease resolved with rotigotine: a case report. Acta Biomed: Atenei Parmensis. 2014;85(3):281–4.

83. Fryml LD, Williams KR, Pelic CG, Fox J, Sahlem G, Robert S, et al. The role of amantadine withdrawal in 3 cases of treatment-refractory altered mental status. J Psychiatr Pract. 2017;23(3):191–9.

84. Whitman CB, Ablordeppey E, Taylor B. Levodopa withdrawal presenting as fever in a critically ill patient receiving concomitant enteral nutrition. J Pharm Pract. 2016;29(6):574–8.

85. Nakamura M, Yasunaga H, Miyata H, Shimada T, Horiguchi H, Matsuda S. Mortality of neuroleptic malignant syndrome induced by typical and atypical antipsychotic drugs: a propensity-matched analysis from the Japanese Diagnosis Procedure Combination database. J Clin Psychiatry. 2012;73(4):427–30.

86. Gurrera RJ. A systematic review of sex and age factors in neuroleptic malignant syndrome diagnosis frequency. Acta Psychiatr Scand. 2017;135(5):398–408.

87. Nielsen RE, Wallenstein Jensen SO, Nielsen J. Neuroleptic malignant syndrome-an 11-year longitudinal case-control study. Can J Psychiatry. 2012;57(8):512–8.

88. Su YP, Chang CK, Hayes RD, Harrison S, Lee W, Broadbent M, et al. Retrospective chart review on exposure to psychotropic medications associated with neuroleptic malignant syndrome. Acta Psychiatr Scand. 2014;130(1):52–60.

89. Keck PE Jr, Pope HG Jr, McElroy SL. Declining frequency of neuroleptic malignant syndrome in a hospital population. Am J Psychiatr. 1991;148(7):880–2.

90. Viejo LF, Morales V, Punal P, Perez JL, Sancho RA. Risk factors in neuroleptic malignant syndrome. A case-control study. Acta Psychiatr Scand. 2003;107(1):45–9.

91. Sheehan R, Horsfall L, Strydom A, Osborn D, Walters K, Hassiotis A. Movement side effects of antipsychotic drugs in adults with and without intellectual disability: UK population-based cohort study. BMJ Open. 2017;7(8):e017406.

92. Berardi D, Amore M, Keck PE Jr, Troia M, Dell'Atti M. Clinical and pharmacologic risk factors for neuroleptic malignant syndrome: a case-control study. Biol Psychiatry. 1998;44(8):748–54.

93. Sachdev P, Mason C, Hadzi-Pavlovic D. Case-control study of neuroleptic malignant syndrome. Am J Psychiatr. 1997;154(8):1156–8.

94. Ciranni MA, Kearney TE, Olson KR. Comparing acute toxicity of first- and second-generation antipsychotic drugs: a 10-year, retrospective cohort study. J Clin Psychiatry. 2009;70(1):122–9.

95. Nisijima K, Ishiguro T. Cerebrospinal fluid levels of monoamine metabolites and gamma-aminobutyric acid in neuroleptic malignant syndrome. J Psychiatr Res. 1995;29(3):233–44.

96. Serrano-Duenas M. Neuroleptic malignant syndrome-like, or--dopaminergic malignant syndrome--due to levodopa therapy withdrawal. Clinical features in 11 patients. Parkinsonism Relat Disord. 2003;9(3):175–8.

97. Gordon PH, Frucht SJ. Neuroleptic malignant syndrome in advanced Parkinson's disease. Mov Disord. 2001;16(5):960–2.

98. Nisijima K, Shioda K, Iwamura T. Neuroleptic malignant syndrome and serotonin syndrome. Prog Brain Res. 2007;162:81–104.

99. Gurrera RJ. Sympathoadrenal hyperactivity and the etiology of neuroleptic malignant syndrome. Am J Psychiatr. 1999;156(2):169–80.

100. Levenson JL. Neuroleptic malignant syndrome. Am J Psychiatr. 1985;142(10):1137–45.

101. Karamustafalioglu N, Kalelioglu T, Celikel G, Genc A, Emul M. Clinical utility of neutrophil-lymphocyte ratio in the diagnosis of neuroleptic malignant syndrome. Nord J Psychiatry. 2019;73(4–5):288–92.

102. Gurrera RJ, Mortillaro G, Velamoor V, Caroff SN. A validation study of the international consensus diagnostic criteria for neuroleptic malignant syndrome. J Clin Psychopharmacol. 2017;37(1):67–71.

103. Gurrera RJ, Caroff SN, Cohen A, Carroll BT, DeRoos F, Francis A, et al. An international consensus study of neuroleptic malignant syndrome diagnostic criteria using the Delphi method. J Clin Psychiatry. 2011;72(9):1222–8.

104. Caroff SN, Mann SC. Neuroleptic malignant syndrome. Psychopharmacol Bull. 1988;24(1):25–9.

105. Modi S, Dharaiya D, Schultz L, Varelas P. Neuroleptic malignant syndrome: complications, outcomes, and mortality. Neurocrit Care. 2016;24(1):97–103.

106. Sachdev PS. A rating scale for neuroleptic malignant syndrome. Psychiatry Res. 2005;135(3):249–56.

107. Yacoub A, Francis A. Neuroleptic malignant syndrome induced by atypical neuroleptics and responsive to lorazepam. Neuropsychiatr Dis Treat. 2006;(2):235–40.

108. Pelonero AL, Levenson JL, Pandurangi AK. Neuroleptic malignant syndrome: a review. Psychiatr Serv. 1998;49(9):1163–72.

109. Strawn JR, Keck PE Jr, Caroff SN. Neuroleptic malignant syndrome. Am J Psychiatr. 2007;164(6):870–6.

110. Ghaziuddin N, Hendriks M, Patel P, Wachtel LE, Dhossche DM. Neuroleptic malignant syndrome/malignant catatonia in child psychiatry: literature review and a case series. J Child Adolesc Psychopharmacol. 2017;27(4):359–65.

111. Luchini F, Lattanzi L, Bartolommei N, Cosentino L, Litta A, Kansky C, et al. Catatonia and neuroleptic malignant syndrome: two disorders on a same spectrum? Four case reports. J Nerv Ment Dis. 2013;201(1):36–42.

112. Lang FU, Lang S, Becker T, Jager M. Neuroleptic malignant syndrome or catatonia? Trying to solve the catatonic dilemma. Psychopharmacology. 2015;232(1):1–5.

113. Nagamine M, Yoshino A, Sakurai Y, Sanga M, Takahashi R, Nomura S. Exacerbating factors in neuroleptic malignant syndrome: comparisons between cases with death, sequelae, and full recovery. J Clin Psychopharmacol. 2005;25(5):499–501.

114. Caroff SN, Mann SC, Keck PE Jr. Specific treatment of the neuroleptic malignant syndrome. Biol Psychiatry. 1998;44(6):378–81.

115. Krause T, Gerbershagen MU, Fiege M, Weisshorn R, Wappler F. Dantrolene--a review of its pharmacology, therapeutic use and new developments. Anaesthesia. 2004;59(4):364–73.

116. Sakkas P, Davis JM, Janicak PG, Wang ZY. Drug treatment of the neuroleptic malignant syndrome. Psychopharmacol Bull. 1991;27(3):381–4.

117. Rosenberg MR, Green M. Neuroleptic malignant syndrome. Review of response to therapy. Arch Intern Med. 1989;149(9):1927–31.

118. van Rensburg R, Decloedt EH. An approach to the pharmacotherapy of neuroleptic malignant syndrome. Psychopharmacol Bull. 2019;49(1):84–91.

119. Schreiner NM, Windham S, Barker A. Atypical neuroleptic malignant syndrome: diagnosis and proposal for an expanded treatment algorithm: a case report. A A Case Rep. 2017;9(12):339–43.

120. Nisijima K, Noguti M, Ishiguro T. Intravenous injection of levodopa is more effective than dantrolene as therapy for neuroleptic malignant syndrome. Biol Psychiatry. 1997;41(8):913–4.

121. Avarello TP, Cottone S. Serotonin syndrome: a reported case. Neurol Sci. 2002;23(Suppl 2):S55–6.

122. Sandyk R. L-dopa induced "serotonin syndrome" in a parkinsonian patient on bromocriptine. J Clin Psychopharmacol. 1986;6(3):194–5.

123. Cheng P-L, Hung S-W, Lin L-W, Chong C-F, Lau C-I. Amantadine-induced serotonin syndrome in a patient with renal failure. Am J Emerg Med. 2008;26(1):112.e5–6.

124. Trollor JN, Sachdev PS. Electroconvulsive treatment of neuroleptic malignant syndrome: a review and report of cases. Aust N Z J Psychiatry. 1999;33:650–9.

125. Scheftner WAMD, Shulman RBMD. Treatment choice in neuroleptic malignant syndrome. Convuls Ther. 1992;8(4):267–79.

126. Ruth-Sahd LA, Rodrigues D, Shreve E. Neuroleptic malignant syndrome: a case report. Nursing. 2020;50(4):32–8.

127. San Gabriel MC, Eddula-Changala B, Tan Y, Longshore CT. Electroconvulsive in a schizophrenic patient with neuroleptic malignant syndrome and rhabdomyolysis. J ECT. 2015;31(3):197–200.

128. Casamassima F, Lattanzi L, Perlis RH, Litta A, Fui E, Bonuccelli U, et al. Neuroleptic malignant syndrome: further lessons from a case report. Psychosomatics. 2010;51(4):349–54.

129. Chiou YJ, Lee Y, Lin CC, Huang TL. A case report of catatonia and neuroleptic malignant syndrome with multiple treatment modalities: short communication and literature review. Medicine. 2015;94(43):e1752.

130. Hashim H, Zebun N, Alrukn SA, Al Madani AA. Drug resistant neuroleptic malignant syndrome and the role of electroconvulsive therapy. JPMA: J Pak Med Assoc. 2014;64(4):471–3.

131. Denborough MA, Forster JF, Lovell RR, Maplestone PA, Villiers JD. Anaesthetic deaths in a family. Br J Anaesth. 1962;34:395–6.

132. Dexter F, Epstein RH, Wachtel RE, Rosenberg H. Estimate of the relative risk of succinylcholine for triggering malignant hyperthermia. Anesth Analg. 2013;116(1):118–22.

133. Hopkins PM. Malignant hyperthermia: pharmacology of triggering. Br J Anaesth. 2011;107(1):48–56.

134. Larach MG, Klumpner TT, Brandom BW, Vaughn MT, Belani KG, Herlich A, et al. Succinylcholine use and dantrolene availability for malignant hyperthermia treatment: database analyses and systematic review. Anesthesiology. 2019;130(1):41–54.

135. Migita T, Mukaida K, Kobayashi M, Hamada H, Kawamoto M. The severity of sevoflurane-induced malignant hyperthermia. Acta Anaesthesiol Scand. 2012;56(3):351–6.

136. Riazi S, Larach MG, Hu C, Wijeysundera D, Massey C, Kraeva N. Malignant hyperthermia in Canada: characteristics of index anesthetics in 129 malignant hyperthermia susceptible probands. Anesth Analg. 2014;118(2):381–7.

137. Rosenberg H, Davis M, James D, Pollock N, Stowell K. Malignant hyperthermia. Orphanet J Rare Dis. 2007;2:21.

138. Bachand M, Vachon N, Boisvert M, Mayer FM, Chartrand D. Clinical reassessment of malignant hyperthermia in Abitibi-Temiscamingue. Can J Anaesth. 1997;44(7):696–701.

139. Ording H. Incidence of malignant hyperthermia in Denmark. Anesth Analg. 1985;64(7):700–4.

140. Brady JESM, Sun LSMD, Rosenberg HMD, Li GMDD. Prevalence of malignant hyperthermia due to anesthesia in New York state, 2001–2005. Anesth Analg. 2009;109(4):1162–6.

141. Litman RS, Rosenberg H. Malignant hyperthermia: update on susceptibility testing. JAMA. 2005;293(23):2918–24.

142. Litman RSDO, Rosenberg HMD. Malignant hyperthermia-associated diseases: state of the art uncertainty. Anesth Analg. 2009;109(4):1004–5.

143. Amburgey K, Bailey A, Hwang JH, Tarnopolsky MA, Bonnemann CG, Medne L, et al. Genotype-phenotype correlations in recessive RYR1-related myopathies. Orphanet J Rare Dis. 2013;8:117.

144. Brandom BW, Bina S, Wong CA, Wallace T, Visoiu M, Isackson PJ, et al. Ryanodine receptor type 1 gene variants in the malignant hyperthermia-susceptible population of the United States. Anesth Analg. 2013;116(5):1078–86.

145. Gillies RL, Bjorksten AR, Du Sart D, Hockey BM. Analysis of the entire ryanodine receptor type 1 and alpha 1 subunit of the dihydropyridine receptor (CACNA1S) coding regions for variants associated with malignant hyperthermia in Australian families. Anaesth Intensive Care. 2015;43(2):157–66.

146. Gomez AC, Holford TW, Yamaguchi N. Malignant hyperthermia-associated mutations in the S2-S3 cytoplasmic loop of type 1 ryanodine receptor calcium channel impair calcium-dependent inactivation. Am J Physiol Cell Physiol. 2016;311(5):C749–c57.

147. Gonsalves SG, Ng D, Johnston JJ, Teer JK, Stenson PD, Cooper DN, et al. Using exome data to identify malignant hyperthermia susceptibility mutations. Anesthesiology. 2013;119(5):1043–53.

148. Haraki T, Yasuda T, Mukaida K, Migita T, Hamada H, Kawamoto M. Mutated p.4894 RyR1 function related to malignant hyperthermia and congenital neuromuscular disease with uniform type 1 fiber (CNMDU1). Anesth Analg. 2011;113(6):1461–7.

149. Ibarra Moreno CA, Hu S, Kraeva N, Schuster F, Johannsen S, Rueffert H, et al. An assessment of penetrance and clinical expression of malignant hyperthermia in individuals carrying diagnostic ryanodine receptor 1 gene mutations. Anesthesiology. 2019;131(5):983–91.

150. Rosenberg H, Pollock N, Schiemann A, Bulger T, Stowell K. Malignant hyperthermia: a review. Orphanet J Rare Dis. 2015;10:93.

151. Klingler WMD, Rueffert HMD, Lehmann-Horn FMD, Girard TMD, Hopkins PMMD. Core myopathies and risk of malignant hyperthermia. Anesth Analg. 2009;109(4):1167–73.

152. Alkhunaizi E, Shuster S, Shannon P, Siu VM, Darilek S, Mohila CA, et al. Homozygous/compound heterozygote RYR1 gene variants: expanding the clinical spectrum. Am J Med Genet A. 2019;179(3):386–96.

153. Bamaga AK, Riazi S, Amburgey K, Ong S, Halliday W, Diamandis P, et al. Neuromuscular conditions associated with malignant hyperthermia in paediatric patients: a 25-year retrospective study. Neuromuscul Disord: NMD. 2016;26(3):201–6.

154. Brislin RP, Theroux MC. Core myopathies and malignant hyperthermia susceptibility: a review. Paediatr Anaesth. 2013;23(9):834–41.

155. De Wel B, Claeys KG. Malignant hyperthermia: still an issue for neuromuscular diseases? Curr Opin Neurol. 2018;31(5):628–34.

156. Hedenmalm K, Granberg AG, Dahl ML. Statin-induced muscle toxicity and susceptibility to malignant hyperthermia and other muscle diseases: a population-based case-control study including 1st and 2nd degree relatives. Eur J Clin Pharmacol. 2015;71(1):117–24.

157. Nelson P, Litman RS. Malignant hyperthermia in children: an analysis of the North American malignant hyperthermia registry. Anesth Analg. 2014;118(2):369–74.

158. Salazar JH, Yang J, Shen L, Abdullah F, Kim TW. Pediatric malignant hyperthermia: risk factors, morbidity, and mortality identified from the Nationwide Inpatient Sample and Kids' Inpatient Database. Paediatr Anaesth. 2014;24(12):1212–6.

159. Broman M, Heinecke K, Islander G, Schuster F, Glahn K, Bodelsson M, et al. Screening of the ryanodine 1 gene for malignant hyperthermia causative mutations by high resolution melt curve analysis. Anesth Analg. 2011;113(5):1120–8.

160. JSA guideline for the management of malignant hyperthermia crisis 2016. J Anesth. 2017;31(2):307–17.

161. Glahn KP, Ellis FR, Halsall PJ, Müller CR, Snoeck MM, Urwyler A, et al. Recognizing and managing a malignant hyperthermia crisis: guidelines from the European Malignant Hyperthermia Group. Br J Anaesth. 2010;105(4):417–20.

162. Litman RS, Smith VI, Larach MG, Mayes L, Shukry M, Theroux MC, et al. Consensus statement of the malignant hyperthermia association of the United States on unresolved clinical questions concerning the management of patients with malignant hyperthermia. Anesth Analg. 2019;128(4):652–9.

163. Amano T, Fukami T, Ogiso T, Hirose D, Jones JP, Taniguchi T, et al. Identification of enzymes responsible for dantrolene metabolism in the human liver: a clue to uncover the cause of liver injury. Biochem Pharmacol. 2018;151:69–78.

164. Brandom BW, Larach MG, Chen MS, Young MC. Complications associated with the administration of dantrolene 1987 to 2006: a report from the North American Malignant Hyperthermia Registry of the Malignant Hyperthermia Association of the United States. Anesth Analg. 2011;112(5):1115–23.

165. Kaku DA, Lowenstein DH. Emergence of recreational drug abuse as a major risk factor for stroke in young adults. Ann Intern Med. 1990;113(11):821–7.

166. Devgun J, Rasin A, Kim T, Mycyk M, Bryant S, Wahl M, et al. An outbreak of severe coagulopathy from synthetic cannabinoids tainted with long-acting anticoagulant rodenticides. Clin Toxicol (Philadelphia, Pa). 2019:1–8.

167. Courts J, Maskill V, Gray A, Glue P. Signs and symptoms associated with synthetic cannabinoid toxicity: systematic review. Australas Psychiatry. 2016;24(6):598–601.

168. Freeman MJ, Rose DZ, Myers MA, Gooch CL, Bozeman AC, Burgin WS. Ischemic stroke after use of the synthetic marijuana "spice". Neurology. 2013;81(24):2090–3.

169. Tait RJ, Caldicott D, Mountain D, Hill SL, Lenton S. A systematic review of adverse events arising from the use of synthetic cannabinoids and their associated treatment. Clin Toxicol (Philadelphia, Pa). 2016;54(1):1–13.

170. Piano MR. Cannabis smoking and cardiovascular health: It's complicated. Clin Pharmacol Ther. 2017;102(2):191–3.

171. Wolff V, Jouanjus E. Strokes are possible complications of cannabinoids use. Epilepsy Behav: E&B. 2017;70(Pt B):355–63.

172. Wolff V, Armspach JP, Beaujeux R, Manisor M, Rouyer O, Lauer V, et al. High frequency of intracranial arterial stenosis and cannabis use in ischaemic stroke in the young. Cerebrovasc Dis (Basel, Switzerland). 2014;37(6):438–43.

173. Warner EA. Cocaine abuse. Ann Intern Med. 1993;119(3):226–35.

174. Van Dyke C, Barash PG, Jatlow P, Byck R. Cocaine: plasma concentrations after intranasal application in man. Science. 1976;191(4229):859–61.

175. Jenkins AJ, Keenan RM, Henningfield JE, Cone EJ. Correlation between pharmacological effects and plasma cocaine concentrations after smoked administration. J Anal Toxicol. 2002;26(7):382–92.

176. Fleming JA, Byck R, Barash PG. Pharmacology and therapeutic applications of cocaine. Anesthesiology. 1990;73(3):518–31.

177. Dean RA, Christian CD, Sample RH, Bosron WF. Human liver cocaine esterases: ethanol-mediated formation of ethylcocaine. FASEB J. 1991;5(12):2735–9.

178. Brust JC, Richter RW. Stroke associated with cocaine abuse--? N Y State J Med. 1977,77(9).1473–5.

179. Westover AN, McBride S, Haley RW. Stroke in young adults who abuse amphetamines or cocaine: a population-based study of hospitalized patients. Arch Gen Psychiatry. 2007;64(4):495–502.

180. Sloan MAM, Kittner SJMM, Feeser BRMM, Gardner JM, Epstein A, Wozniak MAMDP, et al. Illicit drug-associated ischemic stroke in the Baltimore-Washington Young Stroke Study. Neurology. 1998;50(6):1688–93.

181. Kaufman MJ, Levin JM, Ross MH, Lange N, Rose SL, Kukes TJ, et al. Cocaine-induced cerebral vasoconstriction detected in humans with magnetic resonance angiography. JAMA. 1998;279(5):376–80.

182. He GQ, Zhang A, Altura BT, Altura BM. Cocaine-induced cerebrovasospasm and its possible mechanism of action. J Pharmacol Exp Ther. 1994;268(3):1532–9.

183. Du C, Yu M, Volkow ND, Koretsky AP, Fowler JS, Benveniste H. Cocaine increases the intracellular calcium concentration in brain independently of its cerebrovascular effects. J Neurosci. 2006;26(45):11522–31.

184. Brown E, Prager J, Lee HY, Ramsey RG. CNS complications of cocaine abuse: prevalence, pathophysiology, and neuroradiology. AJR: Am J Roentgenol. 1992;159(1):137–47.

185. Büttner A. Neuropathological alterations in cocaine abuse. Curr Med Chem. 2012;19(33):5597–600.

186. Jacobs IG, Roszler MH, Kelly JK, Klein MA, Kling GA. Cocaine abuse: neurovascular complications. Radiology. 1989;170(1 Pt 1):223–7.

187. Lowenstein DH, Massa SM, Rowbotham MC, Collins SD, McKinney HE, Simon RP. Acute neurologic and psychiatric complications associated with cocaine abuse. Am J Med. 1987;83(5):841–6.

188. Levine SR, Brust JC, Futrell N, Ho KL, Blake D, Millikan CH, et al. Cerebrovascular complications of the use of the "crack" form of alkaloidal cocaine. N Engl J Med. 1990;323(11):699–704.

189. Levine SR, Brust JC, Futrell N, Brass LM, Blake D, Fayad P, et al. A comparative study of the cerebrovascular complications of cocaine: alkaloidal versus hydrochloride--a review. Neurology. 1991;41(8):1173–7.

190. Mody CK, Miller BL, McIntyre HB, Cobb SK, Goldberg MA. Neurologic complications of cocaine abuse. Neurology. 1988;38(8):1189–93.

191. Konzen JP, Levine SR, Garcia JH. Vasospasm and thrombus formation as possible mechanisms of stroke related to alkaloidal cocaine. Stroke. 1995;26(6):1114–8.

192. Togna G, Tempesta E, Togna AR, Dolci N, Cebo B, Caprino L. Platelet responsiveness and biosynthesis of thromboxane and prostacyclin in response to in vitro cocaine treatment. Haemostasis. 1985;15(2):100–7.

193. Klonoff DC, Andrews BT, Obana WG. Stroke associated with cocaine use. Arch Neurol. 1989;46(9):989–93.

194. Kaye BR, Fainstat M. Cerebral vasculitis associated with cocaine abuse. JAMA. 1987;258(15):2104–6.

195. Krendel DA, Ditter SM, Frankel MR, Ross WK. Biopsy-proven cerebral vasculitis associated with cocaine abuse. Neurology. 1990;40(7):1092–4.

196. Sloan MA, Mattioni TA. Concurrent myocardial and cerebral infarctions after intranasal cocaine use. Stroke. 1992;23(3):427–30.

197. Sauer CM. Recurrent embolic stroke and cocaine-related cardiomyopathy. Stroke. 1991;22(9):1203–5.

198. Kibayashi K, Mastri AR, Hirsch CS. Cocaine induced intracerebral hemorrhage: analysis of predisposing factors and mechanisms causing hemorrhagic strokes. Hum Pathol. 1995;26(6):659–63.

199. Kelley PA, Sharkey J, Philip R, Ritchie IM. Acute cocaine alters cerebrovascular autoregulation in the rat neocortex. Brain Res Bull. 1993;31(5):581–5.

200. Treadwell SD, Robinson TG. Cocaine use and stroke. Postgrad Med J. 2007;83(980):389–94.

201. Martin-Schild SMDP, Albright KCDOMPH, Misra VMD, Philip MMD, Barreto ADMD, Hallevi HMD, et al. Intravenous tissue plasminogen activator in

patients with cocaine-associated acute ischemic stroke. Stroke. 2009;40(11):3635–7.

202. Ramoska E, Sacchetti AD. Propranolol-induced hypertension in treatment of cocaine intoxication. Ann Emerg Med. 1985;14(11):1112–3.

203. Catravas JD, Waters IW. Acute cocaine intoxication in the conscious dog: studies on the mechanism of lethality. J Pharmacol Exp Ther. 1981;217(2):350–6.

204. Richards JR, Garber D, Laurin EG, Albertson TE, Derlet RW, Amsterdam EA, et al. Treatment of cocaine cardiovascular toxicity: a systematic review. Clin Toxicol (Philadelphia, Pa). 2016;54(5):345–64.

205. O'Connor AD, Rusyniak DE, Bruno A. Cerebrovascular and cardiovascular complications of alcohol and sympathomimetic drug abuse. Med Clin N Am. 2005;89(6):1343–58.

206. Ho EL, Josephson SA, Lee HS, Smith WS. Cerebrovascular complications of methamphetamine abuse. Neurocrit Care. 2009;10(3):295–305.

207. Edwards KR. Hemorrhagic complications of cerebral arteritis. Arch Neurol. 1977;34(9):549–52.

208. Selmi F, Davies KG, Sharma RR, Neal JW. Intracerebral haemorrhage due to amphetamine abuse: report of two cases with underlying arteriovenous malformations. Br J Neurosurg. 1995;9(1):93–6.

209. Harrington H, Heller HA, Dawson D, Caplan L, Rumbaugh C. Intracerebral hemorrhage and oral amphetamine. Arch Neurol. 1983;40(8):503–7.

210. Hondebrink L, Nugteren-van Lonkhuyzen JJ, Rietjens SJ, Brunt TM, Venhuis B, Soerdjbalie-Maikoe V, et al. Fatalities, cerebral hemorrhage, and severe cardiovascular toxicity after exposure to the new psychoactive substance 4-fluoroamphetamine: a prospective cohort study. Ann Emerg Med. 2018;71(3):294–305.

211. Le Roux G, Bruneau C, Lelièvre B, Bretaudeau Deguigne M, Turcant A, Harry P, et al. Recreational phenethylamine poisonings reported to a French poison control center. Drug Alcohol Depend. 2015;154:46–53.

212. McGee SMMD, McGee DNPB, McGee MBMD. Spontaneous intracerebral hemorrhage related to methamphetamine abuse: autopsy findings and clinical correlation. Am J Forensic Med Pathol. 2004;25(4):334–7.

213. Lappin JM, Darke S, Farrell M. Stroke and methamphetamine use in young adults: a review. J Neurol Neurosurg Psychiatry. 2017;88(12):1079–91.

214. Auer J, Berent R, Weber T, Lassnig E, Eber B. Subarachnoid haemorrhage with "Ecstasy" abuse in a young adult. Neurol Sci. 2002;23(4):199–201.

215. McEvoy AW, Kitchen ND, Thomas DG. Intracerebral haemorrhage and drug abuse in young adults. Br J Neurosurg. 2000;14(5):449–54.

216. De Silva DA, Wong MC, Lee MP, Chen CL-H, Chang HM. Amphetamine-associated ischemic stroke: clinical presentation and proposed pathogenesis. J Stroke Cerebrovasc Dis. 2007;16(4):185–6.

217. Manchanda S, Connolly MJ. Cerebral infarction in association with Ecstasy abuse. Postgrad Med J. 1993;69(817):874–5.

218. McDonald ES, Lane JI. Dietary supplements and stroke. Mayo Clin Proc. 2005;80(3):315.

219. Chen C, Biller J, Willing SJ, Lopez AM. Ischemic stroke after using over the counter products containing ephedra. J Neurol Sci. 2004;217(1):55–60.

220. Yoon BWMDP, Bae HJMDP, Hong KSMDP, Lee SMP, Park BJMDP, Yu KHMDP, et al. Phenylpropanolamine contained in cold remedies and risk of hemorrhagic stroke. Neurology. 2007;68(2):146–9.

221. Kernan WN, Viscoli CM, Brass LM, Broderick JP, Brott T, Feldmann E, et al. Phenylpropanolamine and the risk of hemorrhagic stroke. N Engl J Med. 2000;343(25):1826–32.

222. Cantu C, Arauz A, Murillo-Bonilla LM, Lopez M, Barinagarrementeria F. Stroke associated with sympathomimetics contained in over-the-counter cough and cold drugs. Stroke. 2003;34(7):1667–72.

223. Wills B, Theeler BJ, Ney JP. Drug- and toxin-associated seizures. In: Dobbs MR, editor. Clinical neurotoxicology: syndromes, substances, environments. Philadelphia: Saunders Elsevier; 2009. p. 131–50.

224. McGarvey CK, Rusyniak DE. Neurotoxicology. In: Biller J, editor. Practical neurology. 3rd ed. Philadelphia: Lippincott, Williams, & Wilkins; 2009. p. 745–63.

225. Thundiyil JG, Kearney TE, Olson KR. Evolving epidemiology of drug-induced seizures reported to a Poison Control Center System. J Med Toxicol. 2007;3(1):15–9.

226. Cock H. Drug-induced status epilepticus. Epilepsy Behav: E&B. 2015:76–82.

227. Sutter R, Ruegg S, Tschudin-Sutter S. Seizures as adverse events of antibiotic drugs; a systematic review. Neurology. 2015;85(15):1332–41.

228. Druschky K, Bleich S, Grohmann R, Engel R, Neyazi A, Stubner S, et al. Seizure rates under treatment with antipsychotic drugs: data from the AMSP project. World J Biol Psychiatry. 2019;20(9):732–41.

229. Riley AL, Nelson KH, To P, Lopez-Arnau R, Xu P, Wang D, et al. Abuse potential and toxicity of the synthetic cathinones (i.e., "Bath salts"). Neurosci Biobehav Rev. 2020;110:150–73.

230. Frommer DA, Kulig KW, Marx JA, Rumack B. Tricyclic antidepressant overdose. A review. JAMA. 1987;257(4):521–6.

231. Boehnert MT, Lovejoy FH Jr. Value of the QRS duration versus the serum drug level in predicting seizures and ventricular arrhythmias after an acute overdose of tricyclic antidepressants. N Engl J Med. 1985;313(8):474–9.

232. Hulten BA, Adams R, Askenasi R, Dallos V, Dawling S, Volans G, et al. Predicting severity of tricyclic antidepressant overdose. J Toxicol Clin Toxicol. 1992;30(2):161–70.

233. Brust JCM. Seizures and substance abuse: treatment considerations. Neurology. 2006;67(12 Suppl 4):S45–8.

234. Kofler M, Arturo Leis A. Prolonged seizure activity after baclofen withdrawal. Neurology. 1992;42(3 Pt 1):697–8.

235. Boison D. Methylxanthines, seizures, and excitotoxicity. Handb Exp Pharmacol. 2011;200:251–66.

236. Chen HY, Albertson TE, Olsen KR. Treatment of drug-induced seizures. Br J Clin Pharmacol. 2016;81(3):412–9.

237. D'Onofrio G, Rathlev NK, Ulrich AS, Fish SS, Freedland ES. Lorazepam for the prevention of recurrent seizures related to alcohol. N Engl J Med. 1999;340(12):915–9.

238. Rathlev NK, D'Onofrio G, Fish SS, Harrison PM, Bernstein E, Hossack RW, et al. The lack of efficacy of phenytoin in the prevention of recurrent alcohol-related seizures. Ann Emerg Med. 1994;23(3):513–8.

239. Starr P, Klein-Schwartz W, Spiller H, Kern P, Ekleberry SE, Kunkel S. Incidence and onset of delayed seizures after overdoses of extended-release bupropion. Am J Emerg Med. 2009;27(8):911–5.

240. Paloucek FP, Rodvold KA. Evaluation of theophylline overdoses and toxicities. Ann Emerg Med. 1988;17(2):135–44.

241. Zwillich CW, Sutton FD, Neff TA, Cohn WM, Matthay RA, Weinberger MM. Theophylline-induced seizures in adults. Correlation with serum concentrations. Ann Intern Med. 1975;82(6):784–7.

242. Wills B, Erickson T. Drug- and toxin-associated seizures. Med Clin N Am. 2005;89(6):1297–321.

243. Lee T, Warrick BJ, Sarangarm P, Alunday RL, Bussmann S, Smolinske SC, et al. Levetiracetam in toxic seizures. Clin Toxicol (Philadelphia, Pa). 2018;56(3):175–81.

244. Juurlink DN, Gosselin S, Kielstein JT, Ghannoum M, Lavergne V, Nolin TD, et al. Extracorporeal treatment for salicylate poisoning: systematic review and recommendations from the EXTRIP workgroup. Ann Emerg Med. 2015;66(2):165–81.

245. Ghannoum M, Wiegand TJ, Liu KD, Calello DP, Godin M, Lavergne V, et al. Extracorporeal treatment for theophylline poisoning: systematic review and recommendations from the EXTRIP workgroup. Clin Toxicol (Philadelphia, Pa). 2015;53(4):215–29.

246. Decker BS, Goldfarb DS, Dargan PI, Friesen M, Gosselin S, Hoffman RS, et al. Extracorporeal treatment for lithium poisoning: systematic review and recommendations from the EXTRIP workgroup. Clin J Am Soc Nephrol: CJASN. 2015;10(5):875–87.

247. Lawrence DT, Kirk MA. Chemical terrorism attacks: update on antidotes. Emerg Med Clin North Am. 2007;25(2):567–95; abstract xi.

248. Black RE, Gunn RA. Hypersensitivity reactions associated with botulinal antitoxin. Am J Med. 1980;69(4):567–70.

249. Nelson BK. Snake envenomation. Incidence, clinical presentation and management. Med Toxicol Adverse Drug Exp. 1989;4(1):17–31.

250. Lawrence D, McLinskey N, Huff S, Holstege CP. Toxin-induced neurologic emergencies. In: Dobbs MR, editor. Clinical neurotoxicology: syndromes, substances, environments. Philadelphia: Saunders Elsevier; 2009. p. 30–46.

251. Chamberlain JM, Klein BL. A comprehensive review of naloxone for the emergency physician. Am J Emerg Med. 1994;12(6):650–60.

252. Clarke SFJ, Dargan PI, Jones AL. Naloxone in opioid poisoning: walking the tightrope. Emerg Med J. 2005;22(9):612–6.

253. Watkins JW, Schwarz ES, Arroyo-Plasencia AM, Mullins ME, Toxicology Investigators Consortium Investigators. Toxicology the use of physostigmine by toxicologists in anticholinergic toxicity. J Med Toxicol. 2015;11(2):179–84.

254. Arens AM, Shah K, Al-Abri S, Olson KR, Kearney T. Safety and effectiveness of physostigmine: a 10-year retrospective review. Clin Toxicol (Philadelphia, Pa). 2018;56(2):101–7.

255. Boley SP, Stellpflug SJ. A comparison of resource utilization in the management of anticholinergic delirium between physostigmine and nonantidote therapy. Ann Pharmacother. 2019;53(10):1026–32.

256. Boley SP, Olives TD, Bangh SA, Fahrner S, Cole JB. Physostigmine is superior to non-antidote therapy in the management of antimuscarinic delirium: a prospective study from a regional poison center. Clin Toxicol (Philadelphia, Pa). 2019;57(1):50–5.

257. Burns MJ, Linden CH, Graudins A, Brown RM, Fletcher KE. A comparison of physostigmine and benzodiazepines for the treatment of anticholinergic poisoning. Ann Emerg Med. 2000;35(4):374–81.

258. Dawson AH, Buckley NA. Pharmacological management of anticholinergic delirium - theory, evidence and practice. Br J Clin Pharmacol. 2016;81(3):516–24.

259. Nilsson E. Physostigmine treatment in various drug-induced intoxications. Ann Clin Res. 1982;14(4):165–72.

Correction to: Acute Visual Loss

Jane H. Lock, Cédric Lamirel, Nancy J. Newman, and Valérie Biousse

Correction to: Chapter 5 in: K. L. Roos (ed.), Emergency Neurology, https://doi.org/10.1007/978-3-030-75778-6_5

Figure 5.10 had an error in the published version of the book, and the term Pseudopapilledema (in the middle grey box) has now been corrected to Papilledema. The updated figure is provided below.

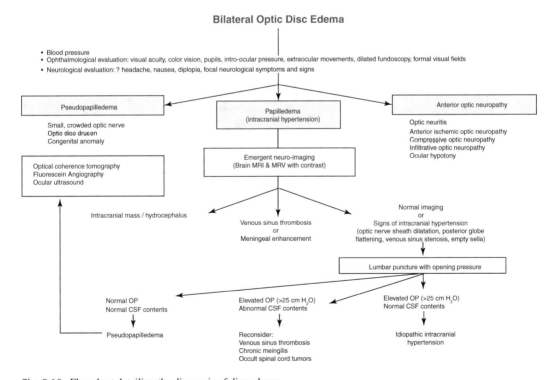

Fig. 5.10 Flowchart detailing the diagnosis of disc edema

The updated version of this chapter can be found at
https://doi.org/10.1007/978-3-030-75778-6_5

Index

Printed in the United States
by Baker & Taylor Publisher Services